Oxford Specialist Handbook of
Paediatric
Respiratory
Medicine

Published and forthcoming Oxford Specialist Handbooks

Oxford Specialist Handbooks in Paediatrics
Paediatric Nephrology (Rees, Webb, and Brogan)
Paediatric Neurology (Forsyth and Newton eds.)
Paediatric Gastroenterology, Hepatology, and Nutrition
    (Beattie, Dhawan, and Puntis eds.)
Oncology and Haematology (Bailey and Skinner eds.)

Oxford Specialist Handbooks in Cardiology
Echocardiology (Leeson, Mitchell, and Becher eds.)
Cardiac Catheterization and Coronary Angiography
    (Mitchell, Leeson, West, and Banning)
Heart Failure (Gardner, McDonagh, and Walker)
Pacing and Implantable ICDs
    (Timperley, Leeson, Mitchell, and Betts eds.)

Oxford Specialist Handbooks in Surgery
Vascular Surgery (Hands, Murphy, Sharp, and Ray Chaudry)
Plastic Surgery (Giele and Cassell eds.)
Urology (Reynard, Sullivan, Turner, Feneley, Armenakas, and Mark eds.)

Oxford Specialist Handbooks in Neurology
Parkinson's Disease and Other Movement Disorders
    (Edwards, Quinn, and Bhatia)
Epilepsy (Alarcon, Nashaf, Cross, and Nightingale)

Oxford Specialist Handbook of **Paediatric Respiratory Medicine**

Jeremy Hull

Consultant in Paediatric Respiratory Medicine,
Oxford Children's Hospital, Oxford, UK

Julian Forton

Clinical Lecturer, Department of Paediatrics,
Oxford University, Oxford, UK

Anne H. Thompson

Consultant in Paediatric Respiratory Medicine,
Oxford Children's Hospital, Oxford, UK

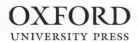

OXFORD
UNIVERSITY PRESS

OXFORD
UNIVERSITY PRESS

Great Clarendon Street, Oxford OX2 6DP

Oxford University Press is a department of the University of Oxford.
It furthers the University's objective of excellence in research, scholarship,
and education by publishing worldwide in

Oxford New York

Auckland Cape Town Dar es Salaam Hong Kong Karachi
Kuala Lumpur Madrid Melbourne Mexico City Nairobi
New Delhi Shanghai Taipei Toronto

With offices in

Argentina Austria Brazil Chile Czech Republic France Greece
Guatemala Hungary Italy Japan Poland Portugal Singapore
South Korea Switzerland Thailand Turkey Ukraine Vietnam

Oxford is a registered trade mark of Oxford University Press
in the UK and in certain other countries

Published in the United States
by Oxford University Press Inc., New York

© Jeremy Hull, Julian Forton, Anne Thomson 2008

The moral rights of the authors have been asserted
Database right Oxford University Press (maker)

First published 2008

British Library Cataloguing in Publication Data

Data available

Library of Congress Cataloging in Publication Data

Data available

Typeset by Newgen Imaging Systems (P) Ltd., Chennai, India
Printed in China through
Asia Pacific Offset

ISBN 978–0–19–920484–7

10 9 8 7 6 5 4 3 2 1

Preface

In writing this handbook our aim has been to provide a practical guide to paediatric respiratory medicine that will be a useful first point of reference for paediatricians faced with children with acute or chronic respiratory problems.

The book has been written for use by general paediatricians and by specialists in paediatric respiratory medicine at both consultant and trainee level. It deals with common problems seen by all paediatricians and rarer conditions more often seen at specialist centres, but managed in collaboration with general paediatricians. The information is in a readily accessible format, with extensive use of bullet points. The focus is on clinical presentation, diagnosis, and management of respiratory problems. There is less emphasis on background information, such as epidemiology and pathogenesis, but this is sufficient where necessary to provide insight into clinical presentation and management, or where this information would be helpful for parents.

The book is divided into four parts. Part 1 provides a practical approach to acute and non-acute clinical problems. Part 2, the bulk of the book, provides detailed information about common and not-so-common clinical conditions. Part 3 provides useful information on supportive care, including, for example, use of non-invasive ventilation and the care of a child with a tracheostomy. Part 4 gives details on how to perform several practical procedures, such as ciliary brush biopsy, flexible bronchoscopy, and inserting a chest drain. Finally, the appendices provide information on lung function testing and tables of age-corrected normal values for several respiratory parameters.

The book has been written by two consultants who work in a tertiary respiratory unit and by a respiratory trainee. This combination of authors has provided the experience necessary to deal with topics where there is an absence of published evidence and to present the information in a format that both consultants and trainees will find useful.

JH, JF, and AHT July 2007

Foreword

So why would anyone want to buy a book in the 21st century, when a profusion of information is available at the touch of a computer key? Cough in children yields more than 6,500 references on a PubMed search, so why would anyone want to read a 5 page section on the same subject in this book? One of the most misquoted phrases in English poetry, 'a little *learning* is a dangerous thing' could now be adapted as 'a lot of PubMed is a dangerous thing', and unless the searcher has a sound grounding in the subject searched, it is likely to lead to confusion in mind, an unbalanced perspective, and ultimately, inappropriate management of children. A view of the woods is an essential prelude to a detailed study of an individual tree.

And that is where this book will be so valuable to all in the field of paediatric respiratory medicine, from the raw young tyro to the elderly professorial dodderer, and all stages in between. The reader will find a clear account of the subject, from both a problem-based and a disease-based approach. It gives a commonsense overview of all the important topics in the field, with crisp tables and bullet points, written in clear English. There are a few, up-to-date papers, reviews and websites as a basis for further learning, and the authors have fully achieved their aim, of writing a practical handbook in line with the long tradition of the *Oxford* series. The trainee can rapidly acquire a good grasp of the subject, and can then safely dive into PubMed for more advanced studies, particulary of pathophysiology. Few if any of the allegedly trained will read this without finding something to learn, or some new idea not previously thought of, to try when next a problem arises. Few will agree with absolutely every statement, but that is inevitable and part of the intrinsic beauty of the subject—and in any event, medicine is learned by doing, and cannot be learned solely from books, whatever the views of those currently changing medical training with all the natural talent of a hippopotamus playing the piccolo.

So in summary, who can benefit from this book, and how? The trainee will certainly not outgrow it—even the most experienced paediatrician, seeing a child with an uncommon condition, or preparing a teaching session on a common one, will benefit from taking a surreptitious peek at the relevant section here, to ensure nothing has been forgotten. For example, I would challenge the reader to list the totality of the associated conditions which need to be detected in a baby with a PHOX2b mutation before turning to Chapter 26. Review copies of books come into three categories: 'throw away', 'give away' and 'chain it to the wall'—this Handbook is definitely in the last category. Departmental thieves, hands off!

Andy Bush
Professor of Paediatric Respirology
Royal Brompton Hospital
London

Acknowledgements

We gratefully acknowledge the skill and patience of Professor Sir David Hull who drew most of the figures.

Contents

Appendices

Symbols and abbreviations

>	greater than
<	less than
ABPA	allergic bronchopulmonary aspergillosis
AIDS	acquired immunodeficiency syndrome
ANA	anti-nuclear antibody
ANCA	anti-neutrophil cytoplasmic antibody
ARDS	acute respiratory distress syndrome
ATS	American Thoracic Society
BAL	broncho-alveolar lavage
BCG	Bacille Calmette Guérin
BIPAP	bilevel positive airways pressure
BO	bronchiolitis obliterans
BPD	bronchopulmonary dysplasia
BTS	British Thoracic Society
CAP	community acquired pneumonia
CF	cystic fibrosis
CFTR	cystic fibrosis transmembrane conductance regulator
CMV	cytomegalovirus
CNS	central nervous system
CO	carbon monoxide
CPAP	continuous positive airways pressure
CT	computerized tomogram
CXR	chest x-ray
DIP	diffuse interstitial pneumonitis
DLCO	diffusion capacity for carbon monoxide—same as TLCO
EBV	Ebstein-Barr virus
ECG	electro-cardiograph
ELISA	enzyme linked immuno-assay
EMG	electromyogram
ENT	ear nose and throat
ERS	European Respiratory Society
ESR	erythrocyte sedimentation rate
FBC	full blood count
FEV1	forced expiratory volume in one second
FiO2	fractional inspired oxygen
FRC	function residual capacity

FVC	forced vital capacity
g	gram
GI	gastro-intestinal
GOR	gastro-oesophageal reflux
Hb	haemoglobin
HIV	human immunodeficiency virus
HLA	human leucocyte antigen
HRCT	high resolution computerised tomogram
ICU	intensive care unit
IgA	immunoglobulin A
IgE	immunoglobulin E
IgG	immunoglobulin G
IgM	immunoglobulin M
ILD	interstitial lung disease
IM	intramuscular
ITU	intensive therapy unit
IV	intravenous
IVC	inferior vena cava
kCO	CO transfer factor corrected for alveolar volume
L	litre
LCH	Langerhans cell histiocytosis
LFTs	liver function tests
LIP	lymphoid interstitial pneumonitis
LRTI	lower respiratory tract infection
LTOT	long term oxygen therapy
MDI	metered-dose inhaled
MDR-TB	multi-drug resistant tuberculosis
mcg	microgram
mg	milligram
min	minute
MTB	*Mycobacterium tuberculosis*
ng	nanogram
NIPPV	non-invasive positive pressure ventilation
NIV	non-invasive ventilation
NO	nitric oxide
NSAID	non-steroidal anti-inflammatory drug
NSIP	non-specific interstitial pneumonitis
OSA	obstructive sleep apnoea
PCP	Pneumocystis pneumonia
PCR	polymerase chain reaction
PEEP	positive end expiratory pressure
PEFR	peak expiratory flow rate

PFTs	pulmonary function tests
PHT	pulmonary hypertension
PSG	polysomnography
RAST	radioallergosorbent test
REM	rapid eye movement
RSV	respiratory syncytial virus
RT-PCR	reverse-transcriptase polymerase chain reaction
RV	residual volume
SARS	severe acquired respiratory syndrome
SLE	systemic lupus erythematosus
TB	tuberculosis
Th2	T-helper 2 cell
TLC	total lung capacity
TLCO	total lung carbon monoxide transfer factor
U&E	urea and electrolytes
URT	upper respiratory tract
URTI	upper respiratory tract infection
V/Q	ventilation/perfusion
VATS	video-assisted thorascopic surgery
WHO	World Health Organisation

Part I

Approach to clinical problems

Chapter 1

Examining the respiratory system

Introduction

Examining the chest is part of the routine physical examination of all children who are unwell. Most doctors are expert at identifying the abnormal signs that indicate disease. This short section provides the background to a common language so that clear descriptions can be given to colleagues.

Clubbing

- Gross clubbing is easy to recognize. Early clubbing is more subtle with an impression of fullness and 'floating' of the root of the nail bed on compression.
- The mechanisms that underlie the development of clubbing remain unclear. Possibilities include circulating mediators of vasodilatation released in response to hypoxia, and effects of the vagal nerve, resulting from the observation of the association between clubbing and disease in organs with vagal innervation.
- In children with respiratory symptoms, clubbing usually suggests suppurative lung disease or hypoxic cardiac disease. It can also be seen in interstitial lung disease and with bronchiolitis obliterans, and in children with chronic hypoxia from a respiratory cause.

Chest shape

- Fixed deformities of the chest are relatively common in children, affecting 0.5% of the population. They usually have no significant functional consequences. The commonest deformity is pectus excavatum (see 📖 Chapter 40).
- Hyperinflation (Fig. 1.1) is a reversible change in chest shape, and indicates air-trapping, usually as a result of small airways obstruction. In the context of asthma it suggests poor control. It is most easily seen from the side.
- Harrison's sulci (Fig. 1.2) refers to the indentation of the lower chest wall with the apparent splaying of the costal margins. They may be seen in association with hyperinflation. They are associated with chronic respiratory disease associated with increased work of breathing and may be caused by the necessarily increased power of diaphragmatic contraction on relatively soft costal cartilage.

Palpation

- Placing the hands on the chest can give valuable information about the presence of secretions and wheeze. It can also help determine whether chest expansion is equal.
- In older children who can perform a vital capacity manoeuvre, measuring the chest expansion, using a tape measure at the level of the xiphoid cartilage, can be predictive of lung volumes measured by spirometry. Depending on the height and sex of the subject, normal values for chest expansion can range from 3cm to 9cm.

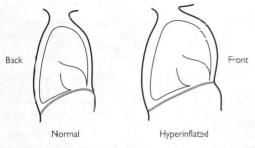

Back   Front

Normal   Hyperinflated

Fig. 1.1 Lateral view of the normal and hyperinflated chest.

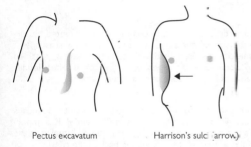

Pectus excavatum   Harrison's sulci (arrow)

Fig. 1.2 Anterior views of pectus excavatum and Harrison's sulci.

Percussion

Despite occasional views to the contrary it is always useful to percuss the chest in children. A dull percussion note is consistent with extensive consolidation or pleural disease, either pleural thickening or pleural fluid.

Stridor

Stridor (from the Latin *stridere*, to make harsh sounds) is a harsh monophonic noise that comes from the trachea or larynx as a result of narrowing. It may be heard with or without a stethoscope. When the extra-thoracic airway is affected the noise always has an inspiratory component but can be biphasic if the narrowing is severe. When the intra-thoracic trachea is affected, the stridor will usually be biphasic with a relatively loud expiratory phase. A purely inspiratory stridor indicates narrowing of the extrathoracic airway. Stridor is louder when airflows are increased such as with crying or exertion and quieter when flows are reduced, e.g. during sleep .

Stertor

This term is used to describe the harsh coarse noises generated by turbulent airflow in the supraglottic space. It may be caused by spasticity of the pharyngeal muscles, e.g. in a child with cerebral palsy, by retained secretions, or by adeno-tonsillar hypertrophy. Stertor is often louder during sleep because of reduced tone of pharyngeal muscles.

Auscultation

A clear description of breath sounds and any added adventitial sounds is much more informative than the often used term 'air entry'. It is important to listen to all of the lobes of each lung. This means listening at the apices and the axillae as well as at the front and back of the chest.

Breath sounds

Breath sounds are generated by air moving though the trachea and large bronchi. When listening at the midline over the trachea, the breath sounds are loud with a full inspiratory and expiratory phase with the inspiratory phase usually being louder. There is no pause between the 2 phases. Breath sounds with these characteristics are called bronchial.

- Vesicular breath sounds. When listening at the periphery of the lung, the breath sounds are quieter and only the inspiratory phase and the initial part of expiration can be heard. There is a short pause between the 2 phases.
- Bronchial breathing. If there is consolidation of the lung, the sound from the large airways passes more easily through the solid material and bronchial breath sounds are heard at the periphery.

When there is airway narrowing, the expiratory phase of the breath sounds heard at the periphery may become louder and more prolonged. This sign may be present before obvious wheeze is heard.

Adventitial noises

- Wheeze—a whistling 'musical' noise, caused by turbulent airflow passing through narrowed medium-sized airways If present, wheezes always occur predominantly in expiration but may be present on inspiration as well when airways obstruction is severe.
- Crepitations or crackles—sharp noises, usually heard on inspiration, can be coarse or fine depending on the pitch and quality of the sound. The mechanism by which the sounds are generated is not well understood. One possibility is that they are caused by fluid clearing rapidly from small airways (coarse) or alveoli (fine) so that pressures on either side of the obstruction suddenly equilibrate resulting in vibrations of the airway wall. It seems likely that these explanations are rather simplistic. Airflow rapidly diminishes as the airway divides, and gas movement in the bronchioles and alveoli is thought to occur by Brownian motion and diffusion. Such low energy movement cannot produce audible sounds. Whatever the origin of the sound, the presence of crepitations does indicate small airway or alveolar disease. When crepitations are present it is helpful to determine if they are cleared by coughing. If they are it suggests that they are caused by secretions and that chest physiotherapy may be a helpful part of management.
- Rattles (also known as ruttles)—noises coming from secretions in medium-sized and large airways.
- Transmitted sounds—noises coming from the upper airway heard when auscultating the chest.

The terms râles or rhonchi are sometimes used and frequently cause confusion. They were coined by the French inventor of the stethoscope, Laennec, in the 19th century. They mean the same thing—râles is the French word and rhonchi is Latin. They were used to describe crackles (râle crépitant), rattles (râle sec sonore), and wheeze (râle sibilant). Some doctors still use the terms sibilant and sonorous rhonchi or râles. For the more modern doctor, it is probably best to stick with wheeze, crepitations, and rattles.

Listen to the cough

Some children will cough spontaneously during their clinic visit. Others may be able to do so if asked. Listening to the nature of the cough can be illuminating.

- Is it dry or productive sounding?
- Is it brassy, croup-like, honking? This type of cough sound originates in the trachea and is consistent with the presence of tracheal narrowing, tracheomalacia, or habit cough.

Further information

Forgacs, P. (1978). The functional basis of pulmonary sounds. *Chest* **73**, 399–405.
Lehrer, S. (2002). Understanding lung sounds (booklet and audio CD). W.B. Saunders Company, Philadelphia.

Poorly controlled asthma

Introduction

Managing children with poorly controlled asthma is a common clinical problem for all doctors who look after children. It is easy to make assumptions about the diagnosis and pattern of illness. When faced with a child with difficult asthma it is helpful to re-evaluate all aspects of the disease. Here we suggest an approach that can be used to do this.

History

There are a number of critical questions to address.

- Is it asthma?
- How is the child currently affected?
- Are there any treatable or avoidable precipitants?
- What treatments is the child using or has tried in the past?
- Are the treatments used appropriately (including use of inhaler devices)?
- Is the child adherent to the prescribed treatment?
- Is the home environment stable and supportive and free of precipitants (smoke and other irritants as well as allergens)?

Establishing that asthma is the correct diagnosis is often the most important part of the assessment.

- A diagnosis of asthma requires a clear description of recurrent wheezing that is relieved by an inhaled bronchodilator. Ideally this should have been corroborated by physical examination during a wheezy episode. Parents understanding of the term 'wheeze' may vary and includes almost any noise coming from the airway. We can all wheeze at low lung volumes, and it can be useful to be able to demonstrate a wheeze to the family by making a forced expiration to FRC.
- Additional information that supports a diagnosis of asthma includes:
  - wheeze in response to likely precipitants (e.g. exercise, allergen exposure, smoke exposure);
  - excessive breathlessness on exertion and exercise limitation;
  - symptoms of wheeze and cough occurring at night;
  - the presence of a predominantly dry cough is also consistent with asthma. Although cough may be the major reported symptom, cough without wheeze is not asthma;
  - the presence of other atopic conditions such as eczema or hay fever;
  - a first-degree relative with asthma.
- A clear description of symptoms, including severity and frequency is required.
  - Does the child wheeze every day?
  - Are they exercise-limited?
  - How often do they have disturbed nights?
  - How much school have they missed?

- The presence of associated symptoms should also be sought. Gastro-oesophageal reflux may contribute to poor control. Symptoms include retrosternal pain, abdominal pain, waterbrash, wheeze in relation to eating, symptoms associated with lying flat. The presence of nasal symptoms and allergic rhinitis may also have an influence on respiratory symptoms; excess nasal secretions can collect in the pharynx during sleep, resulting in night-time coughing (sometimes referred to as 'postnasal drip').
- Is there evidence of steroid resistance? Has a trial of oral steroids been given with appropriate measures of lung function before and afterwards? Steroid resistance is discussed further in 🕮 Chapter 14.

Examination

A full and careful clinical examination is required. Children with severe persistent asthma will usually have a hyperinflated chest, and wheeze either at rest or on forced expiration. A normal chest shape with good chest expansion is reassuring.

Investigation

- Spirometry should be performed in all children who are able to cooperate with the technique. This may reveal airflow obstruction. If this is present, reversibility with a bronchodilator should be demonstrated.
- Tests of bronchial responsiveness using methacholine or hypertonic saline challenge are not likely to be helpful in making a diagnosis of asthma where there is doubt after clinical assessment since these tests are neither sensitive nor specific for clinically significant asthma.
- Exercise tests (see 🕮 Chapter 69) can be more informative and, if exercise causes a significant drop in FEV1 and wheeze is heard, there is little doubt that asthma is present. The test can vary from time to time and is affected by air conditions. A negative test does not exclude asthma. Where there is a clear history of exercise-induced symptoms, an exercise test can be helpful to determine if those symptoms are caused by bronchospasm.
- Where there is clinical suspicion of gastro-oesophageal reflux, appropriate investigation, e.g. oesophageal pH measurement, may be helpful.
- Assessment of allergy, e.g. measurement of total IgE, specific IgE (RAST tests), and skin prick tests, may be helpful as corroborating evidence for a diagnosis of asthma (by demonstrating allergic sensitization), and may direct allergen avoidance programmes where these are undertaken.
- Aspergillus IgE and IgG (precipitin lines).
- Sputum culture or cough swab may be helpful in identifying persistent bacterial endobronchial infection and the presence of Aspergillus may contribute to a diagnosis of allergic bronchopulmonary aspergillosis.
- Fractional exhaled nitric oxide may indicate persistently elevated levels suggesting poorly controlled ongoing airway inflammation.
- Bronchoscopy may be helpful in the refractory severe asthm exclude abnormal airway anatomy or malacia and to perfo to look at cell types present and determine whether there persistent inflammation. Bronchial biopsies may be taken research protocol.

- Where appropriate:
  - sweat test;
  - nasal brush biopsy for cilial evaluation;
  - serum IgG, IgA, and IgM and specific antibody responses to vaccinations;
  - HRCT of the chest—to identify any unexpected bronchiolitis obliterans or bronchiectasis.
- Sometimes a home visit, e.g. by an asthma nurse specialist, can be very helpful. Unexpected social problems leading to poor adherence or exposure to airway irritants or allergens may be discovered.

Alternative or concurrent diagnoses

The following may be mistaken for asthma.
- Postviral cough.
- Habit cough.
- Gastro-oesophageal reflux.
- Vocal cord dysfunction.
- Chronic bronchial infection:
  - primary ciliary dyskinesia;
  - cystic fibrosis;
  - immune deficiency;
  - idiopathic bronchiectasis.
- Aspiration lung disease.
- Inhaled foreign body.
- Allergic bronchopulmonary aspergillosis.
- Tuberculosis.
- Congenital lung anomalies or masses compressing the airways.
- H-type tracheo-oesophageal fistula.
- Rare interstitial lung disease.

One common error is assuming that a persistent cough is likely to be asthma without a clear history of wheeze. Another pitfall is to take a history of wheeze at face value. This can be especially easy to do in children with vocal cord dysfunction (see 📖 Chapter 14). Most of these diagnoses can be excluded by a careful history and examination. If there is doubt, further investigation, including exercise testing, CXR, CT scan, or bronchoscopy may be needed. Many of the respiratory diseases listed above can cause wheeze. Asthma is common, and may be present as a second problem, or exacerbated by another coexisting condition. A poor response to standard asthma therapy should prompt a careful review rather than simply prompt an increase in asthma therapy.

Treatment

Treatment of poorly controlled asthma will depend on the results of the approach outlined above. It is very important to consider both adherence to therapy and alternative diagnoses or conditions that may be contributing to asthma severity before escalating asthma drug treatment. Options for treating severe asthma are discussed in 📖 Chapter 14.

Recurrent or persistent 'chest infection'

History

One of the most common presentations to a respiratory clinic is the child who has recurrent chestiness or (as it is often reported) chest infection. A good history is essential in order to understand the problem.

- What do the parents mean by chestiness or chest infection?
  - Cough? Is it dry or does it sound productive?
  - Fever?
  - Wheeze? Is it persistent or intermittent and what precipitates it?
  - Upper airway rattle?
  - Breathlessness?
- Are the symptoms there all the time or do they come and go?
- What is the longest time between symptoms?
- What precipitates symptoms?
- What is the pattern of an episode?
- Do the symptoms bother the child or just the parents?
- What happens with exercise?
- Do symptoms stop the child from doing anything?
- Are there any accompanying symptoms?
  - Runny nose?
  - Discharging ears?
  - Ear infections?
  - Failure to thrive?
  - Loose stools?
  - Infections elsewhere?
  - Heartburn or waterbrash?
- Is there a history of early or neonatal respiratory symptoms?

Examination

- Is the child well-nourished and growing normally?
- Is the child making any respiratory noise?
- If the child is quiet in clinic can parents copy any respiratory noise they are concerned about for you?
- Is there:
  - clubbing;
  - tachypnoea;
  - hyperinflation;
  - any signs of respiratory distress?
- Does the child have a cough whilst they are in the clinic?
- Are there any signs on auscultation of the chest?
- Are there any focal signs?
- Are there any signs of systemic disease such as eczema or muscle weakness?

Investigation and diagnosis

A CXR is likely to be necessary unless there is a previously normal CXR available. Thereafter, the history and examination should permit the redefinition of chestiness into one of 5 groups of symptoms (as below) and investigation and management can be directed on this basis.

- Many children who present to secondary care with recurrent chestiness will be normal children with recurrent viral infections. These are usually pre-school children with frequent coryzal symptoms and intermittent cough. The clues that these are normal children without underlying pathology are that:
  - they are thriving;
  - although their symptoms seem continuous to the parents, on careful questioning they are actually distinct illnesses;
  - the respiratory symptoms are always accompanied by a runny nose and possibly a sore throat;
  - on examination there is nothing abnormal to find;
  - the CXR if done is normal.
- Upper airway noises. Consider:
  - inspiratory stridor—possibly laryngomalacia, but other conditions may need excluding;
  - biphasic stridor—always needs further investigation with laryngo-bronchoscopy;
  - a rattle (ruttle) transiently cleared by swallowing—usually no further investigation needed.
- Chronic productive cough. Consider:
  - chronic endobronchial infection;
  - primary ciliary dyskinesia;
  - cystic fibrosis;
  - immunodeficiency;
  - aspiration lung disease.
- Recurrent cough and wheeze. Consider:
  - wheeze associated with viral illnesses;
  - atopic asthma;
  - aspiration lung disease.
- Persistent wheeze. Consider:
  - asthma;
  - structural airway disease, either because of external compression from bronchogenic cyst, vascular ring, etc.; an airway wall abnormality such as bronchomalacia; or internal obstruction by either a foreign body or airway granuloma. If structural airway disease is suspected, a bronchoscopy and chest CT will be needed;
  - aspiration lung disease.
- Recurrent or persistent infection with or without CXR changes. Consider
  - middle lobe syndrome (see below);
  - immunodeficiency;
  - structural airway disease (as above);
  - cardiac disease, usually left to right shunting;
  - aspiration lung disease;
  - poor cough clearance, possibly reflecting bulbar dysfunction or muscular weakness;
  - tuberculosis.

Uncommon and rare conditions

Most respiratory specialists will have one or two children with these conditions under their care, but very few will have experience of all of these disorders. Some will present with either recurrent chestiness or with a diagnosis of 'atypical asthma'.

- Post-infectious bronchiolitis obliterans.
- Hypersensitivity pneumonitis.
- Pulmonary infiltrates with eosinophilia.
- Rare interstitial lung disease, including:
  - disorders of surfactant function;
  - connective tissue disease;
  - pulmonary vasculitides.
- Other rare lung diseases:
  - pulmonary haemosiderosis;
  - pulmonary alveolar proteinosis;
  - sarcoidosis;
  - disorders of the pulmonary lymphatics.

Further details on all the conditions mentioned in this chapter can be found in the relevant chapters later in the book.

Middle lobe syndrome

- Middle lobe syndrome (MLS) refers to persistent or recurrent respiratory symptoms associated with right middle lobe or lingula consolidation on CXR in the context of normal anatomy.
- It predominantly affects pre-school children. Accurate incidence data are not available, but reports in the literature suggest that many centres see 2–5 affected children each year.
- The middle lobe is thought to be prone to recurrent or persistent collapse and consolidation for the following reasons.
  - The bronchus to the right middle lobe has a small diameter and an acute take-off angle from the right main bronchus, which may increase its probability of becoming obstructed.
  - The bronchus may be particularly at risk of compression by hilar lymph nodes.
  - The middle lobe has poor collateral ventilation, which means that, when it has collapsed, it is is less likely to re-expand than other areas of the lung.
- Symptoms are rather non-specific but in most series include cough, which is usually productive sounding. Wheeze is present in 50–70% of affected children. Occasionally MLS will be asymptomatic and identified on incidental CXR.
- There may be a pre-existing diagnosis of asthma and mucus plugging from related airway inflammation may be an important mechanism. Asthma is probably less common than was previously thought. Some studies suggest that only around 25% of affected children show symptoms of asthma at follow-up.
- 50–70% have positive bacterial culture of bronchoalveolar lavage (BAL) fluid, usually *Haemophilus influenzae*.
- Occasionally the right middle lobe bronchus will be obstructed with unsuspected foreign body or airway tumour.

Investigations
- CXR.
- Bronchoscopy and BAL.
- CT scan if CXR changes and symptoms persist despite aggressive management.

Management
- Early intervention, within 6 months of symptoms, is likely to result in a better outcome. Although the chances of finding anatomical abnormality of the airway is very low, it is well worth carrying out the bronchoscopy and lavage sooner rather than later. The lavage process itself may help improve patency of the bronchus.
- After investigations are complete, management consists of a combination of prolonged courses of antibiotics, chest physiotherapy, bronchodilators, and inhaled steroids. In children with wheeze and positive BAL cultures, all 4 interventions can be used.

Outcome
- Outcome is usually good, with resolution of symptoms and CXR changes in 60% and improvement in a further 30%.
- In 10%, symptoms and CXR changes persist These children are more likely to have had long-standing symptoms before aggressive therapy was started, and are also more likely to have CT evidence of bronchiectasis.

Further information
De Boeck, K., Willems, T., van Gysel, D., Corbeel, L., and Eeckels, R. (1995). Outcome after right middle lobe syndrome. *Chest* **108**, 150–2.

Priftis, K.N., Anthracopoulos, M.B., Mermiri, D., Papadopoulou, A., Xepapacaki, P., Tsakanika, C., and Nicolaidou, P. (2006). Bronchial hyperresponsiveness, atopy, and bronchoalveolar lavage eosinophils in persistent middle lobe syndrome. Pediatr. *Pulmonol.* **41**, 805–11.

Priftis, K.N., Mermiri, D., Papadopoulou, A., Anthraco pouos, M.B., Vaos, G., and Nicolaidou. P. (2005). The role of timely intervention in middle lobe syndrome in children. *Chest* **128**, 2504–10.

Springer, C., Avital, A., Noviski, N., et al. (1992). Role of infection in the middle lobe syndrome in asthma. *Arch. Dis. Child.* **57**, 592–4.

Chronic cough

Definition

- A cough that has been persistent for 6 weeks or more is unlikely to be purely related to common viral infections and can be considered a chronic cough.
- Clues to the aetiology lie primarily in:
  - the history;
  - the nature of the cough (dry or productive);
  - (ideally) hearing the cough.

History

- When did the cough start?
- What happened at the start, e.g. was there a respiratory tract infection or a choking episode?
- What has the pattern been?
  - Getting worse/better/staying the same?
  - Episodic/paroxysmal/nocturnal?
  - Periods without cough?
- Is cough dry or productive?
- What precipitates the cough, e.g. eating or exercise?
- Does the cough occur at night?
- Any other associated symptoms, e.g. wheeze?
- Any previous chest symptoms?
- Any other infections?
- Any other symptoms particularly symptoms of:
  - dyspepsia, suggesting gastro-oesophageal reflux;
  - loose stools or failure to thrive, suggesting cystic fibrosis.
- Are there upper respiratory tract symptoms (may suggest ciliary dyskinesia)?
  - Rhinitis?
  - Ear infections?
  - Glue ear?
- Early history:
  - prematurity;
  - early neonatal lung disease.
- Family history of cough/chest illness.
- School history of symptoms in other children, e.g. pertussis infection.

Examination

A full and careful clinical examination is required particularly of upper respiratory tract including ears (Arnold's ear-cough) and chest. If chest is hyperexpanded and/or wheeze is heard asthma becomes more likely.

Ask the child to cough and ask the parents if the cough you have heard is typical. Is the cough paroxysmal or dry/tickly or wet/productive or barking/tracheal/laryngeal?

Causes of a dry chronic cough

- Reactive airways disease (asthma). Clues are:
  - presence of wheeze
  - presence of exercise intolerance
  - allergen or exercise precipitants for cough
  - cough at night
- Gastro-oesophageal reflux. Clues are:
  - upper abdominal pain
  - cough after meals
- Post-viral or post-pertussis. Clues are:
  - paroxysmal nature, associated with going red in the face or vomiting
  - history of acute illness at onset
- Habit cough. Clues are:
  - loud barking cough
  - absent at night
  - often distractable
- Postnasal drip. Clues are:
  - usually pre-school child not yet able to effectively blow their nose
  - cough occurs at night shortly after going to bed
- Tracheo-bronchomalacia. Clue is loud barking cough from early life
- Arnold's ear–cough reflex. If the auricular branch of the vagus nerve is present, ear inflammation can cause cough
- Drugs, usually ACE inhibitors. Clue is that cough resolves when medication stopped
- Non-specific cough. No cause identified

Causes of a productive-sounding chronic cough

- Cystic fibrosis. Clues are:
  - abnormal bowel habit or failure to thrive
  - family history
- Primary ciliary dyskinesia. Clues are:
  - recurrent ear or sinus infection
  - neonatal respiratory distress
  - persistent nasal discharge
  - situs inversus in 50% of cases
- Immune deficiency. Clue is infections elsewhere.
- Chronic endobronchial infection. Clues are:
  - otherwise well
  - normal physical examination
  - normal or near normal CXR
  - response to 2–6 weeks antibiotics and physiotherapy
- Aspiration lung disease. Clues are:
  - neurologically abnormal
  - may be wheeze as well
  - abnormal CXR
- Inhaled foreign body. Clue is history of choking episode

Investigation

Investigation is directed by type and severity of cough. If the cough has not been heard in clinic or the parents feel the cough produced is atypical then ask them to record the cough at home on audio or videotape and bring to next appointment. It may also be useful for a symptom diary card to be kept peak flow readings.

Investigations to consider for a dry cough include:
- CXR;
- spirometry;
- exercise test;
- pH study;
- contrast swallow;
- video-fluoroscopy.

Investigations to consider for a productive-sounding cough include:
- CXR;
- cough swab or sputum culture;
- spirometry;
- sweat test;
- ciliary biopsy;
- tests of immune function:
  - full blood count;
  - total immunoglobulins;
  - functional responses to vaccinations.
- CT scan;
- bronchoscopy.

Management

The management is directed to the likely underlying aetiology.

- Post-pertussis cough requires explanation and reassurance only. The family should be warned that the cough is likely to persist for 3 months with gradual improvement but may be exacerbated by any intercurrent URTI.
- Cough associated with asthma responds to asthma treatment.
- Chronic productive-sounding cough in otherwise well children is most likely to be caused be persistent low grade endobronchial infection. This condition has several different names in the literature including chronic bronchitis, chronic endobronchial infection, and persistent bacterial bronchitis. When there are no abnormal physical findings and a normal CXR or one showing mild bronchial wall thickening only and nothing from the history to suggest an alternative diagnosis, it is reasonable to begin treatment with a prolonged course of antibiotics (to ensure no residual bacterial infection driving chronic sputum production) and physiotherapy (to ensure effective airway clearance). Personal practice in Oxford is to give 6 weeks of oral antibiotic combined with chest physiotherapy before review. The vast majority of patients respond to this therapy with no further problems but if symptoms persist or recur then the child should be investigated for an underlying disorder such as cystic fibrosis, immune deficiency, or primary ciliary dyskinesia.
- Habit cough is usually just a habit like any other.
  - A child possibly with very mild tracheomalacia, gets a viral infection that starts them coughing. Because they discover they can make a loud cough, which possibly gets them a bit of attention, this becomes reinforced. Tracheal irritation from the cough itself may also help to perpetuate the cough.
  - There is usually no identifiable underlying psychological problem, nor do the majority of children develop other functional problems once their cough resolves (although it can occasionally happen).
  - Management of a habit cough starts with explanation and reassurance. Teaching the child some breathing exercises to do when they feel like coughing can also be useful. The majority settle without further action but occasionally help from a psychologist is needed.
  - The now famous 'cough and bedsheet' approach is rarely used in practice, but alternative distracting therapies, such as sipping warm water when the child feels the desire to cough, may be equally effective.
- Cough associated with other individual conditions is managed according to the cause—each is dealt with in later chapters.

Further information

Chang, A.B. (2005). Cough: are children really different to adults? *Cough* **1** 7.

Lavigne, J.V., Davis, A.T., and Fauber, R. (1991). Behavioral management of psychogenic cough: alternative to the "bedsheet" and other aversive techniques. *Pediatric.* **37**, 532–7.

Marchant, J.M., Masters, I.B., Taylor, S.M., Cox, N.C., Seymour, G.J., and Chang, A.B. (2006). Evaluation and outcome of young children with chronic cough. *Chest* **129**, 1132–41.

1 Cohlan, S.Q. and Stone, S.M. (1984). The cough and the bedsheet. *Pediatrics* **74**, 11–15.

Chapter 5

Stridor

Definition

- Stridor (from the latin *stridere*—to make harsh sounds) is a harsh monophonic noise that comes from the trachea or larynx as a result of narrowing. It may be heard with or without a stethoscope.
- When the *extrathoracic* airway is affected, the noise always has an inspiratory component, as the extrathoracic airway is at its narrowest, but it can be biphasic if the narrowing is severe.
- When the *intrathoracic* trachea is affected, the stridor will usually be biphasic with a relatively loud expiratory phase.
- A purely inspiratory stridor indicates narrowing of the extrathoracic airway.
- Stridor should be distinguished from the coarse low-pitched stertor and/or snoring that come from the naso/oropharynx.

Acute presentation

In a previously well child presenting acutely with stridor the differential diagnosis is as follows.

- Viral croup. A very common viral illness most often caused by parainfluenza virus. Spring and autumn seasons. Generally preceding history of a mild URTI. Classically the child wakes at night stridulous with barking cough, hoarse voice, and mild fever.
- Epiglottitis. A rare condition since the introduction of universal HiB vaccination. The child is septicaemic and very unwell with a high temperature, soft stridor, and little cough and may be drooling as unable to handle oral secretions.
- Inhaled foreign body. Generally there is a clear history of an inhalation episode. Laryngeal foreign bodies usually cause complete airways obstruction and the child seldom survives long enough to reach hospital. Most objects small enough to fit through the larynx will pass to the main bronchi and, once the coughing has settled, cause minimal if any respiratory distress. Rarely, a linear foreign body such as a fish bone or piece of plastic can become lodged in the larynx whilst continuing to allow adequate ventilation.
- Acute allergic reaction. Generally good history of precipitant.
- Other infections, e.g. retropharyngeal abscess. Preceding history of sore throat/tonsillitis, high fever.
- Airway burns (smoke) and scalds (steam).

Assess stridor severity

- Is the stridor present at rest or only when agitated?
- Is the stridor purely inspiratory or biphasic?
- Is there nasal flaring?
- What is the extent of chest wall indrawing/work of breathing?
- What is the child's position? The child with severe stridor will sit leaning forward, propped on arms with chin extended.
- Is there cyanosis or desaturation?
- What are the chest expansion and breath sounds like? Is there air entry with every respiratory effort or only when a large inspiratory effort is made?

Management of acute severe stridor, independent of underlying cause

- Keep the parent and child as calm as possible. Crying causes the airflow to become more turbulent, increasing resistance to flow, and may precipitate complete obstruction.
- Give the parent an oxygen mask to hold near to the child.
- Call for urgent help from someone with paediatric airway expertise—usually an anaesthetist.
- Give nebulized adrenaline while waiting for anaesthetist to arrive (give IM adrenaline as well if acute severe anaphylaxis is suspected).
- If the airway is still insufficient for effective ventilation after the adrenaline, the anaesthetist will usually give inhalational anaesthetic and intubate the child. IV access can then be obtained.

Persistent or recurrent stridor in infants

The common causes to consider are shown in the box.

History

- Is the child developing and growing normally?
- Is the stridor continuous or episodic?
  - If episodic, is it variable with position, feeding, excitement, sleeping?
- Are there any associated features?
- Is there a history of birth trauma?
- Are there any cranial nerve anomalies?
- Is there a history of cardiac/thoracic surgery?
- Are there any cutaneous haemangiomata? 50% of patients with subglottic haemangioma will have a cutaneous haemangioma, usually in the beard distribution of the face.
- Are there any swallowing difficulties? May suggest bulbar dysfunction.

Examination

- Is the stridor inspiratory or biphasic? This is most important—if the stridor is inspiratory only then the cause is extrathoracic.
- Is the stridor positional?
- Is the work of breathing increased?
- Are there chest expansion and breath sounds on auscultation with every respiratory effort?
- Are there any cutaneous haemangiomata?

Investigations

The most likely cause for stridor in early infancy is laryngomalacia. Where there is a mild intermittent purely inspiratory stridor starting soon after birth in an otherwise well and thriving infant, an expectant approach can be taken. If there is any doubt about the cause of the stridor and certainly if the stridor is biphasic or associated with poor feeding or poor growth or with more than very minor chest wall retraction, further investigation should be carried out. These investigations are:

- CXR: to assess mediastinum and cardiac size and position of aorta;
- laryngo-bronchoscopy: to visualize airway structures;
- blood tests for serum electrolytes: rarely metabolic disorders such as hypocalcaemia and hypomagnesaemia may cause stridor in infancy.

Management depends on cause. The management of specific causes of stridor in infancy is given in 🕮 Chapter 24.

Causes of persistent stridor in infancy

Purely inspiratory
- Laryngomalacia
- Vocal cord palsy
- Supraglottic cyst, laryngeal cyst
- Laryngeal cleft
- Hypocalcaemia or hypomagnesaemia
- Lingual thyroid

Biphasic
- Vocal cord palsy
- Subglottic stenosis
- Subglottic cyst
- Subglottic haemangioma
- Branchial cleft cyst
- Cystic hygroma
- Vascular ring

Persistent or recurrent stridor in the older child

The common causes to consider are shown in the box.

History

Chronic and persistent stridor in a previously normal older child is unusual and the history needs to concentrate on when and how it developed and any variation with activity, eating, and sleep.

Recurrent stridor is more common and may occur in context of:
- recurrent viral croup: there is usually clear history of viral symptoms at or preceding onset and no stridor between episodes;
- allergy: usually the child is known to be atopic. There may be clear precipitating exposures including foodstuffs. There will be no stridor between episodes;
- vocal cord dysfunction: sudden onset often during serious sporting activity. Causes alarm around the child and halts the activity. Usually lasts for minutes only, and again the child is completely well between episodes.

Examination

Unless stridor is present the examination is likely to be completely normal. If stridor is present:
- is it inspiratory or biphasic?
- is there any associated lymphadenopathy?
- are there any neck masses?
- is the throat normal?
- is the child distractable?

Investigation

- Chronic and persistent stridor needs urgent investigation with:
  - spirometry—inspiratory and expiratory loops;
  - CXR;
  - laryngo-bronchoscopy;
  - CT scan of the chest and neck.
- Recurrent viral croup with no symptoms between episodes does not require further investigation.
- The child suspected of having vocal cord dysfunction will have normal CXR and lung function. The symptoms may be reproduced during an exercise test particularly if the child is put under some stress at the time. The diagnosis can be made definitively if laryngoscopy can be done at the time of the stridor—with vocal cord narrowing (to near closure) during inspiration. Vocal cord dysfunction is discussed further at the end of 📖 Chapter 14.

Management

- For chronic and persistent stridor, management depends on aetiology.
- Recurrent viral croup, with no interval symptoms, needs treatment only at time of episodes and parents may be advised to keep oral dexamethasone at home to use on instruction from their general practitioner.

Causes of persistent stridor in older children

- Pharyngeal tumour
- Neck mass/tumour
- Juvenile respiratory papillomatosis
- Foreign body in pharynx, larynx, subglottis, oesophagus, trachea
- External tracheal compression—usually from a tumour, most often a mediastinal lymphoma

Infant apnoea

Introduction

Clinical apnoea is defined as an abnormal respiratory pause of more than 20 seconds or of shorter duration if associated with cyanosis, marked pallor, hypotonia, or bradycardia. Apnoea in infants, particularly pre-term infants, is common, most probably because of immaturity of respiratory control. Young infants have excessive laryngeal reflex-mediated obstruction, diminished ventilatory hypercapnic responses, and hypoxia-induced respiratory depression. Apnoeic events can be obstructive, central, or mixed. Airways obstruction will usually lead to a period of increased effort associated with tachycardia. This may be followed by central apnoea and hypoxic bradycardia. Events may terminate spontaneously, with minor stimulation or, more rarely, only when rescue breaths are given.

History

A detailed description of the event will give the best clues towards identifying the cause. Most usually there will be a clearly defined single event that has caused significant distress in the carer. Less often the events are multiple and observed in hospital.

Background information

- Was infant previously well or had there been any prodromal illness?
- Are there any developmental concerns?
- What is the gestation of the infant?

Details of the event

- Where was the infant?
- In what position?
- Awake or asleep?
- What was the relationship to feeding?
- What caused the parent to look at the infant?
- Was the infant stiff or floppy or jerking?
- Was there any colour change?
- Were there abnormal eye movements?
- Was the infant making efforts to breathe?
- Was there any evidence of choking or vomit in infant's mouth?
- What did the parent/carer do?
- How long did the episode last?
- What happened after the event?

Possible causes

See box. In 40–50% of cases no cause will be found.

- An awake infant who coughs and chokes and has a predominantly obstructive apnoea (continued respiratory effort) is likely to have had an episode of laryngospasm. This may have been triggered directly during feeding or by gastro-oesophageal reflux (GOR). There is some debate about the relationship between GOR disease and apnoea, particularly in pre-term infants. A number of studies using pH monitoring have shown that there is no convincing temporal relationship between apnoea in pre-term infants and acid reflux and these data certainly suggest that anti-reflux treatment should not be routinely given to preterm infants with apnoea. There is also good evidence that placing tiny amounts of milk on to the infant larynx can precipitate dramatic laryngospasm. For single dramatic events with a typical history, GOR is still one of the most likely causes of obstructive apnoea.
- If the infant is described as having had a sudden abnormal cry followed by a change in tone or posture, with or without abnormal movements, they are most likely to be having fits.
- Parental observation of apnoea during sleep may reflect normal physio-logical periodic breathing, which is commonly seen up to the age of 6 months, and in older infants born prematurely. During periodic breathing there may be central pauses of up to 15s, with small falls in saturation (as low as 88%). Pauses beyond 15s are not usually seen in term infants. Warm ambient temperatures, such as those caused by over-wrapping, can increase periodic breathing and apnoea.
- Longer periods of central apnoea during sleep are likely to reflect underlying CNS pathology or central alveolar hypoventilation.

Possible causes of infant apnoea

- Gastro-oesophageal reflux
- Aspiration (primary or secondary to reflux)
- Sepsis
- Respiratory infection, especially RSV or pertussis
- Seizures
- Intracranial haemorrhage
- Metabolic disease
- Undiagnosed neuromuscular weakness
- Central alveolar hypoventilation
- Trauma
- Airway obstruction or H-type tracheo-oesophageal fistula
- Cardiac arrhythmia

Investigations

These will depend on the nature and severity of the event. For a single brief event, without colour change, related to choking on feeds, in a baby who has a completely normal physical examination, it is reasonable to observe without investigations. For other infants, who had more dramatic events or who are unwell, more detailed investigation will be required. These investigations may include:

- septic screen including LP;
- NPA for RSV;
- throat swab for pertussis;
- serum electrolytes and glucose;
- pH study;
- barium oesophagram;
- CXR;
- polysomnography;
- ECG;
- urinary and plasma AA and OA;
- MRI brain;
- EEG;
- laryngobronchoscopy.

Management

Most infants who have had an event that frightened the parents will be admitted to hospital for observation. Feeding patterns can be observed during this period, and common feeding-related events can be witnessed and parents reassured. If the infant is well, investigations are normal, and no events are witnessed over 48h, then these babies can be discharged. Further investigation, follow-up, the need to teach parents basic life support, and the role of monitoring will depend on the severity of the episode and local practice. More information is provided in 📖 Chapter 28.

Cystic fibrosis: poor weight gain

Introduction

Children with cystic fibrosis (CF) will be weighed at every clinic attendance, usually every 2–3 months. Good weight gain and nutrition is
strongly correlated with lung function and survival in CF, and promptly
identifying and dealing with the cause of poor weight gain is an essential
part of the management of these children.

History

Weight gain is dependent on the balance between intake and output in
the child with CF as in other children. Involving the dietician from the
outset is vital. Information needed from the child and/or parents includes
the following.

- Is this an acute problem associated with:
  - a recent chest exacerbation;
  - a gastrointestinal upset;
  - other illness?
- Is this a longstanding problem over several months/years?
- Is there any abdominal pain or discomfort?

Assessment of intake

- Has there been a recent change in appetite/food intake?
- What is the child's/parent's perception of appetite?
- Describe typical daily diet.

If child is pancreatic insufficient then details of pancreatic enzyme supple
mentation are important.

- How many and what type of enzymes are taken (total daily)?
- How are they taken?
  - Opened?
  - Swallowed whole?
  - Crunched?
  - Distribution with food, e.g. all at start of meal or divided through-out?
  - Distribution with fat intake, e.g. how many for pie and chips versus
    salad?
  - What is taken for snacks, e.g. packet of crisps?
  - What happens at school?

Assessment of losses

- Frequency of stool.
- Stool description:
- are stools offensive?
- do they float?
- do they flush away?
- are they greasy?
- is grease left in pan/potty?
- Change in urinary frequency/volume/nocturia/enuresis? May suggest
  development of CF-related diabetes.
- Energy loss. Changes in exercise regime?

Examination

Height and weight will be measured routinely at each clinic visit and comparison made with previous trends and centile charts. An assessment of subcutaneous fat should be made clinically. Abdominal examination includes evidence of :

- distension/bloating (suggestive of malabsorption);
- faecal loading (constipation secondary to poor fibre intake is not uncommon in CF and may lead to secondary decreased appetite);
- right iliac fossa mass (an early sign of distal intestinal obstruction syndrome (DIOS), which may be causing some discomfort and decrease in appetite).

Investigation

- Dietetic assessment. The dietician's assessment of intake may initially be informal in discussion with the family. The aim is for children with CF to achieve an intake of 120% the daily recommended value (DRV) of age- and sex-matched norms. However, it is often useful to proceed to a formal assessment of a 3-day food diary. This may demonstrate to the family where the problem lies. The problem may not be one unique to CF, e.g. the high-volume juice-drinking toddler.
- Stool collection and examination.
    - Visual appearance.
    - Fat content. Microscopic examination for fat globules (i.e. no excess/moderate excess/gross excess) can be very helpful as a crude indicator of steatorrhoea. Laboratories will now rarely perform a 3-day faecal fat estimation.
    - If the child was previously pancreatic sufficient then a stool elastase should be performed (levels < 150mcg/g indicate pancreatic insufficiency).
- Depending on duration/severity of the problem blood tests looking for evidence of malnutrition and/or other diagnoses may be considered, e.g. serum albumin, total protein, iron, folate, endomysial antibodies, etc.
- If cystic fibrosis related diabetes (CFRD) is a possibility, then a fasting blood glucose and either a glucose tolerance test (GTT) or a glucose series (finger prick blood glucose 2h after breakfast, lunch, and dinner over 2–3 days) should be performed. HbA1c levels can be normal in early CFRD.

Management

Inadequate intake

The most common reason for poor weight gain is inadequate energy intake. It is important to consider and address where possible the reasons for this, including family and emotional difficulties or problems at school. Recent school emphasis on healthy eating has not been helpful for the child with CF who does not want to be seen to be different from their contemporaries but needs more than a piece of fruit at break time. Strategies to address poor intake include the following.

- Dietary adjustment.
- Dietary supplementation:
  - calories to drinks (e.g. Calogen);
  - CHO-based fruit drinks (e.g. Enlive);
  - milk mixed high calory drinks (e.g. Scandishake).
- For refractory intake problems nasogastric or gastrotomy feeding may be needed (see Chapter 15).

Excess energy losses

Enzyme supplementation may need adjustment in timing or total. The aim is not to exceed a total daily intake of 10 000 units of lipase/kg body weight. If the daily intake is near or above this with evidence of malabsorption then excess acid in the upper small intestine may be inhibiting optimal enzyme release. Strategies include:

- use of an H2 blocker such as ranitidine;
- use of a proton pump inhibitor such as omeprazole (it is worth remembering that omeprazole has a short half-life and, when used for this purpose, may need to be taken twice daily).

CF-related diabetes

Usually requires treatment with insulin. See 📖 Chapter 15.

Other diagnoses

Children with CF may have non-CF-related reasons for poor weight gain such as lactose intolerance, cow's milk protein intolerance, or coeliac disease.

Cystic fibrosis: loss of lung function

Introduction

In most centres lung function tests will be carried out every 2–3 months on all children with CF who are able to perform simple spirometry. Evaluating changes in lung function is part of the routine assessment of these children. When there is a fall in lung function it will often be associated with a clinically obvious infective exacerbation of lung disease. On other occasions the cause of the fall in lung function is less obvious. Correct identification and prompt treatment of the cause will ensure that affected children have the best possible long-term outcomes.

History

- Has the loss of lung function been associated with an upper respiratory tract infection or other viral illness?
- Is there an increase or change in cough?
- Is there a change in sputum volume/consistency/colour?
- Has the child been wheezing?
- Are there associated symptoms:
  - poor appetite;
  - weight loss;
  - tiredness;
  - polyuria or polydipsia?

Examination

- Is there a change in respiratory signs:
  - hyperinflation;
  - respiratory distress;
  - wheeze;
  - crackles?
- Are there focal signs?
- Is the child systemically unwell?
- Is the child hypoxic?

Investigation and management

The commonest cause for loss of lung function is infection.

- A cough or sputum specimen should be sent for culture and first-line antibiotics started (dependent on previous microbiology).
- If the child is systemically unwell or hypoxic these antibiotics should be given IV.
- If there are focal signs a CXR should be performed.

If there is no response or a poor response to appropriate treatment with first-line antibiotics to which the organism is sensitive then continue IV antibiotics and consider the following.

- Is there another infective organism?
  - Repeat the sputum culture after discussion with the microbiology lab to ensure extended culture and plating for unusual organisms.
  - Culture for atypical mycobacteria.
  - If it is difficult to obtain sputum consider induced sputum techniques or bronchoscopy with bronchoalveolar lavage.

- Perform or repeat the CXR.
  - Are there new changes?
  - Does the CXR suggest infection?
  - Are there pulmonary infiltrates suggestive of allergic bronchopulmonary aspergillosis (ABPA)?
- Other investigations to consider when there is failure to improve:
  - FBC: is there neutrophilia (suggesting infection) or eosinophilia (suggesting ABPA);
  - CRP;
  - immunology: total IgE; aspergillus precipitins; specific IgE to aspergillus;
  - virology: from airway secretions;
  - fasting blood glucose and blood glucose series to investigate whether CFRD is associated with the change in lung function.
- The development of ABPA should always be considered if there is an unexplained loss of lung function. Often there will be other clues such as wheeze or the development of exercise intolerance, and infiltrates on CXR but the onset can be insidious. A total Ig E > 1000IU along with some evidence of a specific immunological response to Aspergillus is diagnostic in a child with unexplained loss of Lung function. Treatment is with oral steroids initially oral itraconazole. Further details can be found in 📖 Chapter 15.
- The development of CFRD is frequently insidious with an increase in respiratory symptoms and loss of lung function described up to 3 years before frank diabetes develops. Children > 12 years of age should have an annual assessment of glucose handling either by a glucose tolerance test or by a series of blood glucose tests taken 2h after normal meals. An unexpected and unexplained fall in lung function should precipitate a further assessment. Further details can be found in 📖 Chapter 15.
- It is not unusual for a viral infection to precipitate a bacterial exacerbation in CF and for there to be a slow return of lung function after appropriate antibiotic treatment. After assessment for the presence of other complicating factors, treatment with a short course of oral steroids may accelerate the return of lung function to normal levels.

Chest pain

Introduction

Chest pain occurs at all ages but is most common in late childhood and adolescence. Unlike in adults, it is not usually a manifestation of organic disease and is rarely cardiac in nature. Chest pain in younger children is more likely to have an organic aetiology.

History

A careful history regarding the character of the pain and associated symptoms should help elicit the cause of pain in most cases.

- Is the pain acute or chronic?
- How frequent is the pain?
- How long does the pain last?
- Is it well localized?
- Is it related to exertion?
- Is it exacerbated by chest wall palpation?
- Is it exacerbated by deep inspiration or coughing?
- Does the pain radiate anywhere?
- Is the patient febrile?
- What relationship is there to mealtimes and to sleeping?
- Are there associated symptoms (lightheadedness, palpations, nausea, sweating, fainting, tingling fingers)?
- Use of oral contraceptive pill; history of smoking; cocaine use.
- Past history of underlying chronic disease (asthma, CF, cardiac disease, sickle cell disease, SLE).
- Family history of arrhythmia, cardiomyopathy, sudden death, Marfan's syndrome, or peptic ulcer disease.
- Is there a relative with recent chest pain or heart attack? Other psychological factors that may be important are relatives with chronic pain, the recent loss of a relative, family dynamics, and school progress.

Causes

Lists of possible causes of chest pain are given in the boxes.

Musculoskeletal

Musculoskeletal causes are the most common and can usually be reproduced by palpation of the chest.

Psychogenic

- Psychogenic pain is the second most common cause of chest pain in children (accounting for 30%).
- It is a diagnosis of exclusion.

Pulmonary

- Pulmonary chest pain may originate from the parietal pleura, diaphragm, chest wall, or main airways.
- Lung parenchyma and visceral pleura are insensitive to pain.
- Pleuritic chest pain is characterized by sharp localized pain that is worse on inspiration or coughing. It may be associated with low tidal volume breathing, secondary tachypnoea, and a positional scoliosis to limit expansion on the affected side.

- Pain from irritation of the upper parietal pleura is usually well localized, but lower parietal and diaphragmatic pleural irritation may localize to the abdomen.
- The phrenic nerve (C3–C5) innervates the central component of the diaphragm. Irritation here may manifest as ipsilateral shoulder tip pain.
- Pain from the major airways is usually retrosternal.
- Pain from pneumonia will be accompanied by tachypnoea and fever, but classic signs of consolidation may be absent.
- Empyema may present with fever and abdominal pain.
- Spontaneous pneumothorax often presents with a sharp unilateral pain followed by a dull discomfort and associated with a feeling of breathlessness.
- Pneumomediastinum is not an uncommon complication of severe acute asthma and may be associated with surgical emphysema and/or musculoskeletal pain from prolonged coughing. The condition is usually non-progressive and recovery is uneventful.

Gastrointestinal

- A gastrointestinal cause is suggested by association with eating or posture. The pain may be at the lung bases, shoulder-tip from diaphragmatic irritation, or retrosternal pain.
- The pain usually reflects inflammation in the oesophagus, stomach, liver, gall bladder, or pancreas.

Cardiac

- Pallor, sweating, and breathlessness associated with chest pain imply cardiovascular compromise.
- Ischaemic heart disease is extremely rare in children. Cocaine use and vasculitis may precipitate angina pectoris. Myocardial ischaemia from anomalous origin of the left coronary artery from the pulmonary artery may present with severe persistent irritability in infants.
- Older children with a history of Kawasaki disease may be at risk of coronary artery thromboembolic disease from coronary artery aneurysms.
- Pericarditis presents with sharp stabbing pain across the precordium, is classically exacerbated by inspiration and coughing, and is relieved by leaning forward. Physical findings are dependent on the degree of pericardial fluid accumulation. A pericardial friction rub may be heard if little fluid is present; a silent precordium with muffled heart sounds, neck vein distension, and increased pulsus paradoxus implies fluid accumulation and the risk of tamponade.
- Acute myocarditis is typically associated with central stabbing chest pain on exertion, and may be associated with a gallop rhythm and signs of congestive cardiac failure.

Possible causes of chest pain: 1

Musculoskeletal
- Tietze's syndrome (costochondritis)
- Precordial catch syndrome (intercostal muscle cramps)
- Rib fracture
- Slipping rib syndrome

Psychogenic

Pulmonary
- Pleuritic chest pain:
  - pneumonia with/without parapneumonic effusion
  - empyema
  - pneumothorax
  - pneumomediastinum
  - pleurodynia (Coxsackie virus)
  - pulmonary infarction (after embolism)
  - sickle cell disease (acute chest syndrome)
- Retrosternal chest pain:
  - tracheobronchitis
  - bronchopneumonia
  - bronchospasm
  - foreign body

Possible causes of chest pain: 2

Gastrointestinal
- Gastro-oesophageal reflux
- Peptic ulcer disease
- Oesophageal foreign body
- Cholecystitis
- Pancreatitis
- Acute viral hepatitis
- Subphrenic abscess

Cardiac
- Pericardial disease:
  - acute pericarditis
  - post-pericardiotomy syndrome
- Cardiac ischaemia:
  - Kawasaki disease
  - anomalous coronary arteries
  - sympathomimetic ingestion (e.g. cocaine)
  - tachyarrhythmias
  - familial hypercholesterolaemia
- Acute myocarditis
- Cardiomyopathy
- Aortic dissection
- Mitral valve prolapse

Neurogenic
- Dermatomal shingles (pain may precede rash)
- Spinal cord or nerve root compression

Investigations

In the majority of cases, the cause of chest pain is clear and no investigation is required. CXR will help define most acute respiratory causes of chest pain and an ECG will help in excluding cardiac causes. An exercise test may be useful if the pain is brought on by exercise or if the child has been stopped from doing exercise as a result of family anxiety about the pain. Further investigations may include pleural aspiration, V/Q scan, HRCT chest, and autoantibody profile. If the pain is thought to be cardiac in origin, cardiology referral is indicated.

Haemoptysis

Introduction

Haemoptysis is defined as expectoration of blood or blood-stained sputum. It is relatively rare in children. Care must be taken to distinguish it from haematemesis and epistaxis. Haemoptysis results from bleeding from the bronchial or pulmonary vessels into lungs or airways. Blood that is expectorated from the lung or airways is generally bright red and alkaline (as opposed to haematemesis blood, which is usually dark red and acid). It is useful to divide possible causes into focal bleeding (either from the lung parenchyma or airways) and diffuse bleeding (nearly always from the alveolar bed). These causes are listed in the boxes.

The commonest clinical situation is small volume haemoptysis, usually streaked within purulent sputum. This is consistent with mucosal bleeding in a child with bronchiectasis. These children will have a long history of productive cough and will in most cases have been seen and investigated for this symptom. More rarely, similar mucosal bleeding can be seen in acute airways infection.

Haemoptysis as a presenting symptom is rare in children. If the blood is genuinely coming from the airways or lungs and there is nothing to suggest acute or chronic infection, the bleeding is likely either to be due to an airway lesion, pulmonary thromboembolism, or one of the causes of diffuse alveolar haemorrhage.

Possible causes of focal pulmonary haemorrhage

- Infection:
  - viral or bacterial tracheobronchitis
  - pneumonia
  - tuberculosis
  - atypical mycobacterial infection
  - parasitic infection (e.g. echinococcosis)
- Bronchiectasis:
  - cystic fibrosis
  - primary ciliary dyskinesia
  - allergic bronchopulmonary aspergillosis
  - immunodeficiency (antibody)
- Cavitatory lesions, including congenital lung anomalies
- Pulmonary vascular problems:
  - pulmonary thromboembolism
  - pulmonary artery aneurysm (idiopathic or associated with Behçet and other vasculitides)
- Foreign body
- Arteriovenous malformation
- Haemangiomata
- Neoplasms
- Tracheostomy-related:
  - granuloma around stoma
  - mucosal erosion from chronic suctioning

Possible causes of diffuse pulmonary haemorrhage

- Pulmonary haemosiderosis:
    - idiopathic or with pulmonary capillaritis
    - associated with glomerulonephritis (Goodpasture's syndrome)
- Systemic vasculitis:
    - Wegener's granulomatosis
    - Henoch–Schorlein purpura (very rarely and mainly in adults)
    - Churg–Strauss
    - microscopic angiitis
- Collagen vascular disease:
    - systemic lupus erythematosus
    - Behçet disease
- Cardiac:
    - left-sided obstructive lesions
    - high pulmonary flow (left to right shunts)
    - heart failure
    - myocarditis
- Diffuse alveolar injury:
    - drug toxicity (penicillamine, nitrofurantoin)
    - insecticides
    - smoke inhalation
    - radiation
    - oxygen toxicity
    - mechanical ventilation
- Bleeding diathesis

History

Ask about the following.

- Nature of the blood: bright red? mixed with sputum?
- Situation in which haemoptysis occurred.
- Other bleeding problems—including nose bleeds.
- Number of episodes of haemoptysis.
- Previous history of similar episodes.
- Related respiratory symptoms:
    - bubbling sensation in the chest—may help localize bronchial bleeding;
    - chest pain (?pleuritic);
    - cough (dry or productive);
    - breathlessness;
    - exercise tolerance.
- Related non-respiratory symptoms:
    - ear infections, nasal symptoms;
    - rash;
    - joint pain;
    - dark urine;
    - red or sore eyes;
    - change in behaviour or psychological problems.

- Weight loss, sweats.
- Foreign travel, exposure to animals.
- Drug history—including oral contraceptive use.
- Family history of TB, connective tissue disease, vasculitis.

Examination

Look for:
- finger clubbing;
- pallor;
- rash;
- joint swelling or tenderness;
- eye redness;
- lymphadenopathy;
- otitis media;
- heart murmur;
- pulses;
- evidence of respiratory distress;
- presence of crackles on auscultation.

Investigations

These will depend on the history and examination but may include:
- blood for:
  - FBC, clotting;
  - inflammatory markers and auto-antibodies.
- imaging: CXR and CT scan (Fig. 10.1);
- cardiac evaluation, including ECG and echo;
- bronchoscopy;
- lung biopsy.

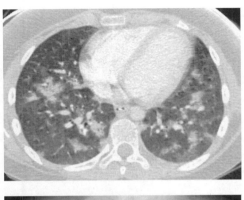

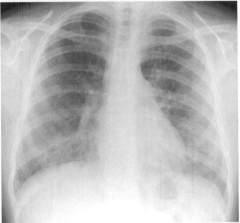

Fig. 10.1 CXR (upper) and CT scan (lower) of a 10-year-old girl with connective tissue disease who developed haemoptysis. She was not breathless and had preserved lung function. The CT shows scattered ground-glass airspace changes. At bronchoscopy bright pink blood was returned by the lavage procedure. The cytospin of the lavage fluid was positive for haemosiderin-laden macrophages.

The immuno-compromised child

Introduction

In this short section we propose an approach to respiratory assessment of a child who is known to have some form of immunocompromise. This will usually be a child who is receiving some form of immunosuppressive medication (usually for malignancy or post-transplantation) or a child with known primary immune deficiency.

The commonest reason for carrying out a respiratory assessment will be either that the child has developed a persistent or recurrent cough (with or without CXR changes) or because the child has developed an acute respiratory illness, usually with breathlessness and an oxygen requirement.

Differential diagnosis

- The most likely reason for respiratory illness in this group of children will be infection. The infection may be a typical viral or bacterial illness, but opportunistic infection needs to be considered.
  - CMV pneumonitis (more likely in children after solid organ or stem cell transplantation; rare in children on standard chemotherapy for malignancy). See 📖 Chapter 19.
  - Pneumocystis pneumonitis (more likely in children with severe combined immune deficiency, children on chemotherapy who have stopped their co-trimoxazole prophylaxis, and in children with HIV infection). See 📖 Chapter 20.
  - Fungal lung infection (more likely if there has been prolonged severe neutropenia or > 3 weeks high dose systemic steroid treatment as part of a chemotherapy regimen). See 📖 Chapter 20.
  - Tuberculosis (more likely in children in high-risk groups for exposure). See 📖 Chapter 22.
- Infection may be persistent or recurrent because there is underlying bronchiectasis. This is more likely in children with long-standing immune deficiency
- Non-infective causes of respiratory problems include the following.
  - Drug-induced pneumonitis. This can occur at any time from within a few hours of administration of the responsible drug to several months later. Likely candidates include bleomycin, DNA alkylating agents, and methotrexate. See 📖 Chapter 50.
  - Radiation pneumonitis. Acute radiation pneumonitis can develop within 2–3 weeks of radiotherapy and can spread out of the radiation field to give diffuse lung disease. See 📖 Chapter 50.
  - Cardiac dysfunction: drug-induced or related to infection.
  - A direct effect of the underlying disease, e.g. leukaemic or lymphomatous infiltration of the lung, or an effect secondary to airway compression.
  - A secondary effect of pain in the thoracic cage: infiltration or fracture of ribs or thoracic vertebrae.
  - Pleural disease: pleural effusion, haemothorax, or pneumothorax.

History

- Determine nature and duration of immunocompromise, including recent or prolonged previous use of systemic steroids.
- What medications is the child currently taking?
- What was the relationship of the onset of symptoms to any chemotherapy or radiotherapy the child had received?
- What is the nature of the current illness:
  - duration;
  - symptoms: cough, stridor, breathlessness, wheeze, pain;
  - severity;
  - rate of progression;
  - treatments already tried.
- Have there been previous episodes of opportunistic infection with CMV, fungi, or Pneumocystis?
- Is the child at risk of TB exposure or re-activation?

Examination

- Assess severity of respiratory distress.
- Carry out a full respiratory examination.

Investigations

- Imaging.
  - CXR will be needed in all cases.
  - HRCT is often very useful. Contrast should be given if fungal infection is suspected. There may be evidence of a diffuse infiltrate, local consolidation, cavitation, tumour infiltrate, airway compression, or bronchiectasis.
- Blood:
  - CMV PCR.
  - TB interferon-gamma release assay.
- Urine.
  - CMV PCR.
  - Nasopharyngeal aspirate can be sent for respiratory virus assessment, usually by PCR.
  - Sputum or cough swab can be sent for culture.
  - Bronchoscopy is often required to obtain lower airway samples by bronchoalveolar lavage, which can be sent for bacterial, viral, and fungal assessment. Cytological examination may be helpful if malignant infiltration is suspected.

Diagnosis and treatment

Diagnosis and treatment will depend on the clinical findings and results of investigations. Whilst awaiting investigations it is likely that broad spectrum antibiotics will be started. Depending on the severity and/or duration of the illness and the clinical situation, antifungal, anti-tuberculous, and antiviral drugs may be added. A diagnosis of drug-induced pneumonitis is one of exclusion and usually requires a typical infiltrative change seen on CT, a likely causative drug, and negative cultures.

Muscle weakness

Introduction

The respiratory paediatrician is increasingly involved in the management of children with neuromuscular weakness. Occasionally a respiratory specialist may be asked to assess a child presenting with an acute illness, e.g. a child with Guillain–Barré syndrome, to determine whether they need immediate respiratory support. A more common situation will be the respiratory assessment of an infant or child with a chronic or congenital disorder affecting respiratory muscle strength.

History

- Is the name of the disorder known? This information may be useful in determining the likelihood of respiratory compromise and the rate of progression of the condition.
- How weak is the child?
  - Can they walk, with or without support?
  - Can they stand, with or without support?
  - Can they sit, with or without support?
  - Can they talk?
  - Can they eat?
  - Can they swallow secretions and saliva?
- How effective is their cough?
- Can they handle their secretions when awake and when asleep?
- How frequent are chest infections?
- What happens when they have a chest infection?
- Have they ever needed respiratory support?
- Have they had episodes of stridor?
- Do they sleep well? Do they need turning at night?
- Do they snore/have noisy breathing at night?
- Do they have symptoms of hypoventilation (see box)?
- Are they getting weaker?
- How rapid is the progression?
- Do they have scoliosis?

Symptoms of nocturnal hypoventilation

- Fatigue
- Morning headache
- Morning anorexia/vomiting
- Multiple nocturnal arousals/awakening with dyspnoea
- Daytime sleepiness
- Poor concentration
- Irritability
- Nocturnal urinary frequency

Examination

It is important to examine the infant or child sitting, standing, and lying down.
- Do they have good and equal chest expansion?
- Is chest expansion asymmetrical, suggesting either significant scoliosis or unilateral diaphragmatic weakness?
- Are they using accessory muscles either for respiration or accessory abdominal muscles to aid expiration?
- Do they have paradoxical respiration on lying, suggesting significant intercostal weakness?
- Are they using their glottis to maintain lung volume until end expiration?
- Listen to the cough or huff.
- Can they clear respiratory secretions?
- Which muscle groups are involved in the weakness?
  - Intercostals?
  - Diaphragm?
  - Bulbar?

Investigation

- An assessment of lung capacity can be made using standard spirometry in the mildly weak, changing to using a slow vital capacity manoeuvre in the moderately and severely weak child. Depending on the pattern of muscle weakness there may be a large difference between the VC achieved in the upright position and that achieved when supine; the supine measurement correlates better with nocturnal hypoventilation. Children with a supine slow VC of 40% predicted should be assessed for nocturnal hypoventilation. Children with some forms of congenital muscular dystrophy and structural myopathies are associated with a rigid spine and early respiratory compromise. These children should be expectantly investigated for nocturnal hypoventilation.
- Mouthpieces with lip seals may be needed for lung function testing.
- In older children and adults a cough peak flow rate correlates with ability to clear secretions (cough peak flow needs to exceed 160L/min for effective secretion clearance).

- Assessment of gas exchange during wakefulness:
  - end tidal CO_2 or capillary CO_2 during wakefulness—daytime hypercapnia is a definitive indicator of need for nocturnal ventilatory support;
  - oxygen saturation.
- Assessment of gas exchange during sleep:
- End tidal or transcutaneous CO_2 during sleep and oxygen saturation are the minimum measurements required. Measurement of abdominal and chest wall excursion and/or airflow help confirm the presence of hypoventilation.

Management

- Secretion management.
  - In children with intact bulbar function the mainstay of management is chest physiotherapy to mobilize and clear airway secretions. Postural drainage and percussion are combined with deep breathing (sometimes aided) and cough or huff. Manually assisted coughing can be used. In very weak children the cough in/exsufflator or cough-assist machine is a very useful aid.
  - Aggressive treatment of chest infection is indicated with antibiotics started at onset of any viral URTI or, in some children, low dose antibiotics used throughout the winter months.
  - If there is some bulbar weakness then consideration needs to be given to decreasing the amount of oral secretions by pharmacological or surgical intervention. There are 2 choices for reducing salivary secretions: botulinum toxin injections of the salivary glands or surgery, usually salivary duct ligation. Hyoscine patches, whilst easy to use, tend to increase the stickiness of secretions, which are then harder to clear, and should be used with caution.
- Ventilatory support.
  - Where there is evidence of nocturnal hypoventilation with daytime symptoms, non-invasive ventilatory support is indicated. Generally a nasal/facemask interface is used and there is now a large selection of interfaces available. The secret of success is to find a comfortable interface that is acceptable to the child. Occasionally non-invasive negative pressure jacket ventilation is the best solution.
  - Where there is diurnal ventilatory failure and/or severe bulbar weakness then consideration must be given to long-term ventilatory support via tracheostomy.

More details on individual neuromuscular conditions and management are available in 📖 Chapter 48.

Pneumonia on the intensive care unit

Introduction

Children with critical illness cared for in the intensive care unit (ICU) are a heterogeneous group of individuals with different underlying problems. In this group of children severe pneumonia that is not responding to appropriate treatment for straightforward community-acquired pneumonia should prompt assessment for other contributing aetiology. Important considerations are listed below.

History

- Is this a complicated pneumonia with abscess formation or empyema?
- Is the deterioration associated with systemic infection and shock?
- Are there any indicators of chronic respiratory disease?
  - History of prematurity and chronic lung disease.
  - Family history of cystic fibrosis (CF).
  - Gastrointestinal symptoms suggestive of malabsorption (suggesting CF).
  - Unexplained respiratory distress at term.
  - Chronic rhinitis and/or recurrent otitis media.
  - Previously diagnosed tracheobronchomalacia (or previous cardiothoracic or tracheal surgery).
  - Chronic cough when well.
- Is there a history of choking suggesting foreign body aspiration?
- Could this be aspiration pneumonia?
  - Consider in a child with chronic disability or acute neurological deterioration.
  - Evidence of GORD.
  - Evidence of primary aspiration.
  - Evidence of bulbar palsy, laryngeal cleft, vocal cord palsy, H-type tracheo-oesophageal fistula.
- Does this child have congenital heart disease?
  - Has pneumonia exacerbated pre-existing pulmonary vascular disease?
  - Is the child in cardiac failure?
- Is this a complication of previous cardiothoracic surgery?
  - Phrenic nerve palsy with diaphragmatic dysfunction.
  - Recurrent laryngeal nerve palsy (with history of acquired stridor, weak voice, or weak cough).
  - Chylothorax.
  - Post-pericardiotomy syndrome.
- Is there an underlying congenital abnormality of the lung?
  - Bronchogenic cyst.
  - Congenital cystadenomatoid malformation.
  - Intralobar or extralobar lung sequestration.
  - Diaphragmatic hernia.

- Could the child have immune deficiency?
  - History of previous invasive bacterial infection.
  - Maternal HIV status.
  - Previously affected infants in the family with SCID
  - Consider PCP or CMV pneumonitis.
- Are there any indicators of muscle weakness?
  - Is motor development normal?
  - Is there a family history of muscle disease?
  - Does the child normally have a good cough and strong voice?
  - Does the child have a scoliosis or weakness on examination?
  - Is the child able to clear secretions?
- Is this ventilator-acquired pneumonia?
  - Was the original CXR normal?
  - See 📖 Chapter 18, p. 184.

Other points to consider

- Infants ventilated on ICU during the RSV bronchiolitis season who do not follow the normal timeframe for RSV disease should be investigated for underlying susceptibility to infection or for an alternative diagnosis. Cystic fibrosis, primary ciliary dyskinesia (PCD), or immunodeficiency may result in prolonged RSV disease. Persistent profound hypoxia should prompt consideration of alternative aetiology including CMV or pneumocystis pneumonitis in an immunocompromised child. Heart failure from a significant left to right shunt (e.g. from unsuspected partial anomalous pulmonary venous drainage) also presents in this age group and is a differential diagnosis in the child who is not improving with supportive care.
- Children with underlying PCD are likely to have a strong history of chronic rhinitis and recurrent otitis media and may report a history of unexplained tachypnoea at term delivery. 50% have situs inversus.
- A detailed history of the clinical deterioration should be taken, with particular reference to timing of feeding. Evidence of aspiration pneumonia in the neurologically normal infant should prompt investigation of the airway, to exclude congenital abnormalities including the following.
  - H type tracheo-oesophageal fistula.
  - Laryngeal cleft.
  - Congenital or acquired vocal cord palsy.
  - In the child with neurological deterioration or established neurodisability, bulbar palsy may result in aspiration pneumonia.

- Infants and children with congenital heart disease from longstanding left to right cardiac shunting and increased pulmonary blood flow will have a strong vasoreactive response to hypoventilation and hypoxia. Pneumonia in these children may therefore act to precipitate an increase in pulmonary vascular resistance with consequent right to left shunting or right-sided heart failure. Pulmonary artery pressures may be assessed using echocardiography using tricuspid regurgitant flow as an indicator of pulmonary arterial pressure but cardiac catheter with acute vasodilator testing is the gold standard. Interventions to reduce an acute increase in pulmonary vascular resistance in the ICU setting include the following.
  - High concentrations of oxygen.
  - Inhaled nitric oxide.
  - IV infusions of prostacyclin analogues.
  - Sildenafil, a phosphodiestaerase inhibitor, and bosentan, an endothelin receptor antagonist, may be started as chronic therapy (see 📖 Chapter 51).
- Reduced respiratory function and prolonged ventilation post-cardiothoracic surgery may result from ipsilateral phrenic nerve palsy. Ultrasound can be used to assess real time diaphragmatic function in the ICU. Be aware that the movement of a paralysed diaphragm will not be paradoxical unless the child is self-ventilating. Paradoxical movement of the diaphragm will contribute to:
  - reduced respiratory function;
  - ventilator dependence;
  - failure to effectively clear secretions.
- Surgical injury is usually ischaemia, rather than transection-related, and will recover over 2–6 weeks. Whilst awaiting recovery the child can usually be supported with non-invasive ventilation, either by using negative pressure cuirass ventilation (e.g. using the Medivent RTX) or by using a nasal mask system. Surgical plication of the hemidiaphragm will also usually be effective in allowing the child to be extubated provided there are few or no other complicating factors, such as significant parenchymal lung disease or heart failure.
- Failed extubation post-cardiothoracic surgery may be due to vocal cord dysfunction secondary to recurrent laryngeal nerve palsy. Acute acquired stridor, weak cry, and weak cough may be apparent, and aspiration pneumonia may occur in the postoperative period. Alternatively, the child with postoperative stridor may have laryngeal oedema or acquired subglottic stenosis. Laryngotracheobronchoscopy under sedation without paralysis is indicated to observe active vocal cord function and to inspect the larynx and subglottis.
- Unusual opacity on CXR should prompt assessment for congenital lung anomalies. Bronchogenic cysts, congenital cystadenomatoid malformations, lung sequestrations, and cystic hygromas may all become secondarily infected and present acutely (see 📖 Chapter 41). Other possible causes for unusual CXR opacities include malignancy, progressive mycobacterial disease, or occult congenital diaphragmatic hernia.

- Immune deficiencies should be considered in unusually prolonged or severe illness or when illness is recurrent. FBC and film, total immunoglobulins, functional antibody titres, and HIV test should be performed as first-line screen, if immunodeficiency is suspected clinically. Lymphocyte subsets may be sent with the initial screen if there is a high index of suspicion of cell-mediated immune deficiency. See 📖 Chapter 35.
- Children with muscle weakness are susceptible to recurrent pneumonia with slow recovery. Several factors contribute:
  - low lung volumes and longstanding atelectasis increase risk of infection;
  - bulbar weakness may result in primary aspiration of secretions;
  - weak cough;
  - poor chest excursion and scoliosis compromise efficiency of mucus removal.
- Early extubation of children with muscle weakness often fails as secretions continue to be produced in excess, and may no longer be removed effectively with tracheal suction. Intensive physiotherapy is paramount. Negative pressure ventilation and assisted cough manoeuvres may be used in conjunction with physiotherapy, prior to extubation. This approach enables continued access to tracheal secretions. Extubation should not be attempted until the patient is ventilated in air, and secretion production has fallen. Once extubated, a combination of negative pressure ventilation and non-invasive BIPAP may be used in weaning ventilatory requirement (see 📖 Chapter 48).

Part II

Specific conditions

Asthma

Definition

Asthma is an illness in which there are recurrent episodes of airway narrowing resulting in difficulty breathing and coughing, and in which the airway narrowing is variable or can be improved with an inhaled beta-adrenergic agonist. Not all asthma is allergen-mediated.

Aetiology

The cause of airway narrowing in asthma is a combination of bronchial smooth muscle constriction and obstruction of the lumen by inflammatory exudates and airway wall oedema. The relative contribution of these different components varies with age, between children, and between attacks in the same child. The efficacy of inhaled beta-agonists, which only act on the smooth muscle component, will vary in a similar fashion.

The mechanisms that underlie bronchospasm and airway inflammation are not fully understood. It is likely that both have a primary protective role, attempting to keep noxious substances out of the lung. In susceptible individuals, the balance between protection and damage to the host is tipped towards damage, and the response leads to significantly increased work of breathing and impaired gas exchange.

Immunological mechanisms

- Asthma is a complex immune-mediated multifactorial disease. There is a clear genetic component, more strongly inherited from the mother than the father.
- Several susceptibility loci have been identified. It is not yet known whether any of these are critical to the development of asthma, nor what combination may result in the biggest risk.
- Whatever the mechanism, susceptible individuals tend to develop a wheezing response to airway insults. In young children the commonest trigger is viral respiratory infection. In older children viral infection remains an important trigger, but a higher proportion will have developed allergic sensitization to a range of non-infectious aeroallergens.
- There are well-described differences in immunological responses in children with asthma. Adaptive immunity is divided into that mediated by antibodies, *humoral immunity*, and that mediated by direct cell contact, *cell-mediated immunity*. These responses are controlled by T lymphocytes. Different classes of T cells can direct the immune response towards predominantly humoral or cell-mediated effects. These directing T cells are called T helper (Th) cells. Th1 cells direct a cell-mediated response and Th2 cells direct a humoral response. Each type of response is characterized by the production of specific soluble mediators (cytokines).
- Some of the Th2 cytokines required by B cells to produce antibodies also attract other effector cells to the airway. These include eosinophils and mast cells. If the T helper response is skewed towards Th2, the cytokine environment is thought to promote allergic sensitization, the production of IgE, and the activation and degranulation of eosinophils and mast cells. These cells release a fresh set of soluble mediators, including leukotrienes, which contribute further to airway inflammation and bronchoconstriction.

Epidemiology

- A wide range of studies has been used to estimate the prevalence of asthma. Some are medium-sized cohort studies with detailed follow-up and others are very large international studies, using parental questionnaires.
- When discussing the frequency of asthma in the general population, it is important to be clear about the definitions being used. Many questionnaire surveys use a form of the question 'has your child wheezed at all in the last 12 months' as one measure of current asthma. It is by using these types of questions that the high prevalence rates of 15–20% are found in some Western countries. The frequency of more frequent wheeze that causes interference with lifestyle is much lower (≤ 5%).
- One of the best known studies is the International Study of Asthma and Allergies in Childhood (ISAAC).[1] In phase I of this study, questionnaires were used in 56 countries to estimate asthma prevalence amongst children of school age. It was this study that highlighted the higher incidence of asthma in Western industrialized nations when compared to those in the developing world. Sequential asthma studies in the UK, as well as in other countries, using the same format of questions, have detected a significant increase in asthma over the last 25 years. This increase has been mirrored by increases in asthma admissions to hospital, suggesting that the figures represent a genuine increase in disease. The increase appears to have peaked, and phase III of ISAAC has shown a small fall in the prevalence of asthma in countries with the highest burden of disease (such as New Zealand, Australia, and the UK).

Risk factors

- The reason why some children make a wheezing response to viral respiratory tract infections or aeroallergens and others do not is poorly understood. There are several factors that are associated with altered risk of wheezing illness (see box).
- The genetic component to asthma risk is important, but cannot explain the increased prevalence of wheeze seen in recent years.
- There have been a number of attempts to try and explain some of the epidemiological associations. One of the best known is the 'hygiene hypothesis' which proposes that early life exposure to certain pathogens (particularly those found on farms) can protect against later atopic disease.
- The data supporting this concept are conflicting. For example, Strachan has shown that having large numbers of older siblings seems to be associated with a reduced risk of atopy.[2] If this association is a reflection of increased exposure to infection, then the same effect might be expected from attendance at day-care, which has consistently been shown to increase exposure to respiratory infections. Studies looking at the influence of attendance at day-care have had inconsistent results

1 The International Study of Asthma and Allergies in Childhood: http://isaac.auckland.ac.nz
2 Strachan, D.P. (2000). Family size, infection and atopy: the first decade of the "hygiene hypothesis". *Thorax* 55 (Suppl. 1), S2–10.

with some showing an association with increased risk of asthma. Similarly inconsistent results have been found with the influence of specific infections including the effects of BCG and TB.
• Other hypotheses have suggested that the increase in asthma prevalence is a reflection of indoor or outdoor pollutants, or any of a large number of environmental factors, including herbicides and agricultural fertilizer. None have been proven.

Factors that affect risk of wheezing illness

Increased risk
• Parental asthma or atopy (especially maternal)
• Sibling with asthma or atopy
• Low birth weight
• Prematurity
• Airway calibre
• Parental smoking
• Viral bronchiolitis in early life
• Previous or current eczema

Decreased risk
• Breastfeeding
• Living in a rural location
• Large number of siblings

Patterns of wheeze

- When assessing a child with asthma it is important to get a clear picture of the nature and frequency of the symptoms. This will help with both diagnosis and management. Three patterns of wheezing can be defined.
    - *Infrequent episodic wheeze.* These children have clear episodes of wheeze, usually lasting 1–5 days, between which they are completely well and wheeze- and cough-free day and night. The episodes of wheeze occur at intervals of at least 6 weeks.
    - *Frequent episodic wheeze.* These children have clear episodes of wheeze, usually lasting 1–5 days, between which they are completely well and wheeze- and cough-free day and night. The episodes of wheeze occur every 2–6 weeks.
    - *Persistent wheeze.* These children have wheeze and cough on most days. They will usually also have disturbed nights.
- Within each category the symptoms may vary in severity. For example, a child with infrequent episodic wheeze may have a severe attack requiring hospital admission; conversely a child with persistent wheeze may have never needed hospital care.
- It should be noted that these clinical categories differ from those used in some longitudinal epidemiological studies. One of the best known of these studies is the Tucson Children's Respiratory Study. This study describes a large birth cohort and identifies 3 groups of children with wheeze; those who wheezed before the age of 3 but not after (transient episodic wheeze, TEW); those who wheezed only after the age of 3 years (late onset wheeze, LOW) and those who wheezed before and after the age of 3 years (persistent wheeze, PW). The TEW group were no more likely to be atopic than the non-wheezers, whereas the LOW and PW groups had increased markers of atopy. Similar results have been found using a UK birth cohort—the Avon Longitudinal Study of Parents and Children (ALSPAC).

Viral-associated wheeze

Most exacerbations of asthma in childhood, including children with atopic disease, are associated with respiratory viral infections, even though in older children there may be few signs of coryza. In pre-school children the association is particularly strong, with wheeze only occurring with obvious colds, and frequently no symptoms present at all between viral infections. The episodes of wheeze in this age group often respond poorly to bronchodilators and are not easily prevented using inhaled steroids. These differences, seen in this group compared to older children with asthma, have led to the assumption that this pattern of wheeze is different from 'proper' asthma and has resulted in a common dogma that asthma cannot be diagnosed in a child < 2 years old. It is also often but incorrectly stated that infants do not respond to beta-adrenergic agonists because they have no beta-adrenergic receptors. This has led to inconsistent use of salbutamol and ipratropium bromide in this age group. The following points should help provide clarification.

• Viral-associated wheeze is a more recent and slightly more precise term than wheezy bronchitis, but it means the same thing.
• Most school-age children with significant asthma will have had wheezing in the first 3 years of life, at which time they may have been indistinguishable from children who subsequently stopped wheezing.
• Around 60% of children who have an episode of wheeze in the first 3 years of life will not be wheezing by the age of 6 years. The likelihood is even lower if there is no evidence of other atopic disease, no family history of atopy, and if the parents do not smoke.
• Beta-adrenergic receptors are present in the airway from birth. Poor response to beta-agonists by some infants with viral-associated wheeze may reflect a relatively small contribution to airway narrowing from smooth muscle bronchoconstriction with airways obstruction predominantly due to inflammatory exudate and airway wall thickening. The small size of the airways at this age may also be relevant. There is no evidence that ipratropium bromide works better than salbutamol in this age group.

Some children with viral-associated wheeze will have a good response to bronchodilators and, in those with persistent symptoms, a trial of inhaled steroids or leukotriene receptor antagonists may be justified. Why then is there reticence to call their disease asthma? These children certainly fulfil the definition given at the beginning of the chapter. There are 2 reasons. Firstly, most children with viral-associated wheeze will grow out of their illness by the time they are 6 years old. Secondly, a doctor's diagnosis of asthma, at any time in a person's life, can affect employment. For example, people who wish to work as commercial airline pilots, as commercial divers, in the armed forces or the police, or in some chemical industries will require specific medical examinations and evidence of normal pulmonary function testing if they have previously been diagnosed as asthmatic. It therefore seems reasonable to wait until later childhood before using the diagnostic term 'asthma' since at this stage there is a greater likelihood that symptoms will persist.

History

The first aim of the history should be to try and establish whether the symptoms are consistent with asthma. This requires the presence of variable wheeze, with or without cough. It is essential to establish early on whether what the family mean by wheeze and what you mean by wheeze are the same thing (see ▭ Chapter 2). Important features of the history include the following.

- Age at onset of wheeze.
- Frequency of wheeze (see ▭ p. 94).
- Severity or control of current symptoms (see below).
- Previous treatments tried, including use and frequency of courses of oral steroids.
- Requirement for hospital treatment: duration; need for oxygen; IV treatment; ventilation.
- Current medication: how given; estimate of adherence to therapy.
- Gestation and need for neonatal intensive care.
- Previous history of eczema or hay fever.
- Presence of other allergies, including food allergies.
- Use of peak flow meter.
- Triggers for wheeze and/or cough (see below).
- Family history of asthma and other atopic disease.
- Smoking by parent or other household member (including the child!).
- Nature of housing, especially the child's bedroom.
- Presence of pets.

Measure of severity or control

Current asthma severity can be assessed by 3 questions

- Is there exercise limitation?
- Is there full school attendance?
- Is there night-time disturbance from cough or wheeze?

Satisfactory answers to these questions indicate that the asthma is either mild or well-controlled, depending on the amount of treatment the child is taking. If the answers are unsatisfactory it is important to estimate how badly the child is affected: how much school has been missed; how much exercise can be performed; how much bronchodilator is used ('how long does an inhaler last?' is a good question); how many nights per week are disturbed.

GINA definition of controlled asthma

The Global Initiative for Asthma (GINA) 2006 guidelines[3] define good control as:
- no (twice or less/week) daytime symptoms;
- no limitations of daily activities, including exercise;

3 The Global Initiative for Asthma (GINA) (2006). Global strategy for asthma management and prevention 2006. www.ginasthma.com.

- no nocturnal symptoms or awakening because of asthma;
- no (twice or less/week) need for reliever treatment;
- normal or near-normal lung function results;
- no exacerbations.

Increased use, especially daily use, of reliever medication should be taken as an indicator of deteriorating control and need to re-assess management.

Triggers for wheeze or cough

Any of the following can trigger asthma symptoms.
- Viral respiratory infection.
- Exercise.
- Cold air.
- Allergens:
  - house dust mite;
  - animal dander;
  - grass or tree pollen;
  - straw or hay;
  - foods.
- Cigarette smoke or other irritants such as diesel fumes or perfumes.
- Gastro-oesophageal reflux—either vagally mediated bronchoconstriction or micro-aspiration.
- Acidic fizzy drinks—vagally mediated.

Aspirin-induced asthma is relatively common in adults and is associated with the presence of nasal polyps. In these individuals other NSAIDs can also cause wheeze. Aspirin/NSAID-induced asthma is rare in children. Ibuprofen, which is a valuable analgesic and antipyretic, should not be withheld from febrile asthmatic children unless they have a history of aspirin/NSAID sensitivity.

Cough without wheeze

Recurrent dry cough is common and affects up to 20% of 7-year-olds. It is a poor marker for asthma.
- Although cough may be the predominant symptom in a child with asthma, cough without wheeze is not sufficient for an asthma diagnosis.
- Most isolated dry coughs are postviral. Many persist for several weeks. The majority resolve within 3 months.
- The temptation to carry out a 'therapeutic trial' of inhaled steroids should be resisted. There is a good chance that the cough will resolve spontaneously during the trial, giving a false impression of efficacy, and potentially leading to longer-term and unnecessary steroid use. Worse still, the cough may fail to resolve, leading to increased doses of inhaled steroids being used. When there is normal lung function, this can lead to especially high levels of alveolar absorption and potential adrenal suppression.
- Only a small proportion of children with persistent dry cough will subsequently develop asthma with wheezing.

Examination

This is nearly always normal between exacerbations. In all children check for the following.

- Clubbing (not consistent with a diagnosis of asthma).
- Chest shape—hyperinflation suggests poorly controlled disease.
- Symmetry and degree of chest expansion.
- Nature of the breath sounds.
- Presence of crepitations (not consistent with a diagnosis of asthma).
- Presence of a prolonged expiratory phase to the breathing cycle.
- Presence of wheeze.
- If wheeze is heard, a bronchodilator should be given and its effect noted.

Children with more persistent symptoms often claim to feel well, but on examination may have wheeze at rest. This may only be apparent during prolonged expiration, and it is often useful to listen to the chest as the child carries out a forced expiratory manoeuvre.

Investigations

In most children the diagnosis of asthma can be made by history and examination. If the diagnosis is not in doubt and the symptoms are mild, no investigations are required. In other circumstances, spirometry may be helpful. Most children with asthma will have normal spirometry between exacerbations. Children with active postviral cough will have normal spirometry (unlike most children with active asthma) and this finding can help prevent unnecessary treatment being prescribed. A simple assessment of the extent of symptoms and variability of lung function using home peak flow recordings and symptom diaries over a month or so can be helpful if the family is sufficiently motivated to make the twice daily measurements.

Bronchial provocation tests

- Interpretation of tests of bronchial responsiveness, e.g. induced by inhaled histamine or methacholine or following exercise, is not straightforward.
- Most children with moderate or severe asthma will have very reactive airways. In children with mild asthma (where there is likely to be more diagnostic doubt), up to 50% will give negative tests. About 10% of children with no symptoms will show bronchial reactivity with methacholine.
- Most centres would reserve histamine or methacholine bronchial challenge tests to research studies.
- Exercise testing can be useful in children with exercise-induced symptoms, in whom the diagnosis of asthma is in doubt. A positive exercise test that reproduces the child's symptoms, with relief from inhaled bronchodilator, will provide clarification.
- Not all children with asthma have exercise-induced falls in FEV1; a negative test does not exclude the diagnosis.
- As with histamine or methacholine challenge, normal children with no symptoms of cough or wheeze can show bronchial reactivity on exercise testing. More than 50% of UK children at the ages of 8–10 years showed a 15% fall in peak expiratory flow after 6min of exercise on at least one occasion when tested at monthly intervals for 1 year.[4]

Allergy testing

Tests of allergic sensitization, such as skin prick tests or serum-specific IgE assays, have a limited role in the diagnosis or management of asthma.

- A negative test usually rules out allergic sensitization of the airways to the allergen tested.
- The tests have a false positive rate of around 15%. Thus it is hard to justify getting rid of the cat, for example, without additional evidence that it is a cause of respiratory symptoms.
- Demonstrating allergic sensitization does provide a rationale for allergen avoidance, although the benefits of allergen avoidance are uncertain (see 📖 p. 102).

4 Powell, C.V., White, R.D., and Primhak, R.A. (1996). Longitudinal study of free running exercise challenge: reproducibility. *Arch. Dis. Child.* **74** (2), 108–14.

Exhaled nitric oxide (NO)

NO is produced in the epithelial cells of the bronchial wall. NO production increases during eosinophilic inflammation and is elevated in patients with asthma. Although not yet part of routine outpatient work, fractional exhaled nitric oxide (FENO) may be able to assist in asthma diagnosis and in assessment of steroid treatment efficacy in reducing airway inflammation. Repeated measurements in the same child may also be predictive of imminent deterioration of asthma control. See 📖 Chapter 70 for methods of measuring exhaled NO.

Other investigations

Where there is doubt about the diagnosis, or where asthma is unusually severe or difficult to manage, the following additional investigations should be considered.

- Oesophageal pH study to investigate possible gastro-oesophageal reflux.
- Bronchoscopy to exclude abnormal airway anatomy, including tracheobronchomalacia, and to collect lavage fluid for analysis (eosinophil and neutrophil cell counts and culture).
- Where appropriate:
  - sweat test (to exclude CF);
  - nasal brush biopsy for cilial evaluation (to exclude PCD);
  - serum IgG, IgA, and IgM and specific antibody responses to vaccinations (as a screen for immune deficiency);
  - HRCT of the chest—to identify any unexpected bronchiolitis obliterans or bronchiectasis.
- *Aspergillus* IgE and IgG (precipitin lines) and total IgE, which may indicate the presence of allergic bronchopulmonary aspergillosis.
- Sputum culture or cough swab may be helpful in identifying persistent endobronchial infection or *Aspergillus*.

Outpatient management

The aims of asthma management are to

- control symptoms, allowing normal levels of activity, undisturbed sleep, and full school attendance
- prevent exacerbations
- maintain normal lung function
- use the minimum therapy necessary

In all children a balance between symptom control and drug toxicity needs to be made and this may mean that complete symptom control is not always achieved. The approach used is based on the British Thoracic Society guidelines, and depends on the pattern of asthma symptoms.[5]

Non-pharmacological approaches

Benefits are limited.

- The most critical is to reduce exposure to cigarette smoke.
- Although gastro-oesophageal reflux may be present, and should be treated aggressively if symptoms are found, there is no evidence that treatment for reflux will improve asthma control.
- There is no evidence of sustained benefit for any of the alternative therapies, including homeopathy, herbal medicines, breathing techniques (including the Buteyko method), acupuncture, air ionizers, hypnosis, dietary manipulation, or chiropractice.
- Families may wish to try alternative medicine. There is no evidence of harm, provided that their usual therapies are continued. Some children may find alternative therapies helpful, particularly if the child or family feel more in control of the condition. Breathing exercises may be successful in this way.
- Allergen avoidance is often raised by families and is dealt with in more detail next.

Allergen avoidance

The rationale behind allergen avoidance is straightforward.

- Exposure to allergen is associated with the development of allergic sensitization.
- Sensitized individuals with asthma have more severe symptoms when exposed to high levels of allergen.
- Some strategies to avoid allergens do help, e.g. children with atopic asthma with house dust mite allergy have improved symptom control and lung function when taken from their usual environment to one at high altitude that is virtually mite-free.

---

5 The BTS/SIGN Guideline on Asthma Management, November 2005 Update. Available from the British Thoracic Society website: *www.brit-thoracic.org.uk/guidelines*.

The difficulty is that less drastic approaches to allergen avoidance are less effective at getting the allergen load below the threshold that produces symptoms. It is essential to deal with all sensitizing allergens to get a clinically useful benefit and most atopic children are sensitive to a wide range of allergens. As a consequence, although most studies investigating effects of allergen avoidance show that allergen load can be reduced, the clinical effect is variable, and *there is no evidence of sustained improvement in asthma control*.

Methods of allergen removal that have been tried include those to remove or exclude existing allergen and those to remove the source of the allergen. Pets are often a potential area of conflict. More than half of families in which the child with asthma is sensitized to pet allergens (Fel d1 for cats and Can f1 for dogs) deny that exposure is correlated with symptoms. Furthermore, simply removing the cat or dog from the home is not enough. Allergen levels persist at high levels for months or years unless concerted action to change floor and wall coverings is also taken.

Some families may wish to pursue allergen avoidance, despite the lack of evidence of benefit. Suggested methods that have been tried with inconsistent results include:

- removal of soft furnishing from bedrooms;
- removal of carpets;
- excluding pets from the house;
- complete barrier bed-covering systems (more than a simple mattress cover);
- high temperature washing of bed linen;
- devices to reduce air humidity;
- high-efficiency particle arrest (HEPA) air filters;
- HEFA filter vacuum cleaners;
- chemical agents to kill mites (acaricides) on soft furnishings.

There is also some evidence that primary prevention in high risk infants (those with an affected first degree relative) can reduce the prevalence of asthma in later childhood. The preventive measures recommended include allergen avoidance from birth, combined with avoidance of tobacco smoke and encouragement of breastfeeding.

Pharmacotherapy

This is based on the combination of treatments to relax smooth muscle and to reduce airway inflammation. In general, it is appropriate to start therapy according to the pattern of symptoms. Regular review then allows therapy to be stepped up or down according to response. Occasionally, in children with longstanding poor control, it may be necessary to start at a high level of therapy, such as high dose inhaled steroids or even a course of oral steroids, to gain good control before weaning therapy to maintenance levels. Therapy should be reviewed and reduced if appropriate in any child with asthma who has had good symptom control for 3–6 months. Table 14.1 lists some of the delivery devices available for pharmacotherapy.

Spacer devices

These are properly called valved holding chambers. They increase the airway deposition of inhaled medication from an MDI from around 10% to as much as 25%. Thus it may be possible to get the same benefit from the drug at half the dose. This is particularly important when using high-dose inhaled steroids. The correct method of use requires:

- the valve to be working;
- the device to be held horizontal or in a slightly mouthpiece down position;
- actuations delivered singly into the chamber, each followed by inspiration;
- minimum delay between actuation and starting inspiration;
- slow deep inspirations (tidal breathing is as good but takes more breaths).

Most spacers should not be washed more than once per month. They should be allowed to drip dry to prevent static. Plastic spacers need to be replaced every 6–12 months.

Infrequent episodic wheeze

If the episodes of wheeze occur less frequently than every 6 weeks, and are relatively mild (moderate breathlessness, able to continue with most activities, duration 1–3 days), then intermittent use of a broncho-dilator using an age-appropriate device is appropriate (salbutamol or terbutaline).

Frequent episodic wheeze or persistent wheeze

For more frequent episodes, a preventative therapy is needed.

- In most children with this pattern of asthma the preventive therapy of choice is inhaled steroids using an age-appropriate device.
- There is little to choose between the available inhaled steroids.
- It is important to note that, although different inhaled steroids have similar efficacy, they have different potency. Fluticasone and mometasone have twice the potency of budesonide and beclometasone.
- Inhaled steroids should be given twice daily initially. Once good control is achieved, once daily therapy can be effective. There is no benefit from dosing more frequently than twice daily.
- For families anxious about using inhaled steroids, leukotriene receptor antagonists (montelukast and zafirlukast) can be used. Montelukast may be particularly useful for viral-associated wheeze.
- The effectiveness of sodium cromoglicate and nedocromil in childhood asthma is contentious. Nedocromil may be of some benefit in the control of exercise-induced asthma.

Table 14.1 Delivery devices[*]

Device	Drug	Suitable for
MDI alone	Bronchodilators	Some teenagers
Breath-actuated MDI, e.g. Autohaler or EasiBreathe	Bronchodilators	Some school-age children
MDI & spacer with facemask	Bronchodilators, cromoglicate, & steroids	All children able to use a mouthpiece
Dry powder inhalers	Bronchodilators & steroids	School-age children
Turbohaler	Terbutaline; budesonide; formoterol	
Accuhaler	Salbutamol; salmeterol; fluticasone	
Clickhaler	Salbutamol; beclometasone	
Diskhaler	Salbutamol; salmeterol; beclometasone	
Foradil aerolizer	Formoterol	
Twisthaler	Mometasone	

[*] There is no indication for the use of a nebulizer to deliver maintenance inhaled medication.

Add on therapy

A reasonable starting dose for inhaled steroids would be 200mcg per day of beclometasone or equivalent. If adequate control is not achieved after 6 weeks, or previously well controlled asthma deteriorates, a review is needed to re-assess symptoms and inhaler technique. Thereafter, increased therapy may be needed. Options are as follows.

- Increase inhaled steroids (beclametasone or equivalent) to 400mcg per day.
- Add a long-acting beta agonist (LABA).
- Add a leukotriene receptor antagonist.
- Add oral theophylline.

One approach is to start a LABA and then, if necessary, increase the steroid dose; then add the leukotriene receptor antagonist and, finally, add theophylline. Only a very small proportion of asthmatic children will need more than an inhaled steroid and an inhaled LABA. Lack of control at this stage should prompt a careful review of the symptoms and diagnosis (see 🕮 Chapter 2). There is no evidence that combination inhalers (steroid and LABA) provide better asthma control in children than single inhalers, although they may be more convenient and improve adherence.

If, despite these measures, control is still poor and the diagnosis is certain, increasing doses of inhaled steroids can sometime lead to better control. Use of beclometasone or equivalent is not licensed for the treatment of asthma in children at doses above 400mcg per day and its use at higher doses should only be undertaken by experienced clinicians.

Other medication

- In severe persistent asthma not responding to standard therapies, it may be necessary to gain control with a course of oral steroids. Prednisolone can be started at high dose (1–2mg/kg/day) and then weaned over 2–4 weeks to a maintenance level. If possible, an alternate day regime should be used. When control is poor despite oral prednisolone, pulsed methylprednisolone given monthly for 2–6 cycles may help improve control (anecdotal evidence only).
- If high doses of oral steroids are required for control, steroid-sparing drugs may be helpful. There is limited or anecdotal experience for the use of other anti-inflammatory drugs such as methotrexate, ciclosporin, gold, and IV immunoglobulin in children with severe steroid-dependent asthma. Two meta-analyses assessing the benefits of methotrexate in severe asthma found only minor steroid-sparing benefit at the cost of significant adverse effects.
- Bronchoscopic evaluation of inflammation may assist management. If the bronchoscopy is carried out in children with persistent airflow obstruction after a course of high dose systemic steroids, the following interpretations may apply.
  - If there is no evidence of inflammation and no reversibility with beta agonists, the likely diagnosis is bronchiolitis obliterans. There is little value in using high dose steroids in these children and treatment should be symptomatic only.

- If there is eosinophilic inflammation, there is likely to be a degree of steroid resistance, and either high dose steroids or steroid-sparing agents (such as ciclosporin) can be tried.
- If there is neutrophilic inflammation, response to steroids is likely to be poor and these should be weaned to the lowest dose that provides baseline control. There is anecdotal evidence that macrolides (e.g. azithromycin) may be helpful in this group of children.
- Omalizumab is a recombinant humanized monoclonal IgG antibody that binds IgE and reduces free IgE in the serum by over 95% (although total IgE is unaffected or increases). Reduced free IgE is thought to lead to a reduction in IgE-mediated activation of mast cells and other effector cells of the allergic immune response. When given to patients with severe persistent asthma it has been shown to reduce the frequency of exacerbations (2–3 fold reduction). It seems less effective in those requiring maintenance therapy with oral steroids or in those with baseline $FEV_1 > 80\%$ predicted. Current (2007) use in children is limited to those over 12 years of age with persistent asthma who have symptoms despite the use of high dose inhaled steroids and who have:
  - allergy (positive skin prick test or serum specific IgE) to a perennial antigen such as house dust mite);
  - total IgE of 30–700IU/mL (there are no data on those with higher IgE levels, and potentially more side-effects because of immune complex formation).

Steroid-resistant asthma

- A subset of children with asthma responds poorly to both inhaled steroids and oral prednisolone. This relative lack of response is seen even when other likely contributors to poor control (discussed in 📖 Chapter 2) are taken into account.
- In most children the resistance takes the form of decreased sensitivity rather than a complete lack of effect.
- The definition most often used for steroid-resistant asthma is failure to improve FEV_1 by 15% after 14 days of oral prednisolone (dose is variable, but around 1mg/kg). These children must also have a clear diagnosis of asthma, with at least a 15% improvement in FEV1 following inhaled beta agonist.
- The most likely reason for a poor response to oral steroids is non-adherence and this possibility must be pursued. Admission to hospital for a period of evaluation, during which compliance with treatment can be assured, is occasionally helpful.
- Typically children with steroid-resistant asthma will have chronic airflow limitation ($FEV_1 < 70\%$) with daily symptoms and frequent exacerbations.
- Glucocorticoids such as prednisolone diffuse from the blood into cells where they interact directly with the glucocorticoid receptor (GCR). After binding, the receptor moves to the nucleus where it binds to specific DNA sequences called glucocorticoid response elements associated with specific genes. Upon binding to DNA, the receptor can either activate or repress transcription of the associated gene.

- Steroid resistance arises because of:
  - decreased affinity between the GCR and glucocorticoid or between the bound GCR and DNA. In most cases the resistance is acquired rather than genetic, and may be controlled by specific T-cell cytokines (so called type 1 resistance). This resistance is specific to the airway and steroid effects seen in other tissues (including sideeffects) will be observed;
  - decreased numbers of available GCRs (type 2 resistance). This form of steroid resistance affects all tissues and does appear to have a genetic background. These children exhibit very few steroid side effects despite long-term use of high dose oral steroids.
- Type 1 steroid resistance is most common.
- Adults with steroid-resistant asthma show persistence of eosinophilic inflammation despite steroid use. Bronchial biopsies (rather than lavage) may be necessary to demonstrate eosinophils.
- In some countries, prednisone rather than prednisolone is used as the steroid of choice. Prednisone requires metabolism in the liver to form active prednisolone, and this can occasionally be impaired leading to apparent steroid resistance.
- The management of steroid-resistant asthma is the same as for any poorly controlled asthma (see above). Once other aspects of control have been optimized oral steroids may be needed at moderate dose. Occasionally twice daily dosing may be more effective (some children eliminate prednisone faster than others). Other anti-inflammatory drugs such as ciclosporin and methotrexate may be added to try and minimize steroid side-effects and improve asthma control.
- Performing a pharmacokinetic study may be helpful to determine absorption, half-life, and elimination of oral prednisolone. In some centres it may be possible to measure GCR binding efficiency and GCR numbers.

Side-effects of inhaled steroids

- These are often a source of anxiety and may reduce adherence to therapy.
- High-dose inhaled steroids of more than 800mcg per day (beclometasone equivalent) can be associated with adrenal suppression. Children with normal lung function seem to be particularly at risk, presumably because of increased alveolar absorption.
- Synacthen tests to assess adrenal response should be considered in children on prolonged high-dose inhaled steroids.
- Children with adrenal suppression should receive corticosteroid cover during episodes of stress, and oral hydrocortisone replacement should be used when attempting to wean the inhaled steroid dose.
- Temporary reduction in growth velocity commonly occurs with inhaled steroids, but there is no effect on final height even with longterm use of inhaled steroids at standard doses ($\leq$ 400mcg per day). Higher doses may have an effect on final height, although this has not been proven.

- Bone mineral density may be reduced following long-term use of high dose inhaled steroids. Measurements of bone mineral density in children are difficult to interpret. No studies have shown an increased fracture risk.
- High doses may also be associated with a hoarse voice and, rarely, oral *Candida*. These effects can be minimized by using a spacer device and/or mouth rinsing after each dose.

Asthma management plans

All children with asthma should have a written asthma management plan. The long-term value of using written plans is difficult to establish, and it is likely that many are lost on the journey home from the hospital. Nevertheless, the process of going over the rationale of using preventers and relievers, and what to do for exacerbations and in emergencies is very valuable. Provision of a written plan without discussion is unlikely to have the desired effect.

Allergen-specific immunotherapy

- Immunotherapy has been used in the treatment of allergic disease for many years. It is based on the development of immune tolerance to specific allergens, which is induced by a series of exposures to increasing doses of the allergen, traditionally by SC injection and, more recently, by sublingual therapy.
- To be effective a single, well-defined clinically relevant allergen needs to be identified against which the immunotherapy will be directed. There is no evidence that multiple allergen immunotherapy is effective and this significantly limits its use in atopic children who are frequently allergic to a wide range of allergens.
- A Cochrane review, mainly of adult studies, of 75 randomized trials of single allergen immunotherapy showed that it is effective in reducing symptom scores, medication use, and both allergen and non-specific bronchial hyperresponsiveness.[6]
- The benefits of immunotherapy are modest. They have not been compared with the effects of pharmacotherapy in a head-to-head trial.
- There are risks associated with immunotherapy (including anaphylaxis) as well as the inconvenience of regular injections, which need to be carried out in a safe environment with resuscitation equipment available. Sublingual immunotherapy can be given at home.
- Immunotherapy is generally only considered for older children with allergic asthma who have a single predominant allergen trigger and who have poor control despite strict allergen avoidance and adequate pharmacotherapy. It is not widely available in the UK. There is greater use in mainland Europe and the USA.
- Immunotherapy for allergic rhinitis is discussed in 📖 Chapter 43.

6 Abramson, M.J., Puy, R.M., and Weiner, J.M. (2003). Allergen immunotherapy for asthma. *Cochrane Database Syst. Rev.* **2003** (4), CD001186.

Hospital management of acute asthma exacerbation

Treatment of an acute exacerbation starts with an assessment of severity. The BTS guidelines should be followed.

Mild attack

SaO_2 over 92% in air, vocalizing without difficulty, mild chest wall recession, moderate tachypnoea. Bilateral wheeze on auscultation.
   Treat as follows.
- Salbutamol 4 puffs via MDI and spacer.
- Reassess after 10min.
- If not improved, give 10 puffs of salbutamol via MDI and spacer.
- Oral prednisolone 2mg/kg (maximum 40mg) daily for 3 days.
- Reassess and repeat salbutamol up to 4 hourly as needed.

Moderate attack

SaO_2 less than 92% in air, obviously breathless, moderate chest wall recession. Bilateral wheeze on auscultation.
   Treat as follows.
- High flow facemask oxygen.
- Nebulized salbutamol (2.5mg for < 5 years; otherwise 5mg).
- Reassess after 10min.
- If not improved give nebulized salbutamol and ipratropium bromide (250mcg)—mixed in nebulizer chamber.
- Reassess after 10min.
- If not improved give further nebulized salbutamol and ipratropium bromide—mixed in nebulizer chamber.
- Oral prednisolone 2mg/kg (maximum 40mg) for 3 days.

Most children will respond well to back-to-back nebulized treatment. At this stage they should be given oral prednisolone. If they remain wheeze-free after 3 hours observation, they can be discharged.

Life-threatening asthma or failure to respond to nebulized therapy

Severe life-threatening asthma is associated with marked hypoxia, severe chest wall recession, decreased effort in exhausted children, confusion, and collapse.
- Start continuous nebulizer salbutamol.
- High flow facemask oxygen.
- Attach cardiac monitor.
- Consider IV therapy. Salbutamol 15mcg/kg slow bolus or aminophylline 5mg/kg over 20min followed by infusion at 1mg/kg/h (omit loading dose if on oral theophylline).
- Hydrocortisone 4mg/kg IV.
- Get the help of someone skilled in airway management (usually either an anaesthetist or intensivist).
- Unless there is rapid improvement, transfer to an ICU.

Other therapies

For sick children with asthma responding poorly to treatment, additional therapies that may be helpful include the following.

- Salbutamol infusion 1–5mcg/kg/min (monitor electrolytes).
- Magnesium sulphate 40mg/kg (maximum 2g) IV over 20min.
- Ketamine infusion 0.5–1mg/kg/h: can have additive bronchodilator effects.
- Once a child has been intubated and ventilated, sevoflurane (2–3%) has useful bronchodilator effects. Adding volatile agents to the ventilator circuit requires anaesthetic expertise.
- Nebulized magnesium sulphate (2.5mL of 7.5% solution with 2.5mg salbutamol in 0.5mL) appears to have some benefit, but its role in management has not been defined.

Before a child goes home

Discharge can be considered when:
- bronchodilators taken by MDI and spacer are needed no more frequently than 4 hourly;
- oxygen saturations in air are above 92%;
- inhaler technique has been assessed as satisfactory.

A written asthma management plan should be provided, including any adjustment to regular prophylactic therapy, along with follow-up arrangements with the GP and at the hospital.

Vocal cord dysfunction (VCD)

- During inspiration the vocal cords normally abduct to increase the size of the airway.
- In children with VCD, the cords are held in an adducted position, airway size is diminished, and airflow becomes turbulent. This can result in noisy breathing during inspiration and/or expiration, which can be misinterpreted as asthma.
- The condition often coexists with asthma.
- It usually affects school-age children and adolescents; girls are more often affected than boys.
- It may be brought on by exercise, especially in children who take their sport seriously. In other children it comes on spontaneously.
- Rapidly stopping exercise because of VCD can lead to vasovagal symptoms (pallor, light-headedness, and occasionally fainting), which may be misinterpreted as part of the problem.
- VCD is not caused by a conscious voluntary act.
- VCD is usually accompanied by considerable anxiety in the child and parents.
- Often the diagnosis can be made by history. The noise is inspiratory, and tightness is felt in the throat; neither of these symptoms are consistent with asthma.
- In contrast to an asthma attack, child having acute episode of VCD will not have a hyperinflated chest and will have normal oxygen saturation.
- If the symptoms are brought on by exercise, an exercise test can be useful in making the diagnosis.
- Diagnosis is usually based on a suggestive history plus demonstrating flattening of the inspiratory portion of the flow–volume loop during symptomatic episodes. The gold-standard test requires direct laryngo-scopy to show paradoxical vocal fold adduction during inspiration.
- Treatment involves explanation and breathing exercises. An experi-enced physiotherapist or speech and language therapist can provide valuable training sessions to improve breathing and vocal relaxation to control symptoms.
- There are case reports of benefit from the use of ipratropium bromide inhalation prior to exercise in children with exercise-induced VCD.
- Reduction in asthma medication is often possible once VCD has been diagnosed.
- Where VCD occurs in competitive athletes, breathing exercises may help control their symptoms when they occur, but may not prevent them from occurring. Removing stress (including competitive demands by parents) from the sporting activity may be beneficial.
- In some children psychological therapy, in addition to specific relaxation exercises, can be helpful.

Further information

Davies, H., Olson, L., and Gibson, P. (2000). Methotrexate as a steroid sparing agent for asthma in adults. *Cochrane Database Syst. Rev.* **2000** (2), CD000391.

Payne, D. and Bush, A. (2004). Phenotype-specific treatment of difficult asthma in children. *Paediatr. Respir. Rev.* **5**, 116–23.

Sher, E.R., Leung, D.Y.M., et al. (1994). Steroid-resistant asthma. Cellular mechanisms contributing to inadequate response to glucocorticoid therapy. *J. Clin. Invest.* **93**, 33–9.

Waser, M., Michels, K.B., Bielai, C., et al. (2007). Inverse association of farm milk consumption with asthma and allergy in rural and suburban populations across Europe. *Clin. Exp. Allergy* **37**, 661–70.

Cystic fibrosis

Overview

Cystic fibrosis (CF) is an autosomal recessive disease caused by defects in the CF transmembrane conductor gene (*CFTR*). The disease affects several tissues. Most children are severely affected and will develop symptoms in the first year of life—typically poor growth, abnormal stools, and recurrent or persistent coughing. A small proportion, < 10%, have milder disease, with near normal growth and little apparent chest disease. These children may not present clinically until later childhood and occasionally adulthood.

Survival

Life expectancy for people with CF has improved steadily over the last 20 years. It is difficult to estimate accurately the likely survival of an individual child. Available survival figures show 50% survival is 35 years for men and 32 years for women. Median age at death is 26 years for men and 22 years for women. More recent birth cohorts appear to have improved survival.

The lungs

At birth the lungs of children with CF are effectively normal. Occasionally small bronchial casts can be found after bronchoalveolar lavage, but these do not affect lung function. Although there is still some debate in the literature, most evidence suggests that there is no inflammation in the airways before the first infection.

CF airways are prone to infection (see 📖 p. 134). Recurrent and persistent infection sets up a profound inflammatory response, and the combination of bacterial products and host inflammation leads to progressive lung damage. This predominantly affects the airway lining and subsequently the airway walls, resulting in increased mucus production and decreased mucus clearance. This in turn makes further infection more likely and harder to clear. Airway wall inflammation and cellular debris and mucus in the airway lumen cause obstructive lung disease. The profound inflammatory response often makes children feel non-specifically unwell with diminished appetite. The infections are not invasive and fever is rare. Lung disease is responsible for most of the morbidity and mortality in CF.

The pancreas

The site of disease in the pancreas is the pancreatic duct. In 90% of children with CF this becomes completely obstructed during fetal life leading to autolysis of the exocrine pancreas. In these children there is little or no exocrine pancreatic function. The pancreas produces several digestive enzymes as well as bicarbonate. Importantly, the pancreas is the major source of lipase and, as a consequence, children with pancreatic insufficiency fail to digest and absorb fat. Since about half the energy from milk comes from fat, it is not surprising that CF causes marked failure to thrive. About 10% of children with CF retain sufficient pancreatic function to prevent fat malabsorption. As a group, these children are also more likely to have milder lung disease, although there are too many exceptions to make this association useful for prognosis in individual patients. Children with residual pancreatic function are at risk of pancreatitis.

The endocrine pancreas functions normally in young children with CF. In older children, the combination of increasing size with age and progressive pancreas fibrosis can result in glucose intolerance and diabetes. About 20% of children with CF will develop diabetes by the age of 20. The prevalence continues to rise with age thereafter.

The gut

The mucus secreted by the small intestine is abnormally sticky in children with CF. In fetal life this can cause bowel obstruction (meconium ileus) in about 10–15% of affected infants. Outside the neonatal period, obstruction can occur as part of the distal intestinal obstruction syndrome (DIOS). This probably arises through a combination of abnormal mucus and slow intestinal transit times, possibly secondary to steatorrhoea. For reasons that are not clear, CF can also be associated with rectal prolapse. Colon fibrosis, reported in the mid-1990s, was related to high dose pancreatic enzyme use and has not been reported since.

The liver

In the neonatal period CF can be associated with cholestasis, particularly in infants with meconium ileus. The jaundice can persist for as long as 2 months, but eventually clears without treatment. About 30% of children with CF will have elevated alanine or aspartate transaminases, with or without changes in liver texture on ultrasound. The significance of these changes is not clear. 2–5% of patients will develop a form of biliary cirrhosis with portal hypertension. The risk of developing significant liver disease is highest between the ages of 8 and 18 years. It is unlikely that new liver disease will occur in adulthood.

Children with CF have an increased risk of gall stones and biliary sludging. The stones usually contain calcium bilirubinate.

Reproductive tract

More than 98% of men with CF are infertile due to bilateral absence of the vas deferens. In men whose general health is reasonable, libido and sexual performance are normal. Some men with no apparent chest disease, who present with infertility caused by bilateral absence of the vas deferens, have been shown to have 2 CF mutations and thus a form of CF. Surgical sperm retrieval followed by intracytoplasmic sperm injection can offer the possibility of fertility to men with CF.

Women with CF are less fertile than healthy women. This probably results from a combination of poor nutrition leading to anovulatory cycles and more viscid cervical mucus making sperm penetration more difficult.

Genetics

- Mutations in *CFTR* occur in the UK population with a frequency of around 0.04. 1 in 25 people will be heterozygote carriers.
- Assuming random mating, the likelihood of 2 carriers meeting and having children is $1/25 \times 1/25 = 1/625$. Each child will have a 1/4 chance of having CF $1/625 \times 1/4 = 1/2500$. This is very close to the observed birth rate.

- The high frequency of the heterozygous state for a fatal genetic disorder has led to speculation about possible heterozygote survival benefits. No convincing mechanisms have been demonstrated. The most plausible theory relates to reduced fluid loss in diarrhoeal illness.
- CFTR function is disrupted by base changes in the gene sequence. These changes are called mutations. By convention they are named by the amino acid in the protein that is affected or, if they are non-coding, by the base position in the gene. For example, deltaF508 results in the deletion of phenylalanine (F) at position 508 in the protein and R117H results in the replacement of arginine (R) with a histidine (H) at position 117 in the protein. The 1717-1G to A mutation is non-coding (i.e. it does not change an amino acid); rather it affects a splice site 1 base into the intron at position 1717 in the gene.
- 5 different classes of mutation are recognized. Some, which lead to amino acid substitutions, are associated with residual CFTR function and milder disease.
- The commonest mutation in populations of northern European descent is deltaF508. This accounts for 75% of CF mutations in the UK: 57% of patients are deltaF508 homozygotes, 36% have one copy of deltaF508 with another mutation, and 7% of patients have 2 non-deltaF508 mutations.
- By screening for the most frequent 30 mutations, both mutations will be detected in 72% of patients, and less than 2.5% of patients have neither mutation detected.
- After the top 30 mutations, the remaining 1000+ known CF mutations are present in less than 1% of the CF populations, most being found in only one or two families.

CFTR function

CFTR is an ATP-dependent chloride channel. It is present in many different epithelial tissues. ATP is required to open the channel but, once open, chloride moves passively in or out of the cell along electrochemical gradients.

The airway

In the lung CFTR is expressed in airway epithelial cells and the ducts of submucous glands. In addition to acting as a chloride channel, it also has a regulatory function, particularly affecting the activity of the epithelial sodium channel ENaC. When CFTR is defective, ENaC activity is increased, leading to hyperabsorption of sodium. This is thought to reduce the depth of airway surface liquid that supports the mucus layer, allowing the mucus to come into contact with the cells and inhibit cilial function. Adherent plaques of mucus also form sites for persistent airway infection.

The sweat gland

The sweat gland is formed from a single tube, which has a coiled part in the dermis and duct that travels to the skin surface. Sweat production starts in the coiled section and, initially, levels of sodium and chloride are similar to those found in plasma. As the sweat moves up the duct, CFTR provides a channel for chloride absorption. Sodium follows to maintain electrochemical neutrality. The duct is impermeable to water and the resulting sweat is hypotonic. When CFTR is defective, chloride and consequently sodium is not reabsorbed leading to higher sweat concentrations of these ions.

Diagnosis

Where newborn screening is in place, the majority (95%) of children with CF will be diagnosed either by the screening programme or because they have meconium ileus. No screening programme is perfect and children will continue to present symptomatically. The clinical diagnosis of CF requires a combination of likely symptoms, plus either a positive sweat test or 2 identified disease-causing mutations. Isolated sweat tests can be misleading, particularly when carried out in children who are failing to thrive but who do not have typical symptoms of CF. These tests need to be interpreted carefully before a diagnosis is reached. It is good practice to repeat the sweat test or carry out genetic analysis to confirm the diagnosis.

Clinical diagnosis

History

CF should be considered in all children with any combination of:
- productive-sounding cough that is persistent or recurrent;
- failure to thrive;
- bulky, pale, and offensive stool.

Less common presentations include:
- raised intracranial pressure in infants with vitamin A deficiency;
- bleeding in infants with neonatal cholestasis;
- pseudo-Bartter's syndrome;
- rectal prolapse;
- nasal polyps;
- male infertility with bilateral absence of vas deferens.

Examination

Examination may be normal. Signs consistent with CF include:
- finger clubbing;
- hyperinflated chest;
- crepitations on auscultation.

Investigations

Standard investigations would include:
- cough swab, looking for presence of *Staphylococcus aureus*, *Haemophilus influenzae*, or *Pseudomonas aeruginosa*;
- CXR, looking for bronchial wall thickening and hyperinflation;
- sweat test;
- immune-reactive trypsin (IRT) can be useful in neonates.

The sweat test

The sweat test remains the gold standard.
- The sweat test is a quantitative measurement of electrolytes in sweat. Sweat is collected after pilocarpine iontophoresis and accurate results are dependent on careful technique.
- Sweat is collected for 20–30min.
- The sweating rate should exceed $1g/m^2/min$ giving an adequate volume of sweat for analysis: 15µL if collected in a Macroduct system or 100mg weight if collected on filter paper.

- Sweat chloride concentration of > 60mmol/L supports a diagnosis of CF.
- Sweat sodium should not be interpreted without a chloride result. For a test to be considered positive, the sum of chloride and sodium should exceed 120mmol/L and chloride concentration should be greater than the sodium level and > 60mmol/L.
- Sweat conductivity measurement values above 90mEq support a diagnosis of CF but diagnosis should not be based on conductivity levels alone. Chloride concentration should always be measured (usually on the same sample).
- Abnormal sweat tests should always be repeated (unless the diagnosis has been confirmed by genetic analysis).
- Sweat tests can be prone to technical error, the commonest being insufficient collection of sweat, so, where there is clinical doubt, 'normal' sweat tests may also need to be repeated.
- False positives can and do occur, usually for either for technical reasons, again usually insufficient sweat, or because of local skin problems, mainly eczema. There are a number of other conditions that may rarely result in elevated sweat chlorides (see box). Several of these can cause failure to thrive and should be considered if the clinical picture is not typical for CF. Many of the conditions disturb serum electrolytes and this is what is reflected by the sweat test. In atypical presentations, carrying out simultaneous serum electrolyte assays can avoid this pitfall.
- Borderline sweat tests (chloride over 40mmol/L) should also be repeated. Sweat tests are valid from after the first 48h of life, although it can be difficult to get enough sweat from babies under 4kg, and this can delay definitive diagnosis if genetic analysis is inconclusive.
- Sweat chloride levels are lower in normal neonates than in older children and adults. A sweat chloride of 40mmol/L is 4 standard deviations above the mean for the normal neonates (first 4 weeks of life) and levels above 40mmol/L, whilst not considered diagnostic, should prompt further investigation in this age group.

Causes of false positive sweat test

- Technical error:
  - insufficient sweat volume
  - evaporation caused by excessive collection time
  - inadequately cleaned skin surface
- Abnormal skin—serous exudates have high salt content:
  - eczema
  - ectodermal dysplasia
- Electrolyte problems:
  - adrenal insufficiency (aldosterone acts on sweat gland, and low levels result in increased salt loss)
  - pseudo-hypoaldosteronism (peripheral resistance to aldosterone—may also have a wet-sounding cough)
  - diabetes insipidus (high sodium, high chloride, high osmolarity—usually nephrogenic if presenting in first year of life)
  - anorexia nervosa
  - hypoparathyroidism
  - severe malnutrition
  - severe dehydration
- Other metabolic diseases (mechanism unclear):
  - fucosidosis
  - glucose-6-phosphate dehydrogenase deficiency
  - glycogen storage disease type 1
  - mucopolysaccharidosis type 1
  - familial cholestasis
- Miscellaneous (mechanism unclear):
  - Down's syndrome
  - Klinefelter's syndrome

Immune–reactive trypsin

Immune–reactive trypsin present in the blood is an indication of pancreatic injury and is high in neonates with CF.

- A high IRT (> 99.5 percentile for the population) is found in 98% of infants with CF. By definition it will also be found in 0.5% of the unaffected population.
- IRT falls rapidly over the first few weeks of life. If a second IRT measured at 21–28 days is also high (> 95 percentile), the likelihood of CF is increased. About 20% of normal infants with a high initial IRT will have a high subsequent IRT; for infants with CF the figure is around 90%.
- Measurement of IRT forms an essential part of most national screening programmes but has limited value as a diagnostic test because of lack of specificity.
- For reasons that are not clear neonates with meconium ileus can give false negative IRT test results. Bowel surgery can cause elevated IRT levels and measurements taken postoperatively can falsely indicate a diagnosis of CF (false positive results). For both these reasons diagnosis of CF in neonates with meconium ileus will be based either on genetic analysis or, when it is technically feasible, a sweat test.

Additional investigations

Where the diagnosis of CF is in doubt, additional investigations include the following.

- Fecal pancreatic elastase. This enzyme is produced by the pancreas and is a useful indicator of exocrine pancreatic function Levels under 200mcg/g suggest pancreatic insufficiency.
- Chest CT scan looking for evidence of bronchiectasis.
- Nasal potential difference—only available in a few specialist centres. Patients with CF have a higher nasal potential difference (lumen negative) than non-CF subjects. The potential difference is amiloride sensitive, and subsequently fails to respond to manoeuvres designed to increase chloride secretion. This test is difficult to perform in adults and impossible in uncooperative children.
- Nasal nitric oxide. For reasons that are not clear, nasal NO levels are low in children with CF. There is overlap with normal children, children with blocked noses, and children with primary ciliary dyskinesia. For the moment, nasal NO measurements remain a research tool.

Genetic analysis

Genetic analysis can be used as a diagnostic test and will confirm the diagnosis in 70% of patients (of northern European descent). In the remainder, only one or occasionally no CF mutations will be found. This does not mean the patient does not have CF and the majority of these patients will have abnormal sweat tests. The very occasional patients with mild disease and normal sweat test values in whom CF is still suspected are likely to be the patients with rare mutations that will not be picked up by genetic analysis. For these reasons genetic analysis as a diagnostic test is generally reserved for neonates who are too small (< 4kg) to provide adequate volumes of sweat, in whom confirmation of the diagnosis is needed quickly. In other patients, the sweat test is a preferable diagnostic test. All patients diagnosed with CF should have blood sent for genetic analysis, both to allow genetic counselling and to provide information that may become important when considering novel therapies.

Newborn screening

- The majority of children with CF will have symptoms in the first year of life and 85% would be diagnosed on the basis of symptoms before the age of 2 years in most health-care systems.
- There is increasing evidence that children with CF identified by screening programmes have better outcomes than those presenting symptomatically. The best evidence for improved outcome is related to growth and nutritional status, but it probably also applies to lung function and survival.
- Several different screening protocols are used. Most use an elevated (> 99.5th centile) immune-reactive trypsin measured on a blood spot taken at 5–7 days of age as the starting point. This is then followed by a genetic analysis on the same spot of blood. Detection of 2 disease-causing mutations leads to confirmatory investigation, usually repeat genetic testing, and a sweat test. Programmes differ as to how many mutations are tested, how heterozygotes are handled, and whether a second IRT at 21–28 days is used as part of the algorithm. In the

UK infants with a high initial IRT and one identified mutation will have a second IRT performed. If this is below the cut-off level the infant is said to be screen negative. If the IRT is above the cut-off level the infant is referred for a sweat test. Second IRTs are also carried out in infants who have no CF mutations detected but who had initial IRT values above the 99.9th centile.

- No screening programme will identify all children with CF. Most will miss about 3% of cases, either because they do not have an initial IRT above the cut-off chosen, or because they have 2 rare mutations not included in the screening panel. Specific mutation frequencies vary in different ethnic populations and this may affect both the choice of mutations used in the screening programme and the effectiveness of screening in different ethnic groups.
- For all screening methods, a negative result from the newborn screening programme does not exclude CF in a child who presents with likely symptoms.

Explaining the diagnosis

Following diagnosis, the first critical part of management is to explain the diagnosis to the family and to inform the child's GP. It is often useful to include a standard letter to the GP outlining general CF management and introducing the local CF team. Information to give to the family at the first meeting may include:

- a brief description of the effects of CF on the lungs and pancreas;
- the genetic nature of the condition;
- that it is a serious and life-shortening condition;
- that there are many therapies available to improve the outcome;
- the treatments that need to start immediately—usually physiotherapy, prophylactic antibiotics, high energy diet, and pancreatic enzymes;
- that regular hospital visits will be required throughout the child's life;
- that with good care children with CF will go to school and play sport normally.

The family should meet with the local CF nurse, dietitian, and physiotherapist as soon after diagnosis as possible. An appointment with the regional CF centre for annual review should be made.

Physiotherapy

- A twice daily chest physiotherapy regime is one of the mainstays of CF therapy. It aims to keep airway secretions to a minimum thereby decreasing airways obstruction, clearing inflammatory mediators, and reducing opportunities for infection.
- There are no randomized controlled trials showing that physiotherapy has long-term benefits, but there is plenty of anecdotal evidence indicating that stopping physiotherapy in patients with moderate disease can lead to rapid deterioration.
- Even if benefits in children with mild disease are difficult to demonstrate, it is important to have a regular physiotherapy regime so that physiotherapy is used promptly and effectively during respiratory exacerbations.
- Most UK CF centres would recommend that physiotherapy be started immediately after diagnosis and carried out twice daily thereafter.
- Parents should be taught how to carry out effective chest physiotherapy by an experienced CF physiotherapist.
- In infants, tilting head down during physiotherapy may worsen gastro-oesophageal reflux. Most physiotherapy regimes avoid this position in infants. The value of head down position in older children has also been questioned.
- Airway clearance techniques are discussed in detail in 📖 Chapter 58.

Exercise All children, but particularly those with CF, should be encouraged to exercise. Children with $FEV_1 > 60\%$ predicted should be able to undertake exercise to the same level as their normal peer group. Exercise programmes should aim to increase cardiovascular fitness, and include 20–30min of exercise 3–4 times per week.

Mucolytics and DNase

Airway secretions in CF are often very tenacious and difficult to mobilize and expectorate. Three different inhaled treatments are available to reduce the stickiness of the secretions and improve mucociliary clearance.

- Hypertonic sodium chloride (3–7%). This can be inhaled twice daily with some evidence of benefit. It can induce bronchospasm in some children (pre-treatment with salbutamol can help) and the swallowed solution can cause vomiting.
- Acetylcysteine. This has been used in a nebulized form in the past as a mucolytic (it disrupts disulphide bonds between mucin molecules) but relatively frequent bronchospasm has limited its use. A derivative called Nacystelyn has been developed as a metered dose inhaler, but has not yet reached the market.
- DNAase or dornase alfa is the most widely used agent with the best evidence base. In a large RCT DNase was shown to improve FEV_1 by around 8% over a 6 month period. Follow-up studies have shown that the improvement is maintained, provided the treatment is continued. It has also been shown to result in small (2–3%) but significant improvements in lung function (FEF_{25-75}) in 6–10-year-old children over a 2 year period and to reduce the number of infective exacerbations. These children all had near-normal lung function at start of trial.

DNAase is expensive, around £6500 per year. The trial data show that some patients have dramatic benefits, most show modest improvement, and a smaller number of children either have no benefit or deteriorate. Before starting DNAase it is important to optimize other treatments. It is essential that effective, regular physiotherapy is carried out. The benefits of DNAase should be assessed in each patient after 3–6 months to determine whether there is value in continuing the drug in the longer term.

Nutrition

Children with CF have the potential for normal growth. They are at risk of malnutrition because of:
- fat malabsorption;
- increased energy requirements when unwell;
- poor appetite—probably a combination of the systemic effects of pulmonary inflammation and swallowed sputum.

Monitoring growth
- Height and weight should be checked at every clinic visit and plotted on a centile chart.
- Estimates of nutritional status should be made annually, either by calculating BMI or weight for height percentage.

   BMI = weight(kg)/height(m^2)

   %wt/ht = weight/expected weight for height
- Anthropometric measurements to estimate body composition, such as skinfold thickness and mid-arm circumference are not reliable in CF.

General advice
- Although the energy needs of patients with CF vary, a high energy, high fat diet providing 120–150% of the estimated average requirement for energy is recommended.
- Breastfeeding should be encouraged for infants with CF.
- All families should be seen by a dietitian at diagnosis and frequently thereafter to provide advice on the types of foods that can provide the child's nutritional requirements. About 40% of energy requirements will need to come from fat.

Poor weight gain
Poor nutrition can be assessed both by serial measurements and by calculation of %wt/ht. Levels under 85% indicate the need for dietary intervention. The first step is to maximize energy density of meals, ensure appropriate use of pancreatic enzymes, aggressively treat airway infection, and exclude CF-related diabetes. If weight gain remains poor, nutritional supplements may be needed.

Oral supplements
- Glucose and fat powders. Powders, such as Maxijul, Duocal, and Polycose, can be used for all ages. They are useful to enhance energy density without increasing volume of fluid/food.
- High calorie milkshakes, fortified milk, and juice-based drinks. Supplements are additional to regular meals and should only be given after meals or as snacks. They include milkshakes and yoghurt-style and juice-based drinks. Enzymes are required for all the milk-based supplements but are not normally required for the juice-based drinks.

Enteral feeding Some children with CF have very poor appetites and great difficulty in taking regular supplements. After careful review of diet and optimizing treatment for airway infection, consider enteral feeding if:
- weight has fallen two centile positions;

- no weight gain for 6 months;
- weight for height is < 85%.

Enteral feeding is usually via a gastrostomy. Nasogastric tubes can be used for short-term feeding, e.g. to supplement feeding during infective exacerbations or to demonstrate benefits of enteral feeding when child or family uncertain about having a gastrostomy. A range of suitable feeds is available with energy densities of 1–1.5kcal/ml. Most need pancreatic enzyme supplements. Hydrolysed feeds like Emsogen that have a high proportion of medium chain triglycerides that can be absorbed directly may be used without enzymes.

Pancreatic enzyme supplements

- Oral pancreatic enzyme supplements should be started immediately after diagnosis in all children with CF with evidence of malabsorption.
- In well infants detected by newborn screening and older children with mild disease an assessment of pancreatic status, by looking for fecal fat globules and measuring fecal pancreatic elastase, should be undertaken.
- For infants with meconium ileus who have undergone bowel surgery, it is best to start enzyme supplementation and re-assess pancreatic status once child has fully recovered. Enzymes should be started once child reaches half-feeds.
- Infants can be given the enteric coated granules with a spoon of milk or pureed fruit. The usual starting dose is 2500u lipase per feed (1/4 of a 10 000 unit capsule).
- Total daily dose should not exceed 10 000u lipase/kg body weight as higher doses have been associated with fibrosing colonopathy.
- Pancreatic enzymes need to be used for all foods containing fat. They should be taken at the beginning and during the meal.
- Children who are pancreatic sufficient in early life can become insufficient as they get older.
- The enteric coating on enzyme granules prevents loss of activity in the acid environment of the stomach. The coating requires an alkaline environment to dissolve. The major source of bicarbonate in the duodenum is the pancreas. In some children with CF the upper part of the small bowel can remain acidic, reducing the effectiveness of pancreatic enzyme supplements. H_2 antagonists or proton pump inhibitors can overcome this problem and should be tried if fat malabsorption persists despite an apparent adequate dose of enzymes.

Fat soluble vitamins

- Malabsorption of fat is associated with malabsorption of the fat soluble vitamins, A, D, E, and K.
- Pancreatic enzyme supplementation is not sufficient to prevent malabsorption of vitamins A, D, and E and these vitamins need to be routinely supplemented in children with CF.
- Plasma levels of vitamins A, D, and E should be assessed annually.
- Assess vitamin K status by annual check of PT. Give supplements to children with prolonged PT and/or evidence of liver disease. Give children undergoing surgery who are not on vitamin K oral doses in the week before surgery or a dose IV if the surgery is urgent.

Airway infection

- The CF airway is predisposed to infection.
- The infections are prolonged and associated with a profound neutrophil-dominated inflammatory host response.
- Once neutrophils enter the airway lumen, they cannot return to the circulation and when they die they release a wide range of oxidants and enzymes that damage host cells.
- Neutrophils also release large quantities of DNA, which adds to the bulk and viscosity of airway secretions.
- The bacteria that infect the CF airway are not especially virulent. They are not invasive and do not elicit a fever.
- The range of different bacterial infection is small; most infections will be caused by *Staphylococcus aureus*, *Haemophilus influenzae*, or *Pseudomonas aeruginosa*.
- The only early sign of airway infection is a productive cough.
- Over months and years, repeated infections destroy the lung.
- Improved outcome for CF depends on early detection and aggressive treatment of airway infection.
- There is no such thing as airway colonization in CF. The bacteria are always causing harm and the infections should always be treated.

Microbiological surveillance

- Frequent and careful cultures to identify the presence of airway infection should be undertaken in all children with CF. These should be taken at every clinic visit, and not less often than every 3 months.
- In children who can expectorate, sputum culture is ideal.
- In younger children or those without productive coughs, a cough swab sample should be collected.
- The cough swab technique requires a short session of chest physiotherapy followed by coughing. The swab is either placed in the posterior pharynx during the cough or the posterior pharyngeal wall is swabbed immediately after the coughing episode.
- Bronchoscopy and BAL are occasionally necessary if other cultures are repeatedly negative in the face of ongoing symptoms.
- All children with positive cultures should be treated with 2 weeks of antibiotics irrespective of symptoms.
- The first isolation of *P. aeruginosa* needs particular attention (see 📖 p. 139).
- Following a course of antibiotics for a positive culture, a repeat airway culture should be obtained to ensure the infection has cleared.

Pulmonary exacerbation

There is no agreed definition of a pulmonary exacerbation in CF. It is important to have a standard definition for research work, but in clinical practice it is better to have a broad symptom-based description so that infections are not missed. Airway infection should be presumed to be present if:

- a child who does not normally cough has a productive sounding cough for 3 days or more;
- a child who has a daily cough has an increase in severity of cough, increase in sputum production, or change in sputum colour to yellow or green.

During exacerbations there may also be:

- loss of appetite;
- decreased exercise tolerance;
- lassitude;
- coughing paroxysms that may lead to vomiting;
- fall in lung function;
- new changes on CXR;
- new signs on auscultation.

Fever is unusual. A cough swab or sputum culture should be obtained, and oral antibiotics should be started.

- All antibiotic courses should be for a minimum of 2 weeks.
- High antibiotic doses are needed, not only to get sufficient antibiotic concentrations in the sputum, but also because renal clearance of antibiotics is more efficient in children with CF.
- First choice antibiotics will depend on what the child has grown in the past.
- The choice of antibiotic can be changed if necessary when the cough-swab or sputum culture results are available. If there is no growth, the antibiotic course should still continue for 2 weeks.
- If there is a poor response, a 3rd week may be necessary. If symptoms persist after 3 weeks oral antibiotics, IV therapy should be considered.

Specific infections

Staphylococcus aureus

- These are often first bacteria to infect the airways of infants with CF.
- Prophylactic flucloxacillin should be used for the first 2 years of life, using a twice daily dose.
- Where there is appropriate monitoring and treatment of *Pseudomonas aeruginosa*, there is no evidence that prophylaxis against *S. aureus* affects age of chronic infection with *P. aeruginosa*.
- Flucloxacillin is the antibiotic of choice for children not on prophylaxis who isolate *S. aureus*.
- In children on prophylactic flucloxacillin who isolate *S. aureus*, increase flucloxacillin to 4 times daily and add a second antibiotic. Suitable choices are fusidic acid, azithromycin, erythromycin, or clindamycin.

- If, on repeat culture, infection not cleared after 2 weeks, add 2nd antibiotic if on monotherapy. Continue for further 4 weeks until infection gone.
- If infection not cleared after 6 weeks of oral treatment, consider IV antibiotics.

MRSA

MRSA is an increasing problem in CF. MRSA is not more virulent than MSSA but it can be more difficult to eradicate. Local hospital policies will vary on how to deal with MRSA patients. If MRSA is grown from an airway culture follow the following procedure.

- Collect swabs from nose, axilla, and groin.
- Screen other family members in the same way.
- Attempt eradication in child and family using local protocols.
- Treat airway infection with 2 oral antibiotics taking into account local MRSA sensitivities. Avoid monotherapy as this rapidly leads to resistance. MRSA may be sensitive to rifampicin, fusidic acid, trimethoprim, tetracycline, or doxycycline.
- Chronically infected patients may be treated with prophylactic nebulized antibiotics: Colomycin® or Tobi®.
- If IV treatment is needed, vancomycin or teicoplanin may be used.

Haemophilus influenzae

- This is the non-encapsulated form. Airway infection is not prevented by the Hib vaccine.
- Treat children with positive cultures with a 2 week course of oral antibiotics. Suitable choices would be amoxicillin, co-amoxiclav, or a second generation cephalosporin.
- If, on repeat culture, infection not cleared after 2 weeks, add 2nd antibiotic if on monotherapy. Continue for further 4 weeks until infection gone.
- If infection not cleared after 6 weeks oral treatment, consider IV antibiotics.

Pseudomonas aeruginosa

Chronic infection with *P. aeruginosa* (more so than that with *S. aureus* or *H. influenzae*) is associated with declining lung function in children with CF. *P. aeruginosa* is a Gram-negative organism found widely in warm damp environments. It has 2 forms, mucoid and non-mucoid. Early infections are usually non-mucoid and can usually be cleared. Mucoid transformation, in which an alginate jelly coat forms around colonies of bacteria and protects them from the host immune response and from antibiotics, makes eradication near-impossible.

P. aeruginosa infects most children with CF at least once by the time they are 3 years old. Early infection is usually with environmental non-mucoid strains and tends to be intermittent. Chronic infection is characterized by a change to a mucoid phenotype resulting from the production of an alginate gel. Colonies of *P. aeruginosa* organisms exist within these alginate biofilms where they are protected from antimicrobials and host attack, making this form of *P. aeruginosa* infection impossible to eradicate. Early detection of *P. aeruginosa* infection at the intermittent phase followed by aggressive treatment can delay chronic infection to late teenage years for the majority. Chronic infection has been defined in several ways. A practical definition is the persistence of *P. aeruginosa* on repeat testing over a 12 month period, usually with a mucoid phenotype.

- Eradication of early infection can be achieved in over 80% using a 3 week course of oral ciprofloxacin combined with a 3 week course of nebulized Colomycin®.
- There is some evidence to suggest that extending both the ciprofloxacin and Colomycin® for a 3 month period increases the time before the next positive culture (18 months for the 3 month course versus 9 months for the short course). Several centres now recommend this approach.
- If after 3 months the culture is still positive options are to either:
  - try to eradicate with a 2 week course of IV antibiotics;
  - try to eradicate using 1 month of inhaled Tobi®;
  - continue with the colomycin or Tobi® indefinitely.
- Trials of early eradication using Tobi® suggest that monotherapy with Tobi® may be less effective that the combination of ciprofloxacin and Colomycin®. Studies of the efficacy of Tobi® plus ciprofloxacin are underway.
- Early eradication protocols should be followed each time *P. aeruginosa* is isolated unless chronic infection has become established.

Chronic *P. aeruginosa* infection should be treated with inhaled antibiotics: either Colomycin® or TOBI®. Exacerbations should be treated with a 2 week course of oral ciprofloxacin. Children who do not improve after 2 weeks of ciprofloxacin should be given a 2 week course of IV antibiotics.

Burkholderia cepacia complex

- B. cepacia comprise multiple distinct but closely related genomic species or genomovars.
- All can cause infection in CF, but most clinical problems are associated with genomovar III: *B. cenocepacia*.
- B. cepacia is found widely in the environment, particularly in soil and freshwater sediment.
- Nearly all strains of B. cepacia show multiresistance to antibiotics.
- Some forms of B. cepacia can be highly transmissible particularly the ET12 strain of cenocepacia.
- B. cepacia infection can be followed by rapid loss of lung function and death in as little as 12 months.
- B. cepacia can also cause 'cepacia syndrome', a fulminant infection characterized by high fever, sepsis, raised white count, and severe progressive respiratory failure.
- Some patients with chronic B. cepacia infection remain stable for may years and in others the infection may be transient.
- Accurate identification of B. cepacia species is essential and usually means sending the sample to a reference laboratory.
- Treatment is difficult. It should be based on sensitivity patterns and will usually involve a combination of IV and inhaled antibiotics.
- Strict infection control is needed when dealing with children infected with B. cepacia.

Non-tuberculous mycobacteria (NTM)

- The significance of NTM airway infection in CF depends on the context. Single isolates in a child with mild stable lung disease do not require treatment. Repeated positive cultures, especially when associated with unexplained decline in lung function, new radiographic abnormalities, or recurrent fever, should probably be treated, although response to treatment is variable.
- Infection is usually with *M. avium* complex or *M. abscessus*, although infection with several other strains (such as *M. fortuitum*, *M. kansaii*, and *M. chelonae*) can occur.
- The prevalence of NTM (defined as 3 positive cultures over a 12 month period) is 3–5% in pre-adolescent children. The prevalence increases with age to > 30% in older adult patients.
- In most children the clinical impact of NTM infection is difficult to determine. Where there are repeated positive cultures, particularly with *M. abscessus*, there may be an increase in the annual rate of decline of lung function.
- Long-term azithromycin therapy is associated with NTM macrolide resistance, which makes treatment of possible future NTM infection more difficult. Children and adults treated with long-term macrolides should have regular cultures for NTM. If NTM infection is detected, regular macrolide should probably be stopped.
- Annual screening on sputum culture for NTM infection is recommended for all children with CF.
- If treatment for NTM infection is needed, it will need to be taken for several months. A combination of clarithromycin, rifampicin, and ethambutol taken for 12–18 months can be effective. Combinations of macrolides and ciprofloxacin alone can lead to resistance. *M. abscessus* is particularly difficult to treat effectively and IV treatment with amikacin and ceftazidime plus an oral macrolide may be needed for several weeks before there is a clinical response. Oral therapy will then need to be continued for several months.
- Infection with NTM can adversely affect outcome of lung transplantation, particularly infection with *M. abscessus*. Vigorous efforts should be made to treat and eradicate this infection if transplantation is being considered. Untreated infection with *M. abscessus* is a contraindication to transplantation in most units.

Other infections

- The number of different types of unusual bacteria and fungi infecting the airways of patients with CF is increasing. This probably results from a combination of increased use of antibiotics and better organism identification.
- These organisms include:
  - fungi: *Scedosporium apiospermum; Fusarium* species;
  - bacteria: *Stenotrophomonas maltiphilia, Alcaligenes xylosoxidans, and certain Ralstonia* species.
- The consequences of many of these infections are unknown.
- The bacteria are often environmental pathogens that show multidrug resistance.

- In the absence of symptoms, it is reasonable to carry out repeat cultures over a period of 3–6 months. Many of these infections will be transient and, in the absence of symptoms, do not usually require treatment.
- They may have more significance in patients undergoing lung transplantation and advice should be sought from the transplant centre.

Intravenous antibiotics

- IV antibiotics are indicated in CF for:
  - respiratory exacerbations not responding to oral antibiotics;
  - part of *P. aeruginosa* eradication protocol;
  - some children with persistent symptoms who seem to benefit from regular 3-monthly IV treatment, usually those who have previously required 2–3 courses of IV antibiotics per year on clinical grounds.
- IV antibiotic regimes should always use a combination of 2 antibiotics to avoid development of resistance.
- Usually airway cultures will have grown *P. aeruginosa*, but even if they have not it is sensible to cover this organism.
- Although antibiotic sensitivities can be helpful, first-line IV therapy is nearly always a combination of:
  - an aminoglycoside and an antipseudomonal cephalosporin (such as ceftazidime) *or*
  - an aminoglycoside and anti-pseudomonal penicillin (such as ticarcillin/clavulanic acid).
- Aminoglycosides in CF need to be given in high dose to be effective. Once daily regimes can be used and are often more convenient.
- IV courses are for a minimum of 2 weeks and may be extended if symptoms do not improve.
- Special attention should be paid to chest physiotherapy to maximize the benefit of the IV treatment.
- IV antibiotics can be given successfully at home by family members, either via a peripheral long line or using a portacath device.

Prophylactic antibiotics

- Children treated with prophylactic oral flucloxacillin for the first 2 years of life have fewer infective exacerbations and may have slightly improved lung function. It is important to test for *P. aeruginosa* every 3–4 months and to treat it aggressively if detected. It is reasonable to continue with flucloxacillin beyond 2 years of age if airway cultures have grown *S. aureus* repeatedly.
- Children with chronic *P. aeruginosa* infection should be treated with continuous nebulized antibiotics. Since these are given after the infection has occurred they are not strictly prophylactic, but are given to prevent, as much as possible, further lung damage. The choice of antibiotic lies between Colomycin® and Tobi®. The evidence base for Tobi® is better, but it is more expensive.

- There are 3 RCTs that show that azithromycin given 3 times per week can improve lung function and decrease the number of infective exacerbations in children and adults with moderate lung disease and chronic *P. aeruginosa* infection.[1,2,3] Azithromycin may have antiinflammatory as well as antibiotic activity. As mentioned above (see 🕮 p. 140), children on long-term macrolides should be screened for non-tuberculous mycobacterial infection before azithromycin is started and at least annually thereafter.

Infection control

- Most strains of *P. aeruginosa* that infect the airways of children with CF are acquired from the environment.
- Patient to patient spread has been well documented. For most strains it requires prolonged close contact, e.g. sharing a room during inpatient care.
- For most strains transmission requires either large droplet spread or direct contact with infected secretions. Large droplet spread does not extend more than a few feet from the source.
- Some strains of *P. aeruginosa* are highly transmissible.
- *B. cepacia* is more likely to be transmissible than *P. aeruginosa* and the consequences of infection are more serious.

For these reasons it is important to minimize the chances of patient to patient spread.

- Good hygiene is essential: hand washing; use of well ventilated rooms; cleaning of surfaces and equipment after each use.
- Regular assessments of the number of positive airway cultures in the CF clinic population to determine if there is an unexpected increase, suggesting the presence of a transmissible strain.
- 6 monthly typing of *P. aeruginosa* strains to assess for any evidence of 2 or more patients sharing the same strain, which might suggest transmission.
- Segregation of patients infected with transmissible strains of *P. aeruginosa*.
- Segregation of patients infected with any strain of *B. cepacia*.
- Some centres also advocate segregating *P. aeruginosa* positive from *P. aeruginosa* negative patients. Whilst this has some merit it raises difficulties in knowing when to transfer a patient from one clinic to another. Furthermore, since most children infected with *P. aeruginosa* will have their own unique strain, they are at as much risk of being infected by children with other strains of *P. aeruginosa* as children who are *P. aeruginosa* negative.

1 Equi A. Balfour-Lynn IM, Bus A, Rosenthal M. Long term azithromycin in children with cystic fibrosis: a randomised, placebo-controlled crossover trial. *Lancet* 2002; **360**: 978–84.

2 Saiman L, Marsall BC, Mayer-Hamblett N, Burns JL, Quittner AL, Cibene DA, Coquilltte S, Fieberg AY, Accurso FJ, Campbell PW 3rd; Macrolide Study Group, Azithromycin in patients with cystic fibrosis chronically infected with Pseudomonas aeruginosa: a randomized controlled trial. *JAMA*. 2003; **290**: 1749–56.

3 Wolter J, Seeney S, Bell S, Bowler S, Masel P, McCormack J. Effect of long term treatment with azithromycin on disease parameters in cystic fibrosis: a randomised trial. *Thorax*. 2002; **57**: 212–6.

- If segregation is to be carried out, best practice is for each patient to be segregated from every other patient. This is easier said than done. It requires that children with CF do not occupy the same room at the same time (this includes the waiting area), and that the clinic rooms and physiotherapy rooms are left unoccupied for a period of 30min between CF patients.
- Children with CF should not mix socially with other children or adults with the disease.
- Children with CF needing inpatient care should be isolated from other children with CF.

Complications

Allergic bronchopulmonary aspergillosis

Aspergillus fumigatus is a fungus found in the airway secretions of about 30% of children with CF. In most instances it is not thought to be a significant pathogen. 1–10% of children with CF can develop a vigorous allergic immune response to *Aspergillus*. This can cause deterioration in lung function and progression of bronchiectasis. ABPA can be difficult to diagnose with certainty, but should be considered in cases of:
• new or worsening wheeze;
• increased cough productive of brown sputum;
• new infiltrates on CXR (Fig. 15.1);
• unexplained fall in lung function.

Investigations that support the diagnosis are:
• serum total IgE > 500iu/L or a rapid 4-fold rise;
• presence of IgG precipitins to *Aspergillus*;
• *Aspergillus*-specific IgE;
• eosinophil count > 0.5×10^9/L.

It is hard to be precise about the number of criteria needed to make the diagnosis. If there is a clinical suspicion, a trial of prednisolone is worthwhile. An improvement in symptoms and/or radiological signs with a fall in total IgE would be consistent with the diagnosis. Rarely, ABPA may be associated with infection with *A. niger*. This may affect the results of the specific IgE and IgG precipitins, which are usually specific for *A. fumigatus*.

Treatment
• Corticosteroids. Prednisolone (non-enteric coated is needed in CF to get adequate absorption) at 1mg/kg per day for 2 weeks. If there has been clinical improvement, the steroid dose can be reduced to 0.5mg/kg per day for a further 2 weeks, then weaned further to alternate day treatment. After 8 weeks treatment, repeat clinical assessment, CXR, and IgE. A fall in total IgE of 35% suggests remission. The dose can then be weaned over the next 2–4 months. Inhaled steroids have not been shown to be effective in treating ABPA.
• Itraconazole. This can either be used from the onset, or added after 2 weeks if there has been a poor response. The use of itraconazole oral solution formulation is preferred in patients with CF, as higher itraconazole blood concentrations are achieved than with the capsule formulation. The absorption of the solution is more rapid in the fasting state. Itraconazole needs an acid environment to be absorbed and, in children taking antacids, this may be achieved by using citrus drinks or cola to take the itraconazole. Itraconazole can cause liver dysfunction and this needs to be monitored.
• In children with severe or recurrent ABPA not responding to steroids and itraconazole, other treatments with oral voriconazole, nebulized amphotericin, and high dose inhaled steroids should be considered. There are case reports of benefits of pulsed methylprednisolone for resistant or recurrent ABPA. Despite apparently good oral bioavailability, serum levels of voriconazole may be subtherapeutic in children

with CF. Where there is poor response to treatment, particularly if *Aspergillus* continues to grow on sputum samples, it is worth checking serum voriconazole levels and adjusting the dose if necessary. Rarely, IV therapy is required.

- Children with CF should avoid environments with high spore counts such as stables and other places with rotting vegetation. *Aspergillus* species are also found in pepper and other dry spices.

Children on long-term prednisolone should be:
- monitored for:
  - glucose intolerance (urine dipstick);
  - high blood pressure;
  - subcapsular cataract formation;
  - poor growth (minimized on alternate day regime, dose taken in the morning.
- Warned of the increased risk of infection. Children who have not had an obvious episode of chicken pox should have their varicella zoster titres measured. If these are not protective give appropriate advice should they come into contact with chicken pox.

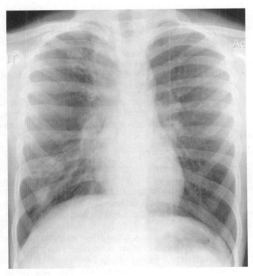

Fig 15.1 CXR of a 10-year-old boy with CF whose lung function had fallen from an FEV1 of 95% predicted to an FEV_1 of 80% predicted. He had a dry cough but was otherwise asymptomatic. The CXR shows new opacification in the right lower zone. His total IgE was 3000 and his sputum grew *Aspergillus fumigatus*. His lung function recovered after 6 weeks of prednisolone and itraconazole.

Arthritis

Joint pain affects 5–10% of older children with CF. There are 2 patterns of disease.

CF-associated arthritis

- Affects the large joints: ankle; knee; hip; elbow; shoulder.
- Usually lasts less than 7 days.
- Can be disabling—some children may find difficulty in walking.
- Can be associated with a rash and fever.
- Can be associated with pulmonary exacerbations.
- May be caused by circulating immune complexes.
- Is more likely in children with more severe pulmonary disease.
- Is self-limiting and very rarely associated with radiographic changes or with joint erosion.
- May be recurrent.

This form of joint pain usually responds to NSAIDs. Occasionally a short course of prednisolone may be needed.

Hypertrophic osteoarthropathy

- Part of the same process that causes clubbing.
- Usually occurs in young adults with an insidious onset.
- Can cause swelling and tenderness at the end of long bones.
- Can cause joint swelling with effusion: usually wrist, knees, or ankles.
- Is usually symmetrical.
- May flare up with pulmonary exacerbations.
- May be associated with radiographic changes—periosteal elevation with layers of new bone formation

Symptomatic treatment with NSAIDs may be sufficient. Occasionally prednisolone with or without steroid-sparing drugs such as methotrexate or azathioprine may be needed. Clubbing and hypertrophic osteoarthropathy can regress after lung transplantation.

CF-related diabetes (CFRD)

- CFRD or impaired glucose tolerance occurs in 5–10% of children with CF.
- The prevalence increases significantly with age; 50% of patients will develop CFRD by 30 years of age. The median age of onset is 21 years.
- Use of oral corticosteroids will increase the tendency to develop impaired glucose tolerance, but this may be reversible when the steroids are stopped.
- Onset of CFRD is often insidious. It can cause weight loss, fatigue, and poor appetite. Polyuria, nocturia, and polydypsia are uncommon.
- CFRD can be associated with loss of lung function, which appears to be independent of weight loss and general ill-health. Lung function can be improved by treating CFRD.

- CFRD can be detected using the oral glucose tolerance test (OGTT). 1.75g/kg glucose (maximum 75g) is taken orally. Blood glucose is measured 2 hours later. A level under 7.8mmol/L is normal, 7.8–11mmol/L is impaired glucose tolerance, and > 11.1mmol/L is diabetic.
- Home monitoring may be a more sensitive method of detecting CFRD. Home monitoring can be carried out over 3 days, with blood glucose measurements taken before and after meals.
- HbA1c is not reliable as it may give false negative results.
- All children over 12 years should have an annual assessment of glucose tolerance, either by home monitoring or an OGTT.
- Patients with CFRD are at risk of all the microvascular complications of diabetes.
- Ketoacidosis can occur, but it is rare in children with CFRD because of residual insulin production. If it occurs it should be managed according to normal diabetes protocols.
- Diet in CFRD is different from that in regular type I diabetes. The opinion of an experienced dietitian should be sought. In general, the CF diet remains unchanged and insulin therapy is adjusted to compensate. Sugary drinks should be avoided
- Insulin therapy is the treatment of choice for CFRD. Oral hypoglycaemic agents are generally ineffective.
- A basal bolus regime gives the best flexibility to cope with the CF diet.
- Blood sugar levels should be monitored at home, ideally 4 times per day, although this is seldom achieved in practice. Monitoring should be more intensive during periods of illness or steroid use when insulin requirements may increase.
- Children with CFRD should have annual monitoring for retinal disease, blood pressure, microalbuminuria, and renal function.

CF-related liver disease

- Neonatal cholestasis affects 2–5% of infants with CF. It can cause prolonged jaundice, which needs to be investigated in the usual way. Cholestasis due to CF resolves spontaneously. It is essential that these infants receive a parenteral dose of vitamin K.
- Transient elevation of serum transaminases is common (about 30% of children), with or without changes in liver texture or ultrasound or an enlarged liver clinically.
- Ursodeoxycholic acid is a bile salt that can improve bile flow. It may affect the natural history of CF liver disease, although this has not been shown. One suggestion is that it should be started in children who have either 2 liver abnormalities (ultrasound, transaminases, or palpable liver) or one abnormality in 2 consecutive years. Ursodeoxycholic acid treatment does usually lower transaminase levels.

- Gall stones are found in around 5% of children with CF. Asymptomatic stones should be treated with ursodeoxycholic acid.
- Cirrhosis affects 2–5% of children. The consequences of associated portal hypertension—hypersplenism, varices, and ascites—are more common than synthetic liver failure.
- Regular oral vitamin K should be given to all children with liver disease.
- NSAIDs should be avoided in children with portal hypertension to reduce the risk of gastrointestinal haemorrhage (see box).
- There is no evidence that screening endoscopy for identification and treatment of asymptomatic oesophageal or gastric varices affects risk of bleeding in children with CF-related liver disease.
- Liver transplantation should be considered in children with hepatocellular failure or uncontrolled portal hypertension with recurrent variceal bleeding. Following liver transplantation some patients have improvement in their lung function. To be able to cope with the stress of liver transplantation, the child's FEV1 must be 65% or better. In children with more severe lung disease a combined lung and liver transplant may give a better outcome.

Emergency treatment of GI haemorrhage

- Haematemesis is most often due to bleeding oesophageal or gastric varices. Melaena follows but may be delayed for up to 24h.
- Primary treatment is to maintain circulating volume, initially with crystalloid and then with packed red blood cell transfusion.
- Give vitamin K (2–5mg slow IV) and 10–20mL/kg fresh frozen plasma
- Give IV ranitidine to reduce any acid-related bleeding.
- Pass an NG tube. This can be used to assess ongoing bleeding.
- If conscious level is diminished, consider intubation to protect the airway.
- Vasopressin may help persistent bleeding. Discuss urgently with local liver unit.
- Most episodes will settle spontaneously. If bleeding persists, urgent endoscopy and variceal sclerosis or banding may be needed.
- The high protein content of the blood meal that results from variceal bleeding may precipitate an encephalopathy. The severity can be reduced by giving lactulose or macrogols to clear the bowel more rapidly and metronidazole to decrease the numbers of ammonia-producing colonic bacteria.
- Once varices have bled, a programme of endoscopic treatments should be arranged in consultation with the nearest paediatric liver unit.

Delayed puberty

- Puberty is often delayed in boys and girls with CF.
- Average delay is around 2 years.
- Chronic illness and poor nutrition are important, but delay can still occur in well-nourished children with apparently mild disease.
- Delayed puberty can have important psychological effects and provide a further reminder to the child that they are different from their peers.
- Puberty is a time when bone density increases as a result of the action of sex steroids. Delayed puberty may adversely affect this process leading to poorly mineralized bones with increased risk of fractures.
- If there are no signs of the onset of puberty by age 13 years in girls or 14 years in boys, consider treatment with sex steroids (ethinyloestradiol for girls, testosterone for boys) in conjunction with a paediatric endocrinologist.

Distal intestinal obstruction syndrome (DIOS)

- This condition, previously known as 'meconium ileus equivalent', is characterized by partial or complete obstruction of the distal ileum. It affects around 10% of children with CF.
- Its cause is not understood but may be related to slow intestinal transit time associated with persistent steatorrhoea.
- Symptoms may be acute or chronic.
- Most often there is colicky abdominal pain, which may be brought on by eating.
- Examination reveals a palpable mass in the right lower quadrant.
- In the acute form there may be abdominal distension and vomiting.
- Important differential diagnoses include:
  - obstruction from adhesions in children who have had previous laparotomy;
  - appendicitis;
  - intussusception;
  - volvulus;
  - constipation.
- Abdominal radiograph shows fecal material with a bubbly or granular appearance in the right flank.

Management of DIOS

Outpatient management of chronic low grade symptoms can be effective using oral macrogols, such as Movicol, twice daily. Acute DIOS can also be managed with oral or more usually nasogastric macrogols such as Klean-Prep, provided there is no evidence of complete obstruction. The following protocol can be used.

- An IV line should be sited so that IV fluids can be given if dehydration occurs.
- If at any stage of the lavage there are signs of complete obstruction (increasing vomiting especially bile-stained vomiting or worsening abdominal distension), the lavage should be stopped and the NG tube left on drainage. Consider repeat AXR and seek a surgical opinion.
- Start early in the morning and continue until the stools are yellow, watery, and free of solid matter.
- 3 litres is usually enough, although more may be needed in larger children. See Table 15.1.
- Children can have clear fluids to drink, but no solids.
- If success is not achieved in 12h, stop, give a light evening meal, and resume the following morning. Electrolyte disturbance is rare and it is not usually necessary to check blood electrolyte levels.

Caution

- If there are fluid levels on plain abdominal radiograph, do not use bowel lavage.
- If there is persistent vomiting, stop the bowel lavage.
- Consider other possible causes, especially adhesions.
- If DIOS is still most likely, then gastrograffin enemas may be helpful. Gastrograffin is hypertonic and by drawing water into the bowel can help dislodge inspissated material.
- To be successful, the gastrograffin must penetrate the obstructing fecal material.
- Significant fluid shifts can occur. IV access should be established before using gastrograffin. Monitor for electrolyte disturbance and hypovolaemia.
- Always inform the surgical team before using gastrograffin enemas.

Table 15.1 Volumes of bowel lavage

	Body weight		
	< 15kg	15–30kg	> 30kg
1st hour	50mL/h	100mL/h	200mL/h
2nd hour	100mL/h	200mL/h	400mL/h
Thereafter	200mL/h	400mL/h	600mL/h

Electrolyte disturbance

- The commonest problem results from excess sodium loss through sweat with secondary hyperaldosteronism.
  - Infants are most at risk, but any age group can be affected, particularly in hot weather.
  - Typical history will be one of listlessness and poor weight gain.
  - Occasionally, especially during prolonged hot weather, there may be an acute illness with signs of dehydration and hypovolaemia.
  - Serum sodium will often be in the lower end of the normal range or a little lower; serum potassium will be low. There will often be associated hypochloraemia and metabolic alkalosis.
  - Urinary sodium will be low and urinary potassium will be high.
  - This combination of electrolyte disturbance is sometimes called pseudo-Bartter's syndrome.
  - Treatment requires sodium and potassium replacement. In infants this may need to be continued for several weeks. A common mistake is to replace potassium without sodium. This fails to correct the problem and the potassium is quickly lost in the urine.
- The other likely cause of electrolyte disturbance is aminoglycoside-induced nephrotoxicity.
- Many children with CF are exposed to recurrent courses of aminoglycosides. Even with careful monitoring of drug levels, some will develop renal injury. This can result in a decrease in the glomerular filtration rate. It can also affect renal tubular re-absorption of electrolytes.
- Typically these children will have hypokalaemia, hypocalcaemia, and hypomagnesaemia and high losses of sodium, potassium, and magnesium in the urine. Occasionally, this is severe enough to cause tetany.
- Treatment is with oral replacement, and is usually required long term. Further use of aminoglycosides needs to be carefully considered.

Haemoptysis

- Haemoptysis can either represent minor mucosal injury due to inflammation and coughing or arterial bleeding from eroded bronchial arteries.
- Mucosal injury will cause streaks of blood within expectorated sputum. It is not a cause for alarm. It usually occurs during an infective exacerbation and the exacerbation should be treated in the usual way.
- Bronchial artery bleeding results in varying volumes of frank haemoptysis. Often the child will feel a bubbling sensation in the chest before coughing up the blood and this may help localize the site of bleeding.
- Bronchial artery bleeding occurs in around 1% of older children with CF per year.
- Bronchial artery erosion occurs in children with moderate to severe lung disease. The bronchial arteries become enlarged and tortuous and can erode through the bronchial walls
- Most episodes will resolve spontaneously. More rarely they can become massive, with a risk of exsanguination, or persistence over several days.
- Massive haemoptysis is associated with an increased 2 year mortality and loss of lung function.

Management of frank haemoptysis

- Admit to hospital.
- Site a secure IV cannula (2 if major haemoptysis) and cross-match 2 units of blood.
- Volume resuscitate if necessary. This is very rarely required.
- Check clotting, FBC, and electrolytes.
- Give IV vitamin K.
- Start IV antibiotics for presumed chest exacerbation.
- Review medication and stop any that interfere with clotting, such as NSAIDs and ticarcillin.
- Positioning for chest physiotherapy can precipitate a bleed and physiotherapy should be confined to simple huffing manoeuvres until major bleeding has settled.
- DNAase can be continued.
- If the bleeding persists, blood transfusion may be needed. Recheck the clotting and give fresh frozen plasma if it is deranged.
- Anecdotal evidence suggests that antifibrinolytic drugs such as tranexamic acid can be beneficial in preventing re-bleeding.
- In most cases the bleeding will settle spontaneously.
- In cases where bleeding is massive or prolonged over several days, bronchial artery embolization should be considered. It is often impossible to localize the site of bleeding and in practice all abnormal tortuous bronchial arteries should be embolized. The procedure can take several hours, and sometimes needs to be carried out on successive days. There is a risk of spinal artery embolization. There is also a risk of massive bleeding during induction of anaesthesia.
- Bronchial artery embolization has a very high (> 90%) immediate success rate in stopping the bleeding.
- After bronchial artery embolization there may be pleural and oesophageal pain and dysphagia due to altered blood supply to these structures.
- Re-bleeding after bronchial artery embolization occurs in 40% of patients within 5 years.
- Very rarely, emergency lobectomy may be required. The site of bleeding must have been unequivocally demonstrated.

Nasal polyps

- Nasal polyps occur in 10% of children with CF.
- There may be associated sinusitis.
- The polyps cause nasal obstruction and, more rarely persistent nasal discharge or postnasal drip with constant throat clearing.
- They can be bilateral.
- Nasal steroids are usually effective, using drops initially if nasal obstruction is complete and changing to maintenance treatment with an aerosol spray.
- Surgery will give immediate relief of obstruction but regrowth of the polyps is common.

Osteoporosis and CF-related low bone mineral density

- The relationship between bone mineral density (BMD) and fracture risk has not been established in CF, and the term CF-related low BMD is preferred, unless there have been fragility fractures in which case the term osteoporosis should be used.
- Measurements of bone density using dual energy X-ray absorptiometry (DEXA) scans in most children with CF are not different from those in normal controls, except in those treated with long-term oral steroids.
- Significantly reduced BMD is seen in around 30% of adults with CF. The incidence of fragility fractures is not known, but is clearly increased in this group. Typical fractures are rib fractures and crush fractures of the vertebrae.
- Pain from rib fractures reduces effectiveness of airway clearance techniques. Affected patients will need hospital admission for treatment.
    - CXR to exclude pneumothorax as the cause of pain.
    - Adequate analgesia, starting with nonsteroidal agents, but including nerve blocks and opiate infusions if necessary. SC calcitonin has been reported to give rapid pain relief in some patients with rib fractures.
    - IV antibiotics should be started to minimize the effects of any infective exacerbations.
    - If DNAase is not being used it should be started to aid sputum clearance whilst the fracture heals.
    - Percussion techniques may not be possible and vigorous percussion should in any case be used with caution in patients at risk of fracture. Other physiotherapy techniques, including PEP mask, vibrating jackets, or breathing and huffing techniques, should be used.
- Risk factors for low bone mineral density are:
    - low BMI;
    - delayed puberty;
    - CF-related diabetes;
    - CF-related liver disease;
    - corticosteroid use;
    - low levels of physical activity (often a result of poor lung function).
- 40% of adult bone mass is accumulated during the pubertal growth spurt, and inadequate mass cannot be made up later.
- Good nutrition throughout childhood is the best preventive treatment, combined with adequate vitamin D supplements.

- Regular exercise may also be protective. Exercise capacity and BMI are strong predictors of bone mineral density.
- Vitamin D levels can be measured at annual review, and it seems reasonable to aim for a 25-hydroxyvitamin D level in the upper part of the normal range (aim for 75–150nmol/L).
- Vitamin K also plays a role in bone metabolism. Although there are no long-term outcome data, some CF centres now recommend routine replacement with daily oral vitamin K in older children with CF to promote stronger bone growth.
- There may be a role for carrying out DEXA scans in all children with CF at 10 years of age and then every 1–3 years thereafter to identify children at risk of developing low bone mineral density. Special attention can then be directed towards these children to ensure adequate calcium intake, adequate vitamin D and K supplementation, and possibly a programme of weight-bearing physical activity. Any delayed puberty should also be treated.
- Bisphosphonate treatment is recommended in adults with CF who have had fragility fractures, or who have very low DEXA scores or medium low scores in patients who are starting a long course of oral corticosteroids. The role of bisphosphonates is children is less clear, and in most centres is currently limited to those with fragility fractures.

Pneumothorax

- Pneumothorax is a serious and potentially life-threatening complication of CF. It occurs in about 1% of older children with CF each year.
- It is more likely in children with more severe lung disease (FEV_1 < 40%).
- Recurrence is common (about 50%) on both the ipsilateral and contralateral sides.
- Most seem to be caused by ruptured subpleural blebs in the upper lobes.
- Typical symptoms are sudden onset of chest pain and breathlessness. There may be less specific symptoms such as unexplained loss of lung function. A high index of suspicion is needed.
- A CXR is usually sufficient to make the diagnosis, but is not definitive. If there is any doubt, a chest CT scan will be needed.
- Tension pneumothorax can occur without complete collapse of the lung because of the abnormal stiffness of the CF lung.
- All children with CF who have a pneumothorax should be admitted to hospital, even if the pneumothorax is small and symptoms are minor.
- 10–30% of small pneumothoraces (< 20% of hemithorax) will resolve spontaneously.
- For larger or symptomatic pneumothoraces, a chest drain should be placed and suction applied. A small (10–14F) pigtail drain is usually sufficient. It is essential that the lung fully re-inflates after placing the drain, so that the visceral and parietal pleura come into contact. If the pneumothorax remains after the chest drain has been sited, the leak is unlikely to heal spontaneously and the possibility of re-siting the drain or placing a second drain should be considered. Most air leaks arise from the upper lobes, and placing the drain at the 2nd intercostal space in the midclavicular line may be most successful at fully-reinflating the lung.

- PEP physiotherapy should be avoided.
- Sputum clearance will be less effective because of chest pain, and IV antibiotics should be started.
- If the pneumothorax fails to resolve after 3 days, thoroscopic surgery, with partial pleurectomy or pleural abrasion, is the most reliable treatment.
- Chemical pleurodesis should be reserved for children who cannot tolerate or who refuse surgery.
- Chemical pleurodesis or surgical treatment of pneumothorax does not significantly alter outcome after lung transplantation, although it does make the surgery more difficult. Previous pleurodesis should not be a barrier to consideration for transplantation.
- Pneumothorax is associated with an increased 2 year mortality at all levels of lung function. It can cause immediate mortality in children with severe lung disease, especially if the drain cannot be removed after 5 days. Despite this, the average age at death of CF patients who had pneumothorax is not different to that of those who did not, which reflects the incidence of pneumothorax in older age groups.

Rectal prolapse

- Rectal prolapse is usually a problem in young children with CF.
- It can be a presenting feature of CF.
- There is usually a history of a red swelling visible only during defecation. Occasionally the parent may need to reduce the prolapse manually.
- The cause is not clear, but may be related to the passage of frequent bulky stools.
- It can usually be treated conservatively by ensuring adequate pancreatic enzyme supplementation and using a mild osmotic laxative, such as lactulose, to prevent the child straining at stool.
- Occasionally rectal prolapse does not respond to conservative treatment. In these children it is important to inspect the anus and rectum endo-scopically to exclude other problems such as rectal polyps or mucosal inflammation. If necessary, rectal prolapse can be treated surgically, e.g. by injection sclerotherapy.

Stress incontinence

- Regular urinary incontinence—more than 2 episodes per month—is reported by 25% of adult women with CF.
- Stress incontinence also occurs in adolescent girls with CF and in a smaller proportion of adolescent boys.
- Stresses that can lead to incontinence include coughing, laughing, and physical activity.
- Frequent stress incontinence can lead to poor compliance with physiotherapy and cough suppression.
- Pelvic floor exercises can help control this distressing symptom.

Respiratory failure
- Lung disease in most patients with CF will eventually result in respiratory failure.
- This is likely to occur once the FEV1 falls below 30%.
- There will be poor exercise tolerance with breathlessness either at rest or brought on by minimal activity.
- Mild to moderate hypoxia will occur. As with most lung disease, this will first be evident during sleep and overnight saturation studies should be carried out 6 monthly in patients with severe lung disease (FEV_1 < 50%). Supplemental oxygen should be used if night-time saturations are below 90% for more than 5% of the night.
- Right heart failure may occur resulting in fluid retention and hepatic tenderness.
- Discussions with the family about transplantation and end of life issues should be undertaken when the child still has relatively stable disease.
- In children with end-stage disease, non-invasive ventilation can be used to improve quality of life and, in some cases, to prolong life whilst waiting for a transplant.
- Intubation and ventilation for end-stage disease is in most cases fruitless. The child will almost certainly die on the ventilator before a lung donor is found. Death on the ICU is usually more difficult to cope with for the family than death in the ward or at home.

Lung transplantation

- Lung transplantation can be a successful treatment for children with end-stage lung disease.
- The 1 year survival is 80–90%, the 5 year survival is 50–75%, and the 10 year survival is around 40%.
- The 1 month mortality is 5–20%
- Two techniques can be used, heart–lung or bilateral sequential lung (BSLT) transplantation. The choice of operation varies between surgeons, centres, and countries. Most centres favour.
- About 30–50% of children listed for transplantation will die on the waiting list.
- Waiting for a transplant is an extremely stressful period for child and family. A pager must be carried at all times, and there may be false alarms.

When to refer for transplant assessment

Timing is important. If referral is left too late, the child will be in a poor state to deal with the transplant and has a higher chance of dying on the waiting list. If the family and child are positive about transplantation, early referral is preferable. The child may not be listed after the first visit, but there will be time to address some of the issues that may arise, such as optimizing nutrition and treating any persistent infections. Most centres agree that, when transplantation is an option and the child and family are committed to the procedure, it should be carried out when the median survival is estimated to be 2 years. Usual criteria are as follows.
- $FEV_1 < 30\%$ predicted.
- Requirement for 24h/day oxygen.
- Impaired quality of life:
  - unable to attend school/work;
  - poor exercise tolerance.

Contraindications for transplantation

These vary from centre to centre, but often include:
- other organ failure;
- untreated *Mycobacteria tuberculosis* infection;
- untreated *Mycobacteria abscessus* infection;
- invasive pulmonary aspergillosis;
- some non-pulmonary infections such as hepatitis β or C, HIV;
- malignancy;
- child does not want the procedure.

Other important factors that may affect the success of the transplant procedure are the following.
- Previous thoracic surgery. Pleurodesis will make the procedure more difficult.
- The presence of multiresistant organisms, e.g. *B. cepacia*, MRSA, panresistant *P. aeruginosa*.
- Chronic infection with NBM. Post-transplantation invasive disease may occur even on treatment and may contribute to post-transplant mortality.
- Severe osteoporosis.

- Poor psychosocial/family support.
- Non-adherence to current treatment. This is strongly correlated with non-adherence after transplantation.
- Long-term high dose steroid use (> 5mg/day) significantly increases the risk of wound dehiscence.

Complications

Surgical
- Stenosis or dehiscence of bronchial anastomosis.
- Wound infection or breakdown.
- Phrenic nerve injury.
- Thoracic empyema.
- Pericardial effusion.

Infection
- Infections are the major cause of morbidity following transplantation.
- Organisms that infected the lungs and sinuses of children before transplantation frequently occur after transplantation in the donor lungs. It is essential to treat all such infections as aggressively as possible before transplantation. This includes infection with *Mycobacteria* and fungi, including *Fusarium*, *Scedosporium*, and *Aspergillus* species.
- Opportunistic infection with CMV and *Pneumocystis carinii*.
- *Clostridium difficile* toxin colitis.

Organ rejection
Lung function in the first month is often relatively low (50–60% predicted), but increases steadily over the first 12 months. Mean values for FEV_1 1 year after transplant should be > 80% predicted. Lung function can be affected by both acute and chronic rejection (as well as infection).

Acute rejection
- Most patients develop at least one episode of rejection, usually within the first 3 weeks following transplantation.
- Symptoms can include dyspnoea, fever, and hypoxia.
- Mild rejection can be asymptomatic.
- Pulmonary function testing may show a decrease in FEV_1 and VC.
- CXR is normal in about half of cases, but may show non-specific changes.
- Transbronchial biopsy is usually performed to establish the diagnosis and exclude infection.
- There is often a dramatic response to treatment with corticosteroids and increased immunosuppression is observed within 24h. Any CXR changes due to rejection should clear within 48h.

Chronic rejection
- Chronic rejection, usually in the form of obliterative bronchiolitis, is the major obstacle to long-term survival following lung transplantation.
- It affects 50–80% of patients by 5 years post-transplantation.
- Obliterative bronchiolitis has a variable course t may plateau or progress gradually or in a stepwise fashion.
- Symptoms are usually caused by airflow obstruction: breathlessness and wheeze. There may be a low grade fever.

- Lung function testing shows an obstructive pattern with a fall in FEV_1 that is not responsive to bronchodilators.
- The diagnosis is usually made clinically without lung biopsy.
- Acute rejection episodes are a risk factor for subsequent obliterative bronchiolitis and some centres carry out surveillance transbronchial biopsies to allow treatment of asymptomatic acute rejection.
- CMV infection also seems to be a risk factor. Using prophylactic ganciclovir in the immediate post-transplant period may be helpful.
- Treatment for established obliterative bronchiolitis is difficult and nothing is particularly effective. Most attempted treatments involve increasing or changing immunosuppressive drugs.

Other medical complications
- Diabetes.
- Chronic renal failure.
- Hypertension.
- Seizures.

Annual review

The development of CF treatment centres where there is a concentration of medical nursing and allied health professionals with expertise in looking after children with CF has been associated with improved outcomes in this disease. The usual pattern of care is one of close liaison between local centres near to where the child lives and a regional CF centre. Each child is seen once a year at the CF centre for an annual review. Children with difficult problems may be seen more frequently. Annual assessment typically includes the following.

- Physiotherapy review by experienced physiotherapist: observation and adjustment of physiotherapy technique with suggestion of different age-appropriate techniques, assessment of exercise tolerance (e.g. shuttle test).
- Dietary review: assessment of diet (e.g. using a 3 day food diary), advice on selecting food types and use of pancreatic enzymes and vitamins. Provision of supplements if necessary.
- CF nurse specialist: time available to give advice on dealing with day to day issues of care.
- Social worker: time available to give advice on benefits and coping strategies.
- Psychologist: time available to discuss concerns or anxieties about looking after a child with a chronic illness.
- Medical review with paediatrician with a special interest in CF. Should cover all aspects of care including:
  - assessment of growth: height, weight, and ht/wt% or BMI;
  - school attendance;
  - exercise tolerance;
  - nature and frequency of any cough, sputum, and wheeze;
  - nature and frequency of bowel habit and any abdominal pain;
  - number of chest exacerbations;
  - antibiotic use and use of other medications;
  - assessment of adherence with therapy;
  - full physical examination;
  - discussion of progress and any concerns of child or family.
- Lung function:
  - FEV_1, FVC, RV, RV/TLC ratio.
- Sputum or cough swab culture. Microbiology lab need to have protocols for setting up the necessary selective media for CF pathogens.
- Blood investigations:
  - FBC, renal function; liver function; HbA1c; clotting; vitamin A, E, and D levels; total IgE; Aspergillus precipitins; and specific IgE.
- Assessment for CFRD in children over 12 years—either by glucose tolerance test or 3 day blood sugar monitoring.
- Radiology:
  - CXR;
  - abdominal ultrasound (assessment of liver, spleen, and portal vein).

Data from the CF clinic visit should be submitted to the national CF registry—after taking consent from the child and family.

Further information

Green, A. and Kirk, J. (2007). Guidelines development Group. Guidelines for the performance of the sweat test for the diagnosis of cystic fibrosis. *Ann. Clin. Biochem.* **44**, 25–34.

Esther, C.R.Jr, Henry, M.M., Molina, P.L., and Leigh, M.W. (2005) Nontuberculous mycobacterial nfection in young children with cystic fibrosis. *Pediatr. Pulmonol.* **40**, 39–44.

Ravzi, S. and Saiman, L. (2007). Nontuberculous mycobacteria in cystic fibrosis. *Pediatr. Infect. Dis. J.* **26**, 263–4.

Cystic Fibrosis Trust consensus documents are written by UK experts on cystic fibrosis. The following are the current documents. All documents are available as pdf files at the CF Trust website: www.cftrust.org.uk.

Bone mineralisation in cystic fibrosis. February 2007.

The Burkholderia cepacia complex—suggestions for prevention and infection control, 2nd edn., September 2004.

Standards of care—standards for the clinical care of children and adults with cystic fibrosis in the UK 2001. May 2001.

Pseudomonas aeruginosa infection in people with cystic fibrosis. Suggestions for prevention and infection control, 2nd edn. November 2004.

National consensus standards for the nursing management of cystic fibrosis. May 2001.

Clinical guidelines for the physiotherapy management of cystic fibrosis. January 2002.

Nutritional management of cystic fibrosis. April 2002.

Antibiotic treatment for cystic fibrosis, 2nd edition. September 2002.

Addendum for antibiotic treatment for cystic fibrosis, 2nd edn. 2002.

Management of cystic fibrosis-related diabetes mellitus. June 2004.

Respiratory pathogens

Introduction

It is sometimes a little daunting to try and keep a full list of possible respiratory pathogens in mind when faced with a child with an acute respiratory illness, particularly when a rational approach to investigation is needed. This section provides a framework of most of the common and less common pathogens that can cause respiratory tract infection (including infection of the pharynx and larynx) in children.

Viruses

A large range of viruses can cause respiratory tract disease. They can usefully be divided according to their families. Several of the specific infections are considered in 📖 Chapter 19. For others there are short notes about the type of respiratory disease they can cause.

Paramyxoviridae

Enveloped single-stranded negative-sense RNA viruses, including:
- parainfluenza viruses 1 to 4;
- respiratory syncytial virus;
- measles virus;
- human metapneumovirus.

All these viruses can cause coryzal illness, bronchiolitis, and pneumonia. Parainfluenza viruses also cause croup.

Orthomyxoviridae

Enveloped single-stranded negative-sense RNA viruses, including influenza A, B, and C.

Herpesviridae

Enveloped double-stranded DNA viruses, including the following.
- Cytomegalovirus.
- Varicella zoster virus.
- Herpes simplex virus: can cause pneumonia in immunocompromised hosts, either during primary infection or reactivation. Pneumonia may occur during viraemia or as direct spread of oral lesions into the airway. Mortality is high despite treatment with aciclovir.
- Epstein–Barr virus: can cause pharyngitis and cervical adenopathy as part of a glandular fever illness and rarely primary EBV pneumonia. In immunodeficient children it can also be associated with lympho-proliferative disease, which can involve the lung.
- Human herpes virus 6: causes erythema subitum (roseola infantum), which can include coryzal symptoms and cervical adenopathy.

Picornaviruses

Non-enveloped single-stranded positive-sense RNA viruses, including the following.

- Enteroviruses. Non-polio enteroviruses are very common causes of infection in children and may cause acute febrile illnesses with coryzal and flu-like symptoms. The incidence of infection peaks in late summer and early autumn and enteroviruses are the most likely cause of 'summer colds'. Specific illnesses include: herpangina; hand, foot, and mouth disease; meningitis; and myocarditis. The following viruses are included in this family:
  - coxsackie viruses;
  - echo viruses;
  - enteroviruses 68–71;
  - polio viruses.
- Rhinovirus. Most common cause of the common cold.

Adenoviridae

Non-enveloped double-stranded DNA viruses, including adenovirus.

Coronaviridae

Enveloped single-stranded positive-sense RNA viruses, including:
- severe acute respiratory syndrome-associated coronavirus (SARS-CoV);
- other coronaviruses can cause coryzal symptoms.

Papovaviridae Non-enveloped double-stranded DNA viruses, including human papilloma virus, which causes laryngeal, tracheal, and bronchial papillomatosis.

Parvoviridae

Enveloped single-stranded DNA viruses.
- Parvovirus B19 causes fifth disease (erythema infectiosum), which does not involve the lungs.
- Human bocavirus: a newly discovered parvovirus that accounts for 1–3% of LRTI in infants.

Bunyaviridae

Enveloped RNA viruses. These include hantaviruses, which are transmitted to humans from rodents and can cause endothelial damage and capillary leak usually resulting in haemorrhagic fever with renal failure. Some strains of hantavirus also cause lung disease characterized by non-cardiogenic pulmonary oedema often with pleural effusions. Hantavirus infection is seen in many parts of the world, but the pulmonary disease appears to be limited to North and South America.

Bacteria

Bacterial pathogens can cause upper and lower respiratory tract disease. The conditions are described in ☐ Chapter 18.

Streptococci
- S. pneumoniae.
- S. pyogenes (group A streptococci).
- Group B strectcocci.
- S. milleri (including S. viridans).

Staphylococci
- S. aureus.

Haemophilus influenzae
- Encapsulated type B (Hib).
- Non-encapsulated—a common cause of bronchial infection.

Klebsiella pneumoniae
Mycoplasma pneumoniae
Chlamydiaceae
- Chlamyophila pneumoniae.
- Chlamyophila psittaci.
- Chlamydia trachomata.

Legionella pneumoniae
Moraxella species
Pseudomonas species
Burkholderia species
- Infection with Burkholderia cepacia complex bacteria is largely confined to patients with cystic fibrosis.
- Burkholderia pseudomallei is the cause of Meliodosis, which is a multiorgan infection seen mainly in South-east Asia and Northern Australia. Meliodosis often first presents with lung disease, which may be an acute pneumonia or more chronic lung disease sometimes resembling tuberculosis. CXR can show a variety of changes including lobar consolidation, pleural effusions, and abscess cavities.

Nocardia species
Nocardia are aerobic, branching filamentous, Gram-positive, weakly acid-fast, soil-associated bacteria that can cause pulmonary infection in immuno-compromised children. There may be acute or more chronic presentation. CXR and CT typically show single multiple nodules, sometimes with cavitation. There may be pleural effusion or empyema. Diagnosis is by microscopy and culture of airways secretions (including BAL fluid). Treatment is with co-trimoxazole.

Actinomyces

Actinomyces are facultative anaerobic Gram-positive bacteria that are commensals of the human oropharynx and GI tract. Pulmonary actinomycosis is very rare and is probably caused by aspiration of oropharyngeal secretions. It is more frequent in patients with HIV, and those on steroids or chemotherapy. It usually presents as a chronic debilitating illness that mimics tuberculosis. There may be soft tissue infection of the head and neck and cavitating lesions may be seen on CXR. Treatment is with penicillin.

Coxiella burneti

Acute Q fever occurs throughout the world, mainly in children. It is transmitted by inhalation or ingestion of infected particles. 3 weeks after inhalation a flu-like illness develops that can include a dry cough and diffuse CXR changes. It is usually a self-limiting illness lasting 2–3 weeks. The possible benefits of giving antibiotics have not been evaluated.

Mycobacterial pathogens

- Mycobacterium tuberculosis.
- Atypical mycobacteria:
  - M. avium-intracellulare complex;
  - M. fortuitum;
  - M. chelonae;
  - M. abscessus;
  - M. kansasii;
  - M. marinum;
  - several others.

Cystic fibrosis-related pathogens

In addition to some of those mentioned above, the following organisms may infect the airways of children with cystic fibrosis:

- Burkholderia cepacia complex;
- Stenotrophomonas maltiphilia;
- Alcaligenes xylosoxidans;
- Ralstonia species.

Fungi

Fungal infection of the lung is unusual in temperate climates and usually indicates underlying immunodeficiency. In the Americas a number of endemic fungal infections can occur. Both types of infection are dealt with in 📖 Chapter 20. Fungi that can cause human infection include the following.

- Pneumocystis jiroveci.
- Candida albicans.
- Aspergillus species.
- Zygomycetes group:
  - Z. rhizopus;
  - Z. mucor.

- *Scedosporium* species.
- *Fusarium solani.*
- *Cryptococcus neoformans.*
- Endemic mycoses:
  - histoplasmosis;
  - coccidioidmycosis;
  - blastomycosis;
  - paracoccidioidomycosis;
  - penicilliosis.

Parasites
- Direct lung disease:
  - *Echinococcus* (hydatid);
  - *Dirofilaria repens* (pulmonary dirofilariasis);
  - *Paragonimus westermani* (paragonimiasis);
  - schistosomiasis.
- Eosinophilic lung disease:
  - *Ascaris*;
  - *Angcylostoma*;
  - *Toxocara*;
  - *Strongyloides*;
  - *Angcylostoma.*

Protozoa
- *Toxoplasma gondii.*
- *Entamoeba histolytica.*

Community-acquired pneumonia

Overview

The term pneumonia means inflammation of the lungs caused by infection. From a histological standpoint it is interchangeable with the term pneumonitis. In clinical practice the term pneumonia is used to describe an illness in a child with fever and respiratory symptoms or signs who has evidence of consolidation on CXR. Where a CXR is not performed and diagnosis is based on symptoms and signs alone, the term acute lower respiratory tract infection is preferred.

Typical and atypical pneumonia

The terms typical pneumonia and atypical pneumonia derive from the late 1800s when it was first realized that pneumonia was caused by a bacterial agent. The first causative bacterium identified was *Streptococcus pneumoniae* and the infection caused by this bacterium had a well-recognized clinical course and radiological and pathological appearance. When it subsequently became clear that other bacteria could cause pneumonia, some with a milder clinical course and with different CXR findings, the terms typical and atypical pneumonias were introduced. It is now appreciated that atypical disease is commoner and that 'atypical bacteria' can cause disease that is similar to typical pneumonia. Thus the terms are not clinically useful and should probably be consigned to the history books.

Pathophysiology

- The development of pneumonia requires a causative pathogen to reach the alveoli and to overcome the host's protective immunity. Most pneumonia is acquired by inhalation of infected particles, either from exogenous sources or from colonization of the nasopharynx or sinuses. More rarely, pneumonia will be acquired following aspiration or from haematogenous spread.
- Local host defence mechanisms include:
  - innate responses: mucociliary clearance and coughing, phagocytosis by alveolar macrophages and neutrophils, and antiviral and antibacterial molecules such as defensins, lysozyme, and interferons produced by the airway epithelium;
  - acquired immunity: surface antibodies and rapid T-cell responses.
- Factors that predispose to pneumonia are:
  - exposure to virulent organisms;
  - high inoculum;
  - impaired innate response;
  - impaired acquired immunity.
- Viral infections are more infectious and transmissible than bacterial pneumonias. It is likely that most community-acquired bacterial pneumonias arise following endogenous spread of organisms from the upper airway after local host responses have been damaged by recent or concurrent viral respiratory infection.

Incidence

- For children under 5 years of age, incidence in developed countries is 40/1000 children per year.
- For children over 5 years of age, incidence in developed countries is 20/1000 children per year.

Causes

- The nature of the causative pathogen depends on the age of the child and the definition of pneumonia used.
- Most epidemiological surveys are hospital-based and require radiological evidence of consolidation, which includes both dense consolidation and increased interstitial markings. An illness in a young child resulting in wheeze and fever and increased markings on CXR would therefore be included in this definition of pneumonia, as would illness in an infant with clinical features of bronchiolitis and patchy consolidation on CXR.
- In up to 40% of children no cause for the pneumonia can be found despite the use of PCR and serology.
- Bearing in mind these limitations and definitions and that there is variation between surveys, approximate proportions of causal organisms are as follows.
  - In children under 5 years viral infections (mainly RSV) account for 60%, Streptococcus pneumoniae 20%, Chlamydophila pneumoniae and Mycoplasma pneumoniae together around 10%, unknown 30–40%. Mixed infections occur in up to 30%.
  - In children over 5 years, Streptococcus pneumoniae 30%, Mycoplasma pneumoniae 30%, Chlamydophila pneumoniae 20% viral infections 30%, unknown 20%. Mixed infections occur in up to 30%.
  - In children under 2 years, viral infections are found in as many as 80%.
  - Streptococcus pneumoniae is the most important bacterial cause in all age groups.
  - The high incidence of mixed infection is usually a combination of viral and bacterial pathogens, probably reflecting the prior role that viral infection has in establishing bacterial pneumonia.
  - The contribution of viral infection to pneumonia will increase significantly during influenza epidemics.

Pathogens causing community-acquired pneumonia

Viral
- Respiratory syncytial virus
- Influenza A, B, and C
- Parainfluenza types 1–4
- Human metapneumovirus
- Adenovirus
- Rhinovirus
- Varicella zoster virus
- Cytomegalovirus
- Enteroviruses
- Measles virus

Bacterial—typical
- *Streptococcus pneumoniae*
- *Staphylococcus aureus*
- *Streptococcus pyogenes* (group A streptococci)
- *Klebsiella* species

Bacteria—atypical
- *Mycoplasma pneumoniae*
- *Chlamydophila pneumoniae*
- *Legionella pneumoniae*
- *Moraxella* species

Bacterial—mycobacteria
- *Mycobacterium tuberculosis*
- Atypical mycobacteria (*M. avium-intracellulare* complex, *M. fortuitum chelonae*, *M. abscessus*, *M. kansasii*, *M. marinum*, and several others)

Symptoms and signs

The likely symptoms and signs of pneumonia depend on the age of the child and the extent of disease. Widespread bilateral disease is more likely to cause breathlessness and signs of respiratory distress. Focal infection may cause fever and lethargy, often with nothing specific to find on examination to suggest a pneumonia.

Possible symptoms include:
- fever;
- lethargy;
- breathlessness;
- cough;
- chest pain—which may result in a reactive scoliosis;
- abdominal pain—usually from a lower lobe pneumonia—which may be severe enough to mimic appendicitis.

Possible signs include:
- fever;
- tachycardia;
- tachypnoea;
- desaturation;
- chest wall recession;
- use of accessory muscles of respiration;
- abnormal findings on auscultation:
  - bronchial breathing;
  - crepitations;
  - wheeze.

Investigations and diagnosis

In many children the diagnosis is made clinically in the primary care setting and investigation is unnecessary. For sicker children requiring hospital treatment (because of poor feeding, oxygen requirement, severe malaise), the following investigations are indicated.
- CXR. Most useful in young children with a fever of unknown origin or in children with severe respiratory distress. It should not be used in an attempt to distinguish viral from bacterial infection (see below).
- Blood for:
  - culture—positive in ≤ 10% of children with pneumonia;
  - FBC—it is helpful to know the haemoglobin in children with an oxygen requirement. The white count is a poor guide to causal pathogen;
  - U & E—children with severe pneumonia can develop a syndrome of inappropriate antidiuretic hormone production;
  - serum—to be saved and used for serological analysis once a convalescent sample has been taken after 10 days.
- Nasopharyngeal aspirate for viral analysis in the under 2 year olds.
- If there is a significant collection of pleural fluid, this can be sent for culture.
- PCR tests where available can be used on blood or respiratory secretions for *Mycoplasma*, *Chlamydophila*, *Pneumococcus* (pneumolysin), and several viruses.

Bacterial or viral?

It is difficult to distinguish bacterial from viral pneumonia in many children. Viruses, mycoplasma, and chlamydophila can all cause focal consolidation. Invasive viruses such as influenza and adenovirus can cause high neutrophil counts and impressively elevated acute phase reactants. Mixed infection occurs in up to 30% of children. Despite these difficulties, some general guidance can be given.

- Bilateral wheeze is perhaps the strongest indicator that any LRTI that may be present is atypical or viral in aetiology.
- Truly focal disease, confined to a single lobe, is not likely to be due to virus.
- Unilateral pleural effusion with adjacent consolidation indicates a bacterial cause.

Management

The majority of children with pneumonia can be cared for in the community. Criteria for admission to hospital include the presence of marked breathlessness and desaturation.

Antibiotics

- The decision to use antibiotics or not depends on the clinical picture and the age of the child.
- Children with mild symptoms, particularly if there are bilateral signs (especially wheeze), are likely to have viral or atypical pneumonia, and it would be reasonable not to treat with antibiotics. The clinical response of mycoplasma and chlamydophila pneumonia to macrolide antibiotics in most children is difficult to demonstrate and, when symptoms are mild, there is probably little to gain from their use.
- Children with more severe disease, including chest pain, high persistent fever, and breathlessness, or those with focal disease clinically or radiologically are more likely to have typical bacterial pneumonia and so benefit from antibiotic treatment.
- Where *S. pneumoniae* is the likely organism then antibiotic treatment should be with penicillin (or amoxicillin) at any age.
- Whilst the efficacy of macrolide treatment against mycoplasma and chlamydophila pneumonia is questionable, there may be benefits in reducing carriage, and they will be effective against most strains of *Streptococcus pneumoniae*. Thus a rational choice of antibiotics would be:
  - amoxicillin in children under 5 years (mycoplasma and chlamydophila are relatively uncommon);
  - macrolide antibiotic for children over 5 years—any of the macrolides will do, although erythromycin has a higher rate of GI side-effects.

Typical CXR appearances of lobar consolidation (Figs 17.1–17.6)

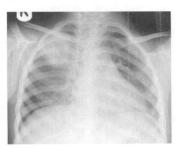

Fig. 17.1 Right upper lobe consolidation.

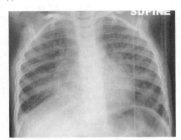

Fig. 17.2 Right middle lobe consolidation—the smooth outline of the right heart border is lost.

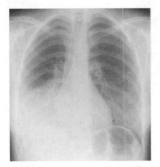

Fig. 17.3 Right lower lobe consolidation—the clear outline of the right hemidiaphragm is lost.

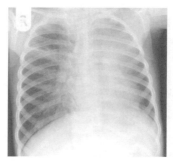

Fig. 17.4 Left upper lobe collapse/consolidation. When the left upper lobe collapses there is usually an indistinct lower border, giving a veil-like appearance.

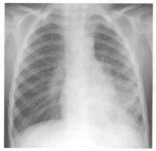

Fig. 17.5 Left lingular consolidation—the smooth outline of the left heart border is lost.

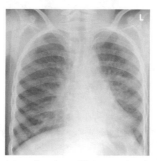

Fig. 17.6 Left lower lobe collapse/consolidation—a triangular appearance behind the heart with loss of outline of the diaphragm.

- Use of narrow-spectrum rather than broad-spectrum antibiotics will reduce the likelihood of the development of antibiotic resistance.
- Oral antibiotics are as effective as parenteral antibiotics for otherwise well children with mild to moderate disease even if they require admission to hospital for supportive care.[1] For very sick children (those with shock or oxygen saturation < 85%) or with complicated pneumonia (e.g. with an effusion), the parenteral route should be used.
- For lobar pneumonia, many units prefer to use penicillin or amoxicillin, rather than a macrolide, as the first-line antibiotic for all age groups. For very sick children and infants, second-line antibiotics with broader spectrum include co-amoxiclav, cefuroxime, and cefotaxime.
- For simple pneumonia 7 days antibiotic treatment is usually adequate.
- If IV antibiotics are used, they can be changed to oral once the child is afebrile.

Additional supportive therapy
This includes the following.
- Oxygen.
- Fluids, NG or IV—usually in very breathless infants.
- Analgesia.

Chest physiotherapy is not helpful.

Failure to respond to treatment
Most children with bacterial pneumonia will respond rapidly to treatment and significant improvement, with resolution of fever, will be seen within 48h. Failure to improve may result from the following.
- Development of an empyema or, more rarely, a lung abscess.
- Underlying disease, such as CF, immunodeficiency, inhaled foreign body, or cystic adenomatoid malformation.
- Infection with antibiotic-resistant bacteria.
- Inappropriately low antibiotic dose.
- Viral or atypical infection can be severe and will not respond to antibiotics.
- Infection with *M. tuberculosis*.
- Fungal infection in the child with previously unrecognized immunodeficiency.
- Extensive bacterial infection. This can take several days to improve on appropriate therapy.

1 Atkinson, M., Lakhanpaul, M., Smyth, A., Vyas, H., Weston, V. Sithole, J., Owen V., Halliday, K., Sammons, H., Crane. J., Guntupalli, N., Walton, L., Ninan, T., Morjaria, A., and Stephenson, T. (2007). A multicentre randomised controlled equivalence trial comparing oral amoxicillin and intravenous benzyl penicillin for community acquired pneumonia in children: PIVOT Trial. *Thorax* (2007 June—epub).

Where there is failure to improve or deterioration, careful clinical reevaluation is necessary. Further investigations can be helpful.
• CXR looking for pleural disease.
• Ultrasound looking for pleural collection.
• Repeated attempts to identify the causative organism from blood or respiratory fluid.
• Occasionally, where CXR and ultrasound have been unhelpful, chest CT scan can identify collections and lung abscesses.
• Tests for immune deficiency.

A change of antibiotics is rarely helpful on its own. Pneumonia caused by streptococcal strains that show *in vitro* resistance responds to standard antibiotic therapy just as well as that caused by fully sensitive strains, probably because the *in vivo* antibiotic concentrations exceed the levels required to kill even the resistant strains. Checking that the dose is adequate is usually more rewarding.

Outcome and follow-up

The vast majority of children, even those with severe disease, recover fully from pneumonia, irrespective of the cause. A tiny proportion will be left with lung damage, either focal bronchiectasis, or bronchiolitis obliterans.

Routine follow-up and repeat CXRs are not required, unless there are atypical features. Children with round pneumonias (which could be confused with tumour masses) or who had lobar collapse should have a repeat CXR after 6 weeks to ensure resolution. Children who have had lung abscess should have a follow-up CT scan to determine if there is an underlying abnormality of the lung (usually a cystic adenomatoid malformation).

Further information
British Thoracic Society Standards of Care Committee (2002). British Thoracic Society Guidelines for the management of community acquired pneumonia in childhood. *Thorax* **57** (Suppl. 1), 1–24.

Bacterial infections

Epiglottitis

- Epiglottitis refers to acute inflammation of the epiglottis and surrounding structures.
- Prior to the introduction of effective vaccination, the majority of cases were caused by *Haemophilus influenzae* type b (Hib), and affected pre-school children.
- In populations vaccinated against Hib, epiglottitis is now rare (< 1 episode per 100 000 children per year). It is more likely to be caused by other bacteria (notably *Streptococcus pyogenes* and *S. pneumoniae* as well as *Staphylococcus aureus*) and to occur in older children and adults. Hib can still cause epiglottitis in non-vaccinated children and where the vaccine has failed.
- Spread from the site of colonization (nasopharynx) to the supraglottic structures is via the blood.

History

Epiglottitis is abrupt in onset and children usually present within 24h of becoming unwell. Typical symptoms include:
- high fever;
- very painful throat;
- unable to swallow;
- progressive stridor;
- cough is usually absent (unlike croup).

Examination

As in all children with unsafe airways, a calm approach is required. Undue distress to the child will cause unnecessarily turbulent inspiratory airflow with consequent reduction in flow rates, and may precipitate complete airways obstruction. Painful or distressing procedures, including examination of the throat, should be avoided until the airway is secure. Typical findings on examination are:
- an agitated and distressed child;
- fever;
- drooling (unable to swallow secretions);
- stridor with chest wall recession (may be absent in exhausted child);
- possible desaturation and cyanosis—ominous signs of severe hypoventilation.

Investigations and diagnosis

The diagnosis is clinical. The appearance of the epiglottis at intubation provides confirmation. No investigations should be carried out until the airway has been secured. Once this has been achieved, the following investigations are helpful:
- blood cultures;
- upper airway swab for culture.

Lateral X-rays of the neck should be avoided. They seldom contribute to the diagnosis and delay definitive management of the airway.

The differential diagnosis includes:

- croup;
- anaphylaxis;
- trauma or burns, including chemical injury, affecting the pharynx and larynx;
- laryngeal foreign body;
- retropharyngeal abscess.

Management

- Securing a safe airway is the first priority.
- Unlike croup where an expectant approach can be used, in children with epiglottitis the risk of loss of the airway is very high and an artificial airway should always be established.
- Whilst waiting for the necessary equipment and personnel to be assembled the child can rest in whichever position they find most comfortable, and receive humidified oxygen if tolerated.
- The procedure for intubating children with epiglottitis varies with local experience. In some centres ICU staff may feel confident to intubate after gaseous induction of anaesthesia in the ICU. In other centres, the procedure will be carried out in an operating theatre with an ENT surgeon available to perform a tracheostomy if intubation is unsuccessful.
- If obstruction occurs suddenly, abdominal thrusts or chest compressions may clear any obstructing secretions. Long firm breaths delivered with a resuscitation bag and mask system may also provide some degree of oxygenation, with chest compression to aid expiration. If oxygenation is not achieved, a needle cricothyroidotomy should be performed. Wall oxygen is usually pressured to 4 atmospheres, and this pressure (rather than that from a bag) is needed to drive the oxygen though the cricothyroid cannula. Ventilation will not be possible, but oxygenation should improve for a few minutes (see 📖 Chapter 63 for more details).
- Once the airway is secure, blood can be taken for culture, and antibiotics, usually a third generation cephalosporin, can be started and given for between 3 and 7 days.
- Close contacts of children with Hib infection should be given antibiotic prophylaxis.

Outcome and complications

- Recovery is usually rapid, with extubation usually possible after 48h.
- Complications are usually associated with hypoxic damage in children where intubation is delayed.
- Occasionally there may be additional foci of infection. Otitis media, pneumonia, and meningitis have all been reported.
- If the infection occurred as a result of Hib vaccination failure, tests of immunity including response to other vaccinations should be made.

Bacterial tracheitis

- Bacterial infection of the larynx and trachea causing purulent inflammation is rare.
- Any age child can be affected, but most are > 5 years of age.
- Bacterial tracheitis occurs most often as secondary infection after viral croup.
- It is usually caused by *Staphylococcus aureus*, *Streptococcus pyogenes*, *Moraxella catarrhalis*, and *Haemophilus influenzae* type b (non-vaccinated or vaccine failure).

History

Symptoms usually arise over 2–3 days (unlike the abrupt onset of epiglottitis):
- prodromal coryzal illness;
- barking cough;
- noisy breathing.

Followed by:
- worsening fever;
- lethargy and anorexia;
- dysphagia and pain may occur.

Examination

- Fever.
- Stridor with evidence of respiratory distress.

Diagnosis

- Bacterial tracheitis is suspected clinically when a child with croup has an expectedly long illness with persisting high fevers. The diagnosis can only be confirmed by direct inspection of the airways, which in practice is only performed in children who have required intubation.
- A high blood neutrophil count is consistent with the diagnosis.
- If the child is intubated, tracheal secretions should be sent for culture.
- Blood culture may be helpful.

Management

- Bacterial tracheitis can be severe enough to cause airways obstruction requiring intubation. The obstruction, as in croup, is usually worst at the subglottis.
- Appropriate antibiotics, such as second or third generation cephalosporins, should be given.
- Systemic corticosteroids will usually already have been given in the 'croup-like' phase of the illness. If the child is intubated, further doses may help with extubation.
- Illness usually lasts 5–10 days.

Retropharyngeal and peritonsillar abscesses

Retropharyngeal abscess

- Infection of the space between the pharynx and cervical spine usually starts as inflammation of the small lymph nodes in this area. Occasionally, as elsewhere, the lymph nodes may be overwhelmed by infection and break down forming an abscess. Rarely the infection may arise because of penetrating trauma (usually a pencil).
- The usual pathogens are *Staphylococcus aureus*, *Streptococcus pyogenes*, and *Haemophilus influenzae* type b (non-immunized children).
- Typical history is of:
  - fever;
  - neck pain, especially on extension, possibly with torticollis;
  - dysphagia.
- Airway compression is relatively unusual (5–20%).
- Examination findings may include:
  - external neck swelling;
  - mass in posterior pharyngeal wall seen by inspecting the throat.
- Diagnosis is usually by direct inspection of the throat. It can be confirmed by a lateral neck X-ray that shows widening of the pre-vertebral space or by contrast-enhanced CT scan. Investigations should only be carried out once the airway has been assessed and made safe.
- Where there is airway compromise, the abscess should be drained, usually via the mouth. Care should be taken not to allow aspiration of released pus.
- If there is no airway compromise, treatment with IV antibiotics is usually sufficient.
- Outcome is usually good. Abscess rupture and aspiration of pus can lead to pneumonitis. Rarely, the abscess may be associated with thrombosis of neck veins or erosion into the carotid artery.

Peritonsillar abscess

- Abscess formation adjacent to the tonsillar capsule usually occurs as a complication of acute tonsillitis or pharyngitis.
- It is most often caused by *S. pyogenes* or *S. viridans*.
- It causes worsening pain, fever, and dysphagia in a child already suffering from tonsillitis.
- Occasionally the swelling may be severe enough to cause airway obstruction and stridor.
- Rupture of the abscess may lead to aspiration of pus and an infective pneumonitis.
- In the absence of respiratory compromise, treatment with IV antibiotics alone is usually sufficient.
- Where there is airway obstruction, drainage, either by needle aspiration or incision, is necessary.

Streptococcal pneumonia

- Streptococci are Gram-positive bacteria occurring as diplococci or in chains.
- They are classified by the pattern of haemolysis seen after culture on blood agar plates. Streptococci showing beta-haemolysis are further classified using serological methods (the Lancefield grouping). These different methods of classification are potentially confusing.
- *Streptococcus pneumoniae* is alpha-haemolytic and so does not have a Lancefield grouping.
- *S. pyogenes* shows beta-haemolytic growth and is also known as Lancefield group A streptococcus.
- *S. agalactiae* shows beta-haemolytic growth and is nearly always known as Lancefield group B streptococcus.
- The viridans group of streptococci shows alpha-haemolytic growth. They commonly colonize the mouth and can cause pneumonia following aspiration events.

Streptococcus pneumoniae

- *S. pneumoniae* is the commonest cause of typical bacterial pneumonia. It can also cause otitis media, meningitis, and septicaemia.
- There are over 90 *S. pneumoniae* serotypes, with a smaller number of virulent strains that cause disease. The strains that cause invasive disease (meningitis and septicaemia) may be different from those that cause pneumonia and otitis media.
- Carriage of *S. pneumoniae* in the nasopharynx is common and will occur in nearly all children at some stage in early life.
- Pneumonia occurs as a result of inhalation of bacteria from the nasopharynx and often follows a viral LRTI that has damaged local defence mechanisms. Despite this probable mechanism of infection the *S. pneumoniae* colonizing the nasopharynx may be a different strain to that causing the pneumonia in the same child and throat culture is not helpful in diagnosis.
- Invasion into the blood is relatively uncommon in children with pneumonia; blood cultures are positive in ≤ 10% of affected children.
- Rates of resistance to penicillin vary according to location. In the UK resistance is found in 5–10% of invasive isolates. *In vitro* resistance to penicillin does not always predict lack of clinical response, and this seems to be the case for pneumococcal pneumonia. In the UK, penicillin is still the first-line antibiotic for suspected pneumococcal pneumonia. Where there is severe septicaemia or meningitis, vancomycin or teicoplanin may be preferred.
- The pneumonia caused by *S. pneumoniae* is usually either a lobar pneumonia or a round pneumonia.
- Severe pneumonia complicated by empyema or cavitating disease (necrotizing pneumonia) due to *S. pneumoniae* appears to be becoming more common. The most commonly isolated serotype from empyema fluid is serotype 1.

- Vaccination in children over 2 years of age can be carried out using the 23-valent Pneumovax. This is a polysaccharide antigen based vaccine and does not work in younger children. Several countries, including the UK, have now included the heptavalent pneumococcal conjugate vaccine in the routine infant immunization schedules. This vaccine provides protection against serotypes 4, 6B, 9V, 14, 19F, 23F, and 18C. It was designed to provide protection against invasive disease (i.e. bacteria entering the blood or CSF) rather than pneumonia. It is associated with a 95% reduction in pneumococcal septicaemia and meningitis and with a 70% reduction in pneumococcal pneumonia. The conjugate vaccine does not include serotype 1. It is possible that this may result in an increase in carriage of this serotype, and consequently increase the incidence of severe forms of pneumococcal pneumonia while decreasing the overall incidence.

Streptococcus pyogenes

- Also called group A streptococcus (GAS).
- Carriage in the nasopharynx is common. Up to 30% of school age children will carry GAS at any one time.
- GAS commonly causes pharyngitis and may also cause serious infection of the upper airway:
  - epiglottitis;
  - retropharyngeal abscess;
  - peritonsillar abscess;
  - bacterial tracheitis.
- It is a relatively rare cause of pneumonia. When pneumonia does occur it is likely to be more severe than most, with necrotizing lung injury and a higher likelihood of lung abscess and empyema.
- During or following GAS infection, non-infectious complications can occur:
  - glomerulonephritis—immune complex mediated;
  - rheumatic fever—immune complex mediated;
  - neuropsychiatric disorders—immune complex mediated;
  - toxic shock syndrome—toxin mediated;
  - scarlet fever—toxin mediated.
- Elevated anti-streptococcal antibodies, most commonly the antistreptolysin O test, indicate previous infection, but are not helpful during the acute illness.
- Treatment is with penicillin. In severe infection, a second generation cephalosporin may be preferred.

Group B streptococcus (S. agalactiae)

- GBS colonize the vagina and GI tract in up to 30% of healthy pregnant women. Infants can acquire infection as they pass through the birth canal.
- Infection in children is limited to the first few months of life.
- Early (0–7 days) and late forms (1–12 weeks) of GBS infection occur.
- Early disease is usually bacteraemia and pneumonia.
- Late disease is usually more severe, causing septicaemia and meningitis.
- Both forms of the disease are rare, despite high maternal carriage rates.
- Treatment is with IV benzyl penicillin.

Staphylococcal pneumonia

- *Staphylococcus aureus* is a Gram-positive coccus that grows in clusters.
- It causes a wide range of pyogenic infections.
- It is a relatively rare cause of pneumonia in children (about 5% of community-acquired pneumonia) and most disease occurs in infants. It is commoner in malnourished populations.
- Like pneumonia caused by *S. pyogenes*, there is an increased risk of severe illness with necrotizing pneumonia, abscess formation, or empyema.
- As with other bacterial pneumonias, infection usually follows inhalation of infectious particles. Lung infection via the blood stream from a distant infective source is more commonly seen in pneumonia caused by *S. aureus* compared with other bacteria, and may cause bilateral, multi-focal cavitating disease.
- Pneumatoceles can form as a result of lung destruction and, although they suggest the presence of *S. aureus*, they are not specific for staphylococcal disease. Even dramatic looking pneumatoceles heal spontaneously once the infection has resolved.
- Treatment is usually with second generation cephalosporin antibiotics.
- Where there is a risk of methicillin resistance or when the infection is severe or fails to respond to conventional treatment, vancomycin is preferred.

Other bacterial pneumonias

Moraxella catarrhalis

- *M. catarrhalis* is a Gram-negative diplococcus that frequently colonizes the nasopharynx in early life (> 50% of infants). Carriage in adults is less common—around 5%.
- It is a common cause of otitis media and sinusitis—third after *Streptococcus pneumoniae* and non-encapsulated *Haemophilus influenzae*.
- Diagnosis is by serology or by culture of respiratory secretions
- *M. catarrhalis* is identified infrequently (1–5%) in children with community-acquired pneumonia. Although patchy consolidation can occur, *M. catarrhalis*, like non-encapsulated *H. influenzae*, tends to cause bronchitis rather than pneumonia. Infection typically occurs either following a viral LRTI, or in children with pre-existing lung disease.
- Treatment is with a macrolide antibiotic.

Klebsiella pneumoniae

- *K. pneumoniae* are Gram-negative rods that can colonize the skin, nasopharynx, and GI tract.
- *K. pneumoniae* is a rare (< 5%) cause of community-acquired bacterial pneumonia in children. It is more likely to cause a hospital-acquired infection.
- It can be associated with necrotizing pneumonia, lung abscess, and empyema.
- In adult life it typically causes pneumonia (Friedländer pneumonia) in debilitated alcoholic middle-aged men.
- CXR may show an apparently swollen consolidated lobe, with a 'bulging fissure'. This sign is not specific for *K. pneumoniae* infection.
- Firm diagnosis usually requires a positive blood or pleural fluid culture. *K. pneumoniae* often show significant antibiotic resistance. Treatment usually requires 3rd generation cephalosporin antibiotics.

Legionella pneumonia

- *Legionella pneumophila* is a Gram-negative rod that requires special culture conditions and special staining to be seen under the microscope.
- It was first identified in 1976 after an outbreak of pneumonia at an American Legion convention in Philadelphia.
- *L. pneumophila* is found widely in stagnant water, and infection is acquired by inhalation.
- It is a very rare (< 1%) cause of community-acquired pneumonia in children.
- It may cause hospital-acquired pneumonia, particularly in immunosuppressed children.
- When infection occurs in children, it resembles the disease in adults, with a risk of severe multifocal necrotizing pneumonia. There is usually significant systemic illness, sometimes with other organ involvement (myocarditis, hepatitis, meningoencephalitis).

- Diagnosis is by culture, usually of respiratory secretions—sputum, bronchoalveolar lavage, or tracheal aspirates.
- Treatment is with macrolide antibiotics, usually azithromycin.
- If *L. pneumophila* is cultured from respiratory secretions, the source of the infection must be identified to prevent further infections.

Mycoplasma infection

- *Mycoplasma pneumoniae* accounts for 10–30% of community-acquired pneumonia in children over the age of 3 years.
- The incidence of infection is highest in children aged 5–9 years, but up to 40% of cases are seen in the 1–5 year age range in some case series.
- Symptomatic infection is uncommon in children < 1 year of age.
- It is spread by droplet and has an incubation period of 1–3 weeks.
- The primary target for *M. pneumoniae* is the respiratory epithelium.
- Infection may spread to more distant sites (see 'Extra pulmonary disease').
- Infection can occur at any time of year.
- Outbreaks may occur where there are large numbers of children in close contact with one another, e.g. in boarding schools.
- Epidemics of *M. pneumoniae* infection tend to occur every 3–4 years.
- The illness usually follows a mild and self-limiting course. < 10% of infections result in symptoms and signs of pneumonia.

Symptoms

- Symptoms usually start gradually, although abrupt onset is possible.
- The illness typically lasts longer than most bacterial pneumonias and can persist for 4 weeks.
- The illness starts with non-specific symptoms of malaise, headache, sore throat, and fever.
- Nasal discharge or ear infection is rare and, when present, suggests a viral aetiology for the respiratory symptoms.
- Cough usually starts a week after the onset of the illness. It may be productive or dry.
- In severe disease there may be breathlessness with/without wheezing.

Signs

- In mild disease there may be nothing to find apart from fever.
- Fever (temperature > 38°C) may be absent in 30% of cases.
- In more extensive disease there may be bilateral inspiratory crepitations with or without wheeze.
- Occasionally more severe disease occurs with tachypnoea and chest wall recession. These children frequently have an oxygen requirement.
- In about 5% of cases there may be bronchial breathing.

Investigation

In most children the clinical picture will be one of a mild community-acquired pneumonia, and no investigations will be required. Where the disease is more severe or there is clinical doubt, the following may be helpful.

- CXR findings are non-specific but are nearly always abnormal.
  - Usually both lungs show increased bronchial markings with patchy consolidation most often in the lower lobes.
  - There may be hilar adenopathy, which can be asymmetrical.

- Lobar consolidation can occur in up to 20% of cases.
- Pleural collections, which are usually small are found in about 5% of cases. Large collections requiring drainage are unusual and may represent secondary infection with *Staphylococcus aureus*.
- *M. pneumoniae* is a tiny rod-like free-living prokaryotic organism that does not have polysaccharide cell wall and as such does not show up on Gram-stain. It is also difficult to culture reliably. Cold-agglutinins (cross-reacting antibodies against human red cells that may be induced by infection with *M. pneumoniae*) are non-specific.
- If definitive diagnosis is required *M. pneumoniae* IgM or paired IgG should be measured in the child's serum. A 4-fold rise in IgG over 2–3 weeks is the gold-standard investigation. Some clinical labs will now offer *M. pneumoniae* PCR (using nasopharyngeal aspirate or throat swab), which seems to be sensitive and specific, although how long the tests remain positive after acute infection is not known.
- FBC may show evidence of haemolytic anaemia (low Hb, possible reticulocytosis). The white count may be normal, elevated, or depressed. There may be a mild thombocytosis.

Treatment

- *M. pneumoniae* is sensitive to macrolide antibiotics *in vitro*, but resistant to penicillins and cephalosporins (since it has no cell wall).
- There is conflicting advice in the major paediatric textbooks as to whether treatment with antibiotics affects the duration or severity of symptoms due to *M. pneumoniae* infection in children.
- Data from adults suggest a marginal benefit: a reduction in illness duration by 1 day.
- A Cochrane review concluded there was no adequate RCT on which to base decisions about the effectiveness of treatment for mycoplasmal infections.[1]
- The trials in children that are available are small and compare macrolide treatment to other antibiotics. In these trials there was no benefit in terms of resolution of symptoms in using a macrolide, but there did seem to be a higher rate of eradication of *M. pneumoniae* from the nasopharynx in those children treated with a macrolide.
- In practice, if a child is unwell with pneumonia and has bilateral disease consistent with atypical infection or has lobar pneumonia with poor clinical response after 48h of beta-lactam antibiotic, it is reasonable on current evidence to give a 5 day course of macrolide antibiotic.
- The efficacy of the different macrolides appears to be similar, but erythromycin is associated with a higher rate of GI upset.

Prevention

During outbreaks in institutions, prophylaxis with azithromycin has been shown to reduce the number of secondary cases.

1 Gavranich, J.B. and Chang, A.B. (2005). Antibiotics for community acquired lower respiratory tract infections (LRTI) secondary to *Mycoplasma pneumoniae* in children. *Cochrane Database Syst. Rev.* 2005 (3), CD004875.

Extrapulmonary disease

These include:
- erythema multiforme and Stevens–Johnson syndrome;
- myocarditis;
- encephalitis;
- Guillain–Barré syndrome;
- transverse myelitis;
- haemolytic anaemia.

Extrapulmonary disease may represent the effects of infection of tissues with *M. pneumoniae* or be due to cross-reacting antibodies. If symptoms occur within 5 days of the onset of prodromal symptoms (fever, malaise, cough) then they are more likely to represent direct infection of tissues. Symptoms occurring after 7 days are more likely to be autoimmune.

Outcome

Pneumonia due to *M. pneumoniae* is usually mild and self-resolving. More rarely, it may be associated with severe disease including acute respiratory distress syndrome, bronchiolitis obliterans, bronchiectasis, and/or organizing pneumonia.

Further information
Othman, N., Isaacs, D., and Kesson, A. (2005). *Mycoplasma pneumoniae* infections in Australian children. *J. Paediatr. Child Health* **41**, 671–6.

Chlamydia infection

- There has been a reorganization of the family of bacteria known as Chlamydiaceae. Two separate genera are now recognized: *Chlamydia* and *Chlamydophila*. The genus *Chlamydia* includes *C. trachmatis*. The genus *Chlamyophila* includes *C. pneumoniae* and *C. psittaci*.
- All Chlamydiaceae are bacterial pathogens that can only divide and multiply inside cells.
- *C. pneumoniae* and *C. trachomatis* are common human pathogens.
- *C. psittaci* can cause infection in humans but is limited to those who have had contact with sick psittacine birds, mainly parrots.

Chlamydophila pneumoniae

C. pneumoniae is a common cause of pneumonia in children of all ages throughout the world. The incidence in children appears to be highest in those aged 5–15 years (causing around 20% of pneumonias), but infection in younger children is not uncommon (15% of pneumonias in 1–5 year olds, and around 5% of pneumonias in those under 12 months). Co-infection with *Mycoplasma pneumoniae* or *Streptococcus pneumoniae* occurs in around 20% of cases.

Symptoms and signs

C. pneumoniae infections cannot reliably be distinguished clinically from those caused by other pathogens. There may be long prodrome of up to 6 weeks, but more acute infection is also possible. Symptoms are similar to those found in viral or *Mycoplasma* infection and include:

- lethargy;
- fever;
- headache;
- sore throat;
- dry cough.

Examination may be relatively normal or reveal severe respiratory distress and hypoxia. Auscultation may be normal or reveal bilateral crepitations or wheeze.

Investigation

- FBC—often normal.
- CXR. As with *Mycoplasma* infections, the CXR often looks more dramatic than the child's clinical condition might suggest. The findings are similar to those described for Mycoplasma infection: usually diffuse bilateral shadowing, with small proportion showing lobar consolidation.
- Serology. Positive IgM or 4-fold rise in IgG titres.
- Culture. Posterior nasopharyngeal swab is often best, but sputum or BAL fluid are alternatives Culture requires inoculation of human cell lines (e.g. HeLa). Check with your lab before you send the test.
- PCR tests are being developed.

Treatment

Macrolides are effective in killing *C. pneumoniae* and a 10 day course of clarithromycin will eradicate nasopharyngeal carriage in 80% of children with symptomatic LRTI. Clinical response, as with *M. pneumoniae*, is more variable.

Outcome

Full recovery occurs in most children. More serious illness has been associated with *C. pneumoniae* infection, including Guillain–Barré syndrome, myocarditits, meningoencephalitis, and reactive arthritis. There are also case reports of chronic lung disease following *C. pneumoniae* infection, similar to those described for *M. pneumoniae*.

Chlamydophila trachomatis

In the developing world *C. trachomatis* causes trachoma, the world's leading cause of blindness. In developed countries *C. trachomatis* is the commonest cause of sexually transmitted disease, causing urethritis in men and cervicitis and salpingitis in women. Infants who are born to infected mothers can develop conjunctivitis and pneumonia.

Neonatal infection

In developed countries, 10–15% of pregnant women will have active chlamydial genital infection. Vaginally delivered infants have around a 50% chance of becoming infected and, in the majority of these, the infection is limited to the nasopharynx where it may cause snuffliness and nasal discharge. Some infants will develop conjunctivitis. Classically this is oedematous and haemorrhagic resulting in contact bleeding when a swab is taken. A smaller proportion will develop pneumonia. The literature suggests that this occurs in as many as 10% of infants born to infected mothers. This would suggest that around 1% of all infants developed symptomatic chlamydial pneumonia, which is certainly much higher than the number of infants being diagnosed. This either means the figures are wrong or the disease is usually very mild and is being treated in the community without being diagnosed as chlamydial.

Symptoms and signs

- Onset is gradual and between 1 and 4 months of age.
- Productive-sounding cough.
- Conjunctivitis only in 15%.
- Breathlessness.
- Apnoea may occur.
- Absence of fever is usual.
- Crepitations, but usually no wheeze.

Investigations

- Peripheral eosinophilia is seen in 50%.
- Nasopharyngeal or conjunctival culture.
- Serology: positive IgM or 4-fold rise in IgG titres.
- CXR: bilateral interstitial markings.

Treatment C. trachomatis conjunctivitis and pneumonia are effectively treated with oral macrolide therapy. A 14 day course of erythromycin is standard, but shorter courses of azithromycin may be as effective. Remember to refer the mother (and father) to an appropriate physician for diagnosis and treatment of genitourinary disease.

Outcome is usually excellent. There are rare case reports of CNS and cardiac infection with *C. trachomatis*.

Pertussis

- Most pertussis or whooping cough is caused by infection with *Bordetella pertussis*. A smaller number of cases are caused by *B. parapertussis*. Bordetellae are Gram-negative cocco-bacilli, and humans are their only host.
- Infection is spread by aeresolized respiratory droplets, and susceptible close contacts have a near 100% risk of acquiring the infection.
- The time between exposure and onset of cough is usually 7–10 days, but very rarely may be as long as 6 weeks.
- Children are infectious for the first 3 weeks of the illness (including the catarrhal stage).
- Successful immunization programmes mean that pertussis is now unusual in infancy. It remains relatively common in school-aged children, despite immunization, where it usually causes a relatively mild but irritating persistent paroxysmal cough.
- The introduction of a pertussis booster immunization at school entry in the UK in 2002 was designed to reduce the incidence of pertussis in the school-aged children and adolescents. A further booster at 18 years, used in some countries, may reduce the burden of disease in the adult population. The acellular pertussis vaccine used in most countries has less reactogenicity than the previous whole-cell vaccine.

Symptoms

- Pertussis starts with a coryzal illness (the catarrhal stage) that is indistinguishable from a viral respiratory tract infection.
- Cough (the paroxysmal stage) develops after 1–2 weeks. The severity and duration of the cough vary considerably. Characteristically it is a dry cough, occurring in attacks of paroxysms of 5 or more coughs without inspiration between coughs. This can lead to facial flushing and vomiting. In severe cases cyanosis can occur. The paroxysm ends with a rapid inspiration that can produce the typical 'whoop'. The cough can persist for as long as 3 months, but more usually lasts 2–6 weeks.
- Half of all children do not develop an inspiratory whoop, and it seldom occurs in infants, in whom inspiratory flow rates are usually insufficient to make much noise.
- Older children and adults may describe a sensation of being unable to breathe or catch their breath after a paroxysm.
- Young infants with pertussis may develop apnoea without severe cough.
- The cough can be precipitated by crying and feeding. Between coughing episodes the child is usually well.
- Infection can be very mild or asymptomatic, but is still infectious (and potentially dangerous to non-immunized infants).

Signs

- Children usually come to medical attention during the paroxysmal stage of the illness. There is usually nothing to find on examination. Occasionally with severe disease, particularly in infants, there may be desaturation during coughing.

- More rarely, there is a complicating bronchopneumonia, which may be caused by *B. pertussis* or by secondary bacterial pathogens. In these children there may be fever, evidence of respiratory distress, and crepitations or bronchial breathing on auscultation.

Investigations

- Diagnosis is often based on clinical suspicion. In relatively well school-aged children with a paroxysmal cough of > 4 weeks duration, who are otherwise well, pertussis is the likely cause in around 30% of children. The only value in confirming recent infection (e.g. by serology) would be to prevent other more costly or unpleasant investigations or treatment. It should be noted that *Bordetella* infection is not the only cause of a pertussis-like illness. *Mycoplasma pneumoniae*, *C. pneumoniae*, adenovirus, parainfluenza virus, and respiratory syncytial virus can all cause a similar illness.
- In sicker children, or those in the earlier phase of their illness where it may be possible to prevent infection in close contacts, attempts should be made to identify the causative organism.
- Culture of nasopharyngeal secretions is specific but not sensitive. The best chance of a positive culture result is in the catarrhal phase of the illness. Even with the best techniques it is rarely positive 3 weeks after the onset of symptoms. Even early in the illness, sensitivity is 40%–80%, dependent on technique and speed of transport to the lab. Naso-pharyngeal secretions are best collected with a swab passed through the nose on a fine wire—the pernasal swab. For the best chance of culturing the organism, the swab should be inoculated directly on to pre-warmed charcoal agar plate at the bedside. Ordinary bacterial throat swabs made of cotton or rayon are inhibitory to *Bordetella* and will be ineffective.
- PCR of nasopharyngeal secretions will give a more rapid result than culture and is more likely to be positive in children who have already had antibiotics. The PCR test also remains positive for longer after the onset illness than culture. Sensitivity ranges from 75% to 100% in the first 3 weeks of the illness. False positive results are rare.
- Detection of *B. pertussis* serum antibodies is the most sensitive test and, of the antibody tests, anti-pertussis toxin IgG is the most specific. A single high titre (>100iu) of anti-pertussis toxin IgG has a sensitivity of 76% and specificity of 99% for diagnosis of acute pertussis. In most children this falls below cut-off levels after 6 months, but may persist for more than 1 year. To be certain that infection is recent, paired sera showing a 4-fold rise in titre are required. Measuring anti-pertussis toxin IgA does not add to diagnostic certainty.
- During the catarrhal stage and early in the paroxysmal phase there is often a marked lymphocytosis that, if present can contribute to the diagnosis.

Management

- Older children with coughs that have been present for more than 3 weeks and who are well between coughs are almost certainly no longer infectious, and the value of investigation or treatment of either the child or contacts of the child are questionable.
- In other children seen earlier in the illness, a 7 day course of macrolide antibiotics can be given. During the catarrhal stage (i.e. first week of illness), this has been shown to reduce disease severity and duration. During the paroxysmal stage, its main purpose is to reduce infectivity by eradicating nasopharyngeal infection. Ideally antibiotics should be given after diagnostic tests (culture or PCR) have been carried out.
- Household contacts of children with known pertussis may benefit from a 14 day course of macrolide antibiotics as prophylaxis if it is given within 3 weeks of onset of symptoms in the index family member. Since protection from infection is not complete and side-effects may occur, antibiotic prophylaxis should probably be reserved for those at risk of severe disease (elderly, young infants, pre-existing lung or heart disease) or those in contact with such persons.
- Management of the coughing episodes is symptomatic. Oxygen and fluids may need to be used. Mechanical ventilation is occasionally required for infants with apnoea (which may be combined with gagging and bradycardia), or children of any age with severe bronchopneumonia and respiratory failure.

Outcome

- In most children, outcome is excellent.
- In infants with severe disease there is a risk of:
  - hypoxic brain injury during cyanotic coughing paroxysms;
  - pulmonary hypertension, which can be fatal;
  - intracerebral or subarachnoid haemorrhage;
  - torn frenulum from tongue protrusion during coughing;
  - inguinal hernias and rectal prolapse caused by raised intra-abdominal pressure during coughing.
- In children with severe pneumonia, caused either by *B. pertussis* or secondary bacterial pathogens, particularly those requiring ventilation, there is a risk of long-term lung injury.

Further information

Crowcroft, N.S. and Pebody, R.G. (2006). Recent developments in pertussis. *Lancet* **7**, 1926–36.

Greenberg, D., Wirsing von Konig, C., and Heininger, U. (2005). Health burden of pertussis in infants and children. *Pediatr. Infect. Dis. J.* **24**, S39–43.

Harnden, A., Grant, C., Harrison, T., Perera, R., Brueggemann, A.B., Mayon-White, R., and Mant. D. (2006). Whooping cough in school age children with persistent cough: prospective cohort study in primary care. *Br. Med. J.* **333**, 174–7.

Ventilator-associated pneumonia

- Ventilator-associated pneumonia (VAP) is defined as pneumonia (usually consolidation on CXR plus fever) acquired more than 48h after intubation and mechanical ventilation. It leads to prolonged stays in ICUs. For the infection to be truly acquired in hospital, the cut-off needs to be more like 7 days, since most infections acquired within that time period are due to organisms already colonizing the child's upper airway.
- VAP is relatively rare in children compared to adults, probably because of shorter periods of ventilation and less comorbidity. An episode of VAP might be expected to occur in around 1 in 20 children ventilated for 5 days or more.
- The most likely causative organisms are:
  - Gram-negative enteric bacteria;
  - *Pseudomonas aeruginosa*;
  - *Staphylococcus aureus*;
  - *Klebsiella pneumoniae*;
  - occasionally viral infections, such as those caused by RSV and adenovirus, may be acquired in the ICU from infected visitors or staff.
- The mechanisms of infection are not well understood, but aspiration of infected secretions, with or without gastro-oesophageal reflux, is most likely for bacterial pathogens.

Symptoms and signs

These are very non-specific, and diagnosis is difficult. Clinically VAP may be recognized by:

- temperature instability;
- new purulent airway secretions;
- cough and increased respiratory effort;
- crepitations or wheeze on auscultation;
- worsening gas exchange.

Risk factors for VAP

- Neuromuscular weakness.
- Prolonged neuromuscular blockade.
- Immunodeficiency or immunosuppression
- Continuous enteral feeds (associated with higher gastric pH and higher levels of gastric bacterial colonization).
- Repeated re-intubations.
- In adults use of nasotracheal tubes is associated with higher risk of VAP, probably because of direct contamination of the lower airway with nasopharyngeal organisms. The effect in children has not been studied, and the need for a stable endotracheal tube may offset any increased risk of VAP.

Investigations

- FBC. Usually shows leucocytosis, occasionally leucopenia.
- Quantitative culture from BAL samples showing $> 10^4$ organisms/mL of lavage fluid. If available protected brush specimens are less likely to be contaminated by upper airway organisms.

Management

Treatment is with appropriate antibiotics, combined with identifying and dealing with any risk factors for infection.

Prevention

- There are small trials showing benefit of decontaminating the GI with oral neomycin or Colomycin® in reducing risk of VAP in children. Sucralfate may help by reducing the likelihood of gastro-oesophageal reflux.
- Use of intermittent rather than continuous feeds may decrease gastric bacterial colonization.

Empyema

Empyema is a rare but well recognized complication of bacterial pneumonia in children. It is defined as the presence of pus in the pleural cavity.

Pathophysiology

Under normal circumstances

- The pleural membranes are separated by a small volume of fluid (0.3mL/kg body weight) with few cells.
- There is a continuous pleural circulation with secretion from apically placed lymphatic channels and absorption through lymphatic pores at the base of the thorax.
- The circulation can cope with greatly increased fluid production.

With infection

- Pleural inflammation leads to an influx of inflammatory cells mediated by cytokines released from mesothelial cells.
- This leads to increased permeability of adjacent capillaries, an increase in pleural fluid production, and the invasion of bacteria across damaged pleural surface.
- A coagulation cascade is activated causing pro-coagulant activity and decreased fibrinolysis leading to deposition of fibrin.
- The pleural lymphatic pores block with debris and inhibit lymphatic drainage.
- Fibrinous stands forming within the pleural fluid further impair the pleural circulation.

The process described above is a continuum and can progress very rapidly. Classically, the effusion is described as being in one of 3 stages.
- Exudative: the underlying pneumonia leads to an inflammatory process with clear, low cellularity fluid in the pleural space.
- Fibropurulent: the fluid thickens due to increased white cell content and becomes overt pus. There is deposition of fibrin in the pleural space leading to septation and loculation.
- Organizational: fibroblasts infiltrate the pleural space and the thin intrapleural fibrin membranes are reorganized into thick non-elastic pleural 'peels'.

Incidence and aetiology

- In the 1990s it was estimated that approximately 0.6% of childhood pneumonias progressed to empyema, giving an incidence of 3.3 per 100 000 children. However, there is good evidence of an increase in empyema in the UK and USA over the past 15 years.
- *Streptococcus pneumoniae* infection remains the most common cause in the developing world.
- Several studies have shown that capsular serotype 1 *Streptococcus pneumoniae* predominates currently and this serotype is not included in the 7-valent pneumococcal infant vaccine.
- *Staphylococcus aureus* remains the most common causative organism in the developing world and TB should also be considered.

Clinical features

- The child presents with symptoms of pneumonia: fever, cough, breathlessness, lethargy, malaise, and exercise intolerance.
- Small parapneumonic effusions are not uncommon and many resolve but warning signs that the parapneumonic effusion is evolving include:
  - swinging fevers;
  - increased dyspnoea;
  - pleuritic chest pain;
  - scoliosis towards the affected side.
- Examination of a child with a pleural effusion reveals:
  - reduced chest expansion;
  - diminished breath sounds;
  - dullness to percussion (stony dull).

Investigations and diagnosis

- Blood culture yields higher than in children with simple pneumonia (10% versus 6.4%).
- Pleural fluid when (if) obtained should be sent for culture and pneumococcal PCR if molecular techniques are available.

CXR (Figs 18.1 and 18.2)

- Shows the extent of the pneumonia and reveals parapneumonic fluid.
- Erect radiograph. Earliest sign is obliteration of the costophrenic angle and a rim of fluid ascending the lateral chest wall (meniscus sign).
- Supine radiograph. May reveal homogeneous increase in opacity over the whole lung field.
- If CXR shows complete 'white out' on one side, it is not always possible to distinguish a completely consolidated lung from a large effusion.
- Radiographs can show whether parapneumonic effusions are changing in size but cannot differentiate an empyema from a parapneumonic effusion.

Chest ultrasonography (Fig. 18.3)

This non-invasive technique is safe, rapid, readily available, requires no sedation, and can be performed at the bedside if necessary. It can:

- size the effusion;
- describe the fluid collection, e.g. clear, hyperechogenic, septated;
- differentiate free from loculated fluid;
- identify pleural thickening;
- permit directional chest tube insertion;
- be repeated as necessary.

Ultrasound appearance is poorly predictive of response to treatment.

CT of the chest

- Not helpful in differentiating between empyema and parapneumonic effusion.
- Radiation dose, depending on technique, is the equivalent of 20–400 CXRs.
- With contrast enhancement it can delineate loculated collections and reveal a lung abscess or mediastinal pathology.
- Valuable in complicated cases not responding to treatment but does not alter management if used routinely.

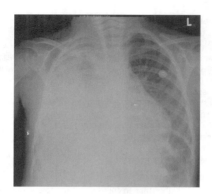

Fig. 18.1 CXR showing large empyema.

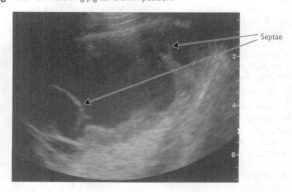

Fig. 18.2 CXR showing pig-tail drain in position.

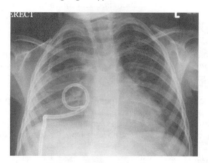

Fig. 18.3 Ultrasound examination showing fluid collection with septation.

Management

The aims of treating empyema are to stop sepsis thus halting the associated inflammatory cascade, and to restore pleural fluid circulation.

Antibiotics
- Antibiotics should be given promptly, IV, and in high dosage.
- Broad-spectrum antibiotics covering the likely organisms, i.e. *S. pneumoniae* and *S. aureus*, should be used.
- Children at risk of aspiration should be covered for anaerobic infection.
- Doses should be high to ensure pleural penetration.

Conservative treatment

Traditionally children with empyema have been treated with antibiotics alone or in combination with simple chest drainage and those failing to improve on this regimen have gone on to an open surgical procedure. Data from many studies indicate a need for surgery in 25–30% and a prolonged hospital stay of 2–3 weeks.

Fibrinolysis (see box)
- There is good evidence that fibrinolytics have a high success rate and reduce hospital stay.
- Urokinase and altepase (tPa) are the most commonly used agents.
- Small-sized soft percutaneous chest drains are used.
- Success rates (judged by no need for surgical intervention) are 90–98%.
- Median hospital stay post-procedure is 5–10 days.

Video-assisted thorascopic surgery (VATS)
- Early thoracotomy using a VATS technique has gained popularity amongst surgeons.
- Postoperative chest drainage averages 3–5 days.
- Median hospital stay is 5–10 days post-procedure.
- Success rate (judged as no further surgical procedure) is 85–100%.
- Operative morbidity is low.
- VATS is an expensive procedure.

Fibrinolysis versus VATS
- Fibrinolytics and VATS are effective and equally efficient in terms of early discharge from hospital.
- The only head to head RCT gives equal failure rates.
- Cost-effectiveness favours fibrinolysis.

Discharge criteria
- Drain removal and discharge should be considered:
  - when apyrexial (temperature < 37.5°C) for 24h; *and*
  - there is minimal pleural drainage (< 100mL/24h).
- The CXR may look very abnormal at discharge but is dramatically improved at 6–8 weeks follow-up.
- Oral antibiotics should be continued for at least 1 week postdischarge.

Outcome

The outcome is excellent. Pleural thickening may persist with gradual improvement over months. Long-term lung function is normal.

Suggested fibrinolytic protocol

- Insert small percutaneous chest drain (10–12FG)
- Urokinase 40 000units in 40mL saline (10 000units in 10mL if < 10kg) given 12 hourly via drain
- Clamp drain and encourage mobility for 4h after urokinase insertion
- Drain on suction −20cmH$_2$O pressure for next 8h
- For pain relief use oral NSAIDs plus bupivacaine (0.25%, 0.5mL/kg) given through the pleural drain with the urokinase

Further information
Balfour-Lynn, I.M., Abrahamson, E., Cohen, G., *et al.* (2005). BTS guidelines for management of pleural infection in children. *Thorax* **60** (Suppl.), 1–21.

Lung abscess

- Lung abscess is formed when there is either destruction of lung tissue by infection or where infection occurs in a pre-existing cavity. Lung destruction resulting in abscess formation is part of the same pathological process that is involved in necrotizing pneumonia.
- In previously normal children, lung abscesses are most commonly caused by *S. aureus*. *S. pyogenes*, or *S pneumoniae* and more rarely by *Klebsiella pneumoniae* and *Pseudomonas aeruginosa*.
- In children prone to aspiration—those with weakness, incoordinate oropharyngeal movements, altered consciousness, or abnormal airway anatomy—the most likely causative organisms are anaerobes from the mouth such as *Bacteroides*, *Fusobacterium* species, *Peptostreptococcus*, and microaerophilic streptococcus.
- Lung abscess may follow inhalation of a foreign body, usually after a period of some weeks.
- Lung abscess may indicate the presence of an underlying congenital lung anomaly, usually a CCAM.
- Mycobacteria, usually tuberculosis, can cause cavitation that resembles abscess formation. Histoplasmosis can also cause cavity formation.
- Rare causes include parasitic infection with hydatid, and invasive aspergillus infection in the severely immunocompromised.

Symptoms and signs

- In most instances the affected child will be previously normal and will present with a severe pneumonia that fails to resolve on appropriate IV antibiotics.
- In children with chronic aspiration lung abscess may cause a low grade illness that persists for several days or weeks before it is recognized. The presence of poor dental hygiene may increase the risk of lung abscess formation in these children.
- Typical findings will be:
  - fever;
  - increased respiratory rate;
  - dullness to percussion with quiet breath sounds.

Investigations

- Lung abscesses are often visible on CXR if there is an air–fluid level (Figs 18.5 and 18.6).
- CT scans are required for definitive diagnosis, particularly to differentiate between lung abscess and empyema with bronchopleural fistula. Typically the CT will show a thick-walled abscess cavity containing mobile fluid. The abscess will be within consolidated lung if it is secondary to pneumonia. CT may also identify predisposing causes such as airway obstruction by a foreign body.
- Blood cultures, as with other bacterial lung infections, are usually negative. Pus obtained by transthoracic aspiration of the abscess will identify the causative organism in around 60% of cases.
- If there is a possibility of inhaled foreign body, bronchoscopy will be necessary to identify and remove it.

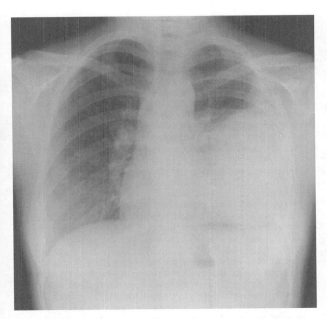

Fig. 18.4 CXR of a 12-year-old girl showing a large left-sided lung abscess.

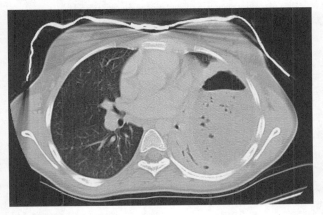

Fig. 18.5 CT scan of the same child showing a thick-walled abscess with an air–fluid level and a collapsed left lower lobe.

Management

- Traditionally the treatment for lung abscess has been prolonged antibiotic therapy. This is effective in 90% of children, although many remain febrile for 2 weeks or more.
- Attempts to drain the abscess have previously thought to carry a high risk of converting the abscess to a pyo-pneumothorax and broncho-pleural fistula, which can persist for several weeks. There are now increasing numbers of reports of success using percutaneous drainage using small percutaneous pigtail catheters. Primary drainage is associated with quicker resolution of fever and shorter hospital stay. There are no reports of pigtail drains resulting in bronchopleural fistula.
- It now seems reasonable to offer either approach:
  - primary drainage using a 10F pigtail catheter combined with IV antibitoics. For some abscesses the drain will need to be placed with CT guidance. The abscess is drained for 2–3 days (no suction, no urokinase) with the expectation of resolution of fever and discharge home within 5–7 days.
  - conservative treatment with IV antibiotics for 1–4 weeks followed by a further 2–4 weeks oral treatment. If the fever fails to settle after 2 weeks, drainage should be considered.
- Antibiotic choice will depend on local practice. Most of the anaerobic bacteria that cause lung abscess are penicillin-sensitive. A common choice of IV therapy would be high dose second generation cephalosporin to cover anaerobes, *S. aureus*, and streptococci. Other combinations that have been used successfully include cefotaxime plus flucloxacillin. Clinda-mycin has theoretical benefits of good tissue penetration and may also be continued orally after the IV stage of treatment; it has also been used successfully. Other oral antibiotics that could be considered for the oral phase of treatment include second generation cephalosporin, co-amoxiclav, or a macrolide.
- Decompression of the abscess may be required acutely in the rare situation when abscess is large enough to cause significant airway compression or mediastinal shift.

Outcome

- Outcome in otherwise healthy children is usually excellent with full clinical, functional, and radiological resolution with whichever treatment regime is used. CT scan 4–6 months after clinical resolution will identify any underlying lung anomaly, which, if present, should usually be excised.
- More rarely, usually in children with comorbidity, there may be perma-nent destruction of lung tissue, which may become a site for subsequent infection. Surgical resection of this part of the lung should then be considered.

Further information

Patradoon-Ho, P. and Fitzgerald, D.A. (2007). Lung abscess in children. *Paediatr. Respir. Rev.* **8** (1), 67–76.

Zuhdi, M.K., Spear, R.M., Worthen, H.M., and Peterson, B.M. (1996). Percutaneous catheter drainage of tension pneumatocele, secondarily infected pneumatocele, and lung abscess in children. *Crit. Care Med.* **24**, 330–3.

Viral infections

The common cold

- Recurrent viral infection of the pharynx, nasal passages, and ears occurs in all children.
- Symptoms include:
  - nasal discharge, which is initially clear and profuse and which becomes thicker and yellow or green after a few days;
  - sneezing;
  - painful throat;
  - sore ears;
  - fever may be present, and is commoner under the age of 4 years;
  - headache and malaise;
  - dry cough can occur, from stimulation of cough receptors in the pharynx. A productive sounding cough indicates LRTI.
- Signs include:
  - often nothing to find;
  - a reddened pharynx, sometimes with pus;
  - bilateral injection of the tympanic membranes.
- Symptoms usually persist for 7 days, although in young children they may continue for 2 weeks.
- Yellow or green discharge reflects the presence of neutrophils (the colour is derived from neutrophil myeloperoxidase, an iron-containing enzyme) and not bacteria. Neutrophils are attracted to the upper airway by virus-induced cytokine release.
- Epidemiological surveys have indicated that children between 1 and 5 years of age suffer an average of 6–8 viral URTIs each year and some have as many as 12. Attendance at day care is a risk factor. The number of infections decreases after 5 years of age, and adolescents and adults have 2–4 colds per year.
- The commonest causative virus is rhinovirus. Others include enteroviruses, coronaviruses, respiratory syncytial virus (RSV), human metapneumovirus (HMP), human bocavirus (a new parvovirus identified in 2005), and parainfluenza viruses (PIV). Adenovirus and influenza virus are also common but usually cause more severe illness.
- Infection is spread by droplets or direct contact, and the incubation period is usually between 2 and 4 days.
- There is no evidence that exposure to cold wet conditions predisposes to URTI.
- Colds are commoner in the winter months in temperate climates, when RSV, HMP, and PIV are the usual causes, but can occur at any time of year.
- No investigations are required.
- There is no effective treatment.

Croup

- Croup or laryngotracheobronchitis is caused by viral infection of the supraglottic, glottic, and subglottic airway.
- Parainfluenza viruses are responsible for 75% of croup episodes. The remainder are caused by any of the other respiratory viruses. *Mycoplasma pneumoniae* may rarely cause croup.
- Croup tends to occur in epidemics in the autumn and winter in temperate climates.
- Most affected children will have their first episode of croup before the age of 5 years, with a peak incidence at around 2 years of age.
- Croup is common and up to 5% of 2-year-olds will have at least one episode for which their parents seek medical attention. Most episodes are mild and only a minority of affected children require hospital treatment.
- Symptoms arise because of narrowing of the subglottic space caused by viral-induced inflammation and oedema. Young children are probably principally affected because narrowing caused by airway wall swelling has a proportionately greater effect on airways resistance when the starting airway size is small.

Symptoms and signs

Croup usually starts with a coryzal illness, often with a fever that is usually low grade but can be as high as 40°C. After 1–2 days croup symptoms develop and usually last 3–7 days, but occasionally persist for as long as 2 weeks. Typical symptoms are:
- hoarse voice;
- barking cough;
- stridor.

Signs are those of subglottic airway obstruction with respiratory distress.
- Stridor, usually inspiratory but biphasic in severe disease.
- Chest wall recession.
- Tachypnoea and tachycardia.
- Desaturation can occur and, in the context of a child with marked respiratory distress, is an ominous sign since it indicates hypoventilation and accompanying CO_2 retention. Urgent steps should be taken to improve the airway in children with hypoxia. Giving oxygen alone will not prevent a respiratory arrest. Occasionally hypoxia will be seen in children with only mild respiratory distress, possibly reflecting secretion retention, patchy atelectasis, and resulting ventilation perfusion mismatch.

A number of croup scores are available to indicate croup severity. They are useful in research studies but of limited value in clinical practice.

Spasmodic croup

The term spasmodic croup is used for children who present with croup-like episodes that typically come on suddenly without preceding coryzal illness. Attacks often occur at night. Affected children tend to be older than those with typical croup and are more likely to have recurrent episodes. Recovery is usually quicker, and often symptoms have gone within 12h. Children with spasmodic croup are said to be more likely to be atopic and this has led to speculation that the airway oedema arises through allergy-mediated inflammation. The treatment of each episode is identical to that of other forms of croup.

Differential diagnosis

The differential diagnosis for a child with new onset stridor includes other causes of acute airways obstruction and causes of pre-existing airway narrowing that have become more obvious during an acute viral respiratory tract infection. In practice the diagnosis is usually straightforward in a previously well child who has a typical clinical course. When the illness is atypical, e.g. in children > 5 years of age or with significant systemic illness, or without a coryzal prodrome, or with pre-existing noisy breathing, other causes should be considered.

Other causes of acute airways obstruction are the following.

- Laryngeal oedema caused by:
  - bacterial infection—epiglottitis or tracheitis;
  - irritants—aspirated caustic chemicals or smoke;
  - allergy—anaphylactic reactions;
  - C1 esterase deficiency—angioedema.
- Laryngeal foreign body. Fortunately this is rare. Objects small enough to fit through the vocal cords are usually small enough to pass to the main bronchi. Linear foreign bodies such as fish bones may become lodged in the larynx and still allow some air entry and cause croup-like symptoms. Larger objects such as grapes will usually cause complete laryngeal obstruction.
- Airway compression by:
  - retropharyngeal abscess;
  - haemorrhage into cystic hygroma;
  - mediastinal lymph nodes, usually in the context of lymphoma;
  - trauma.

Possible pre-existing conditions are:

- subglottic stenosis;
- tracheal haemangioma;
- vascular ring.

Investigation

- For typical episodes of croup, no investigations are required. The diagnosis is clinical.
- The commonest clinical question is whether children who have either prolonged illness or recurrent episodes of croup have underlying pre-disposing conditions requiring evaluation by bronchoscopy.
  - In practice when there are no interval symptoms (i.e. between episodes of croup or before the current episode started, the child had completely quiet breathing, even on exertion, and a normal voice) the likelihood of detecting any important airway pathology is extremely low, and bronchoscopy is not required.

- An exception to this rule is when 'croup' occurs in infants < 6 months of age. This group has a higher likelihood of underlying airway pathology.
- As in all children, where there is doubt, the safest option is always to look.

Treatment

- Most children have mild disease with a barking cough and a runny nose. There may be mild chest wall retractions but the child is otherwise well and there is no stridor at rest. These children can be looked after at home. No specific treatment is needed, although regular paracetamol may be helpful if there is fever or a sore throat. Use of a single dose of oral corticosteroids is optional and varies with local practice. Parents should be warned that the disease can worsen, particularly at night, and that medical review may be required.
- Children with moderate disease, characterized by stridor at rest, benefit from a dose of systemic (oral in most cases) corticosteroids (either 0.15mg/kg dexamethasone or 1mg/kg prednisolone; dexamethasone is more effective with lower rates of re-presentation to emergency departments). These children need to be observed in hospital until the stridor at rest has resolved. In some children this will happen within 4h, although the average is closer to 7h.
- Children with severe disease, with stridor at rest associated with marked chest wall recession and tachycardia, should be treated with nebulized adrenaline plus systemic corticosteroids. Despite concerns in the past, there is no evidence that adrenaline results in worsening rebound of symptoms when its effects wear off. Using adrenaline improves the airway and gives time for the corticosteroids to work. A number of studies have shown that children showing significant improvement can be safely discharged from the emergency department 3–4h after being given nebulized adrenaline.
- Standard L-adrenaline, available in most hospitals, seems to work as well as racemic adrenaline. The usual dose of L-adrenaline is 0.5mL/kg of 1 in 1000 adrenaline nebulized neat, up to a maximum of 5mL. It can be repeated after 30min. The effects last 2–3h.
- Humidified air does not help in moderate and severe croup. There are insufficient data on mild croup to be able to tell if it has an effect or not. Use of steam at home can be hazardous. Overall the balance is in favour of not using it.
- Nebulized budesonide has an onset of action within 30min compared to 60min for oral dexamethasone. It is slightly less effective and more expensive.

Outcome

- In the vast majority of children croup is a mild disease with an excellent outcome. For most children symptoms will have sufficiently improved to allow discharge from hospital within 24h. In others stridor at rest can persist for as long as 2 weeks.
- Deaths from airway obstruction at home are now very rare.

- Up to 20% of children will have recurrent episodes. In the absence of interval symptoms, no further investigation is usually required.
- In about 1 in 50 children admitted to hospital with croup, airway obstruction progresses despite treatment. These children become agitated and poorly perfused associated with worsening hypercarbia and hypoxia. Intubation is required. Once intubated ventilation requirements are usually minimal. Occasionally negative pressure pulmonary oedema can complicate severe croup. Mean duration of intubation is 5–7 days. Most units will use daily corticosteroids in this group of children and wait for a leak to develop around the endotracheal tube before extubation. If extubation fails, subsequent attempts should be carried out in an operating theatre with an ENT surgeon available to inspect the airway to determine if there is significant underlying pathology.

Further information

Moore, M and Little P. (2006). Humidified air inhalation for treating croup. *Cochrane Database Syst. Rev.* **2006** (3), CD002870.

Fitzgerald, D.A. (2006) The assessment and management of croup. *Paediatr. Respir. Rev.* **7** (1), 73–81.

Sparrow, A. and Geelhoed, G. (2006). Prednisolone versus dexamethasone in croup: a randomised equivalence trial. *Arch. Dis. Child.* **91** (7), 580–3.

Juvenile onset recurrent respiratory papillomatosis

Epidemiology

- Juvenile onset recurrent respiratory papillomatosis (JORRP) is caused by infection with the human papilloma virus (HPV), usually HPV subtypes 6 or 11. HPV-11 is associated with more aggressive disease.
- It is relatively rare, with a childhood incidence of 4–5/100 000.
- The majority of children present before the age of 5 years and, of these, 25% develop symptoms in infancy. It can rarely present in adolescence. The adult form of the disease is most common in the 3rd decade of life.
- Infection is thought to be acquired from the genital tract of infected mothers at the time of delivery. Disease in adolescence and adulthood is probably acquired through sexual activity.
- Risk factors for acquiring disease are:
  - mother with active genital condylomata (warts);
  - teenage mother;
  - first born child;
  - vaginal delivery.
- In 50% of children the papillomata are confined to the larynx, most around the vocal folds. In the remainder, infection can spread to the lower airways and lung parenchyma.
- The papillomata are benign neoplasms. There is an undefined risk of malignant transformation to squamous cell carcinoma. For disease limited to the upper airway, risk is low (< 5%). The risk is probably higher in the more aggressive disease that has spread to the lower airway.

Symptoms and signs

- Usual symptoms are hoarseness and/or stridor.
- Decompensation of a compromised airway may occur over a few days and children may present with acute severe respiratory distress. These children can have a nearly complete occluded larynx and require emergency tracheostomy.
- There is often a delay in diagnosis—an average of just over 12 months.
- Other modes of presentation include:
  - cough;
  - recurrent pneumonia;
  - dysphagia;
  - failure to thrive.

Differential diagnosis

The differential for child with stridor with/without hoarse voice includes:
- vocal cord palsy, caused by trauma, malignancy, or brainstem compression;
- recurrent croup;
- vascular ring;
- airway haemangioma;
- cystic hygroma;

- laryngeal web;
- subglottic stenosis.

These children may also have been misdiagnosed as having asthma or recurrent chest infection.

Investigations

- Diagnosis is made by laryngoscopy revealing typical cauliflower-like warts. If laryngeal papillomata are seen, further instrumentation of the airway should be avoided to prevent dissemination of the disease.
- Biopsy of one of the lesions will allow histological confirmation of papilloma and to look for malignant change. PCR or the tissue can be used to identify and type the virus.
- CXR is usually normal. It may show small nodules if there is disease in the lung parenchyma. If a bronchus has become obstructed there may areas of collapse or consolidation.
- CT of the chest can be useful in identifying papillomata in the trachea and bronchi and within the lung parenchyma. Healed papillomata can appear as cystic lesions.
- If there is extensive lower airway disease, investigations to exclude immunodeficiency should be carried out.
- A staging system is available and can help to track response to treatment. It assesses symptoms (stridor and hoarseness) frequency of recurrence, and number and distribution of lesions (graded as surface raised or bulky).

Treatment

- Treatment is difficult because of the propensity of the papillomata to recur. The rate and frequency of recurrence varies widely. Some children need only 1–2 excision procedures per year, others need treatment every few weeks.
- Tracheostomy should be avoided if possible because of risk of spreading the disease into the lower trachea. If a tracheostomy is needed it should be removed as soon as the airway has been made safe
- The most widely used treatment is surgical excision. The goals of treatment are to provide a safe airway whilst preserving the voice. Excision can be by direct resection or with a CO_2 laser. If a laser is used special precautions must be used to protect staff from the virus which can be released into the air during the procedure.
- Eradication by surgery is not possible and overly aggressive surgery can lead to permanent damage to the airway or voice.
- Adjuvant therapy is needed in around 10% of children. It should be considered if:
  - more than 4 surgical procedures are needed each year;
  - there is significant disease in the lower airways or lung parenchyma;
  - there is rapid re-growth with airway compromise.

- Alpha-interferon, given daily for 1 month, then 3 times per week for 6 months, can reduce the severity of the disease during treatment, but the papillomata often recur once treatment has stopped. Alternatives include indole-3-carbinol and cidofovir. The long-term safety of cidofovir is not known but it does seem to be effective in some children, given either IV or as intralesional injections, when other treatments have failed.

Prevention

- Delivery by Caesarean section in women with active genital condylomata probably reduces risk, but does not prevent the disease completely.
- Vaccination of women against HPV is the most likely effective treatment. Effective vaccines have been developed against HPV-16 and HPV-18, the 2 most common subtypes associated with cervical cancer.

Outcome

- Short- and medium-term quality of life for children with frequently recurring disease is poor. Multiple hospital visits for treatment severely disrupt family life and education.
- Remission can occur after several years, usually around the time of puberty.
- A small proportion of children will develop malignant squamous cell carcinoma, which has a poor prognosis.

Further information

Shah, K.V., Stern, W.F., Shah, F.K., Bishai, D., and Kashima, H.K. (1998). Risk factors for juvenile onset recurrent respiratory papillomatosis. *Pediatr. Infect. Dis. J.* **17**, 372–6.

Acute viral bronchiolitis

Acute viral bronchiolitis is an LRTI of infants characterized by:
- preceding coryzal symptoms;
- progressive breathlessness with associated poor feeding;
- cough;
- evidence of respiratory distress, including chest wall recession and desaturation;
- presence of inspiratory crepitations and/or wheeze on auscultation of the chest.

Pathophysiology

Viral infection of the lower airways provokes a host response that results in airway oedema, the production of inflammatory exudate, increased airway mucus, and a varying degree of bronchospasm. Taken together these result in obstruction of the small airways and increased respiratory work.

Epidemiology

- The majority (60–70%) of episodes of bronchiolitis are caused by the respiratory syncytial virus (RSV). Other viruses that can cause bronchiolitis are human metapneumovirus (HMP), adenovirus, influenza virus, parainfluenza virus (PIV), and human bocavirus (HBoV).
- RSV bronchiolitis is the single most important cause of severe LRTI in infants worldwide. The WHO estimates that 64 million children suffer from the infection each year of whom 160 000 die.
- In industrialized countries, 1–3% of infected infants develop severe bronchiolitis and need hospital admission, usually for oxygen therapy and assistance with feeding.
- In temperate climates, bronchiolitis occurs in winter epidemics. In tropical climates, bronchiolitis occurs year round but is more prevalent in the rainy season.
- The mean age of affected infants is 4–6 months with an equal sex incidence.
- In developing countries RSV accounts for ca. 40% of LRTI in infants.
- RSV is highly infectious and nearly all children will have been infected by the virus by the end of their second RSV season. Spread is by respiratory droplets or direct contact with respiratory secretions. The first member of most households who becomes infected is a child attending daycare or school. If there is an infant in the family, their likelihood of becoming infected after the virus is introduced is around 60–70%.
- Nearly all infants will be symptomatic with coryzal symptoms and 50–80% will develop a cough. 1–3% will develop more severe lower respiratory tract disease requiring hospital admission.
- The incubation period for RSV bronchiolitis is 3–7 days. Duration of viral shedding is variable. In infants, shedding lasts on average for 10 days, but may continue for as long as 30 days. In older children and adults, duration of viral shedding is shorter (2–4 days) but again occasionally can be prolonged.

- Some of the known risk factors for developing severe bronchiolitis are:
  - prematurity (probably because of lack of transfer of passive immunity in the third trimester);
  - pre-existing heart or lung disease;
  - older siblings and attendance at daycare—resulting in exposure to a higher viral load;
  - parental smoking.
- Viral strain (RSV A compared to RSV B) does not seem to be important in determining disease severity.
- Most infants who are admitted to hospital with severe disease are previously healthy infants born at full term, and the reasons why these infants develop severe disease are not fully understood. Genetic predisposition may play a role.
- Following severe bronchiolitis 60% of infants will have subsequent wheezing episodes. In most studies the effect of previous bronchiolitis on the risk of wheezing is lost by the age of 5–12 years. The interaction between early bronchiolitis and subsequent atopy is controversial and a topic of active research.

Clinical features

- The typical history is of a young infant who develops a 'snuffly' nose with some nasal discharge and sneezing. This progresses to episodes of coughing and fast breathing that together prevent normal feeding. There may be a fever but this is not always present.
- In infants under 6 weeks, and older infants who were born prematurely, there is a risk of apnoea, which may be the presenting problem before there is noticeable respiratory distress.
- Examination will usually show:
  - evidence of respiratory distress (tachypnoea, chest wall recession, use of accessory muscles, tachycardia);
  - desaturation, which is common in infants with bronchiolitis severe enough to cause chest wall recession;
  - fever, usually low grade (< 38.5°C);
  - inspiratory crepitations on auscultation, with or without expiratory wheeze.

Differential diagnosis

- Relatively rapid onset of respiratory distress in infants is likely to be caused by infection in a previously normal child. Occasionally there will be an important underlying cause that may first come to medical attention as an apparent episode of bronchiolitis. These conditions include:
  - heart failure—usually associated with a left to right shunt, and more rarely with supraventricular tachycardia or a cardiomyopathy;
  - cystic fibrosis;
  - immune deficiency, often severe combined immunodeficiency;
  - congenital lung anomaly such as congenital lobar emphysema.
- Careful evaluation of the infant's health before the acute episode may give clues to a pre-existing condition. When these are present, affected infants usually take longer to recover. Infants with prolonged or recurrent episodes of 'bronchiolitis' should be subject to further investigation.

Investigations

- Bronchiolitis is a clinical diagnosis. No investigations are needed routinely.
- Nasopharyngeal aspirates can be used to identify the causative virus. Analysis can be by ELISA, PCR, or cell culture. Multiplex PCR can assess for several viruses in the same test. Identifying the causative virus can provide some reassurance of the likely clinical course but given that RSV is highly prevalent, finding it in the upper respiratory tract does not mean that it is the sole cause of the infant's respiratory distress. Viral identification can be useful in cohorting infected infants within hospitals and identifying new infection acquired after admission.
- CXR is not needed routinely as it will not affect management. Where the illness is atypical or prolonged, CXR may help identify underlying pathology. If CXR is performed, findings consistent with bronchiolitis include:
  - hyperinflation;
  - patchy atelectasis;
  - perihilar bronchial wall thickening.
- Blood investigations are not normally required. Blood gas analysis will be needed in infants who are struggling despite supplementary O_2. The point at which the CO_2 and pH are checked will vary with local practice, but will usually be required in infants needing more than 50% O_2.

Treatment

- Hospital treatment will be needed for infants who are too breathless to feed or who are hypoxic (saturations < 92%) in room air. Hospital admission should also be considered in less ill infants who are at heightened risk of developing severe disease, e.g. those born prematurely, those with pre-existing heart or lung disease, and those < 12 weeks of age.
- No intervention has been shown to shorten the illness. Treatment is supportive.
- Feeding assistance is given by tube feeds or IV fluids. Choice depends on local practice and disease severity. Some infants who are unable to feed will tolerate tube feeds (ideally orogastric rather than NG). When respiratory distress is severe, tube feeding can make it worse and increase the risk of aspiration. At this point IV fluids will be needed.
- Oxygen can be given by nasal cannulae or, if high concentrations are needed, by head-box (see 📖 Chapter 56).
- Sick infants with bronchiolitis (as with other acute conditions) should be handled as little as possible. Being placed in the prone position seems to reduce respiratory workload for some infants.
- The use of inhaled beta-2 agonists and anti-cholinergic agent has been the subject of a Cochrane review.[1] Neither is recommended for routine use. In older infants (> 8 months) with coryza and wheeze there is an overlap between true bronchiolitis (an LRTI) and wheeze associated with a viral URTI. In this group it may be reasonable to try a bronchodilator and observe for benefit.

1 Kellner J.D., Ohlsson, A., Gadomski, A.M., and Wang, E.E. (2000). Bronchodilators for bronchiolitis. *Cochrane Database Syst. Rev.* **2000** (2), CD001266.

- Nebulized adrenaline does seem to have short-term benefit, with temporary improvement in oxygen saturation and reduction of respiratory effort. There is no effect on duration of illness or need for mechanical ventilation. On this basis, it is not recommended for routine use. It may be of some value in sick infants whilst arrangements are made for review by ICU staff.
- Corticosteroids, either orally or inhaled, do not affect the course of the acute disease, nor the likelihood of subsequent wheezing illness and their use is not indicated.
- Nebulized ribavirin is effective at killing RSV and reducing viral load in infected infants. Unfortunately, it does not significantly affect the clinical course of the illness, and this combined with difficulties of administration (it needs to be nebulized 18h in every 24h) means that it is not used routinely. In some high risk patients, particularly those with immunodeficiency, it still has a role.
- Antibiotics are not indicated routinely. The rate of dual infection with a bacterial pathogen is low. The presence of patchy consolidation on CXR is *not* an indication for prescribing antibiotics. In infants requiring mechanical ventilation, BAL studies have indicated the presence of lower airway bacteria in 20% of intubated infants, and antibiotics are routinely prescribed for ventilated infants with bronchiolitis in some ICUs. Incidental serious bacterial infection, most commonly UTI, can occur in infants with bronchiolitis, usually in the context of unusual or persistent fever. For these infants further investigation will be required.
- Nasal CPAP seems to be beneficial in some infants with severe disease in terms of reducing respiratory work and O_2 requirement. Whether it reduces the need for intubation and ventilation has not been subject to an RCT.
- Mechanical ventilation is needed in a small proportion of infants. Indications are either recurrent apnoea or respiratory failure despite 60% head-box oxygen. Duration of ventilation varies, but is typically 2–5 days.

Outcome
- Outcome is usually excellent. Duration of hospital treatment is around 3 days. Some infants have mild hypoxia during feeds or sleep, which can persist for several days after their oxygen saturation during wakefulness has returned to normal and after they have otherwise recovered. It is safe to stop monitoring saturations in these babies and allow them to go home.
- 30–60% of infants who have had severe bronchiolitis will have subsequent episodes of wheeze. Whether these episodes are causally related to the bronchiolitis or represent a shared predisposition remains unclear.
- Deaths from bronchiolitis are rare in developed countries, and when they occur nearly always do so in children with underlying heart or lung disease.
- Rarely severe bronchiolitis/pneumonitis is associated with post-infectious bronchiolitis obliterans. This is more common with adenoviral infection (see 📖 p. 222).

- Infection with RSV does not generate protective immunity and repeat infections are common. Subsequent infections are usually milder. It is possible, but unusual, for an infant to have 2 distinct episodes of bronchiolitis in a single season.

Prevention

- Strict hand-washing in hospital is required to prevent spread. RSV is easily killed by alcohol and cannot survive for more than a few minutes on dry surfaces.
- Vulnerable babies in hospital and at home should be protected from overattentive coryzal siblings.
- Programmes to develop an RSV vaccine have been active for many years. They suffered a major setback in the 1960s when a formalin-inactivated vaccine resulted in enhanced disease. Newer live vaccines given via the nasal route do seem to provide protection, but not without causing some symptoms themselves. None have yet been licensed.
- Passive immunization with humanized anti-RSV monoclonal antibody (palivizumab) reduces risk of severe disease by 50% in high-risk children. No studies have been powered to detect an effect on mortality. Monthly injections are given for 5 months in temperate climates to provide protection through the RSV season.

Further inforrmation

Monto, A.S. (2002). Epidemiology of viral respiratory infections. *Am. J. Med.* **112** (Suppl. 6A), 4S–12S.
American Academy of Pediatrics (2006). Diagnosis and management of bronchiolitis. *Pediatrics* **118**, 1774–93.

Viral pneumonia

- The terms pneumonia and pneumonitis are often used interchangeably to indicate infection of the lung parenchyma. When CXR findings show areas of consolidation the term pneumonia tends to be used, whereas when there are streaky interstitial changes pneumonitis is more often used. Both patterns can be seen in children with viral LRTI. The distinction between viral bronchiolitis and viral pneumonia is also arbitrary and based on CXR appearance, rather than any distinct clinical features.
- Clinical presentation of viral pneumonia does not differ from other community-acquired pneumonias (see 📖 Chapter 17).
- The likely causative viruses are:
  - RSV;
  - parainfluenza virus;
  - influenza virus;
  - adenovirus;
  - human metapneumovirus;
  - human bocavirus;
  - corona virus.
- In children with immunodeficiency CMV and (to a lesser extent) EBV are also important causes of pneumonia.
- NPA analysed by PCR is the most likely method of successfully identifying the causative virus.
- CXR findings are non-specific. Findings nearly always affect more than one lobe, and commonly changes are seen in all lobes. Possible findings include:
  - perihilar bronchial wall thickening;
  - air-trapping with evidence of hyperinflation;
  - airspace disease with areas of consolidation;
  - streaky interstitial changes;
  - pleural effusions are rare.
- CT scans are not often performed, but may be required in the context of investigating children with respiratory disease of uncertain origin. Findings consistent with viral pneumonia are the same as those described for the CXR. In addition small airways disease may result in a mosaic appearance reflecting heterogeneous air-trapping.
- Treatment is supportive. In children with immunodeficiency, specific antiviral drugs such as ribavirin or ganciclovir may be indicated.
- Outcome is usually excellent. Rarely, persistent airway or lung damage may occur resulting in long-term oxygen requirement and wheeze (see also 📖 Chapter 36).

Cytomegalovirus pneumonia

Infection with CMV is common. The prevalence of seropositive individuals increases with age and varies widely according to socioeconomic status, race, and geographical area. In the UK about 50% of adults are infected. Recurrent infection or reactivation can also occur. The majority (95%) of infections in normal individuals are asymptomatic.

Spread of infection

Normal children

After primary infection in normal children CMV is excreted from multiple sites (e.g. tears, urine, saliva) for months to years. CMV particles can remain infectious on plastic surfaces for several hours. Toddlers in day care frequently transmit CMV to each other and to adults with whom they have contact.

Mother to infant

CMV may be transmitted across the placenta and results in congenital infection in around 1% of live born infants. The risk of infection and of symptomatic infection is highest in mothers who acquire primary CMV infection during pregnancy. Most infected infants are asymptomatic, but around 10% suffer CNS damage.

Immunocompromised children

In immunocompromised children most clinically significant CMV disease is transmitted by blood products and transplanted tissue. Re-infection with a different strain of CMV and reactivation of latent infection can both occur in the immunocompromised. Spread of CMV in hospital by other routes is rare. Risk of CMV pneumonitis depends on the cause of immunosuppression. CMV pneumonitis is:

- very common following lung transplantation. It can be difficult to sepa-rate CMV pneumonitis as a distinct infection from effects of rejection and other infections. Highest risk (90–100%) occurs when donor is CMV-positive and recipient is CMV-negative; reactivation disease in recipient CMV-positive patients with a CMV-positive or CMV-negative donor is also common (60%).
- common (10%) in allogeneic bone marrow or stem cell transplant recipients and has a high mortality (70%). Usually occurs 7–10 weeks after transplantation.
- unusual in renal and liver transplants (around 2–5%) because of prophylactic and pre-emptive treatment.
- rare and often mild in HIV infected children.
- very rare in children receiving chemotherapy for leukaemia and other childhood malignancies.

Symptoms and signs

Normal children

- CMV infection is usually clinically silent.
- When symptoms do occur, they present 9–60 days after primary infection.

- Symptomatic cases are clinically indistinguishable from EBV infection, with fatigue, fever (up to 40°C), lymphadenopathy hepatomegaly, splenomegaly, and lymphocytosis with atypical lymphocytes.
- The illness can last several weeks. Hepatitis and atypical lymphocytes usually disappear after 6 weeks.
- Lower respiratory tract involvement is very rare and if found, strongly suggests the presence of immunosuppression.

Neonates and young infants

- Congenital infection, when symptomatic, may cause intrauterine growth retardation, hepatosplenomegaly, petechiae, jaundice, microcephaly, and intracranial calcification.
- Pneumonitis as part of congenital infection is rare and when present should prompt a thorough search for other causes.
- Common laboratory abnormalities in congenital infection include hyperbilirubinaemia, increased hepatocellular enzymes, thrombocytopenia, and increased CSF protein. Neonates with symptomatic congenital infection have high rates of subsequent learning difficulties.
- Acquired disease in infancy may be similar, but with a lower incidence of CNS disturbance. Occasionally otherwise normal infants who acquire CMV infection postnatally (usually from breast milk) may present as miserable babies with tachypnoea, poor feeding, and poor weight gain. A careful search for underlying primary immunodeficiency should be made.
- Disease may be acquired from breast milk in preterm babies who are still relatively immunosuppressed.

Immunocompromised children

CMV seroconversion and excretion of CMV in body fluids is commonly found after receipt of CMV-positive transplanted tissue or blood. The occurrence and severity of disease are variable.

Important factors determining disease severity are as follows.

- Primary infection versus re-infection or reactivation. Primary infection (occurring in a previously CMV negative child) is more severe.
- Degree of immunosuppression. Patients deficient in cell-mediated immunity are at greatest risk of developing CMV disease.
- Reason for immunosuppression. Children who have had organ transplantation, especially lung and bone marrow, are at greatest risk—see above.

Symptoms and signs include:

- fever, malaise, arthralgia;
- macular rash;
- hepatosplenomegaly.

Complications include:

- retinitis;
- gastrointestinal ulceration and enterocolitis;
- hepatitis;
- pneumonitis;
- encephalitis;
- graft rejection.

Pneumonia

When it does occur, CMV pneumonia has the following characteristics.
- Breathlessness and a non-productive cough.
- Severity ranges from mild dyspnoea to severe respiratory insufficiency.
- There may be an insidious onset, in which case there may be no fever.
- Signs include tachypnoea, with or without chest wall recession and desaturation.
- Breath sounds may be normal, or there may be inspiratory crackles.
- CXR shows bilateral diffuse interstitial changes.
- CT findings are non-specific, commonly showing small nodules and patchy consolidation, particularly in the lower lobes.

Diagnosis (see box)

Diagnosis requires answers to the following 3 questions.
- Is there evidence of CMV infection?
- Is there evidence of CMV in the lungs?
- Is the CMV in the lungs causing the disease?

The answer to the first question can be obtained by looking for CMV in the urine, saliva, and blood.
- Tests for CMV include the following.
  - Culture methods, which can be combined with immunofluorescence to allow early detection (this test is sometimes called the 'shell vial' assay).
  - Detection of CMV antigen in peripheral blood mononuclear cells (PBMCs)—this test is called the pp65 antigen test. The antigenaemia test is semiquantitative, according to the proportion of PBMCs that are stained for the CMV antigen.
  - CMV PCR tests in the past had poor specificity, but now appear to be reliable and sensitive, and are often the detection method of choice.
  - Serology is generally only useful in determining previous exposure to CMV, although CMV-specific IgM has been used to indicate recent infection.
- CMV excretion in the saliva and urine is common in patients who are immunocompromised and is generally of little consequence.
- The significance of CMV viraemia depends on the context and the level of viraemia. In allogeneic marrow transplant patients, any level of viraemia is significant, warrants treatment, and will be associated with CMV pneumonia in 60–70%.
- Following organ transplant, up to 50% of patients can have low levels of viraemia. The presence of viraemia identifies those at greatest risk for CMV pneumonia. Pre-emptive treatment is started at a threshold level of CMV antigenaemia, e.g. 25 positive cells/2×10^5 PBMC.
- The absence of CMV virus in the bloodstream has a high negative predictive value for CMV disease, including pneumonia.
- Negative tests for CMV in urine do not exclude lung infection, but make it less likely.
- CMV detection in the lungs requires BAL, transbronchial biopsy, or open lung biopsy. Lower airway brushing can improve the yield of BAL alone.

- Expectorated sputum or ETT aspirates are not acceptable. They will probably be contaminated with mouth and upper respiratory tract secretions where CMV is commonly found.
- CMV may be found in the lung of 5–10% of normal adult subjects. The likelihood of CMV disease depends on the setting. Quantification of viral load using PCR techniques can also predict disease. Higher viral loads in blood and lung are more likely to be associated with pneumonia.

Prevention and treatment
- In immunosuppressed CMV-negative children CMV-negative leucocyte-depleted blood should be used.
- In transplant patients it is usually not possible to avoid CMV-positive organs because of limited supply.
- High dose prophylactic aciclovir and pre-emptive ganciclovir (when CMV is detected in routine blood samples) can be used in CMV-negative patients receiving CMV-positive tissue.
- Treatment of CMV infection is with ganciclovir, with or without CMV immunoglobulin. Both CMV infection and ganciclovir depress neutrophil count and increase risk of fungal infection. Duration of therapy is 2–5 weeks.
- Foscarnet or cidofovir can be used if ganciclovir is ineffective.

- Most methods for diagnosing CMV pneumonia have a poor positive predictive value
- In immunosuppressed children, CMV pneumonia is a diagnosis based on:
  - the clinical picture *plus*
  - pulmonary infiltrates on CXR or CT scan *plus*
  - evidence of CMV in BAL and often in the blood *plus*
  - the absence of other opportunistic pathogens such as *Pneumocystis iroveci* or *Candida* species, or EBV

Varicella pneumonia

- Primary infection with varicella zoster virus (VZV) causes clinically recognizable chickenpox in over 90% of subjects.
- The incubation period is usually 10–14 days, but can be as long as 21 days.
- Children are infectious from 1–2 days before the rash appears until the last spot has scabbed over or 5 days after the rash appeared, whichever is the longer.
- Varicella zoster spreads mainly by airborne droplets. The respiratory tract is the point of entry.
- The virus replicates in local lymph glands for several days before dissemination via the bloodstream to the viscera and skin. Spread back to the lungs occurs at this stage and the child becomes infectious through the production of varicella-containing airborne droplets.
- Primary varicella pneumonia can occur in immunocompetent individuals. It is more common in adults than children.
- Pneumonia usually occurs 2–5 days after the appearance of the rash; rarely it precedes the rash.
- The presence of pneumonia is an indication of high levels of viraemia and may be associated with other organ involvement: hepatitis; arthritis; myocarditis; encephalitis.
- Pneumonia is more likely in neonatal disease and in immunocompromised children, including those on long-term oral steroid therapy.
- Secondary bacterial infection, particularly invasive group A streptococcus and *Staphylococcus aureus*, are important alternative causes of respiratory distress in a child with chickenpox. Both can cause pneumonia and empyema.

Symptoms

Minor cough and coryza are common in chickenpox. More persistent coughing and breathlessness suggest pneumonia.

Signs

Tachypnoea and, occasionally, inspiratory crepitations. Cyanosis may be present.

Investigation

- The diagnosis of chickenpox is usually made clinically. If confirmation is required in high-risk patients, immunostaining of vesicular fluid is possible.
- When pneumonia is present, CXR will show diffuse bilateral nodular densities with bilateral linear opacities. After recovery the nodules may calcify.
- Lobar pneumonia or pleural collection is more likely to be caused by either group A streptococcus or *Staphylococcus aureus*.

Treatment

IV aciclovir for 10–14 days should be used in children with immunosuppression. Evidence of benefit in immunocompetent children is lacking, but most paediatricians would probably use it.

Prevention

- An effective vaccine is now available, and should be given to all children, when there is time, before immunosuppression occurs. In children < 13 years, a single dose is needed. For older children, 2 doses 4–8 weeks apart, should be given.
- Post-exposure zoster immune globulin (ZIG) is effective in prevention or ameliorating chickenpox when given within 72h of exposure. ZIG is in short supply in some regions and its rational use requires knowledge of the levels of anti-zoster IgG in the patient's blood. If the immune status of the child is not known, this may need to be checked before ZIG is given.

Outcome

In previously healthy children, clinically apparent pneumonia is rare and outcomes are generally good. In immunosuppressed children with varicella pneumonia, mortality can be as high as 10%.

Adenovirus pneumonia

- Large population-based surveys have suggested that adenovirus accounts for 5–10% of upper and lower respiratory tract infections in infants and children.
- Most infections are asymptomatic or very mild and by 4 years of age about half of all children will have serological evidence of previous adenovirus infection.
- Severe pneumonia can occur. It is more common in infants and in immunocompromised children, when it can be fatal.
- Infections also occur in older children and young adults, particularly in crowded, stressful conditions. Up to 20% of military recruits develop symptomatic adenoviral respiratory infection requiring hospital treatment.
- 51 different adenovirus serotypes have been described, divided into 6 subgroups, A–F, based on their DNA sequence and their ability to agglutinate erythrocytes. Immunity appears to be serotype specific.
- Adenovirus type 7 (Ad7), a group B virus, like all adenovirus types, usually causes mild URTI, but is also the most frequently isolated type from patients with severe or fatal respiratory infection.
- Adenovirus can infect epithelial cells from many different tissues, usually causing cell lysis. Occasionally chronic latent infection occurs, especially in lymphoid tissue, and adenovirus may be cultured from the pharynx and stool of asymptomatic children.

Symptoms and signs

Symptomatic adenoviral infection can cause a wide-variety of symptoms, generally not lasting more than 7 days. Infections can affect the upper and lower airway, causing simple colds, croup, bronchiolitis, or pneumonia. Most respiratory infection is caused by serotypes 3, 4, and 7. Respiratory symptoms include:

- runny nose;
- cough;
- fever;
- sore throat;
- croup;
- conjunctivitis;
- breathlessness.

The physical signs are those seen in any viral respiratory tract infection and depend on the nature and severity of the infection. Acute conjunctivitis and exudative tonsillitis are more commonly seen with adenoviral infection than most of the other respiratory viruses, and may provide a clue to the diagnosis. It affects both eyes (usually one then the other), and usually causes only mild discomfort. A more severe keratoconjunctivitis (caused predominantly by serotypes 8, 19, and 37) can occur, causing a red, painful eye for several weeks.

Other illnesses caused by adenovirus include watery diarrhoea, especially in infants, intussusception, haemorrhagic cystitis, hepatitis, and encephalitis.

Investigations

- Imaging studies: CXR and chest CT scans in children with acute adenoviral LRTI show non-specific bilateral reticulo-nodular shadowing. In children with severe pneumonia that has become prolonged, mosaic air-trapping may be seen, consistent with small airways obstruction. Pleural effusions can occur as part of the acute systemic illness.
- The presence of adenovirus in respiratory secretions (NPA or BAL) can be detected by culture combined with immunofluorescence or by PCR. Both are reliable tests. As noted above adenovirus may be cultured from asymptomatic children, and detected adenovirus may not necessarily be the cause of respiratory symptoms, although in the absence of other causes it is a reasonable assumption, particularly in a child under the age of 5 years.
- Serology is often unhelpful. Most clinical laboratory tests will not provide the serotype and, without paired sera 4 weeks apart, it is hard to interpret the results. It may be worth storing sera for later analysis.
- Blood investigations may show:
  - decreased white cell count;
  - anaemia;
  - elevated transaminases;
  - deranged coagulation.

Treatment

- Treatment is supportive. Some children will progress to respiratory failure and require mechanical ventilation.
- In immunodeficient children antiviral agents such as ribavirin and cidofovir, sometimes combined with pooled human immunoglobulin, have been used with variable success.

Prevention

Adenovirus vaccines have been developed by the US military and appear to be effective. These live attenuated virus vaccines were given orally and resulted in a significant reduction in outbreaks of adenoviral infection amongst army personnel, although for financial reasons production ceased in 1996. Adenoviral vaccine is not available for use in children.

Outcome

- Adenoviral infections are usually mild self-limiting illnesses.
- Adenovirus is more likely to cause severe lung disease than most of the other respiratory viruses, including disease severe enough to cause respiratory failure. A small number of these children, especially neonates and immunocompromised children, will die from their pneumonia and a proportion will be left with long-term lung damage, usually in the form of bronchiolitis obliterans.

Measles pneumonia

- Measles virus is a paramyxovirus, the same family that includes RSV, human metapneumovirus, and parainfluenza viruses.
- Measles is spread by respiratory droplets. The incubation period is 10–14 days. Initial infection and viral replication takes place in airway epithelial cells of the upper and lower respiratory tract. After 2–4 days infection there is a primary viraemia after which infection spreads to the lymph nodes and generalized lymphadenopathy develops. After a further period of replication, secondary viraemia occurs with dissemination of the virus to various organs, including back to the lungs and the skin causing the typical rash.
- Measles virus infection is exclusive to humans—there is no animal host. In immunized communities it is commonest in 2–3 year olds. In non-immunized communities incidence peaks at 5–10 years of age. It tends to occur in seasonal epidemics, usually in the early spring in temperate climates. Attack rates are very high and 90% of susceptible individuals will become infected after exposure to the virus.
- Measles infection is associated with depression of host immunity, including lymphopenia, which can last for weeks to months after the infection and which predisposes to subsequent bacterial infection, most commonly, otitis media and bronchitis or pneumonia.
- Typical measles symptoms are as follows.
  - A prodrome of fever, runny nose, conjunctivitis, dry cough occurs during the initial respiratory tract infection and is indistinguishable from any viral coryza, except that Koplik's spots may be seen on the buccal mucosa. A croup-like illness can occur.
  - After 2–4 days a florid macula blanching red rash appears, spreading downwards from the head and neck to cover the whole body. The initial spots are discrete and pinpoint, but as they become more numerous they enlarge and become confluent.
  - The rash usually lasts around 3 days after which fever settles and the rash resolves.
  - Common complications are bacterial bronchitis and pneumonia and otitis media. Diarrhoea is also common particularly in poorly nourished children, as is corneal ulceration associated with vitamin A deficiency. Encephalitis occurs in 1 in 5000. Subacute sclerosing panencephalitis is very rare and occurs 4–10 years after the initial infection.
- Diagnosis is often made on symptoms and signs. Confirmation can be obtained by measuring measles IgM, which will be positive in all children 4 days after the onset of the rash, and often earlier. PCR is also sensitive and specific, either from naspharyngeal samples, throat swabs, or urine (90% of children excrete measles virus in the urine) collected any time from illness onset to 12 days after the rash has resolved.

Pneumonia

- The first site of infection with measles is the respiratory tract and measles always causes respiratory disease. Often this is confined to coryzal symptoms or croup during the prodrome, but the damaged airway epithelium is prone to secondary bacterial infection, causing a more persistent bronchitis. Small airways can be obstructed by inflammatory debris resulting in areas of collapse that can also develop secondary bacterial pneumonia. Likely bacteria causing secondary pneumonia are *Staphylococcus aureus*, *Streptococcus pyogenes*, and *Pneumococcus*.

- Primary measles pneumonia can also occur with infection of alveolar cells and interstitial cells with measles virus. Adjacent infected cells can fuse together forming syncytial giant cells. Giant cell formation is not isolated to measles pneumonia and can be seen with RSV and parainfluenza pneumonia.
- Primary pneumonia will occur during the early course of the disease, within 2 days of the onset of the rash. Secondary bacterial infection often occurs after the initial fever and rash have resolved and is accompanied by recurrence of fever and systemic disturbance.
- When pneumonia occurs it is usually associated with widespread airway epithelial cell damage and consequent airway wall oedema and airways obstruction. This will contribute to increased respiratory work.
- CXR is usually typical of a viral pneumonia, with increased perihilar bronchial wall thickening, evidence of air-trapping, and patchy atelectasis. There may also be evidence of hilar adenopathy. Secondary bacterial infection may cause lobar consolidation.
- Occasionally, measles pneumonia may occur in a child who does not have a typical measles rash.

Treatment

Treatment is supportive. Antibiotics should be used for secondary bacterial infection. The antibiotic selected should cover *Staphylococcus aureus* and *Streptococcal* species.

In malnourished children, high dose vitamin A reduces morbidity and mortality associated with measles.

Prevention

- Effective vaccination is available. Since measles has only one strain and only infects humans, it should be possible to eradicate it from human populations in the same way that small pox has been eradicated.
- Where there are effective national vaccine programmes against measles, the annual incidence is very low, and most of these cases are due to immigration of non-vaccinated individuals.

Outcome

Measles is usually a self-limiting disease. Most children are miserable and unwell for 3–5 days, following which they make a full recovery. It is hard to estimate the frequency of respiratory complications. Pneumonia has been reported to affect 3–30% of infected children. Of those with pneumonia, 5–10% will develop respiratory failure and some will die. Mortality is much higher in malnourished children in resource-poor communities. In 1999 measles accounted for 800 000 deaths per year worldwide. In 2004 this figure had halved since the more widespread use of measles vaccine.

Influenza

- Influenza infection causes an illness characterized by:
  - fever;
  - muscle aches;
  - headache;
  - cough.
- Several different respiratory viruses, as well as bacteria such as *Mycoplasma* and *Chlamydophila*, can cause a flu-like illness that is impossible to distinguish clinically from influenza infection
- Influenza is a seasonal illness with the majority of cases occurring in a 6–8 week period during the winter months. The incidence of infection varies widely from year to year, affecting between 0 and 45% of the childhood population. On average, 5–10% of children are infected each winter. Attack rates are highest in children.
- Immunity is strain-specific. Influenza strains vary from year to year, based on alteration of the surface glycoproteins haemagglutinin and neuraminidase. As a consequence repeated infection often occurs several times in an individual's life. Previous infection or vaccination may provide some protection against related strains and limit the severity of illness. When a completely new strain arises there will be no existing protection within the population and a pandemic is more likely.
- Three major subgroups of influenza are recognized, A, B, and C. Influenza A and B both cause epidemic flu. Influenza A infection tends to be more severe. Influenza C causes sporadic infection. Influenza A viruses are further divided according to the haemagglutinin (H1–H9) and neuraminidase (N1–3) types. Each year one or two subtypes of influenza A may be in circulation with one type of influenza B.
- Infection is by respiratory droplets, either directly or via contact with a contaminated object. Influenza viruses can survive on environmental surfaces, especially non-porous materials, for up to 48h. Symptoms appear 1–3 days after infection. Viral shedding and infectivity persist for 5–7 days. Infectivity is highest in the 24h after symptoms appear.
- Influenza viruses are easily killed by washing with soap and water, alcohol-based cleaners, and cleaning with normal household detergents.

Symptoms and signs

- Influenza infection nearly always results in a noticeable illness. In the majority of children it is not debilitating but usually worse than a regular cold.
- Symptoms typically start abruptly usually with fever, sore throat, chills, aches, and headache. A feeling of weakness and fatigue is common. Although rhinitis can occur, it is not usually a predominant symptom. There may be a dry cough and conjunctivitis. Influenza infections are less distinctive from other respiratory tract infections in younger children.
- In addition to the typical flu-like illness, influenza infection can cause bronchiolitis, pneumonia, and croup.
- Examination findings are usually limited to fever and a red throat. There may be evidence of croup or pneumonia.

- Young infants may present with severe illness resembling bacterial septicaemia.
- In a typical illness fever will last 2–4 days. Return to full health may take several days or weeks. Cough may also persist for several days.

Diagnosis

- During the flu season, the diagnosis of flu-like illness is made on the basis of clinical signs and symptoms.
- Confirmation of influenza infection can be obtained from NPA or throat swab. These can be processed by viral culture, direct immunofluorescence, or by PCR. Near-patient testing kits are available but have limited specificity and add little to the clinical diagnosis.

Complications

- Secondary bacterial pneumonia is the most common complication and responsible for most deaths. Infection arises because of viral-mediated damage to the airway surface and usually occurs 3–4 days after the onset of symptoms. The most likely bacterial pathogens are *Staphyloccocus aureus* and *Streptococcus pyogenes*. Secondary bacterial infections should be suspected when there is prolonged fever, recrudescence of fever, or worsening respiratory distress.
- Primary influenza pneumonia is relatively rare, but can cause a severe necrotizing disease resulting in respiratory failure.
- Multiorgan failure with a septicaemia-like illness has been observed with avian influenza infection. This does not appear to represent the consequences of secondary bacterial infection but rather is caused by overwhelming viral disease.
- Myositis with myoglobinuria, encephalitis, and myocarditis may also occur.

Treatment

- For previously healthy children treatment is supportive, with oral fluids, antipyretics, and bed rest.
- For infection in high-risk groups (children with heart disease, lung disease, immunocompromise) antiviral agents should be used. Amantadine (a viral ion channel blocker) is no longer recommended because of readily acquired viral resistance. Two neuraminidase inhibitors are available, oseltamivir (Tamiflu®) and zanamivir (Relenza®). These drugs inhibit the release of virus from infected cells and thus limit the spread of the virus in the airways. To be effective they must be given within 48h of the onset of symptoms. Their use reduces illness duration by 30% (1–1.5 days) and illness severity. Oseltamivir is taken orally either as a capsule or suspension and is licensed for all children > 12 months of age. Zanamivir is a dry powder for inhalation for use in children > 12 years of age.
- For previously healthy children who develop severe illness it is likely that symptoms will have been present for more than 48h and antiviral therapies are unlikely to help. At this stage their disease will be largely due to the consequence of viral damage rather than active viral replication.
- Antibiotics should be used when secondary bacterial infection is suspected. During epidemics of severe disease there may be a role for using antibiotics from the onset of flu-like symptoms to prevent secondary bacterial infection.

- Some children will require intensive care and mechanical ventilation for respiratory failure, usually as a consequence of primary viral or secondary bacterial pneumonia.

Influenza pandemics

- The term seasonal influenza refers to the expected burden of disease each winter. When there are more cases than usual the term 'epidemic' is used; there is no strict boundary when epidemic proportions are reached. It reflects a combination of disease incidence and disease severity. The term 'pandemic' is used when there are widespread epidemics around the world. Pandemics occur when:
  - a new influenza subtype arises for which there is no existing immunity;
  - the new strain infects humans causing serious disease;
  - the new strain spreads easily from person to person.
- There have been 3 pandemics in the last 100 years, in 1918 (Spanish flu), 1957 (Asian flu), and 1968 (Hong Kong flu).
- Avian flu (H5N1) fulfils the first 2 requirements for a pandemic strain, but person to person spread is rare. Nevertheless, some form of a virulent influenza virus crossing the species barrier from birds or pigs to man is the most likely source of the next pandemic strain. It is most likely that this will arise in Asia where cohabitation between livestock, poultry, and people is common.
- Pandemic preparedness plans have been developed in many countries to deal with the next pandemic. The UK plan assumes that 25% of the population will be infected with a case fatality of 0.4–2.5% resulting in 20 000–700 000 excess deaths. A pandemic of this proportion could severely disrupt all major services and businesses. The key elements of the preparedness plan are as follows.
  - Measures to minimize spread of infection. These will include advice about avoiding crowds and staying at home if symptoms develop. There are also likely to be restrictions on national and international travel. Strict hygiene measures will limit spread within homes and hospitals.
  - Provision of necessary medical services. This will include ensuring that health care workers stay well by priority provision of antiviral therapy. Non-essential treatment will be postponed to deal with the large numbers of people who will seek medical attention and non-medical support workers will be trained to triage potential cases and to supply antiviral treatments using simple algorithms. In order that sufficient supplies of antiviral treatment are available countries have stockpiled drugs. In the UK there are sufficient stocks for 25% of the population to receive a 5 day treatment course of oseltamivir. Algorithms to determine access to limited intensive care services may also be required.
- Once a pandemic strain has been identified it will take 4–6 months to produce significant quantities of vaccine. This will not be quick enough to protect most populations from the initial season, but may protect those uninfected for subsequent seasons.

Prevention

- Inactivated influenza vaccine is available (given as an intramuscular injection) and on average provides 70% protection from influenza infection. This varies from year to year and depends on how well matched the vaccine is to the prevalent strain of influenza.
- Each year a new vaccine is designed based on predictions of which strains are most likely to be prevalent. The vaccine usually contains two subtypes of influenza A and one of influenza B. Strain inclusion is determined by a group in the WHO, based on analysis of strains collected over the previous winter and identification of new strains that have the potential to spread. Production of the vaccine starts in March each year and is usually complete by October. The selected vaccine strains are grown using hens' eggs. Children with severe allergy to egg should not be given the vaccine. Protection takes 2 weeks to develop after vaccination.
- The public health value of widespread immunization in otherwise healthy adults and children is debatable and in most seasons it has been hard to show objective evidence of benefit.
- Targeted immunization in at risk groups such as those with chronic lung disease including asthma and cystic fibrosis, seems reasonable (although the benefits have not been proven).
- A live attenuated vaccine given as a nasal spray is also available and has similar efficacy to the inactivated formulations made with the same strains of virus.
- Neuraminidase inhibitors can provide 2–5-fold protection against influenza infection when taken daily during the influenza season. In most countries (including the UK and US) they are not recommended for use in this way, even in high risk groups. Although viral resistance to neuraminidase inhibitors is rare, widespread prophylactic use may increase the likelihood of a pandemic of a resistant strain.

Outcome

The prognosis for children with seasonal Influenza infection is excellent. The majority of the mortality from seasonal influenza is in the elderly (in the UK there are an estimated 12 000 excess influenza-related deaths each year). During the 1918 pandemic the majority of the morbidity and mortality was in young adults of working age. This may reflect both the virulence of that particular strain and possible partial immunity in older people because of repeated prior influenza infection. The 1957 and 1968 pandemics more closely resembled the impact of seasonal influenza with the greatest effects on the elderly. The virulence and severity of the next pandemic strain is hard to predict. The avian influenza strain (H5N1) has a case fatality of 30–50%.

Further information

Jefferson, T. (2006). Influenza vaccination: policy versus evidence. *Br. Med. J.* **333**, 912–15.
Health Protection Agency Influenza Pandemic Contingency Plan: www.hpa.org.uk/infections/topics_az /influenza/pandemic/fluplan.
Department of Health UK: www.dh.gov.uk/PolicyAndGuidance EmergencyPlanning/PandemicFlu.

Severe acute respiratory syndrome (SARS)

- SARS is caused by a novel coronavirus (SARS-CoV). Closely related viruses have been found in animals, and it has been suggested that SARS-CoV arose through mutation of one of these viruses allowing it to cross the species barrier and infect humans.
- SARS was first identified as an epidemic that occurred in 2003. 8000 people became unwell and 774 died. The index case was a doctor from China who was visiting Hong Kong. The disease spread to Singapore and Toronto by air travel. Over 100 health care workers caring for affected patients became infected themselves. Since 2003 there have been no further outbreaks.
- SARS appears to be spread by respiratory droplets, either directly or via fomites.
- The incubation period is 2–10 days. In adults the disease had 3 phases.
  - Phase 1: a flu-like illness with fever, myalgia, headache, coryza, and occasionally diarrhoea. During this phase viral replication occurs. It lasts 2 days and is followed by transient improvement.
  - Phase 2: recurrence or persistence of fever with worsening cough and respiratory distress and developing hypoxia. CXR consistent with bronchopneumonia (bronchial wall thickening plus patchy consolidation). Viral load is already decreasing during this phase, and illness is related to inflammatory host response. Systemic corticosteroids appear to be helpful in this stage.
  - Phase 3: acute respiratory distress syndrome with diffuse alveolar damage sometimes leading to pulmonary fibrosis.
- Children, particularly those under the age of 12 years, were much less severely affected than adults. Very few progressed to phase 3 of the illness. Less than 10% of all those affected by SARS were children, and of these only 5% required hospital treatment, and less than 1% needed mechanical ventilation. No child died. The reasons why children had milder disease are not known.
- Treatment requires early recognition, triage, and cohorting with strict infection control measures to prevent spread of infection. Current recommendations are to use broad-spectrum antibiotics in children with fever and pneumonia to prevent secondary bacterial infection. Systemic corticosteroids should be tried if there is progressively worsening disease. Ribavirin has been tried and found to be ineffective.
- At follow-up about 10% of children requiring hospital care for pneumonia had mild restrictive or obstructive lung disease. Whether this will further improve with time is not known. This outcome is probably not different from that in any severe viral pneumonia.

Further information

Li, A.M. and Ng, P.C. (2005). Severe acute respiratory syndrome (SARS) in neonates and children. *Arch. Dis. Child. Fetal Neonatal Ed.* **90** (6), F461–5.

Fungal infections

Introduction

Fungi can be divided into 2 basic morphological forms, yeasts and hyphae. Yeasts are unicellular fungi that reproduce asexually by blastoconidia formation (budding) or fission. Hyphae are multicellular fungi that reproduce asexually and/or sexually. Dimorphism is the condition whereby a fungus can exhibit either the yeast form or the hyphal form, depending on growth conditions. A mass of hyphal elements is termed the mycelium (synonymous with mould). *Pneumocystis* species are also now classified as fungi, and are dealt with on p. 242.

Fungal infection in healthy children

- Fungal lung infection in otherwise normal children is rare in Europe.
- Surface colonization of the upper airway with *Candida albicans* is common, as is detection of *Aspergillus* species in airway secretions.
- Allergic bronchopulmonary aspergillosis is a condition that arises as a result of an abnormally vigorous IgE-mediated immune response to *Aspergillus* species rather than invasive fungal disease.

Endemic mycoses

This term refers to fungal lung infections that occur in specific geographical locations. They are all caused by dimorphic fungi and can all occur in otherwise normal children. They are all also found in immunosuppressed children, including those with HIV infection, when they tend to be more severe and are more likely to be disseminated.

Histoplasmosis

Caused by *Histoplasma capsulatum*. Occurs mainly in central eastern states of the USA. Infection is asymptomatic in 50%, but can leave long-standing nodular changes on CXR. Acute pulmonary infection causes a flu-like illness with fever, cough, chest pain, and lethargy. CXR shows non-specific patchy consolidation, hilar adenopathy, or pleural effusion. Disseminated potentially fatal disease can occur in children < 2 years old and in children exposed to a very large inoculum. Disseminated disease can affect almost any organ. Chronic pulmonary disease can occur and resembles cavitatory TB. Diagnosis requires cytology and culture of airway sections. Skin tests may also be helpful. Itraconazole and fluconazole are effective for pulmonary disease. Amphotericin B should be used for disseminated disease.

Coccidioidmycosis

Caused by *Coccidioides immitis*. Occurs in southwestern states of USA, Mexico, and in Central and S. America. Outbreaks occur following dust storms, earthquakes, and earth excavation, which favour dispersion of the spores. After inhalation of the spores there is a flu-like illness with fever, cough, chest pain, a transient rash (maculopapular, erythema multiforme, or erythema nodosum), and arthralgia. CXR shows non-specific patchy consolidation, hilar adenopathy, or pleural effusion. Infection can also affect bones, joints, and CNS. 5–10% develop chronic pulmonary disease with pulmonary nodules or cavities. Diagnosis is based on cytology of airway sections and on antibody detection. Itraconazole is effective. For severe illness, amphotericin B should be used.

Blastomycosis

Caused by *Blastomyces dermatitidis*. It occurs in the southern states of USA and mainly affects young adults who spend most of their time in outdoor environments. It can affect children, sometimes in epidemics. It usually causes a chronic illness that mimics TB, with fever, night sweats, weight loss, and lethargy. CXR shows local consolidation. Diagnosis requires cytology and culture of airway secretions. Itraconazole is effective. For severe illness, amphotericin B should be used.

Paracoccidioidomycosis

Caused by *Paracoccidioides brasiliensis*. Found in Central and S. America. Rare in children.

Penicilliosis

Caused by *Penicillum marneffei*. Found in China and Southeast Asia. Although it can occur in normal children it is now most commonly found in children with HIV infection and is an AIDS-defining illness in this setting. It can cause local and systemic infection. The lung is the usual portal of entry.

Cryptococcosis

- *Cryptococcus neoformans* is a yeast found in soil contaminated with pigeon droppings. Infection occurs by inhalation.
- Serological evidence of infection can be found in most children > 2 years of age.
- Symptomatic infection is rare, and most, but not all, occur in children who are in some way immunocompromised.
- Pulmonary infection can cause fever, malaise, chest pain, weight loss, and night sweats.
- Dissemination may occur, usually as meningitis.
- Clinical evidence of meningitis may be very mild, and lumbar puncture should be performed in all children with cryptococcal infection.
- CXR shows non-specific infiltrates or nodules.
- Diagnosis can be difficult. *C. neoformans* can colonize the respiratory tract in normal children. Nevertheless, bronchoalveolar cultures growing *C. neoformans* in a child with pulmonary disease and risk factors (immunosuppression or chronic lung disease) are usually sufficient to initiate treatment.
- Treatment is with fluconazole or amphotericin B.
- Cryptococcal infection is relatively common in adult patients with AIDS, but less so in children with AIDS.
- Other causes of deficient cell-mediated immunity, but not neutropenia or systemic steroids (unlike invasive aspergillosis), are risk factors for cryptococcal infection.

Fungal infections in immunocompromised children

The most important fungal lung infections in this group of children are invasive pulmonary aspergillosis and *Candida* pneumonia. Of these, *Aspergillus* infection is more common. *A. fumigatus* is one of the most widespread airborne fungi, and nearly everyone will inhale several hundred *A. fumigatus* spores every day. It is a major component of compost and other rotting vegetation. Minimizing exposure to environments likely to have high levels of fungus will reduce risk of infection in immunocompromised children. In immunocompromised children with *Aspergillus* infection, the lung is the most common site (90%), followed by the sinuses/nose (15%) and the brain (10%). *Candida* infection can affect almost any organ including liver, spleen, brain, bones, and eyes. The lungs are usually involved as part of disseminated infection. More rarely they may be the main organ involved.

Other fungi that can more rarely infect the airway or lungs of immunosuppressed children are the *Zygomycetes* group (includes *Rhizopus* and *Mucor*), the *Scedosporium* species, and *Fusarium solani*. Cryptococcal infection and the endemic mycoses are all more likely to occur and cause symptoms in immunosuppressed children.

Risk factors for invasive fungal infection

- Severe neutropenia (< 500 neutrophils/μL) for > 10 days in previous 60 days.
- Prolonged (> 3 weeks) high dose corticosteroid treatment as part of a chemotherapy regime in previous 60 days.
- Use of significant immunosuppression agents in previous 30 days. Myelo-ablative chemotherapy associated with allogeneic bone marrow transplantation is a particularly high risk.
- Probable or proven invasive fungal infection during a previous episode of neutropenia.
- Primary immune deficiency affecting neutrophil function, particularly chronic granulomatous disease.

Other specific risk factors for *Candida* infection:
- neonates, especially low birth weight and preterm infants;
- children on prolonged courses of broad-spectrum antibiotics;
- children with longstanding central venous lines.

Clinical features

In high risk patients, temperature instability (< 36°C or > 38°C) for 4 days or more despite broad-spectrum antibacterial therapy suggests the possibility of fungal infection. In addition, there may be:
- cough;
- chest pain;
- haemoptysis;
- breathlessness;
- pleural rub;

Sinus disease may be suggested by:
- nasal discharge or epistaxis;
- nasal or palatal ulceration or necrosis;
- periorbital swelling.

Investigations

Making a definitive diagnosis of fungal lung infection can be very difficult, and requires:
- a tissue sample, such as a fine needle aspirate or an open biopsy, with evidence of fungal infection. Microscopy, showing hyphae or yeast cells, is more sensitive than culture; *or*
- a positive culture, microscopy, or antigen test (e.g. the galactomannan enzyme immunoassay for *Aspergillus*) from a normally sterile site. For invasive lung infection, likely samples would be BAL fluid or sputum or sinus biopsy. Since *Candida* may colonize the upper airway, a positive protected brush sample, obtained with a bronchoscope, is more likely to be specific for LRTI; *plus*
- evidence of tissue damage, either histological on the biopsy or radiological, e.g. bony erosion in the sinuses or abscess formation in the lung seen by CT scan.

The presence of fungaemia in a high-risk child with respiratory signs is also highly suggestive of fungal pneumonia. *Aspergillus* fungaemia is best identified by antigen test or PCR test. Blood culture for *Aspergillus* is unreliable; positive blood cultures for *Aspergillus* may represent serious invasive disease, but are more likely to represent sample contamination. *Candida* fungaemia is more common than *Aspergillus* fungaemia and, in the context of a high risk patient, is likely to represent deep-seated invasive disease, unless the sample was drawn from an indwelling central venous catheter. Contamination of catheters with *Candida* is a problem. A positive culture for *Candida* taken from a central line should be confirmed by a peripheral blood culture. Isolation of *Candida* species from the urine (in the absence of a urinary catheter) in a sick high-risk patient is also usually sufficient for a probable diagnosis and to initiate treatment.

Imaging can help diagnose fungal pneumonia.
- CXR showing any new infiltrate or pleural effusion may be suggestive in a high risk patient with a fever.
- CT findings considered to be strongly suggestive of pulmonary aspergillosis are:
  - halo sign—an area of ground-glass opacity surrounding a nodule or area of consolidation (Fig. 20.1);
  - air-crescent sign—air crescents surrounding soft tissue lesions;
  - cavity within consolidation (differential includes TB)

Invasive fungal infection carries a high mortality. Despite investigation with blood culture, antigen testing, BAL samples, and CT scans, invasive pulmonary fungal infection can be missed and found only at post-mortem. As a consequence, most children who are at high risk for fungal infection will be started on antifungal therapy on the basis of a persistent fever for 48h that has not responded to broad-spectrum antibiotics, without requiring positive identification of fungal organisms.

Treatment

- Amphotericin B is standard first-line therapy for invasive fungal disease in immunocompromised children. It has good activity against most *Aspergillus* and *Candida* species and most other fungi (except *Scedosporium*). The conventional formulation is associated with significant toxicity, including infusion-related events, such as chills, fever, headache, nausea and vomiting, and dose-limiting nephrotoxicity. The liposomal form (ambisome) is significantly less toxic and higher doses can be used.
- The azoles—fluconazole, ketoconazole, itraconazole, and voriconazole—are the other main group of antifungal drugs. They have a wide spectrum of activity against most fungi, including *Candida*, but only itraconazole and voriconazole have activity against *Aspergillus*. IV voriconazole can be used in children with suspected or proven invasive *Aspergillus* infections not responding to amphotericin B. The azoles have poor activity against *Zygomycetes*.
- Flucytosine (5-fluorocytosine) is a pyrimidine drug with good activity against *Candida*, and may be combined with amphotericin B for deep or disseminated *Candida* infections, especially if good penetration into the CNS is required.
- Caspofungin is a newer antifungal. It can be used for invasive *Aspergillus* infections not responding to amphotericin or voriconazole. It has a different mechanism of action than that of voriconazole and there is some evidence of a synergistic effect with this drug.

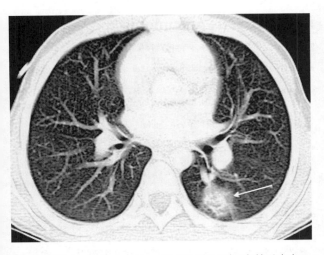

Fig. 20.1 CT scan of a 7-year-old boy with relapsed acute lymphoblastic leukaemia who developed a high spiking fever during an episode of neutropenia that had not responded to broad-spectrum antibiotics. The scan shows a focal area of consolidation (white arrow) with surrounding ground-glass change. BAL of the affected lung segment was negative for fungi. Amphotericin B was not effective, but there was a good response to IV voriconazole.

Pneumocystis pneumonia

- *Pneumocystis jiroveci* (pronounced 'yee row vet zee'), is an opportunistic unicellular fungal pathogen.
- Initially, *Pneumocystis* organisms were thought to be protozoa, but in the late 1980s they were re-classified as fungi.
- *P. jiroveci* was previously known as *P. carinii* and was re-named in 1999 after genetic studies showed that the form of *Pneumocystis* that infects humans is actually different from *P. carinii*, which is predominantly a rat pathogen. The acronym PCP can still be used and now refers to *Pneumocystis* pneumonia.
- *P. jirovecii* does not cause disease in immunocompetent children. *P. jiroveci* is found widely in the environment and is thought to enter the body by inhalation of airborne cysts. Seroconversion studies have shown that almost every child will have been exposed to *P. jiroveci* by the age of 3 years. Disease is thought to occur in immunodeficiency states through re-activation of latent infection.
- Children most at risk of developing *P. jiroveci* pneumonia are those:
  - on immunosuppressant drugs, usually for malignancy;
  - infected by HIV;
  - with severe combined immunodeficiency syndromes.

Symptoms

- Onset is usually insidious over a few weeks.
- Poor growth or weight loss.
- Breathlessness.
- Dry cough.
- Mild fever.

Signs

- Tachypnoea.
- Mild chest wall recession.
- Often normal breath sounds.
- Hypoxia.

Investigations

- CXR (Fig. 20.2) shows bilateral diffuse increase in perihilar interstitial and/or alveolar markings. Pleural effusions are rarely due to *P. jiroveci* and an alternative pathogen should be sought.
- CT scan (may not be needed) will show ground-glass attenuation.
- Induced sputum can be used for fluorescence test or PCR analysis. *Pneumocystis* organisms are at higher levels and hence easier to detect in children with HIV and SCID than in those on immunosuppressive drugs, possibly reflecting severity of the underlying immune deficiency.

- Bronchoscopy and BAL. Cytology should be performed and the cell count determined. There is usually a relatively normal cell count suggesting little inflammation. Presence of foamy macrophages and foamy alveolar casts is typical of *Pneumocystis* infection. *P. jiroveci* organisms cannot be seen with normal stains and Grocott's methenamine silver nitrate is needed to visualize the cysts. A commercial diagnostic PCR for *P. jiroveci* is not available. BAL fluid should also be sent for bacterial, viral, and fungal culture and PCR for respiratory viruses and CMV.
- Gold standard diagnostic test remains lung biopsy. This will show alveoli filled with foamy proteinaceous material and Grocott's methenamine silver nitrate stain will reveal the *Pneumocystis* organisms. Once again there is scant evidence of inflammation.

Treatment

- Standard treatment is with high dose IV co-trimoxazole (trimethoprim–sulfamethoxazole).
- IV pentamidine can be used if co-trimoxazole not tolerated or poor response to treatment (there may be resistance to co-trimoxazole). Pentamidine infusion can be associated with severe hypotension.
- For milder disease not responding to co-trimoxazole, combination therapy with either oral dapsone and trimethoprim or oral clindamycin and primaquine may be effective.
- There may be deterioration in the first 2–3 days after onset of treatment, possibly reflecting worsening inflammation caused by dying *P. jiroveci* organisms.
- Giving systemic corticosteroids with the co-trimoxazole is associated with better outcomes in adults. The effect has not been studied in children or in conditions other then HIV. Steroids may worsen CMV infection, and this should be excluded before steroids are used.

Prevention

All at risk children should receive prophylactic treatment with daily co-trimoxazole. Where this is not tolerated, dapsone, atovaquone, or inhaled pentamidine can be used.

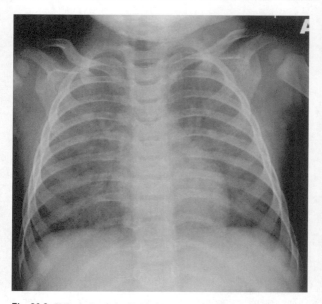

Fig. 20.2 CXR of a 6 month old girl who presented with a 1 month history of cough and a 3 day history of worsening respiratory distress. She developed progressive hypoxia and required mechanical ventilation. Non-bronchoscopic lavage showed foamy macrophages and Grocott's stain was positive for *Pneumocystis* cysts. Further investigation showed she had SCID. Her respiratory distress resolved after treatment with high dose IV co-trimoxazole.

Further information

Ascioglu, S., Rex, J.H., de Pauw, B., et al. (2002). Defining opportunistic invasive fungal infections in immunocompromised patients with cancer and hematopoietic stem cell transplants: an international consensus. *Clin. Infect. Dis.* **34**, 7–14.

Parasitic and protozoal infections

Introduction

- Lung diseases caused by parasites and protozoa are very uncommon in most developed countries, particularly those in Western Europe. Worldwide they remain an important cause of morbidity. Increasing population migration and mobility make it more likely that children with these diseases will be seen in any country, and an awareness of these conditions is important.
- Parasites (multicellular organisms) can cause lung disease either by directly infecting the lung or by inducing eosinophilic lung inflammation. This chapter deals with direct lung infection. Pulmonary infiltrates with eosinophilia are dealt with in 📖 Chapter 52.
- Protozoa are single cell organisms. The 2 most likely to cause lung disease are *Toxoplasma gondii* and *Entamoeba histolytica*.

Parasitic disease

Pulmonary hydatid disease

- Pulmonary hydatid disease is the most common parasitic lung disease worldwide, is geographically widespread, and largely associated with sheep farming.
- It is caused by the tapeworm *Echinococcus*, most commonly *E. granulosus*, which infects domestic livestock, particularly sheep.

Life cycle

- Sheep become infected when they ingest worm eggs from pasture contaminated with dog faeces. The eggs hatch inside the sheep, forming cysts and the life cycle is completed when dogs are infected through eating the offal of infected livestock, particularly the liver and lung. The adult worms live in the dog intestine and eggs are passed into the stool.
- Humans become infected by ingesting eggs as a result of contact with infected dogs. After ingestion the eggs hatch to produce larvae that migrate through the gut wall and enter the portal system and are carried to various organs where they form cysts. Infection cannot be spread from person to person and human infection represents a dead end for the *Echinococcus* life cycle.

Clinical features

- The liver is the most commonly affected organ. Liver cysts are often asymptomatic and may regress spontaneously. Large cysts can cause compression. Rupture of the cysts can be associated with anaphylaxis.
- The lung is the second most common site for hydatid cysts. Symptoms depend on whether the cyst is intact or has ruptured.
- Intact cysts may be asymptomatic and found incidentally on CXR. They may also cause:
  - chest pain;
  - breathlessness;
  - cough.
- Cysts may rupture into a bronchus resulting in coughing up of jelly-like material, bits of cyst membrane, and recurrent haemoptysis. Occasionally there is wheezing or an anaphylactic reaction to the cyst contents. Subsequently the cyst cavity can be the site of secondary infection.
- Cysts may also rupture into the pleural cavity causing pneumothorax, pleural effusion, empyema, or anaphylaxis.

Investigations

- CXR will show homogeneous, dense, round, or oval lesions that have well-defined borders, ranging in size from 2 to 20cm, surrounded by normal lung tissue. There may be a thin rim of calcification in the wall of longstanding cysts. Multiple cysts are seen in 30% of cases, including bilateral disease. If the cyst has ruptured into a bronchus there will be an air–fluid level. The membrane from the partially collapsed cyst may be seen floating on the surface—sometimes called the lily-pad or crescent sign.
- Concurrent liver cysts may occur, but are not usually present.

- CT scan will show similar appearances to CXR but with greater detail. The CT will usually show that the cyst walls are relatively thick consistent with an acquired inflammatory condition. The main differential diagnosis for cysts will be congenital anomalies, particularly congenital cystic adenomatoid malformations. These cysts are thin-walled unless they have been complicated by secondary infection.
- Serology can be helpful but is positive in only 50% of children with hydatid lung disease (it performs better in liver disease where it is positive in 80%). The diagnosis is usually based on clinical suspicion and radiological findings.
- Eosinophilia is present in 25% of infected children.
- The intradermal Casoni test, which has a poor sensitivity, is no longer recommended.

Treatment

- Treatment for cystic pulmonary hydatid disease is surgical removal of all cyst material. At operation the cyst is aspirated and then the cyst membrane is removed. Spillage of cyst contents should be avoided to prevent dissemination of daughter cysts and allergic reactions. The resulting cavity once the cyst has been removed may be obliterated by purse-string sutures (capitonnage) or left to resolve spontaneously.
- Treatment with anthelmintics such as oral mebendazole or albendazole is rarely successful and, even if the parasite is killed, the cyst cavity will remain as a site of future secondary infection.
- If a surgical approach is used, concurrent chemotherapy is not necessary. If there are cysts affecting more than one organ, or if surgery is not possible for other reasons, chemotherapy can be used, and needs to be continued for 3–6 months.
- Incomplete surgical removal can result in recurrence.

Pulmonary dirofilariasis

- *Dirofilaria repens* is a slender thread-like worm transmitted from dogs to man by infected mosquitoes.
- Infection is seen in southern Europe, Asia, Australia, and N. and S. America.
- The larvae migrate via the pulmonary arteries to the lung tissue, where the adult worm becomes surrounded by granulation tissue.
- Most infections are asymptomatic, but may cause chest pain and haemoptysis.
- Imaging shows a single or multiple nodules, less than 3cm in diameter, usually in the periphery of the lung. The nodules may be mistaken for malignancy and the possibility of dirofilariasis needs to be borne in mind in the differential of lung nodules in endemic regions.
- Diagnosis requires excision and histological examination. Treatment is by excision.

Paragonimiasis

- *Paragonimus westermani* is a fluke (worm) that infects human lung tissue.
- It predominantly affects children between 11 and 15 years of age and is found in the Far East, West Africa, and Central and S. America.
- Infection is acquired by ingesting raw freshwater crayfish and crabs.
- After ingestion the larval stages migrate to the lungs where they become adult worms that become encapsulated within the lung tissue and deposit eggs into the bronchioles.
- Most children have a low worm load and are asymptomatic. Higher parasite loads can cause haemoptysis and cough.
- CXR usually shows patchy infiltrates but may be normal. CT scan shows single or multiple nodules in the pleura or lung parenchyma.
- Rarely there may be pneumothorax, pleural effusion, empyema, lung abscess, and bronchiectasis.
- Extrapulmonary disease, e.g. in the brain, can occur.
- Treatment is with a 2 day course of praziquantel.

Schistosomiasis

- Schistosoma parasites are small worms that invade the bloodstream and cause disease as a result of the granulomatous host response to the eggs carried by the bloodstream to the tissues.
- Infection is common in children and occurs in many parts of the world including Africa, the Middle and Far East, the Caribbean, and S. America.
- Infection is acquired from contaminated water, with the snail acting as the intermediate host. The free-living form of the parasite (cercariae) is able to penetrate intact skin.
- Clinical manifestations include an itchy rash at the time of infection and more rarely a febrile illness (Katayama fever) 4–8 weeks after exposure. This illness typically includes:
  - shortness of breath;
  - wheezing;
  - dry cough;
  - fever, myalgia, headache;
  - hepatosplenomegaly and marked eosinophilia.
- Chronic disease is usually associated with either renal involvement (with long-term risk of renal failure and bladder cancer) or liver involvement (with fibrosis and portal hypertension).
- Ectopic migration of the eggs from the portal system can result in deposition in the lung. Here they are associated with a granulomatous reaction that can cause pulmonary fibrosis and pulmonary hypertension.
- When there is pulmonary involvement, chest CT scan will show multiple nodules, sometimes associated with either reticulo-nodular or ground-glass opacity. The appearances can mimic miliary TB, sarcoid, or lung metastases.
- Diagnosis is based on detection of eggs in stool or urine or serology.
- Treatment is with praziquantel.

Protozoal disease

Toxoplasmosis

- *Toxoplasma gondii* is an obligate intracellular protozoan. Infection in children can be congenital or acquired.
- *Toxoplasma* can infect virtually all warm-blooded animals, including farm animals, and uses cats as the definitive host. The incidence of latent human infection identified by positive serology varies widely but in some communities is as high as 80%. Humans are infected by eating undercooked meat or by ingestion of oocytes, which are found in infected cat faeces.
- Congenital infection, acquired by infection crossing the placenta, is often mild or asymptomatic in the neonatal period although nearly all untreated children will develop some symptoms before adolescence, usually due to chorioretinitis. More severe neonatal disease occurs in a minority. This illness can include pneumonitis.
- Acquired disease in immunologically normal children is often asymptomatic. Cervical or occipital lymphadenopathy, the commonest problem, occurs in 10% of infected children. Vary rarely, severe systemic illness occurs, and pneumonitis can be part of this illness.
- Acquired disease in immunocompromised children may be severe, and often affects the CNS. *Toxoplasma* pneumonitis can occur in this group of children, and typically causes breathlessness with diffuse interstitial changes on CXR.
- Investigations.
  - Positive *Toxoplasma* IgG represents previous infection and persists for life. Recent infection results in an elevated IgM.
  - PCR tests for *Toxoplasma* DNA indicate the presence of active infection.
  - Tachyzoites can be identified in tissue sections or body fluid such as BAL or CSF.
  - Eye examination may reveal chorioretinitis.
  - CT scan of the brain may show calcification in congenital infection.
  - CXR will show diffuse bilateral interstitial markings in *Toxoplasma* pneumonitis.
- Treatment is not indicated for asymptomatic acquired disease or acquired disease with lymphadenitis. Congenital infection should always be treated to prevent subsequent illness, as should symptomatic acquired infection, particularly in the immunocompromised child. Treatment requires combination therapy with pyrimethamine, sulphadiazine, and folinic acid, usually for several weeks in acquired disease and for 12 months for congenital disease. Corticosteroids are used when there is CNS disease or disease threatening vision.

Amoebiasis

- *Entamoeba histolytica* infection is endemic in the tropics, but can occur anywhere.
- Spread is by the faecal–oral route. Ingested cysts release trophozoites that invade the mucosal lining of the large intestine.
- Infection is asymptomatic in 90% of children.

- Colitis is the most common disease manifestation and liver abscess is the most likely extraintestinal form of the disease.
- Invasive disease is more common in immunosuppressed children, including those with HIV infection.

Lung disease

- The lung is the second most likely extraintestinal site of amoebic involvement after the liver. Infection usually results from direct extension of a liver abscess, although haematogenous spread can also occur.
- Lung disease usually affects the right lower lobe. Symptoms and signs include:
  - fever;
  - right upper quadrant pain;
  - shoulder tip pain;
  - haemoptysis;
  - hepatomegaly.
- CXR shows an elevated right hemidiaphragm usually with right lower lobe consolidation and a right-sided pleural effusion. Ultrasound will show a liver abscess.

Diagnosis and treatment

- Diagnosis is usually made by detecting trophozoites in fresh stool.
- If there is a pleural collection, trophozoites may be seen in the fluid, which is usually thick and opaque.
- Treatment of invasive disease is with metronidazole. Amoebic empyema requires closed chest drainage.

Further information

Montoya, J.G. and Liesenfeld, O. (2004). Toxoplasmosis. *Lancet* 363, 1965–76.

Kuzucu, A. (2006). Parasitic diseases of the respiratory tract. *Curr. Opin. Pulm. Med.* **12**, 212–21.

Kosar, A., Orki, A., Haciibrahimoglu, G., Kiral, H., and Arman, B. (2006). Effect of capitonnage and cystotomy on outcome of childhood pulmonary hydatid cysts *J. Thorac. Cardiovasc. Surg.* **132**, 560–4.

Tuberculosis

Introduction

In most developed countries TB notifications have fallen steadily over the last 50 years, and in the UK there are now approximately 10 new cases of TB per 100 000 population per year. In other parts of the world TB remains a very significant cause of mortality and morbidity in both children and adults. It has been estimated that one-third of the world's population (2 billion people) has latent TB infection, and that around 10 million people per year will develop TB disease. Population migration will make eradication of TB in any one country impossible, and within many countries there will be geographical variation in TB incidence reflecting the origins of immigrant residents. For example, some London boroughs have a TB incidence of over 100 new cases per 100 000 per year.

Pathogenesis

- The most frequent route of infection by *Mycobacterium tuberculosis* (MTB) is inhalation and in 95% of cases the primary focus is in the lung.
- Once in the alveoli MTB are ingested by alveolar macrophages, and may be killed off at this point without causing further problems. The efficiency with which this occurs depends on the virulence and quantity of MTB present and on host immune competence. Usually the majority of MTB are killed or contained. The site of infection is walled off by epithelial cells and a tubercle forms. In most individuals this primary focus becomes undetectable on CXR. In a proportion of people the lesion may calcify or necrose or caseate. If calcification occurs, the lesion is called a Ghon focus and, in combination with calcified hilar lymph nodes, constitutes the Ghon complex.
- Cell-mediated immunity (CMI) develops slowly during the first weeks of infection in all individuals. Where there is a relatively large number of MTB organisms or the organisms are particularly virulent, the MTB organisms will divide and a more prominent primary focus will develop associated with enlarged mediastinal and paratracheal lymph nodes.
- During the phase of caseation, before CMI is fully developed, MTB multiplication can lead to local extension (progressive primary TB) and distant haematogenous spread of infection. In some cases haematogenous spread will result in symptomatic miliary TB. In the majority, however, the bacilli are contained in tubercles within the tissues in which they lodge where most of the bacilli are killed by effector cells of the CMI response.
- A small number of MTB organisms can lie dormant in the lung and other tissues (e.g. bone, brain, kidney), with a risk of reactivating later in life.

Progressive primary TB

Although the tendency is for primary pulmonary TB to heal, the primary focus can continue to enlarge. There may be local spread, which can include the pleura. The caseous centre can liquefy and empty into bronchi and produce a cavity and cause cavitating primary TB. This is unusual and more likely to occur in young children. Most complications of TB occur during the first few years after infection.

Reactivation TB disease

Adolescence is a time when reactivation can occur with 'adult-type' disease. This occurs twice as often in girls as in boys. Reactivation usually occurs in the apical portion of the lung. Cavities form more readily and liquefied material disseminates through the airways. If untreated, large areas of the lung can be destroyed. Reactivation can also occur in any organ in which TB organisms were deposited during the primary infection. Reactivation of multiple forms of infection can result in miliary TB.

Important concepts

There are a few important concepts that will help in understanding the management of children with TB.

- TB is infectious. Close contacts (usually in the same household) of an individual with open TB are at risk of getting the infection, although the proportion infected is usually < 10%. The presence of infection is detected by either a delayed hypersensitivity response, in the form of the tuberculin skin test (TST), or by interferon-gamma release assays.
- TB *infection* is different from TB *disease*. A positive TST indicates that infection with TB has occurred and an immune response has been made (see 🕮 p. 266). A positive TST plus clinical, radiological, or microbiological abnormalities indicates TB disease.
- After TB infection, small numbers of viable organisms may reside in several tissues for many years without causing symptoms. Reactivation of the disease can occur given the right conditions, e.g. a waning of host immunity. About half of children who develop disease will do so within a few years of the primary infection.
- The risk of TB disease after TB infection varies with age (see Table 22.1). In children under 2 years it is as high as 50%, with most disease occurring within 6 months of the infection. Disease at this age group is also more likely to include miliary disease and tuberculous meningitis (TBM). Because of the high risk in this age group, children under 2 years of age who are in close contact with TB should be protected with chemoprophylaxis as soon as possible after exposure whilst awaiting a TST or T-cell assay.
- In healthy adults disease risk after infection is thought to be about 10% and can occur at any time, sometimes many years after the primary infection. The risk is dependent on the health of the individual involved.
- There are no good data indicating the amount by which the risk of TB infection converting to TB disease is reduced by chemoprophylaxis for any given individual. The best estimates suggest 60–90% protection.
- Some MTB organisms are more virulent than others, both in terms of severity of disease and infectivity.
- BCG is most effective in preventing young children from disseminated disease and TBM (overall reduced relative risk of 0.2–0.5). It is less effective at protecting children and adults from pulmonary TB.
- In contrast to adults who have reactivation disease, young children who have primary TB infection are not highly infectious. They rarely develop cavitating disease and, in the absence of cavitating disease, their sputum carries few organisms. Adolescents can have adult-type reactivation open TB.
- Once chemotherapy has been started for a susceptible organism, an adult with smear-positive TB will usually become non-infectious after 2 weeks.

Table 22.1 Age-specific risk of progression to disease after primary infection with MTB in immunocompetent children. Note that there is a bimodal distribution of pulmonary disease risk—highest in infancy but increasing again in the over 10 year olds. Also note that these are average figures and will vary according the virulence of each particular MTB organism. (Adapted from reference 1)

Age at primary infection (y)	Risk of progression to disease (%)		
	No disease	Pulmonary disease	Miliary disease or TBM
1	50	30–40	10–20
1–2	75–80	10–20	2–5
2–5	95	5	0.5
5–10	98	2	0.5
>10	80–90	10–20	0.5

1 Marais, B.J., Gie, R.P., Schaaf, H.S., Beyers, N., Donald, P.R., and Starke, J.R. (2006). Childhood pulmonary tuberculosis: old wisdom and new challenges. *Am. J. Respir. Crit. Care Med.* **173**, 1078–90.

At-risk groups

Children at increased risk of TB infection are those with a high risk of exposure due to:
- close contact with someone with open disease;
- living in a community with a high incidence of TB infection;
- travel to, or exposure to visitors from countries with high incidence of TB infection.

Children at increased risk of developing TB disease once infected are those:
- with immunodeficiency, including HIV infection;
- <2 years of age.

Children with a high risk of exposure to TB should be vaccinated with BCG in the neonatal period. In countries with a low incidence (<40/100 000) of TB infection, BCG should not be given to infants who are known to have, or who are at high risk of having HIV infection, including infants of HIV positive mothers, because of the increased risk of disseminated infection with BCG.

Symptoms and signs

The majority of primary TB disease in children will be pulmonary. In around 50% of children with a positive TST and an abnormal CXR there will be no symptoms or signs of TB disease. In the remainder, the commonest symptoms are:
- weight loss;
- cough;
- malaise;
- fever.

In some older children who may present with reactivation TB there may also be night sweats. The cough is usually dry. Haemoptysis may occur rarely. Breathlessness only occurs in late disease when there has been extensive lung destruction or when there is a large pleural effusion.

More rarely, the site of primary TB is within the peripheral lymph nodes, mainly the cervical lymph nodes. The enlarged nodes are usually painless with an absence of redness or heat making the classic 'cold abscess'. The overlying skin may become discoloured and sinus formation with discharge can occur. Atypical mycobacterial infection is an important differential diagnosis for this type of cervical lymphadenopathy.

Other forms of TB disease

TB disease affecting other sites can occur at any time after the primary infection, and all forms of TB disease can be seen during childhood.
- Miliary TB. Symptoms are non-specific and of 1–2 weeks duration with malaise and fevers (see 📖 p. 282).
- TB meningitis. Symptoms come on over a period of 2–6 weeks, initially with altered behaviour, poor feeding, and vomiting. Later, irritability, drowsiness, and seizures may occur. There may be focal neurological signs including cranial nerve palsies.
- Bone and joint TB. This most often affects the spine where abscess formation can cause spinal cord or nerve root compression.
- Renal TB may present with dysuria, haematuria, and loin pain. Systemic symptoms are not common,
- Gastrointestinal TB usually causes abdominal pain with a palpable mass. Intestinal obstruction can also occur.

Investigations

Imaging

Chest X-ray findings (see Fig. 22.1) include:
- mediastinal lymph node enlargement;
- areas of parenchymal opacification that may be single or multiple;
- lobar consolidation;
- areas of atelectasis;
- pleural effusion;
- miliary deposits—the size of the lesions can vary;
- calcification, either of hilar nodes or of the parenchymal primary focus.

Most frequent radiological finding in children with primary pulmonary TB is hilar adenopathy without evidence of parenchymal lung disease.

Tuberculin skin tests (TSTs)

- TSTs involve intradermal injections of purified proteins derived from *Mycobacterium tuberculosis* (tuberculin proteins).
- TSTs do **not** measure protective immunity to *M. tuberculosis*. Rather they measure delayed-type hypersensitivity responses to tuberculin.
- Two types of TSTs were previously available in the UK: the Heaf test and the Mantoux test.
  - The Heaf test used a gun with 6 injectors arranged in a circle to drive the tuberculin into the skin. This gun had the advantage of being easy to use, even in wriggling toddlers. The tuberculin used for this test is no longer available so this test is no longer performed.
  - The Mantoux test involves an intradermal injection of tuberculin in volume of 0.1mL using a syringe and 26 gauge needle. It is essential that the injection is intradermal (producing a wheal of 6mm) for the test to be valid. SC injections will leave no wheal and will almost always be negative. The previous standard dose was 10 tuberculin units (TUs). This has now been changed to 2TUs. Lower dose gives the same information but reduces the number of severe reactions. Where there is a high index of suspicion and the test with 2TUs is negative, a repeat test using 10TUs can be carried out. Mantoux tests should be read 48–72h after injection. The size of *induration* (not redness) is measured. Best practice is to measure transverse and longitudinal diameters of induration and calculate the average.
- Interpretation of Mantoux test depends on the clinical situation. Usually children will be tested because of contact with an index case (usually a smear-positive adult) or because they have illness that might be caused by *M. tuberculosis*. In either scenario, children who have not had BCG and who have an induration of 6mm or more following a Mantoux test should be considered to have been infected with *M. tuberculosis*. If BCG has been given (85–90% will have a scar as a result of intradermal BCG vaccination) induration of up to 15mm may represent effects of the BCG rather than TB infection. If child has symptoms consistent with TB, Mantoux responses over 6mm should

be interpreted as indicating possible TB even after BCG vaccination. Induration greater than 15mm indicates TB infection in all situations.

- Exposure to environmental atypical mycobacteria can also contribute to Mantoux reactions of up to 15mm.

- Following BCG vaccination a proportion of children will develop some response to subsequent TSTs. There remains debate in the literature, but the majority view is that the presence of detectable delayed type hypersensitivity by skin tests after BCG does not correlate with protection for TB disease. In most studies, the proportion of children with some measurable response (>1mm induration) to TSTs more than 12 months after neonatal BCG is only 10–20%.

- Delayed-type hypersensitivity response to tuberculosis can take up to 6 weeks to develop after exposure to TB.

- *In immunodeficient children, including those with HIV infection or receiving chemotherapy. TSTs can be negative despite active TB disease. TSTs can also be negative in cases of severe disseminated TB.*

- The size of reaction to a TST does not correlate with either the likelihood of disease (as opposed to TB infection) or with disease severity.

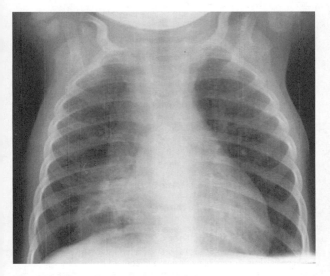

Fig. 22.1 Primary progressive TB. CXR of 9-month-old boy presenting with persistent fever and poor weight gain. CXR shows area of consolidation with cavity formation in right middle lobe and widening of the upper mediastinum consistent with adenopathy. Early morning gastric aspirates were positive for *M. tuberculosis*.

- 'Boosting' refers to an enhanced response to repeat TST as a result of stimulation of immune system by a previous TST. It only occurs in individuals (nearly always adults) who had previous exposure to TB infection, but in whom immune response has waned to such a low level that first TST response is less than 6mm induration. Exposure to the TST reactivates the immune response, so that second TST results in larger reaction. Boosting effects can be seen up to 2 years after first TST. Second TST is the more valid reflection of the person's TB status. The difference between first and second tests must be less than 10mm of induration. A greater change than this is thought to indicate conversion—a result of exposure to TB infection between the 2 tests.

Interferon-gamma release assays (IGRA)

- These tests (such as QuantiFERON-TB gold and T-SPOT TB) measure interferon-gamma production by TB-specific T cells.
- They require white cells from the person being tested to be incubated with peptides derived from specific MTB proteins (so-called RD1 antigens such as ESAT-6 and CFP-10).
- These proteins are not found in BCG or most atypical mycobacteria (with the exception of *M. kansasii* and *M. marinum*) and hence this test is not affected by exposure to these organisms.
- The tests are more sensitive and specific than TSTs and can provide a result in 24–48h.
- The tests have been commercially available since 2005 and can be useful where there is difficulty in interpreting a TST or where the clinical index of suspicion is high and the TST is negative.
- In the new algorithms from the UK's National Institute for Clinical Excellence for assessment and treatment of TB in children it has been suggested that IGRAs be used to confirm all positive TSTs prior to commencing chemoprophylaxis or treatment, on the basis that some positive TSTs will reflect effects of previous BCG vaccination and/or exposure to non-tuberculous mycobacteria[2].
- The clinical significance of a positive IGRA test combined with a negative TST in a well child who has had contact with TB is not known. It is likely that a positive IGRA represents exposure to MTB. However it is not known whether in children who are TST negative this result is predictive of a significant risk of later disease, and therefore the need for chemoprophylaxis.
- IGRA tests, like TSTs, are likely to have a false-negative rate in children with immunodeficiency.

Microscopy, PCR, and culture

- Identification of the infecting MTB organism is important for definitive diagnosis, drug susceptibility testing, and contact tracing.
- In children with TB infection but not TB disease, cultures are very likely to be negative, and treatment will be based on the MTB identified in the index case.
- In children with TB disease, attempts should be made to culture the organism, even if an index case has been identified.

---

2 http://guidance.nice.org.uk/topic/respiratory

- Culture for TB can take 6 weeks or longer.
- PCR tests are available that appear to be both sensitive (95%) and specific (100%) in the diagnosis of TB in both smear-positive and smear-negative adult patients. PCR may then provide a more rapid method of making the diagnosis than culture. Rifampicin resistance can also be identified by the same PCR test (it is commonly due to one or more of several possible mutations of the rpoB gene) and a positive result would indicate the likely presence of MDR-TB.
- Most children with TB disease are not sputum-producers and the likelihood of spontaneous smear-positive sputum is low and age-dependent. In adolescents who are more likely to have reactivation rather than primary disease, about 10% are smear-positive (20% have positive cultures). In children <10 years of age, less than 2% are smear-positive (5% have positive cultures).
- Microscopy and culture of early morning gastric aspirates (see 📖 Chapter 68, p. 787) is the most commonly used method to isolate MTB in children. Samples are taken on 3 consecutive days. Overall about 10–25% of children with suspected TB disease (positive TST, contact, and CXR changes) will have positive gastric aspirate cultures, and about half this number will have acidfast bacilli seen at microscopy of the aspirate.
- Induced sputum can also be used in children, including infants. In one study at least this seemed to be more successful than gastric aspirates—one induced sputum sample had the same success rate as 3 gastric aspirates.
- Bronchoscopy is not usually necessary in children. In high risk children, e.g. those with immune deficiency where a positive diagnosis is needed and TSTs are often false negative, bronchoscopy can be helpful. Lavage can be performed in one lobe of each lung arc, at least in adults, this has been shown to increase the yield of smear and culture results in patients who are sputum smear-negative or not sputum producers.
- In most cases, particularly in young children with primary infection, a presumed diagnosis of TB disease is made on the basis of an abnormal CXR or other clinical findings consistent with TB, plus a positive TST or IGRA, plus a history of contact.

Most children with TB in developed countries will present to a respiratory service as a consequence of contact tracing. More rarely, children will present with TB disease where the index case is unknown.

Contact tracing

For the purposes of contact tracing, the definitions of close and casual contact are not explicit and will vary between centres. For practical purposes, *close* contact can be taken to mean contact for more than an hour or so per day either within the household or elsewhere (e.g. close friends or children in the same class at school) and with a cumulative contact of 8h or more. *Casual* contact can be taken to mean brief contact only outside the household, e.g. attending the same school.

For the purposes of contact tracing, all children who are *close contacts* of an index case will be screened. If the index case is smear-positive (i.e. tubercle bacilli are seen in sputum) *casual contacts* <4 years of age, or any immunocompromised children (or adults) will also be screened. If the index case has been shown to be *highly* infectious (>10% of close contacts infected) all casual contacts (irrespective of age) are screened.

Managing a well child who has been in contact with TB

- Careful history should be taken, including identifying index case and number of people infected. Symptoms suggestive of TB disease (weight loss, cough, malaise, fever, night sweats) should be sought. Child's BCG status, including presence or absence of scar, should be noted.
- Risk factors for MDR-TB: index case previously treated for TB, or has HIV, or is a known contact of MDR-TB, or has prolonged smear-positive disease despite chemotherapy, or has failed to show clinical improvement on treatment.
- The drug sensitivities of the organism should be identified if known.
- A Mantoux test should be performed.
  - If test shows >6mm induration in child without previous BCG vaccination or >15mm in child who had BCG vaccination, CXR should be performed. If CXR is normal and no symptoms suggestive of TB, diagnosis is TB infection without disease and chemoprophylaxis should be given. If CXR is abnormal, or there are symptoms, TB disease should be suspected and treated (see below).
  - If Mantoux test negative, no symptoms suggestive of disease, and child (any age) had previous BCG vaccination, no further action necessary.
  - If Mantoux test negative and the child has not had BCG, management depends on whether index case is smear-positive or not. If index case is smear-negative, BCG vaccination can be offered and no further action is required. If index case is smear-positive, the Mantoux test (or IGRA) should be repeated 6 weeks after last contact with index case. If this test is also negative, BCG vaccination should be offered. If it is now positive, child should be re-evaluated and a CXR performed. If CXR is abnormal, TB disease should be suspected and treated. If it is normal, and child remains asymptomatic, the child should receive chemoprophylaxis.
- There are important differences in the algorithm that should be followed in young children who have been in contact with a smear-positive index case.
  - Children who are aged 4 weeks to 2 years *at the time of exposure* who have **not** previously been given BCG are at increased risk of developing disseminated TB disease. These children need to be protected by chemoprophylaxis (isoniazid monotherapy is adequate) for 6 weeks even if the first Mantoux test is negative and the child is well (it can take this long for TST to become positive). 6 weeks after the last contact with the index case, the Mantoux should be repeated. If this test is negative, then chemoprophylaxis can be stopped and vaccination with BCG should be given. If the Mantoux is now positive (>6mm induration) a CXR should be performed with re-evaluation of any symptoms and signs. If the CXR is abnormal, full treatment is commenced. If the CXR is normal and the child remains well they should complete their course of chemoprophylaxis—a further 4.5 months of isoniazid.

- Children who are aged 4 weeks to 2 years old at the time of exposure who have had previous BCG should have a tuberculin skin test in the usual way. It is likely that protection from BCG takes at least 2–3 weeks to develop and, if contact with TB occurs within this timeframe, children should be managed as if they have **not** been given BCG. If the Mantoux test is negative, no chemoprophylaxis is required, but they should be re-tested after 6 weeks. If this repeated test is now positive (Mantoux >15mm) they should be as-sessed for evidence of TB disease (symptoms, physical examination, CXR). If there is no evidence of TB disease, chemoprophylaxis should be given (see below).
- Neonates (0–4 weeks) do not need the initial Mantoux as it will almost certainly be negative irrespective of whether they have been given BCG, since insufficient time will have elapsed to allow an immune response to develop. Well neonates who have been exposed to TB should be started on chemoprophylaxis (isoniazid monotherapy), and have their Mantoux test after 6 weeks. If this test is negative (<6mm irrespective of BCG status), chemoprophy-laxis can be stopped and BCG given. BCG should also be given to infants who had neonatal BCG since the isoniazid may have affected the effectiveness of the vaccination. If the Mantoux is positive, proceed as above for children not previously given BCG.

Recommended chemoprophylaxis

Chemoprophylaxis for TB infection is either isoniazid alone for 6 months or isoniazid and rifampicin for 3 months. Most centres now use rifampicin and isoniazid for 3 months.

Algorithms for assessment of asymptomatic children

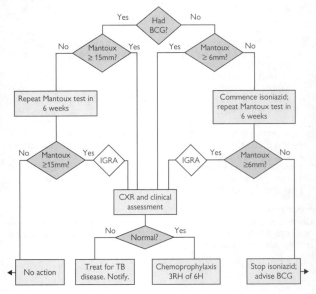

Fig. 22.2 Algorithm for approach to assessment of asymptomatic children between 4 weeks and 2 years of age who have had contact with a person with active TB. 3RH = 3 month treatment with isoniazid and rifampicin; 6H = 6 month treatment with isoniazid. Note: where IRGAs are available they should be used to confirm positive Mantoux tests prior to commencing TB chemoprophylaxis or treatment.

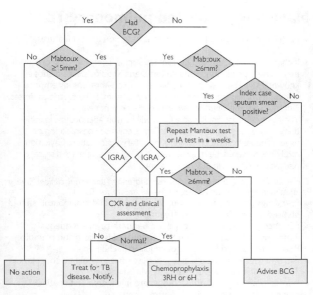

Fig. 22.3 Algorithm for approach to assessment of asymptomatic children >2 years of age who have had contact with a person with active TB. 3RH = 3 month treatment with isoniazid and rifampicin; 6h = 6 month treatment with isoniazid. Note: where IRGAs are available they should be used to confirm positive Mantoux tests prior to commencing TB chemoprophylaxis or treatment.

Managing suspected pulmonary TB

- In children diagnosis of TB infection is based on clinical features, CXR, and TSTs.
- If child has been identified by contact tracing, likely infecting organism may already be identified and cultured and antibiotic sensitivities known. If this is not so or child has systemic symptoms, attempt to obtain the organisms, either by induced sputum or by gastric aspirates. *Inability to identify organism should not delay treatment.*
- The most common finding on a CXR will be hilar adenopathy. In addition there may be segmental or lobar collapse, collapse consolidation or hyperinflation, bronchopneumonia, or miliary opacification. Cavitation is rarely encountered, but may be seen in progressive primary disease, or reactivation disease in older adolescents.

Children with a positive tuberculin test and either abnormal clinical findings or an abnormal CXR should receive full treatment for TB.
- *Four* drugs (rifampicin, isoniazid, pyrazinamide, and ethambutol) should be used in the initial phase of treatment.
- For uncomplicated respiratory TB, a 6-month regime is adequate: 2 months of 4 drugs followed by 4 months of isoniazid and rifampicin. Routine use of pyridoxine is not required in children.
- For other forms of TB disease, specialist advice should be sought. For TB meningitis 12 months treatment will be needed.
- Isoniazid can cause hepatitis. This is rare in children and routine monitoring of liver function is not required.
- Ethambutol can be associated with ocular toxicity. This is very rare (<0.5%) at a dose of 15mg/kg and, when used for only 2 months, routine eye testing is not necessary. For longer-term use in children >5 years of age, visual acuity and colour vision should be assessed at the beginning of treatment and monthly thereafter. This risk of toxicity may be reduced by using a 3 times per week schedule. Children <10 years of age are unlikely to report visual disturbance. If ocular toxity occurs, it is reversible in more than half of cases.
- Children undergoing chemotherapy for TB disease should be reviewed with a repeat CXR after 2 months of treatment. Close attention to compliance is required. If the child is improving the chemotherapy can be adjusted to isoniazid and rifampicin for the final 4 months of treatment. There is no evidence that further follow-up is necessary, but some centres elect to see children at the end of treatment, and this assessment may include a final CXR.

Multidrug resistant TB

- Multidrug resistant TB (MDR-TB) is defined as resistance to rifampicin and isoniazid.
- MDR-TB is rare in the UK accounting for around 1% of infections.
- MDR-TB usually arises in conditions of poor adherence to treatment protocols. There is an increased risk of MDR-TB in children if:
  - the index case is known to have MDR-TB;
  - the index case has previously been treated for TB;
  - the index case has HIV infection;
  - the index case remains smear-positive after 6 weeks of treatment.
- Treatment of MDR-TB is difficult and requires combination chemotherapy that includes quinolones. Patients with MDR-TB need to be treated in isolation facilities. Expert help should be obtained.
- Extreme drug resistance TB (XDT-TB) has now also emerged where there is, in addition, resistance to quinolones.

Complications

Failure to improve

In children with TB disease who fail to improve on apparently adequate therapy, three possibilities should be considered.

- There is an alternative or additional cause for the symptoms or CXR findings.
- The child is not taking their therapy. This likelihood can be minimized by clear instructions to parents at the start of treatment. Directly observed therapy (DOT) is rarely needed for children with TB.
- The disease is caused by MDR-TB.

Paradoxical reaction to treatment

- Worsening of disease and the appearance of new lesions can be part of a so-called 'paradoxical reaction' (PR) to TB treatment, and is seen in around 10% of cases.
- The most likely PR represents heightened cell-mediated immunity directed against MTB resulting in increased local inflammation.
- It usually occurs after 4–6 weeks of treatment, but may occur from a few days to many months after starting treatment.
- There may be new changes on CXR, including pleural effusion, and new symptoms can include fever. There may be bronchial compression from enlarging hilar lymph nodes.
- It is a particular problem in the CNS where enlargement of existing lesions can cause pressure effects, e.g. on the spine.
- It can be difficult to distinguish PR from treatment failure, drug resistance, or another infection. Careful history to establish adherence to therapy and knowledge of the MTB sensitivity are important factors. There is anecdotal evidence for the use of steroids in the treatment of PR and these can be tried for troublesome symptoms. Otherwise, PR will resolve on continuation of standard chemotherapy.

Endobronchial TB

- Enlarged hilar lymph nodes may cause bronchial compression and most usually affect the right middle lobe bronchus.
- Endobronchial TB refers to a more progressive process in which disease has spread from adjacent lymph node tissue into the airway wall and then into the airway lumen.
- Bronchial obstruction may be apparent at diagnosis, and can also occur during the first 6 weeks of therapy as part of a paradoxical response to TB treatment.
- Bronchial compression is usually detected either by the routine repeat CXR after 2 months of treatment (one lung looks hyperinflated, or there are areas of collapse) or by symptoms of breathlessness or wheeze.
- Further investigation should include bronchoscopy or CT scan. At bronchoscopy granulation tissue can be seen within the airway lumen

- Provided the child is taking effective antituberculous chemotherapy, treatment of endobronchial TB with 4–6 weeks of corticosteroids is usually effective (1mg/kg per day orally for the first month, and then weaning over the next 2 weeks).
- Occasionally bronchial stenosis can develop at the site of compression when healing occurs.

Pleural effusion

- Pleural effusions can occur during primary infection with TB, and may be the mode of presentation. They are more frequently seen in older children and are usually unilateral.
- In some countries TB is one of the commonest causes of pleural effusion in children.
- Children with tuberculous pleural effusions (TPE) often present acutely with fever and chest pain. Cases of TPE may be indistinguishable from those of acute bacterial pneumonia with effusion.
- TPE usually complicates primary TB. It arises as a result of an immune response (delayed hypersensitivity) to mycobacterial proteins released into the pleural cavity. Typically this results from rupture of subpleural caseous foci, generally 6–12 weeks after primary infection. Rarely, TPE may represent spread from a tuberculous focus in the spine.
- Occasionally TPE will develop 6–8 weeks after antituberculous treatment has been started—another example of a paradoxical response to chemotherapy (see Fig. 22.4).
- A definitive diagnosis of TPE requires either identification of the bacillus in cultures of pleural fluid or pleural biopsy tissue, the presence of pleural granulomata, or MTB seen on pleural biopsy
- Pleural fluid should be aspirated for analysis. This will show a high protein level and lymphocytosis. MTB organisms are scanty; Ziehl–Neelsen stains are positive in 5% and cultures are positive in only 25–30% of cases. Pleural biopsy may therefore be needed to make the diagnosis; granulomata may be seen and pleural culture for MTB is positive in 60–80%. A finding of high levels (>40U/L) of the enzyme adenosine deaminase (ADA) in pleural fluid is reported to have a high sensitivity (99%) and specificity (93%) for TPE.
- CXR usually shows no abnormality other than the effusion (Fig. 22.4). Pulmonary infiltrates may be visualized in up to 30% of cases. The effusion usually affects less than two-thirds of the hemithorax.
- Antituberculous treatment is given as for primary TB. The effusion will reabsorb slowly and most will be gone by 3 months.
- Chest tube drainage is not usually required unless there is respiratory embarrassment or evidence of tuberculous empyema with the development of thick pus containing MTB organisms. Where there is an empyema, chest tube drainage, with or without intrapleural fibrinolytic treatment will be needed. Pneumothorax may also complicate TPE, and will also need to be treated with a chest drain.

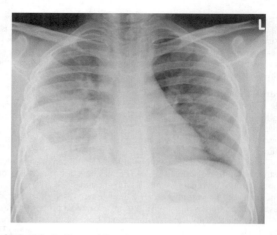

Fig. 22.4 CXR of a 12-year-old boy diagnosed with tuberculosis 6 weeks earlier and started on antituberculous chemotherapy. On clinical review he was found to have a mild fever with signs of an effusion. The CXR shows a right-sided pleural effusion and widening of the right side of the mediastinum. The pleural fluid was tapped and showed a mild lymphocytosis and raised protein. Stain for MTB was negative and the fluid subsequently failed to grow any organisms. The infecting organism had been isolated from an adult index case, was fully sensitive, and the boy was compliant with his treatment. His fever settled on simple antipyretics and his antituberculous therapy was continued. His effusion resolved 3 weeks later and was thought to be part of a paradoxical reaction to therapy.

- There is anecdotal evidence that prednisolone may help to speed resolution of the effusion and fever. There is no evidence that steroid treatment will prevent pleural thickening.
- Pleural thickening can occur in up to 50% of children, and persist for 12 months or more. Rarely, the pleura can contract during healing causing chest wall deformity and scoliosis.

Miliary TB

- Miliary TB refers to generalized disease resulting from haematogenous spread of MTB from the primary focus. In children, miliary TB is usually a complication of the primary TB infection and occurs within 6 months of infection.
- It most commonly occurs in young children (<2 years old) but can occur at any age.
- The history is usually short: 1–2 weeks of lethargy followed by onset of fever. Examination most often shows an obviously ill child with an intermittent fever. Hepatosplenomagaly and enlarged lymph nodes are found in 50% of affected children. Occasionally children can look surprisingly well with little to find.
- The lungs are nearly always involved, although there may be no abnormal physical findings.

- CXR shows widespread multiple lesions. The size of the lesion depends on the extent of the host response. They may be classic milletsized (1–2mm) lesions or much larger (1–2cm). If the CXR is not conclusive, chest CT scan will show well-defined nodules.
- Head CT or MRI may show intracerebral lesions. A lumbar puncture can be carried out after the CT scan to look for evidence of TBM.
- Fundoscopy should be carried out and may show retinal tubercles.
- Untreated miliary TB is always fatal, usually as a result of TBM.
- Progressive respiratory distress can occur, and may result in respiratory failure requiring mechanical ventilation.
- Specialist infectious diseases advice should be sought.
  - Treatment is 4 antituberculous drugs.
  - There is anecdotal evidence that prednisolone may help resolve respiratory distress in children with miliary lung disease.
  - Prednisolone is also recommended during the first 3–6 weeks of treatment of TBM.
  - Rifampicin and isoniazid can be given IV. Pyrazinamide and ethambutol are given orally even in sick patients, using an NG tube if necessary.

Notification/surveillance

All forms of tuberculosis are compulsorily notifiable in the UK under the Public Health (Control of Disease) Act 1984. The doctor making or suspecting the diagnosis is legally responsible for notification. A decision to commence treatment (but not chemoprophylaxis) indicates a level of suspicion that should trigger notification. Notification must be made to the local 'proper officer', usually the consultant in communicable disease control.

Further information

Cheng, V.C., Ho, P.L., Lee, R.A., Chan, K.S., Chan, K.K., Woo, P.C., Lau, S.K., and Yuen, K.Y. (2002). Clinical spectrum of paradoxical deterioration during antituberculosis therapy in non-HIV-infected patients. *Eur. J. Clin. Microbiol. Infect. Dis.* **21**, 803–9.

Clinical diagnosis and management of tuberculosis and measures for its prevention and control; guideline produced by the National Institute of Clinical Excellence. http://www.nice.org.uk

Pai, M., Riley, L.W., and Colford, J.M. Jr. (2004). Interferon-gamma assays in the immunodiagnosis of tuberculosis: a systematic review. *Lancet Infect. Dis.* **4**, 761–76.

Traore, H., van Deun, A., Shamputa, I.C., Rigouts, L., and Portaels, F. (2006). Direct detection of *Mycobacterium tuberculosis* complex DNA and rifampin resistance in clinical specimens from tuberculosis patients by line probe assay. *J. Clin. Microbiol.* **44** (12), 4384–8.

HIV infection

Overview

- Children with HIV infection often present with respiratory illnesses.
- The incidence of HIV infection in children shows strong geographic variability. In some parts of sub-Saharan Africa 10–30% of children are infected. The incidence of HIV infection in children in most Western countries is falling because of effective perinatal prevention of vertical transmission.
- It is important for the respiratory paediatrician to be familiar with the clinical features that may suggest a child has HIV infection. The usual clinical question will be: could this child, who has a respiratory illness, have HIV infection as an underlying aetiology? Respiratory paediatricians may also be involved in the care of children with HIV who develop acute or chronic respiratory illness.

Prevention of vertical transmission

- 85% of HIV infection in children is acquired from the mother in the perinatal period.
- The risk of vertical transmission is 15–20%. There is a further increased risk of around 15% from breastfeeding.
- Combination antiretroviral treatment (ART) given to the mother from 28 weeks gestation, together with IV zidovudine during labour, elective Caesarean section, and abstinence from breastfeeding, reduces the risk of vertical transmission to < 1%.
- A single dose of nevirapine given to mother during labour followed by a single dose to the infant reduces the risk of transmission to around 8%. This is the WHO recommended regime currently practised in most developing countries
- Caesarean section is recommended in the UK.
- Breastfeeding should be avoided where this is possible.
- If the mother requires treatment in her own right because she is symptomatic or has a low CD4 count, ART will be started before 28 weeks. Some mothers will already be on treatment when they become pregnant.
- The long-term safety of ART given during pregnancy is not known but the benefits outweigh the risks.
- If the mother takes ART during pregnancy and has a low viral load, then the infant need only be given zidovudine for 4 weeks postnatally.

Symptoms and diseases in children with HIV infection

The age at presentation of a child with vertically acquired HIV infection is very variable. 50–60% of children will present within the 1st 2 years of life with more rapidly progressive disease. These children generally have a poor prognosis and are at risk of HIV encephalopathy. Some children will remain asymptomatic without treatment for 10 years or more and are known as long-term non-progressors.

The Centres for Disease Control (CDC) in Atlanta USA have developed a classification of symptoms, signs, and diseases for symptomatic HIV disease (see box).

Classification of symptomatic HIV disease

- Category N. Asymptomatic, or only 1 category A problem.
- Category A. Mild disease:
  - lymphadenopathy (> 0.5cm at more than 2 sites)
  - hepatomegaly
  - splenomegaly
  - dermatitis
  - parotitis
  - recurrent or persistent URTI, sinusitis, or otitis media
- Category B. Moderately symptomatic. Respiratory conditions in category B include:
  - bacterial pneumonia (single episode)
  - CMV infection with onset before age 1 month
  - lymphoid interstitial pneumonia
- Category C (AIDS). Severely symptomatic. Respiratory conditions in category C include:
  - *Pneumocystis jiroveci* pneumonia
  - Mycobacterial infection: tuberculosis or atypical
  - CMV infection after 1 month of age

The full list of conditions in each category can be found on the CDC website *(www.cdc.gov/niv)*.

When to start ART

Treatment of children with HIV infection should only be undertaken by experts in this field. The treatment is difficult and there are significant side-effects from ART.

The criteria used to decide when to start ART vary but the following provides a guide.

In infants < 12 months of age (who progress more quickly than older children) treat if symptomatic (A, B, or C) *or* CD4 < 25%, irrespective of viral load.

In children > 12 months of age treat if category C (AIDS) or CD4 count < 15% expected.
  And consider treatment if any of the following is true:
- Mild to moderate symptoms (A or B).
- CD4 count 15–25% expected.
- HIV RNA copy number > 100 000/mL.

Treatment can be deferred in children > 12 months of age if they are asymptomatic or have only category A symptoms **and** their CD4 count is > 25% **and** their HIV RNA copy number < 100 000/mL.

Respiratory problems

Children with HIV most commonly present with the normal bacterial infections of childhood. The infections may not be particularly severe, but they are either persistent or recurrent. Possible presentations with respiratory disease are given below. Details of the infections are given in the relevant chapters elsewhere in the book.

Persistent or recurrent typical pneumonia

Usually caused by *Pneumococcus* or *Haemophilus influenzae*. Pneumonia due to *Staphylococcus aureus*, *Klebsiella*, or *Pseudomonas* species is more frequent in children with HIV than in the general population.

Severe or persistent pneumonitis

- This may be of sudden onset, but more usually comes on over a few weeks.
- Likely causes are viral: RSV, influenza, para-influenza, adenovirus, CMV, EBV, or *Pneumocystis jiroveci*.
- Pneumonitis is a frequent presentation of HIV infection.
- Persistent viral shedding is a clue to underlying immune deficiency, e.g. if a symptomatic infant remains RSV positive for several weeks.

Fungal infection

- Pulmonary fungal infection (excluding *Pneumocystis* pneumonia) in children with HIV infection is rare, and usually occurs late in the illness.
- *Cryptococcus neoformans* infection usually causes meningitis, but will occasionally cause an interstitial pneumonia.
- Oropharyngeal infection with *Candida* is common, but invasive disease is not.
- Infection with *Aspergillus* species is also rare, and when it does occur is usually associated with prolonged high dose courses of systemic corticosteroids.

Mycobacterial infection

- Children with HIV infection are at increased risk of developing TB disease when exposed to infection.
- They are also more likely to develop progressive or disseminated disease.
- The risk of atypical mycobacterial disease is also increased, although respiratory disease is unusual.
- Tuberculin skin tests may be negative, reflecting the deficient immune response to the infection.

Lymphoid interstitial pneumonitis (LIP; Fig. 23.1)

- This affects around 25% of children with HIV infection and usually starts between 2 and 10 years of age.
- It tends to occur when the CD4 count is still relatively high. In the initial stages it is asymptomatic.
- CXR shows reticular nodular shadowing, which may be accompanied by hilar adenopathy.

- After a period of weeks to months, a dry cough and breathlessness develop. The disease may progress and hypoxia can occur.
- Examination shows increased respiratory rate with or without hypoxia. In longstanding disease there may be finger clubbing. Breath sounds are usually normal. Occasionally wheeze may be heard.
- The presence of LIP increases the risk of bacterial pneumonia, and recurrent pneumonias may lead to bronchiectasis.
- Symptomatic LIP may be treated with oral corticosteroids, although there are no trials showing benefit. It may also respond to ART. Bronchodilators may help associated wheezing.
- LIP may be caused by a locally exuberant CD8 response to primary or reactivated EBV infection. LIP can be seen without HIV infection, usually in adults with autoimmune or lymphoproliferative disorders, where it is also associated with EBV infection.

Malignancy

- Kaposi sarcoma is reported in children with HIV, mostly in adolescents. It may affect the airways and present with fever, cough, and breathlessness. CXR shows either a diffuse nodular or interstitial shadowing, sometimes with pleural effusion.
- Lymphomas have been reported in children with HIV infection. May present with breathlessness caused by mediastinal lymphadenopathy.
- LIP can also progress to a pulmonary lymphoproliferative disorder and malignant lymphoma.

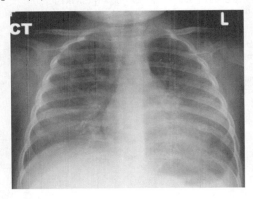

Fig. 23.1 Lymphoid interstitial pneumonitis. CXR of a 2-year-old girl who presented with a 3 week history of respiratory distress and was found to be hypoxic. She had previously been seen for what was thought to be idiopathic immune thrombocytopenia. HIV test was positive; investigation for respiratory infection was negative. Her respiratory illness responded to oral prednisolone.

When to suspect HIV infection

Features in history that increase likelihood of HIV infection
- Child's mother or father is from a region with high incidence of HIV infection.
- Child has:
  - persistent diarrhoea (can be caused either by HIV disease directly or by *Cryptosporidium* infection);
  - growth failure;
  - recurrent or persistent oral *Candida* infection;
  - previous bacterial infections;
  - dermatitis (HIV dermatitis causes a red papular rash);
  - developmental delay—suggesting HIV encephalopathy or CNS infection.

Features in examination that increase likelihood of HIV infection
- Generalized lymphadenopathy—common in early HIV disease.
- Hepatomegaly—found in 70% of children with symptomatic HIV disease.
- Splenomegaly—found in 45%.
- Parotitis—usually painless swelling of parotid glands found in around 30% of children, mainly long-term non-progressors.
- Evidence of heart failure—cardiomyopathy can occur.
- Skin disease:
  - red papular rash (HIV dermatitis);
  - viral warts;
  - *Candida* infection (skin or mouth);
  - impetigo;
  - severe scabies;
  - multidermatomal shingles;
  - widespread molluscum contagiosum.

Investigations, treatment, and outcome

Investigations

- HIV test. ELISA test for antibodies is not reliable in the first 2 years of life in children with HIV-infected mothers because of transplacental maternal antibody. HIV PCR tests should be used. These detect the presence of the HIV RNA and can provide quantification of viral load.
- FBC:
  - 10% will have a consumptive thrombocytopenia that looks like ITP;
  - anaemia is common;
  - neutrophils may be low.
- CD4 count. Combined with viral load the CD4 count gives the best indicator of disease progression.
- Immunoglobulin levels usually go up (hypergammaglobulinaemia) with initial disease progression (HIV to AIDS) and then fall in end-stage disease.
- Liver function and renal function may be deranged.

Treatment

Treat presenting disease. Assess if need to start ART (see p. 297).

Outcome

ART is now effective at controlling symptoms in most children. Recurrent respiratory infection may still occur, with a risk of bronchiectasis. Once treatment has commenced in children with severe immunosuppression, latent respiratory disease (e.g. RSV infection) may become apparent because of immune reconstitution.

Structural problems of upper and lower airways

Nasal obstruction

Congenital abnormalities of nasal structures may lead to obstruction of the nasal airway. Since most babies are obligate nose-breathers these problems often present shortly after birth, sometimes with severe respiratory distress.

Choanal atresia

- Choanal atresia or stenosis, is caused by failure of resorption of the buccopharyngeal membrane during embryonic development.
- It is the commonest congenital form of nasal obstruction and occurs in 1/10 000 births. It is more common in females.
- The atresia can be membranous or bony (Fig. 24.1). Often there is bony stenosis with a membranous covering.
- The atresia can be unilateral (70%) or bilateral (30%).
- 5–40% of affected infants have at least 2 features of the CHARGE association (coloboma–heart defects–atresia choanae–retarded growth and development–genital hypoplasia–ear abnormalities). Infants with bilateral atresia are more likely to have the CHARGE association.

Symptoms and signs

- Unilateral atresia may be asymptomatic in infancy, although infants may have problems during URTIs that block the unaffected nares. Later in childhood unilateral atresia may present with persistent unilateral rhinorrhoea.
- Bilateral atresia can cause severe neonatal respiratory distress. Classically there is cyanosis alleviated by crying.
- Infants with choanal stenosis may present with episodes of primary aspiration during feeds because of difficulty in coordinating sucking and breathing with a partially obstructed nasal airway.

Investigations

- Flexible nasal endoscopy will demonstrate blind-ending nares.
- CT scan can demonstrate bony stenosis or atresia. It can miss mucosal coverings.
- Investigations to identify other features of the CHARGE association should be undertaken.

Treatment and outcome

- Infants with severe respiratory distress where choanal atresia is suspected can be helped with an oropharyngeal airway whilst investigations and definitive treatment are planned.
- Surgery is the definitive treatment using either a transnasal or transpalatal approach.
- Temporary stenting is often needed to prevent re-stenosis.

- Infants with CHARGE association often have very significant problems with feeding, including incoordinate swallowing, aspiration lung disease, and gastro-oesophageal reflux, which arises because of dysfunction of the bulbar nerve supply to the oropharynx. Many affected children need fundoplication and gastrostomy feeding.
- Overall childhood mortality for infants with CHARGE association is high, between 10 and 15%.

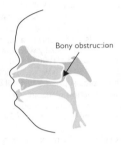

Fig. 24.1 Choanal atresia with bony obstruction.

Further information

Issekutz, K.A., Graham, J.M. Jr, Prasad, C., Smith, I.M., and Blake, K.D. (2005). An epidemiological analysis of CHARGE syndrome: preliminary results from a Canadian study. *Am. J. Med. Genet. A* **133**, 309–17.

Other causes of nasal obstruction

Congenital stenosis of the pyriform aperture

- Defect, sometimes called anterior choanal stenosis, caused by bony overgrowth of nasal lateral process of maxilla during embryogenesis.
- It is considered to be a form of holoprosencephaly. Associated midline defects include a single maxillary central incisor, central diabetes insipidus, and pituitary gland abnormalities.
- Treatment of the nasal obstruction is surgical. Nasal stenting is often needed to prevent re-stenosis.

Dacryocystoceles

- A dacrocystocele (also known as lacrimal sac mucocele) is a cystic dilatation of the nasolacrimal sac that arises because of imperforate valves at the distal end of the duct where it drains into the nasal cavity, under the middle meatus. Usually apparent at birth as bluish swelling below medial canthus of the eye, usually with eye watering (epiphora) or sticky eye. Incidence is around 1/1000 births.
- 75% become infected over the first few months of life. Infection is potentially serious. The orbital septum is not fully formed in early life and there is a risk of the infection spreading to the orbit or CNS.
- Most dacrocystoceles have intranasal component that can cause nasal obstruction. This is second most likely reason for structural nasal obstruction in infants after choanal atresia and can be bilateral.
- Uninfected dacrocystoceles can be managed by massage, but this is often ineffective and probing the nasolacrimal duct is usually required.
- Where there is an intranasal component causing obstruction surgery will be needed, usually an intranasal marsupialization procedure.

Other nasal masses (mostly diagnosed by MRI scan)

Several other congenital masses may rarely cause nasal obstruction, usually in early infancy. These include:

- encephaloceles
- gliomas
- dermoid cysts
- teratomas

Management is usually surgical.

The normal larynx

Figure 24.2 shows the structure of the normal larynx.

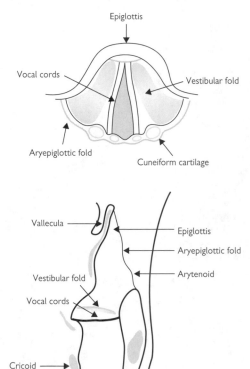

Fig. 24.2 The normal larynx.

Laryngomalacia

- Laryngomalacia is the term used to describe a condition in which there is partial or complete airway closure caused by inward folding of the aryepiglottic folds and epiglottis during inspiration.
- During inspiration the pressure within the airway falls below atmospheric pressure. This provides a force that tends to collapse the airway. This force is usually resisted by rigidity within the airway wall provided by the cartilage and muscular tone.
- The cause of laryngomalacia is not known. The term laryngomalacia implies softening of the laryngeal cartilage, but where it has been examined the cartilage in the larynx of affected infants is not demonstrably different from normal. Three types of laryngomalacia are described (Fig. 24.3):
  - short aryepiglottic folds pull the epiglottis into the typical omega shape with consequent narrowing of the laryngeal opening;
  - loose mucosal tissue overlying the arytenoid cartilages that prolapses into the airway during inspiration;
  - posterior displacement of the epiglottis so that it partially obstructs the larynx;
  - often there is a combination of these types.
- Laryngomalacia is usually a benign condition but can cause failure to thrive and difficulty feeding. It is common and may coexist with lower airway pathology. Thus the presence of laryngomalacia does not exclude other pathologies and should not deter further investigation.
- Laryngomalacia, like other respiratory problems that result in greater negative intrathoracic pressures during inspiration, can be associated with gastro-oesophageal reflux. Reflux to the larynx can cause mucosal oedema, which may worsen the airways obstruction.

Symptoms

- Laryngomalacia results in a purely inspiratory stridor. If there is any expiratory component, seek an alternative diagnosis.
- The stridor may be present from birth or develop over the first few days or weeks.
- It may become louder as inspiratory flow rates increase with age.
- The stridor is staccato and crescendo, increasing in loudness and pitch towards the end of inspiration. It is variable and may be absent during sleep.
- When laryngomalacia is severe there may be failure to thrive and poor feeding.

Signs

- The key physical sign is the nature of the stridor.
- There is often associated chest wall recession.
- Checking adequate growth is an important part of the assessment.
- Look for clues to alternative diagnoses, including haemangiomata, quality of the cry (hoarse cry may indicate vocal cord palsy), cardiac examination.

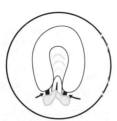

Omega shaped epiglottis with
short aryepiglottic folds

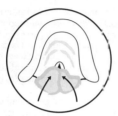

Prolapse of mucosa
over arytenoid cartilages

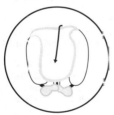

Posterior lapse displacement
of epiglottis

Fig. 24.3 Proposed mechanisms of laryngeal obstruction associated with laryngomalacia.

Differential diagnosis

- The presence of a purely inspiratory stridor indicates a problem that lies above the thoracic inlet. This part of the airway includes the subglottic space as well as the larynx. Possible lesions include:
  - subglottic stenosis;
  - airway wall haemangioma;
  - cysts, e.g. vallecular cyst;
  - laryngeal web.
- Infants with laryngeal cleft may have a stridor that is identical to that in simple laryngomalacia. These infants will also have difficulty feeding with episodes of respiratory distress related to aspiration.

Investigations

- In children with mild laryngomalacia who are thriving, the diagnosis can usually be made clinically and an expectant approach can be taken.
- Certain diagnosis of laryngomalacia requires direct visualization of the larynx during spontaneous ventilation. The typical appearance is that of an omega-shaped epiglottis that is pulled down towards the laryngeal opening during inspiration combined with prolapse of the aryepiglottic folds into the airway. Together these structures obstruct the laryngeal opening.
- When direct visualization is undertaken it is important to fully inspect the lower airway to exclude a second pathology—said to be present in up to 10% of infants. Most commonly this is mild tracheomalacia, which does not require treatment, although subglottic stenosis, laryngeal cysts, and vocal cord paralysis have all been described.

Treatment and outcome

- In most infants laryngomalacia is a self-limiting condition that resolves without intervention, usually by 12–18 months of age (75% resolve within 12 months).
- In infants with moderate or severe disease, a 6 week trial of a proton-pump inhibitor or H2-antagonist may be of benefit to reduce the effects of any laryngeal oedema caused by gastro-oesophageal reflux. If no benefit is seen after 6 weeks, the treatment should be stopped.
- Around 10% of infants have significant failure to thrive and these infants can be helped by surgery. The commonest operation is some form of supraglottoplasty. Where the aryepiglottic folds are short, they can be divided to free up the edges of the epiglottis. Where there is redundant mucosal tissue, this can be resected. Finally, if the posterior attachment of the epiglottis is thought to be contributing to the obstruction, the glossoepiglottic ligament can be divided and the epiglottis sutured to the base of the tongue. Outcome of surgery is usually excellent.

Further information
Olney, D.R., Greinwald, J.H. Jr, Smith, R.J., and Bauman. N.M. (1999). Laryngomalacia and its treatment. *Laryngoscope* **109**, 1770–5.

Laryngeal cleft

Laryngotracheo-oesophageal cleft (LTEC) refers to an abnormal communication between the oesophagus and the larynx and variable parts of the trachea. The oesophagus and trachea start life as a single tube that is divided into the anterior trachea and the posterior oesophagus by the tracheo-oesophageal membrane. The membrane grows from the stomach towards the mouth and LTEC develops when the membrane fails to form completely. Four types of LTEC are recognized, depending on the size of the defect (Fig. 24.4):

- type 1 (30%) affects the interaretynoid musculature only and the cleft is above the vocal cords;
- type 2 (45%) extends down to and includes the cricoid cartilage;
- type 3 (10%) extends down to the mid-trachea;
- type 4 (5%) extends down to the carina.

Although type 1 LTEC does not form a communication with the trachea below the vocal cords, it does significantly reduce the effectiveness of the laryngeal musculature in preventing aspiration.

LTEC is rare, affecting 0.1% of the population. It is associated with other abnormalities, most notably a more distal tracheo-oesophageal fistula and oesophageal atresia (found in 20% of children with LTEC). Other problems include gastro-oesophageal reflux (30–40%), cardiac anomalies, laryngomalacia, and genitourinary abnormalities. It is also associated with 2 described syndromes: G syndrome and Pallister–Hall syndrome.

Symptoms and signs

Symptoms arising from a laryngeal cleft are usually those in relation to aspiration and are usually worse with feeding. Where the cleft is large symptoms will be present from birth. For smaller type 1 clefts, presentation is typically between 6 months and 3 years of age. Symptoms include episodic:

- cough (which may become chronic and persistent);
- cyanosis and other signs of respiratory distress;
- choking after feeds.

In addition there may be:

- stridor;
- poor swallow with increased oral secretions;
- dysphonia or aphonia.

In children who have had tracheo-oesophageal fistula repair who continue to have significant symptoms associated with feeding, the possibility of an undiagnosed LTEC should be considered.

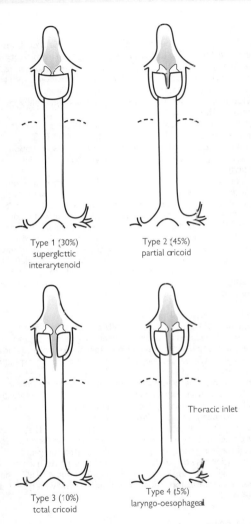

Fig. 24.4 Types of laryngeal cleft.

Investigations

Usually the diagnosis will be unsuspected, in which case likely investigations will be those for infant with recurrent episodes of respiratory distress and possible cyanosis on feeding. These will include the following.

- CXR. Non-specific bilateral increased bronchial markings with patchy areas of increased opacity. Consistent with aspiration.
- pH study. May be abnormal since gastro-oesophageal reflux is common in children with LTEC.
- Contrast swallow to look for hiatus hernia and other structural abnormalities. Likely to be normal in children with LTEC.
- Videofluoroscopy may be performed and may show aspiration into the larynx and trachea. In children with type 1 clefts this investigation may be normal.
- Laryngobronchoscopy. Types 1 and 2 LTEC are *very easy to miss with the flexible bronchoscope*. This is because the passage of the broncho-scopy through the nasopharynx means that it approaches the larynx from a posterior direction and looks at the anterior wall before diving between the cords. If LTEC is a possibility a rigid bronchoscope should be used with laryngeal suspension. This will show the posterior walls of the larynx between the arytenoid cartilage, and will allow this area to be probed to demonstrate the presence (or not) of a cleft. Unless an experienced operator has specifically looked for and excluded a cleft using a rigid bronchoscope, its presence is still a possible cause for respiratory symptoms.

Management

- Management of type 1 defects is usually conservative in the first instance. This includes medical treatment for gastro-oesophageal reflux (motility agents plus proton pump inhibitor), thickened feeds, advice from speech and language therapist, and attention to any aspiration lung disease.
- If conservative management fails after 4–6 months with evidence of persisting aspiration, surgery should be considered. Children with type 1 LTEC may have a primary repair without other intervention. Good results have been reported after endoscopic repair.
- Children with more serious clefts will require surgery. They often require tracheostomy to safeguard the airway whilst the repair is made. If there is gastro-oesophageal reflux, gastrostomy and fundoplication may be needed to prevent refluxing stomach contents from damaging the repair site. Repair of types 3 and 4 LTEC is difficult and recurrent fistula formation is common. Survival with type 4 clefts is unusual.

Further information

Watters, K. and Russell, J. (2003). Diagnosis and management of type 1 laryngeal cleft. *Int. J. Pediatr. Otorhinolaryngol.* **67** (6), 591–6.

Kubba, H., Gibson, D., Bailey, M., and Hartley, B. (2005). Techniques and outcomes of laryngeal cleft repair: an update to the Great Ormond Street Hospital series. *Ann. Otol. Rhinol. Laryngol.* **114** (4), 309–13.

Benjamin, B. and Inglis, A. (1989). Minor congenital laryngeal clefts: diagnosis and classification. *Ann. Otol. Rhinol. Laryngol.* **98** (6), 417–20.

Vocal cord palsy

Vocal cord palsy (failure of vocal cord abduction) in childhood is most often seen either as a congenital problem, or acquired as a direct consequence of cardiac disease or surgery for cardiac disease.

Congenital vocal cord palsy

- 50% are bilateral and 50% are unilateral
- Of the unilateral palsies, most (60%) are on the left, reflecting the longer course of the recurrent laryngeal nerve on the left and its consequent increased risk of injury.
- 40% of both bilateral and unilateral palsies have no identified cause.
- 75% of unilateral and 50% of bilateral palsies recover spontaneously—largely irrespective of the cause of the palsy. If recovery is going to occur, it will nearly always have done so by 2 years of age.
- Bilateral palsy is rare with an annual incidence of around 1 per million births

Causes of congenital vocal cord palsy

Bilateral
- Arnold–Chiari malformation
- Hydrocephalus
- Midbrain or brainstem dysgenesis
- Myasthenia gravis
- Idiopathic

Unilateral
- Birth trauma
- Any cardiac disease resulting in compression injury to laryngeal nerves (Ortner's syndrome)
- Midbrain or brainstem dysgenesis
- Idiopathic

Acquired vocal cord palsy

- Acquired palsy is nearly always unilateral, and usually left-sided.
- The commonest cause is surgical injury, usually associated with aortic arch surgery.
- Brainstem tumours before or after surgery can also cause vocal cord palsy.
- Spontaneous recovery is usual, but its likelihood depends on the cause.
- Vocal cords can become fixed as a result of tethering of the arytenoid cartilages, usually as part of acquired subglottis stenosis. This represents a mechanical problem rather than a true palsy (see 📖 p. 318).

Symptoms and signs

- Bilateral palsy nearly always presents with stridor in the neonatal period. In 50–70% it is severe enough to require an artificial airway. The stridor is often biphasic but louder on inspiration.

- Unilateral palsy causes a husky weak cry. There is no associated airways obstruction and the diagnosis may not be made for some weeks.
- Both unilateral and bilateral palsies increase the risk of aspiration lung disease, which may present with episodes of choking or respiratory distress.

Investigations

- The diagnosis is made by direct inspection of the larynx during spontaneous ventilation (either sedation or very light anaesthesia).
- MRI scan of the head, neck, and thorax to image the full length of the recurrent laryngeal nerves on both sides.
- Videofluoroscopy is useful to determine risk of aspiration. It can help determine the need for intervention, particularly in unilateral palsies.

Treatment and outcome

Bilateral vocal cord palsy

- 50–70% of children with bilateral palsies will need a tracheostomy.
- Spontaneous recovery is less likely in children needing tracheostomy but may still occur in 50%.
- If there has been no improvement in vocal cord function by 2 years of age, surgical options should be considered. The airway can be improved by excising part of the cord on one side or fixing it in abduction. This procedure will adversely affect any prospect for normal vocal function, but may allow decannulation.

Unilateral vocal cord palsy

- Unilateral vocal cord palsy recovers spontaneously in 75% of children. Even where it persists there is often good compensation by the mobile cord to the paralysed side allowing reasonable phonation. Where compensation is inadequate there will be poor phonation and an on-going risk of aspiration lung disease. Function can be improved by increasing the bulk of the paralysed vocal cord using collagen or fat. The bulking is temporary and the material is resorbed over 3–6 months, which may give time for spontaneous function to return.
- Thickening feeds may reduce risk of aspiration, as may the use of NG or gastrostomy feeding. These options are worth trying, often with assistance of speech and language therapists, before laryngeal surgery is considered.

Further information

Miyamoto, R.C., Parikh, S.R., Gallad, W., and Licameli, G.R. (2005). Bilateral congenital vocal cord paralysis: a 16-year institutional review. *Otolaryngol. Head Neck Surg.* **133**, 241–5.

de Gaudemar, I., Roudaire, M., Francois, M., and Narcy. P. (1996). Outcome of laryngeal paralysis in neonates: a long term retrospective study of 113 cases. *Int. J. Pedictr. Otorhinolaryngol.* **34**, 101–10.

Patel, N.J., Kerschner, J.E., and Merati, A.L. (2003). The use of injectable collagen in the management of pediatric vocal unilateral fold paralysis. *Int. J. Pediatr. Otorhinolaryngol.* **67**, 1355–60.

Vascular rings

Aberrant positions of the great arteries can result in compression of the trachea and oesophagus. Vascular rings are relatively rare. A large centre may see 2 or 3 per year. They should always be considered in the differential diagnosis of an infant with noisy breathing or with recurrent respiratory tract infection. Vascular rings may occur with or without underlying congenital heart disease and are not reliably detected by Echocardiography.

Symptoms

- The most prominent symptom caused by vascular rings is noisy breathing as a consequence of the tracheal compression.
- This can range from a harsh inspiratory and expiratory stridor to a less impressive but persistent rattle.
- The symptoms usually worsen during respiratory tract infections and may result in recurrent admission to hospital, often with a diagnosis of 'pneumonia' or croup.
- There may be a persistent barking cough.
- Dysphagia may occur but is relatively uncommon in young children with vascular rings.
- Rarely, infants with vascular rings may present with respiratory failure, usually associated with an LRTI. The diagnosis may be made as part of the evaluation of such an infant who fails to wean from mechanical ventilation.

Diagnosis

- A plain CXR can help exclude parenchymal lung disease and may give a clue to the presence of a right-sided aorta (the trachea will lie in a central or slightly left-sided position).
- In a respiratory centre, the next investigation would be bronchoscopy.
- If this service is not available, a contrast oesophagram can be used to show oesophageal compression. Most rings include the oesophagus and trachea and the posterior part of the oesophagus will be compressed. The pulmonary sling is an exception to this rule. In this condition the anterior wall of the oesophagus is compressed.
- Definitive diagnosis can usually be made with a contrast-enhanced CT scan or MRI scan.
- Cardiac echocardiography will detect any associated congenital heart disease.

Types of ring

- Double aortic arch (50%).
- Right-sided aortic arch and aberrant left subclavian (30%).
- Left-sided aortic arch and aberrant right subclavian (10%).
- Pulmonary sling (5%).
- The remainder is made up of rarer anatomical arrangements.

Normal anatomy and embryology (Fig. 24.5)

The aorta normally originates from the left ventricle just posterior to the main pulmonary artery. The ascending aorta passes in front of the right pulmonary artery, and turns to the left just above the carina. The arch passes in front of the trachea before turning and descending in a posterior direction, behind the main pulmonary artery at the point where it bifurcates. During embryological development there are 2 ventral and 2 dorsal aortae, joined by 6 pairs of brachial arches. The 4th arch forms the aortic arch proper. The 6th arch forms the ductus arteriosus. In the majority of individuals (> 95%), there is a left aortic arch, a left ductus arteriosus, and a left descending aorta. Differing arrangements can give rise to vascular structures that encircle and compress the trachea.

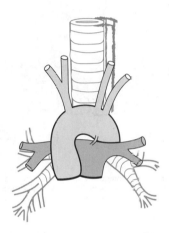

Fig. 24.5 Normal left-sided aorta. The vessels coming off the arch are the innominate artery, the left common carotid artery, and the left subclavian artery in that order.

Double aortic arch

- This is the commonest form of symptomatic vascular ring, and tends to cause the most severe tracheal compression.
- Symptoms are usually obvious from birth.
- A double aortic arch arises because of persistence of both right and left 4th brachial arches. The descending aorta can be left- or right-sided. The left-sided arch passes in front of the trachea. The right-sided arch passes behind the trachea and oesophagus, to join the left-sided arch, completing the ring and forming the descending aorta. The ductus is usually left-sided. See Figs 24.6 and 24.7.
- Both arches are usually patent, and the right is often larger than the left, and will usually give off the right common carotid and right subclavian arteries. Either arch can be atretic or stenosed, usually after the origin of subclavian artery.
- Approximately 20% of children with double aortic arch will also have congenital heart disease, usually Fallot's tetralogy or ventricular septal defect. Up to 20% of affected children will have the 22q11 deletion that is associated with DiGeorge and velocardiofacial syndromes.

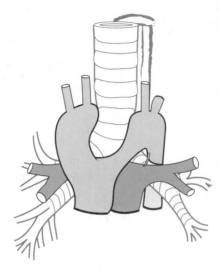

Fig. 24.6 Double aortic arch, anterior view. The figure shows a dominant right arch passing behind the oesophagus, with the right subclavian and right common carotid arising from it. This is the commonest arrangement.

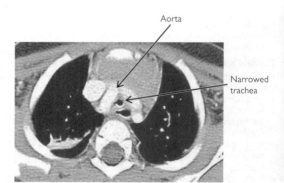

Fig 24.7 Contrast-enhanced CT scan at the level of the aortic arch showing the ascending aorta dividing into right and left arches and a narrowed trachea.

Right-sided arch with aberrant left subclavian artery
(Figs 24.8–24.10)

- When a right-sided arch is present, in 75% of individuals the first vessel arising from the arch is a left innominate, which divides to form the left common carotid and left subclavian. The right common carotid and right subclavian are given off as separate vessels. In 25% of individuals, the first vessel arising from the arch is the left common carotid with the left subclavian arising separately from the descending aorta.

- In most cases with this arrangement, the left-sided duct arises from the aberrant left subclavian artery, and the ring formed is loose and does not cause symptoms.

- Occasionally both left subclavian artery and left ductus arise from a retro-oesophageal diverticulum of the descending aorta, called the diverticulum of Kommerell—an embryological remnant of the left 4th aortic arch, often of the same diameter as the aorta itself. This arrangement forms a tighter ring that can cause tracheal compression. The diverticulum may compresses the oesophagus without significant tracheal narrowing and the predominant symptom may be dysphagia, often only with solid foods. The dysphagia may not present until late childhood.

- Tracheal compression is usually less severe than that seen with double aortic arch, so that symptoms are milder and presentation may be delayed until beyond 6 months of age. Noisy breathing will become more apparent as flow rates increase with increasing age.

Left-sided arch with aberrant right subclavian artery

- An aberrant right subclavian artery, arising from the descending aorta and passing behind the trachea occurs in 0.5% of the population.

- It does not form a ring and seldom causes symptoms.

- Occasionally the aberrant subclavian artery can run between the trachea and oesophagus, rather than behind the oesophagus, and can give rise to dysphagia (so-called dysphagia lusoria). It may not present until adult life.

- This arrangement very rarely produces respiratory symptoms.

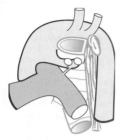

Fig. 24.8 Typical right-sided aorta, left lateral view.

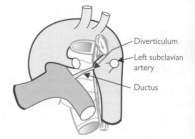

Fig. 24.9 Right arch with aberrant left subclavian artery and ductus arising from the aortic diverticulum

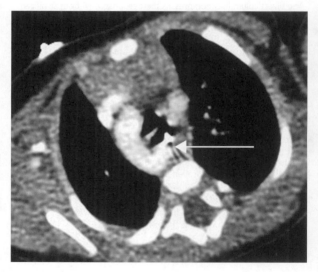

Fig. 24.10 Contrast-enhanced CT scan at the level of the aortic arch showing the aberrant left subclavian artery passing behind the oesophagus (white arrow).

Pulmonary sling

- In this anomaly (Fig. 24.11), the left pulmonary artery originates from the right pulmonary artery and then passes behind the trachea, but in front of the oesophagus towards the left lung.
- The distal end of the trachea and the right main stem bronchus are compressed between the main pulmonary artery and the left pulmonary artery.
- There is no complete ring (hence the term pulmonary sling).
- The respiratory symptoms that arise in these patients are nearly always the consequence of associated *tracheal stenosis* (see 🕮 p. 330).
- The stenosis can affect a significant proportion of the distal trachea and may be associated with a tracheal origin of the right upper lobe bronchus, which can cause confusion at bronchoscopy.

Compression of the trachea by the innominate artery

- The innominate artery, which divides to form the right subclavian artery and the right common carotid, arises from the aortic arch before it crosses in front of the trachea in older children and adults.
- In children < 2 years of age, the origin of the innominate is frequently just to the left of the trachea and the vessel travels across the front of the mid-trachea towards the right arm. In this position it can cause anterior compression of the trachea (Fig. 24.12).
- This is often a normal finding at bronchoscopy, but in some infants the compression is severe enough to cause symptoms of cough and secretion retention. There is no true ring, and tracheal growth can occur.
- The origin of the vessel also tends to moves over to the right side of the trachea with growth.
- Symptoms tend to improve with time, and surgical intervention can usually be avoided.

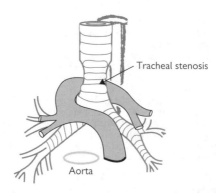

Fig. 24.11 Pulmonary sling. The left pulmonary artery arises from the right pulmonary artery and passes between the trachea and oesophagus. This arrangement may cause compression of the carina and right main bronchus. More often symptoms arise from associated tracheal stenosis and not from the vascular compression.

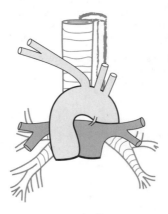

Fig. 24.12 Innominate artery compression. The innominate artery arises from a more distal position than usual and passes in front of the trachea and may cause compression.

Management of vascular rings

- All children with a vascular ring should be seen by a cardiologist to investigate any coexisting congenital heart disease.
- For some defects such as double aortic arch, chromosomes should be sent for 22q11 deletion and serum calcium and lymphocyte numbers and subsets need to be checked. Until these are known to be normal, any blood transfusions must use irradiated blood to prevent possible graft versus host disease.
- The presence of tracheal stenosis, especially in children with pulmonary slings, needs to be carefully evaluated. Simply fixing the sling in these cases will not improve the respiratory symptoms.
- For other vascular rings it is usually necessary only to divide the ring.
- In the case of double aortic arch, this is usually achieved by ligating and dividing the smaller arch as near to the descending aorta as possible, allowing continued proximal flow to the vessels arising from the ligated arch.
- For right-sided arch with aberrant left subclavian artery, there is debate as to whether it is only necessary to divide the left ductus to release the ring or whether the diverticulum of Kommerell also needs to be excised with or without re-implantation of the aberrant left subclavian artery. Bronchoscopy at the time of surgery may help determine whether simple duct division relieves the obstruction. When the main symptom is dysphagia it will usually be necessary to excise the diverticulum to relieve the symptoms.
- In all cases, it is important to counsel the parents that there will be residual segmental tracheomalacia, which can take several months to improve. For simple rings without associated tracheal stenosis, surgical outcomes are excellent with full resolution of symptoms in the majority.
- A small number of children, particularly those with severe compression presenting in the first few weeks of life, will have more significant residual tracheomalacia, requiring longer-term support with positive airway pressure (usually CPAP), with or without a tracheostomy. A small proportion (1–2%) may need further surgery, usually a tracheopexy.

Further information

Backer, C.L., Mavroudis, C., Rigsby, C.K., and Holinger, L.D. (2005). Trends in vascular ring surgery. *Thorac. Cardiovasc. Surg.* **129**, 1339–47.

Backer, C.L., Hillman, N., Mavroudis, C., and Holinger, L.D. (2002). Resection of Kommerell's diverticulum and left subclavian artery transfer for recurrent symptoms after vascular ring division. *Eur. J. Cardiothorac. Surg.* **22**, 64–9.

Subglottic stenosis

In children the subglottic space at the level of the cricoid cartilage is the narrowest part of the airway. See Fig. 24.13.

Acquired subglottic stenosis

- This occurs as a consequence of mucosal damage, most often by endotracheal tubes (ETT). The mucosa overlying the cricoid cartilage is particularly at risk because the cartilage ring here is complete and the mucosa more likely to become ischaemic by ETT compression.
- Risk factors for the development of subglottic stenosis are:
  - long duration of intubation;
  - episodes of hypotension;
  - bacterial airway infection;
  - gastro-oesophageal reflux.
- In the early stages of acquired stenosis, the narrowing is soft and potentially reversible. Later, as fibrosis occurs, the stenosis becomes hard and during this process the stenosis can worsen.
- The stenosis can involve the crico-arytenoid joints and affect the movement of the vocal folds.

Congenital subglottic stenosis

- This occurs in the absence of previous intubation or laryngeal trauma.
- It is caused by failure of the lumen of the larynx to recanalize in embryonic life.
- It can be associated with other abnormalities of the trachea.

Presentation

- The congenital form will cause persistent stridor, usually from birth and worsening with colds, often leading to recurrent admissions with croup.
- The stridor caused by subglottic stenosis is usually biphasic.
- Occasionally the symptoms may be missed or mistaken for laryngo-malacia and these children can present with acute airways obstruction.
- Infants with moderate subglottic stenosis may cope reasonably well but, as they become ambulant toddlers, the subglottic stenosis can limit ventilation and result in exercise intolerance.
- Acquired subglottic stenosis is usually obvious immediately after extubation. It may appear to improve, but then worsen again, often weeks later, as fibrosis progresses.

Management

- Prevention of acquired subglottic stenosis is much easier than the cure. Avoiding lengthy intubations, particularly with oral tubes, which move more easily and cause more trauma, is important. Tracheostomy in children who are likely to need long periods of ventilation (more than 2–3 weeks) should be considered.
- Treating any acid reflux with omeprazole may be helpful.

- When children have failed extubation because of stridor, early involvement of an ENT surgeon is important. Before a second attempt at extubation, 48h of steroids (prednisolone or dexamethasone) can be helpful.
- Resting the larynx by keeping the child as still as possible to prevent ETT movement is important.
- Subsequent extubation carried out under direct vision will allow assessment of the subglottic space. If the airway is still inadequate, and the stenosis is soft, an anterior cricoid split may be indicated.
- If the stenosis is severe, a tracheostomy may be required as part of a staged procedure to get the child extubated.
- If the ETT can be removed safely, the subglottic narrowing may resolve. Early review is necessary and where there is soft scarring of the subglottic space serial debridement with the application of mitomycin C can be helpful.

The management of children with congenital subglottic stenosis, or acquired stenosis presenting days or weeks after extubation, will depend not only on the severity of the stenosis but also the severity of the symptoms.

- Some children can cope with remarkably small airways. It is important to fully inspect the lower airways to exclude a second pathology.
- Where symptoms are mild and the stenosis is < 50–70%, child can be managed expectantly. Congenital stenosis will often improve with time.
- If symptoms are severe and the airway is not safe, then reconstruction will be needed. This may require a tracheostomy in the first instance.
- Several surgical approaches are possible, but reconstruction with costal cartilage grafts is the commonest procedure. If the vocal folds are involved in the stenosis, improving the airway may pose a significant risk to the voice.

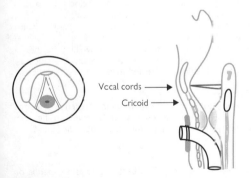

Vocal cords ⟶

Cricoid ⟶

Fig. 24.13 Appearance of subglottic stenosis from above and from the side. In the side-on view there is a tracheostomy tube in place.

Subglottic haemangioma

Haemangiomata are benign vascular tumours characterized by proliferation in infancy (usually between 2 and 9 months of age) followed by slow regression that can take 10–15 years to complete. Cutaneous haemangiomata are common and occur in around 10% of infants. They are 3 times more frequently found in girls and half occur on the head or neck. Occasionally they can be found at other sites, including the liver, lung, brain, mediastinum, and tracheal wall. Complications of cutaneous and visceral lesions include bleeding, ulceration, platelet consumption, and heart failure. In the airway, haemangiomata cause obstruction.

Symptoms and signs

Haemangiomata are usually small or invisible at birth and symptoms are unusual before 6–8 weeks of age. Occasionally presentation may be delayed until 2–3 years of age. 50% of infants with subglottic haemangioma will have cutaneous haemangiomata, usually in the distribution of the beard area of the face. Typical symptoms are:
- biphasic stridor;
- recurrent episodes of croup (but importantly symptoms persist between episodes);
- barking cough;
- difficulty feeding and poor growth.

There are usually no associated medical problems. Examination usually is that of a normal baby with quiet biphasic stridor at rest that worsens on crying. A careful search for cutaneous haemangiomata should be made.

Investigations

- The investigation of choice in an infant with stridor is bronchoscopy. The differential diagnosis includes laryngomalacia, subglottic stenosis, laryngeal web, cysts and laryngoceles, and vocal cord palsy.
- Bronchoscopic appearance is usually of a smooth swelling arising from the wall of the subglottis. Lesions can be unilateral (more commonly found on the left), bilateral, or circumferential. The swelling may be red or bluish depending on the depth of the lesion below the mucosa. A good appreciation of the normal size and shape of the subglottic space is needed to recognize the presence of relatively small circumferential lesions.
- MRI of the neck and chest may be helpful when the presence of a large lesion is suspected, e.g. because the lesion extends down into the trachea or because of additional symptoms such as bounding pulses or a low platelet count.

Treatment

There are several treatment options. The best one to use depends on the size and extent of the haemangioma and on the skill and preference of the ENT surgical team. It is important to remember that the natural history of haemangiomata is resolution and that the treatment should not leave the child worse off in the long run.

- Observation only. If an infant has minor symptoms, e.g. stridor only when crying, and has a haemangioma that occupies ≤ 30% of the airway lumen, a policy of close observation can be followed. In some children, lesion will not progress and no intervention will be required. The possibility of growth of the haemangioma must be considered and the airway re-examined if there is any change in symptom severity.

- Systemic corticosteroids may be useful to buy some time in symptomatic infants whilst definitive treatment plans are established. The dose needed is usually 2 mg/kg per day of prednisolone. In some infants there is a good response that can be sustained at the cost of long-term steroid therapy. Steroids used as monotherapy are usually needed at high dose for 3–4 weeks followed by a long taper over a number of months. They tend to be useful only for the less severe lesions (< 50% obstruction) and carry a significant risk of side-effects.

- Tracheostomy used to be the mainstay of treatment. In most centres it has now been superseded by other interventions (see below). Where there is large haemangioma, the airway above the tracheostomy will usually be insufficient for ventilation. Thus the risks of obstruction of the tracheostomy with secretions resulting in hypoxia or death are high and need to be taken into account when planning care for such infants both in hospital and at home. Tracheostomy is now usually reserved for difficult extensive haemangiomata that are either not suitable for other treatments or have not responded to other treatment modalities.

- Intralesional steroids. Steroids such as triamcinolone can be injected into haemangiomata at bronchoscopy. An over-sized ETT is then left in place, for 5–10 days, to compress the haemangioma. This technique is successful in 70–80% of cases, but needs to be repeated on 2–4 occasions whilst awaiting natural regression of the haemangioma. This results in a total of around 30 intubated days on an ICU, often with muscle paralysis to prevent ETT movement. As a consequence there is related morbidity, mainly due to lower airway infection.

- Laser treatment. Laser treatment is the most widespread successful treatment for unilateral subglottic haemangioma. When it was first used over 20 years ago there were significant complications from subsequent scarring and subglottic stenosis. Newer techniques have improved outcomes, but success is still highly operator dependent. It is most effective for unilateral lesions where the risk of subsequent subglottic stenosis is lower. It is often combined with a course of systemic corticosteroids.

- Open excision and laryngotracheoplasty has been reported by several groups. Cartilage laryngotracheoplasty is usually included as part of the primary surgery to try and prevent subsequent subglottic stenosis. There is a 30% risk of the formation of significant granulation tissue that may require further surgery. It may be an option for infants with circumferential lesions or lesions occupying > 70% of the airway who would otherwise be treated with tracheostomy.

- Interferon. Interferon alpha is an effective treatment for haemangioma, usually daily injections for 3–6 months. There is no benefit in combining interferon with steroids. There are significant side-effects, the most serious of which is spastic diplegia in 5–20% of children, which may be irreversible. Interferon should be reserved for life-threatening massive haemangiomata.
- Vincristine plus corticosteroids. This combination is an alternative for life-threatening haemangiomata. Its role in less severe haemangiomata has not yet been evaluated.

Outcome

Outcome of small- to medium-sized haemangiomata is excellent and most can avoid a tracheostomy. Circumferential lesions or those occupying > 70% of the airway or those associated with extension into the neck or thorax are more challenging. Some of the therapies used to treat these infants can have long-term side-effects. These risks must be balanced against the shorter term benefits. Tracheostomy may be the best option for some children. The absence of a safe airway above the tracheostomy must be taken into account when planning subsequent care for these children.

Further information

Rahbar, R., Nicollas, R., Roger, G., Triglia, J.M., Garabedian, E.N., McGill, T.J., and Healy, G.B. (2004). The biology and management of subglottic hemangioma: past, present, future. *Laryngoscope* **114**, 1880–91.

Tracheobronchomalacia

Definition and respiratory physiology

The cartilage in the walls of the trachea and main bronchi provides support for these structures and prevents their collapse during normal expiration. The posterior wall of the large airways is membranous and lacks cartilage. This allows dynamic narrowing to occur during forced expiration and coughing, which has the effect of accelerating the exhaled air so that it can generate a shearing force to expel mucus.

Tracheobronchomalacia (TBM) is a condition in which large airway wall cartilage is insufficiently strong to splint open the airway and airway collapse occurs more readily during expiration. The presence of small airways obstruction will accentuate this tendency, such that it will occur at higher lung volumes than in the absence of small airway disease. TBM is a disease that nearly always starts in infancy and that may persist into early childhood. Rarely, it may be acquired in later life as a consequence of tracheal chondritis.

Causes

TBM can be primary or secondary. Primary disease is rare. The following conditions are associated with TBM.

- Vascular rings. There is usually a short segment of tracheomalacia at the site of the ring. This frequently causes symptoms that persist after surgical release of the ring.
- Tracheo-oesophageal fistula. There is usually a short segment of tracheomalacia at the site of the fistula.
- Congenital heart disease with cardiomegaly. The mechanism for the TBM seen in these children is not well understood. Compression of the bronchi by a large heart seems to be the main culprit. The effects of the TBM can be worsened by increased airways resistance caused by heart failure or by ventilator-associated injury.
- Bronchopulmonary dysplasia. Many preterm infants with chronic lung disease will have evidence of TBM. The reasons are not clear. It seems likely to be a combination of long-term ventilation of airways with immature cartilage, trauma from repeated intubation and airway suctioning, and the effects of chronic small airways disease tending to cause large airway collapse.

Symptoms

In many infants the symptoms are mild. In others they can be severe and life-threatening and lead to ventilator dependence. In primary TBM symptoms may become apparent at 1–2 months of age. Younger infants tend not to generate sufficient airflows to cause noisy breathing. Symptoms include the following.

- Wheeze. This is usually low pitched. It can be mistaken for bronchiolitis or viral-associated wheeze.
- Cough (may have a brassy or croupy quality).
- Episodes of breathlessness.
- Episodes of cyanosis with poor chest wall movement. These are sometimes called 'malacic spells', 'dying spells', or 'BPD spells'. They

usually occur when the infant is crying and result from complete airway closure, usually at the beginning of expiration. Cyanosis occurs rapidly, probably as a combination of limited respiratory reserve in sick infants and right to left shunting at atrial level because of the high intrathoracic pressures the infant is generating in their attempts to exhale. Bradycardia is also common, which may be mediated either by hypoxia or vagal stimulation. The chest wall does not move. These events most often occur in ventilated infants or infants with tracheostomies, and may require a period of increased ventilatory support (sometimes with a bag-valve-system) and muscle relaxation to overcome the expiratory airway closure.

- Recurrent episodes of LRTI. These arise through a combination of poor secretion clearance by malacic airways, and worsening dynamic airway collapse consequent to small airways disease, often caused by viral infection. They often occur in infants with chronic lung disease who may also have hyperreactive airways.
- There may be symptoms of gastro-oesophageal reflux (vomiting, food refusal, irritability), which often accompanies TBM. Which of these conditions drives the other is not clear. They may both be the consequence of an underlying condition, such as tracheo-oesophageal fistula.
- In ventilated infants the first evidence of TBM may be failure to wean from ventilation. These infants will typically have either chronic lung disease of prematurity or long-term ventilation because of complex congenital heart disease.

Examination

Examination may be normal. Possible findings include:
- low-pitched wheeze, often loudest centrally;
- prolonged expiratory phase;
- hyperinflated chest.

Where there is coexisting disease, such as chronic lung disease, it can be difficult to ascribe symptoms and signs to TBM rather than the underlying condition. TBM should be suspected in infants at risk when their disease is unusually severe or persistent, where there is wheeze that does not respond to bronchodilators, or where there are episodes of unexplained respiratory distress and cyanosis.

Investigations

The diagnosis of TBM requires dynamic assessment of the trachea and bronchi, with demonstration of collapse of the airway in expiration. The examination of choice depends on the clinical situation. For intubated infants there are 3 choices.
- Bronchoscopy is probably the most widely used investigation for TBM. To observe dynamic airway closure the infant must be spontaneously breathing. This can be done by carrying out the bronchoscopy using conscious sedation or by observing the trachea as the child is allowed to wake up from general anaesthesia. This investigation can be carried

out in stable non-ventilated infants as well as those who are intubated. It can be difficult to perform on sick infants with limited respiratory reserve, and in small infants the bronchoscope may splint open the airway reducing the sensitivity of the investigation. In intubated children the ETT may also splint the airway open and tracheomalacia may be missed. Repeat examination via the nose or through a laryngeal mask may be needed.

- Bronchogram. This investigation is suitable for intubated infants. It visualizes the airway by using small (0.2mL) aliquots of contrast injected into the ETT through an airtight port. It has the advantages of allowing the infant to be ventilated without the obstruction caused by a bronchoscopy and of being able to inspect the airways with different levels of CPAP. By determining the level of CPAP that maintains tracheo-bronchial opening, appropriate weaning strategies can be devised. This technique requires experience to be performed well and is not widely available.
- Dynamic CT using high speed scanners is also suitable for intubated infants. This can provide similar information to a bronchogram, but it appears to be less sensitive and carries a higher radiation exposure.

Treatment

- Many infants need no specific treatment for their TBM. Once it has been recognized as contributing to their respiratory symptoms, supportive treatment should be given with the expectation that the TBM will improve with time, which it nearly always does provided that any external compression has been removed. Improvement can take 2–3 years.
- Any small airways disease should be treated aggressively if possible. This may include use of inhaled steroids and bronchodilators (with caution) if there is a reversible component, and possibly the use of prophylactic antibiotics if there are recurrent infections with increased secretions.
- Bronchodilators should be used with caution since they may worsen obstruction from TBM, presumably by affecting the tone of the malacic airways.
- Coexisting illness will often make symptoms from TBM worse. Treatments for cardiac failure should be optimized.
- In infants with more severe symptoms, specific intervention may be required. The options are as follows.
  - Pexy procedures. The most frequent is the aortopexy. In this procedure the aorta is pulled anteriorly by fixing it to the sternum. This in turns pulls the anterior wall of the trachea forward and reduces the likelihood of collapse. This operation is helpful when there is a short defined section of malacia such as occurs in children after tracheo-oesophageal fistula repair. Bronchoscopy at the time of the procedure can guide the surgeon as to the most favourable position in which to fix the aorta. Where there is bronchial involvement it is much less successful (80% failure rate). For predominant involvement of the left main bronchus, pulling the pulmonary artery forward by fixing it to the sternum, or suturing the anterior wall of the left main bronchus to the ligamentum arteriosus may be effective.

- CPAP. Continuous positive airways pressure (usually 5–15cmH$_2$O) can keep the large airways open. It is suitable for children who are intubated. It can also be used in the longer term via tracheostomy. Since it will usually be needed 24h per day, delivery via face mask is not usually an option for long-term support.
- Tracheostomy may be successful for malacia confined to the trachea by physically stenting the airway. Custom-made long tubes can support the majority of the trachea. Tracheostomy combined with CPAP is probably the commonest approach used for severe TBM.
- External airway stents. Hagl's external stent may be effective in short segment tracheomalacia where aortopexy is not possible. However, it is not distensible and once in place determines the maximal size of the airway. External stents are not widely used.
- Internal airway stents. A number of stents are now available, e.g. the Palmaz and Ultraflex nitinol stents. They can be sited in the main bronchi and the trachea. They have many theoretical benefits and often give good short-term results. Unfortunately, there are serious drawbacks, including granuloma formation, stent erosion through the tracheal wall, secretion production and retention, recurrent airway infection, and limitation of final tracheal size. Although the stents are designed to be removable, in practice they become embedded in the tracheal wall and removal is usually not possible. Use of stents should be reserved for intractable TBM not responding to other treatments.
- Tracheal resection of short segment malacia with end to end anastomosis may also be considered. There is a significant risk of stenosis at the anastomosis site and this makes this option unattractive in most circumstances.

Outcome

The impact of TBM on each child will be different and will vary according the presence of other lung or cardiac pathology. The natural history is for improvement, and treatment should be directed towards promoting normal growth whilst this improvement occurs. The possible future development of more effective external airway stents or bioresorbable internal stents may provide safer effective treatments.

Tracheo-oesophageal fistula

Tracheo-oesophageal fistula (TOF) is nearly always congenital, and refers to an abnormal connection between the trachea and oesophagus (Fig. 24.14). In 90% of cases there is oesophageal atresia and a distal TOF. In 5% there is TOF without oesophageal atresia (H-type fistula). TOF is frequently associated with other congenital abnormalities, including the VACTERL association (vertebral–anal–cardiac–TOF–renal–limb).

Presentation

- TOF with oesophageal atresia is associated with polyhydramnios and may be diagnosed *in utero*. If the diagnosis is unsuspected at delivery it usually becomes obvious in the first 12h of life with inability to feed and copious oral secretions, which can lead to aspiration events.
- Infants with H-type fistulae may present later, sometimes after several weeks or months, with episodes of choking or desaturation on feeding or recurrent LRTI.

Diagnosis

- Diagnosis is usually made in the neonatal period on the basis of the clinical picture and a plain CXR showing a coiled nasogastric tube within the thorax suggesting oesophageal atresia, and gas in the stomach consistent with a distal TOF. The CXR may also demonstrate vertebral abnormalities and suggest cardiac defects. The position of the aortic arch should be established. In 5% of infants with TOF it will be right-sided and this will influence the side selected for thoracotomy.
- Where there is doubt about the diagnosis, a small amount of contrast will demonstrate the oesophageal atresia, although there is a real risk of aspiration of contrast during this procedure.
- Bronchoscopy may be used to demonstrate the fistula. H-type fistulae are often in the upper third of the trachea and can be very difficult to demonstrate at bronchoscopy. There may be a visible pit on the posterior wall of the trachea, with surrounding erythema. Rigid bronchoscopy is a more sensitive method of identifying the fistula and may allow a guidewire or catheter to be passed through the fistula. If this is done at the time of surgery it can help guide the surgeon to the correct site for repair.
- H-type fistula can also be demonstrated by prone oesophagram, although false negative results are common. Since these infants are prone to aspiration, contrast oesophagrams can result in desaturation and respiratory distress. A paediatric doctor experienced in resuscitation should be present when an oesophagram is performed.
- Further imaging with CT scan or MRI seldom adds any extra information.

Management

The management of TOF with atresia is surgical repair. If there is a long gap atresia, a temporary gastrostomy may be used to allow the infant to be fed and to grow.

Outcome

Children who have had surgical repair of TOF with oesophageal atresia can have medium- to long-term health problems associated with the condition. The problems include the following.

- Feeding difficulties. A combination of oral aversion because of long delays in commencing oral feeds, oesophageal dysmotility, which is always present, gastro-oesophageal reflux, and possible residual oesophageal stricture. If there is cyanosis with feeds consider the possibility of aspiration, possibly associated with laryngeal cleft.
- Episodes of respiratory distress may occur as a result of segmental tracheomalacia at the site of the fistula. These symptoms may be severe enough to consider surgical intervention. Aortopexy is often successful because the length of malacic trachea is usually short. In this procedure the arch of the aorta is sutured to the sternum to pull it forward. This in turn pulls the anterior wall of the trachea forward and prevents its collapse.
- Parenchymal lung disease. A combination of aspiration, because of an abnormal swallow and worsened by GOR, tracheomalacia, which is almost always present, and the effects of periods of mechanical ventilation and oxygen therapy.

Respiratory and feeding problems can be associated with recurrent fistula formation at the site of the original repair. These can be difficult to diagnose, and careful investigation is needed. Bronchoscopy will be helpful in determining if there is tracheal irritation or malacia. Rarely, functional gastric mucosa can be found in the trachea at the site of the fistula.

If there are feeding problems, the possibility of aspiration needs to be assessed by videofluoroscopy. A gradual programme of introduction of tastes and textures can overcome oral aversion, and early involvement of an experienced speech and language therapist is important. It may be necessary to form a gastrostomy, often combined with anti-reflux surgery, to minimize aspiration whilst providing adequate nutrition. Airway irritation can result in bronchospasm and bronchodilators may help. Early and generous use of antibiotics can minimize secondary damage by low grade infection.

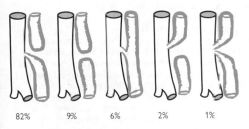

82%   9%   6%   2%   1%

Fig. 24.14 Types of tracheo-oesophageal fistulae.

Tracheal stenosis

Nearly all tracheal stenosis (excluding subglottic stenosis) in children is congenital and will usually present in infancy. Very rarely, tracheal stenosis can be acquired because of airway burns, trauma, poorly fitting tracheostomy tubes, and after tracheal surgery. External compression of the trachea from tumours, particularly lymphoma, is considered in 📖 Chapter 50. Vascular rings are considered separately (📖 p. 310).

- Normal internal tracheal diameter is 3.8mm at birth, 5.5mm at 1 year, and 6.5mm at 2 years.
- Congenital tracheal stenosis is rare. The actual annual incidence is not known, but is around 1/100 000 births.
- 60% of infants with tracheal stenosis will have associated abnormalities, predominantly structural cardiac disease. The most likely cardiac defect is pulmonary sling; others include ASD, VSD, aortic arch lesions, and double-outlet right ventricle. Non-cardiac associated anomalies include:
  - Down's syndrome;
  - absent right lung;
  - oesophageal atresia;
  - anorectal malformation;
  - Crouzon's syndrome.

Symptoms and signs

- Nearly all children with tracheal stenosis will present in early infancy with stridor or respiratory collapse, usually with an intercurrent respiratory infection. Ventilatory support in these children can be very difficult with high pressures required to overcome the airways resistance caused by the stenosis.
- Occasionally milder degrees of stenosis may present in later childhood with recurrent respiratory tract infection associated with noisy breathing.

Investigations

- The diagnosis is usually made with a combination of bronchoscopy and chest CT scan. 3-dimensional CT reconstructions can provide helpful information about the position and extent of the stenosis.
- Echocardiography and cardiac evaluation.
- Bronchograpy can be helpful.
- Investigation needs to determine the following.
  - The severity of the tracheal narrowing. Airways resistance is proportional to the 4th power of the radius of a tube. Thus there is a big functional difference between a 1.5mm and a 2mm trachea.
  - The proportion of trachea affected. If this is more than 2/3 the length of the trachea, the stenosis is classified as long-segment stenosis.
  - The presence of complete tracheal rings. Although these can grow, their presence makes growth and improvement less likely. The presence of complete rings is best assessed by bronchoscopy.
  - The presence of atypical tracheal branching. The most usual variant is a right upper lobe bronchus arising from the trachea. This can affect the surgical technique used.

- The presence of any coexisting tracheobronchomalacia—assessed by bronchoscopy in the sedated child or by bronchography.
- The presence of any cardiac disease.

Treatment

- Where there is short segment stenosis with a reduction in diameter of < 60%, observation alone is often best option. Serial CT scans indicate that in most children with stenosis of this nature, even in the presence of complete tracheal rings, there will be tracheal growth with time.
- For longer or tighter stenoses, tracheal surgery will need to be considered. Tracheal surgery is difficult and associated with significant morbidity and mortality. It should only be carried in large centres with the necessary experience and expertise. In the UK, the national centre is at the Great Ormond Street Hospital for Sick Children in London.
- For very short segment stenosis, resection and end to end anastomosis is usually relatively straightforward and has good results. Balloon dilatation has also been used successfully.
- Where there is long segment stenosis, there is likely to be a difficult postoperative course with the likely need for subsequent repeated tracheal dilatations and an uncertain long-term outcome. Families need to be fully informed and may choose not to have surgery, particularly when there are other complex medical problems.
- The operation of choice for medium and long segment stenosis is now the slide tracheoplasty. Where there is very long segment stenosis involving the bronchi, patch tracheoplasty using pericardium may need to be combined with the slide tracheoplasty.
- Whichever procedure is used, it is essential to fully mobilize the trachea and surrounding structures to prevent any traction on the tracheal anastomoses.

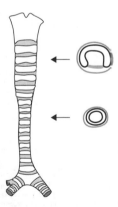

Fig 24.15 Long segment tracheal stenosis. The cartilage segments in the stenosed section are complete, giving a circular appearance to the trachea when viewed with a bronchoscope.

Outcome

- The outcome for short-segment stenosis is good, and largely dependent on the presence of other defects, including tracheomalacia.
- With the advent of multidisciplinary specialist tracheal teams and the more widespread use of the slide tracheoplasty, the outcome for medium- and long-segment stenosis has improved over the last 5 years. The immediate mortality ranges from 3% to 15% in different case series, with a late mortality of 10%.
- Postoperative problems include re-stenosis, granulation tissue at anastomotic sites, anastomotic dehiscence, and severe distal tracheo-bronchomalacia. These problems are complex, require dedicated attention to detail, and often involve repeated and prolonged hospital admissions.

Further information

Backer, C.L., Mavroudis, C., Gerber, M.E., Holinger, L.D. (2001). Tracheal surgery in children: an 18-year review of four techniques. *Eur. J. Cardiothorac. Surg.* **19**, 777–84.

Kocyildirim, E., Kanani, M., Roebuck, D., Wallis, C., McLaren, C., Noctor, C., Pigott, N., Mok, Q., Hartley, B., Dunne, C., Uppal, S., and Elliott, M.J. (2004). Long-segment tracheal stenosis: slide tracheoplasty and a multidisciplinary approach improve outcomes and reduce costs. *J. Thorac. Cardiovasc. Surg.* **128**, 876–82.

Elliott, M., Roebuck, D., Noctor, C., McLaren, C., Hartley, B., Mok, Q., Dunne, C., Pigott, N., Patel, C., Patel, A., and Wallis, C. (2003). The management of congenital tracheal stenosis. *Int. J. Pediatr. Otorhinolaryngol.* **67** (Suppl. 1), S183–92.

Sleep-disordered breathing and other sleep problems

Introduction

- Sleep is a state of reduced consciousness and decreased awareness of external stimuli. Sleep–wake cycles occur over a 24h period, controlled by programmed changes in gene expression of all tissues. This innate cycle of cell activity, which can be seen in human cells grown in the laboratory, has arisen as a result of man's evolution on a planet with a 24h day. Exposure to light and secretion of melatonin by the pineal gland, as well as social factors, all influence when during the 24h cycle sleep is taken.
- Sleep can be divided into rapid eye movement sleep (REM) and non-rapid eye movement (NREM) sleep.
  - REM sleep (also called active sleep) is associated with increased variability in heart rate and reduced tone in most major muscle groups including the intercostal muscles and the muscles of the pharynx, whilst the diaphragm is relatively unaffected.
  - Reduced pharyngeal muscle tone increases the frequency and severity of obstructive events during REM sleep.
  - Reduced intercostal muscle tone makes hypoventilation associated with muscle weakness more apparent during REM sleep.
  - NREM sleep is divided according to EEG findings into stage I (light sleep, 5–10% of sleep time), stage II (40–50% of sleep time), stages III and IV (deep or delta-wave sleep).
  - REM sleep occurs in 4–5 discrete episodes during the night, together accounting for 20–25% of sleep time. REM episodes are longer in the second half of a night's sleep. Waking in the morning is usually from REM sleep.
  - Newborns sleep for 14–16h each day. Sleep in the newborn is characterized by frequent arousals and a high proportion of REM sleep. Unlike older children and adults young infants transition directly from wakefulness to REM sleep. By 6 months this has reduced and consolidated into a night's sleep and one daytime nap.
- Sleep-disordered breathing is common in children. The majority is related to upper airways obstruction. Careful distinction must be made between obstruction and sleep-disordered breathing from central causes, associated with congenital and secondary central hypoventilation syndromes, seizure disorders, and neuromuscular weakness. Those topics are dealt with elsewhere in the book. In this chapter we will deal with principally with obstructive sleep apnoea and other causes of sleep disturbance that may present to the respiratory paediatrician.

Daytime sleepiness and sleep disturbance

Daytime sleepiness or disturbed sleep in a child may be the reason for referral for a respiratory opinion. The usual question will be whether abnormal breathing during the night (obstruction or hypoventilation) is responsible for these symptoms.

Some form of sleep disturbance is very common in childhood and affects up to 30% of children at some time. When considering sleep problems it is useful to try and determine if there is:
- insufficient sleep quality, i.e. disrupted or fragmented sleep; *or*
- insufficient sleep quantity, usually delayed sleep onset or prolonged periods of wakefulness during the night.

Insufficient sleep quantity usually results from behavioural problems related to the absence of a good bedtime routine, sometimes called 'sleep hygiene'. It is worth checking what normally happens at bedtime. Good sleep hygiene requires the following.
- Using a set routine.
- Going to sleep at the same time every night (including weekends).
- Having a wind-down period for 30–60min before bed.
- Going to sleep in the child's own bed (not on the sofa).
- Going to sleep in a darkened room (so there is no alarm in the night when the child wakes up in a darkened room). This means not allowing the child to go to sleep watching television in their own room.
- Avoid using the bedroom for time-out or punishment.

Possible causes of sleep disturbance include:
- parasomnias;
- dyssomnias;
- recurrent nightmares;
- nocturnal epilepsy.

Parasomnias

Parasomnias are disorders characterized by undesirable movements, verbal noises, or experiences that occur in association with sleep or during the sleep–awake transition. They include night-terrors, sleep walking, periodic limb movements, and head-banging.
- Night-terrors. Sleep terrors are disorders of arousal that occur during NREM sleep. There may be apparent extreme panic with screaming and hitting out, sometimes associated with getting out of bed. Recollection of the event is either absent or partial.
- Sleep walking and sleep talking also occur during NREM sleep. Children who sleep walk will often leave their bedrooms and wander aimlessly, sometimes carrying out complex tasks. Once again there is usually no recollection on waking.
- Periodic limb movement in sleep (PLMS).
  - PLMS are repetitive limb movements (usually the legs) during sleep; they can be associated with daytime sleepiness or more often in children with behavioural disturbance including ADHD. When this

association is made the condition is called periodic limb movement disorder (PLMD).

- PLMD is relatively common in adults; the incidence in children is not known.
- PLMD is associated with daytime restless legs syndrome (RLS), a condition where there is an urge to move the legs to relieve discomfort. RLS is often worse in the evening and at night and can cause insomnia. Nearly all adult patients with RLS have periodic limb movements, but only a minority of patients with PLMD also has RLS.
- Since arousal and movement can follow sleep-disturbed breathing, including apparently mild increased upper airways resistance, it is important to exclude this as a possible cause before diagnosing PLMD.
- Children with PLMD have an increased incidence of iron deficiency and, where iron deficiency is found, treatment with iron can improve PLMD.
- There is increased incidence of RLS and PLMD in first-degree relatives.
- Rhythmic movements including head-rocking and head-banging. These can occur at sleep onset and during any stage of sleep. They are commonest in early childhood and usually of no significance.

Dyssomnias

Dyssomnias are characterized by abnormalities in the amount, quality, or timing of sleep. These include primary insomnia and hypersomnia, narcolepsy (see 📖 p. 348), breathing-related sleep disorder (e.g. obstructive sleep apnoea or nocturnal hypoventilation), and circadian rhythm sleep disorder (e.g. jet lag).

Other causes of disturbed sleep

- Nightmares: intense dreams that the sleeper finds unpleasant or frightening. Occasional nightmares are common. Less commonly, recurrent nightmares interfere with sleep sufficiently for the family to seek medical assistance.
- Nocturnal epilepsy (benign partial epilepsy with centro-temporal (rolandic) spikes).
- Depression.
- Anxiety.
- Chronic fatigue syndrome.
- Discomfort related to difficulty moving in children with neuromuscular weakness or cerebral palsy.

Symptoms and signs

It is essential to get a clear description of the problem.

- What is the usual bedtime routine?
- Is there difficulty getting to sleep, or is there frequent wakening?
- How do the child and parents respond when the child wakes up?
- Is there snoring?

- If there is snoring is there other evidence of obstruction such as periods when the snoring stops (but the breathing effort continues) following by snorts or arousals?
- Are there abnormal movements or noises during sleep?
- Does the child have muscular weakness or other predisposing medical condition?
- Does the child feel refreshed in the morning?
- Are there any symptoms of hypoventilation such as morning headache and/or nausea?
- Is there daytime sleepiness?

Examination

Examination is usually normal. Check:
- tonsil size;
- chest shape and expansion;
- for any evidence of muscular weakness.

Investigations

It may be clear from the history that the sleep problem is not related to sleep-disordered breathing. Where there is a possibility that this is the cause, the following investigations should be considered:
- basic spirometry;
- sleep study.

Management

Management depends on the cause. Where no cause is found simple advice on a good sleep routine is a good place to start.

Further information

Simakajornboon, N. (2006). Periodic limb movement disorder in children. *Paediatr. Respir. Rev.* **7** (Suppl. 1), S55–7.

Obstructive sleep apnoea

Definitions

- Obstructive apnoeas (OSA) are events where airflow has ceased, but where there are continued and often vigorous respiratory efforts. These are easily identified using standard polysomnographic recordings. During obstructive episodes, diaphragmatic contraction causes an increase in abdominal volume and a decrease in thoracic volume, resulting in loss of phase in the deflection of signals from chest and abdominal bands.
- Obstructive hypopnoeas are events where a similar pattern of obstruction is seen, but airflow, whilst diminished by at least 50%, is not absent. Some definitions of hypopnoea and apnoea require that desaturation of at least 4% is associated with the event.
- Milder forms of partially obstructed breathing have also been described where there is no change in airflow or oxygen saturation, but a greater effort is needed to overcome the obstruction, as evidenced by a temporal retardation of chest expansion during inspiration. This has been called increased airways resistance syndrome.
- The cause of OSA in children is multifactorial but most studies agree that children with OSA tend to have more collapsible upper airways and larger adenotonsillar tissue. It is also clear that isolated adenotonsillar hypertrophy alone is not sufficient to cause OSA since children with 'kissing' tonsils may be asymptomatic, and OSA can persist after adenotonsillectomy.

Epidemiology

- Snoring is common in children, with estimates suggesting that up to 1 in 5 children snore at some time.
- The true incidence of OSA in children is not known, but it may affect 1–2% of the population.
- The highest incidence is in children in the 2–5 year age group, which may reflect the prominence of tonsillar and adenoidal tissue in this age group.
- At risk groups are:
  - obese children;
  - children of Afro-Caribbean descent;
  - children with craniofacial disorders, particularly those with midface or mandibular hypoplasia;
  - children with Down's syndrome;
  - children with neurological injury associated with spasticity or hypotonia of the pharyngeal muscles.

Symptoms and signs

- The majority (95%) of children with OSA snore every night, and most snore throughout the night.
- Carers may report pauses in breathing during sleep, sometimes followed by loud snorts and changes in position—usually reflecting momentary arousal.
- Children with OSA are often restless during sleep, and may get themselves into unusual postures, presumably in attempts to minimize the obstruction.
- Daytime sleepiness is unusual. There may be behavioural effects such as difficulty in concentration, and effects on cognitive ability.
- Enuresis is associated with OSA and often resolves when OSA is treated.
- Examination of a child with suspected OSA may show:
  - predominant mouth breathing;
  - dysmorphic features, suggesting a craniofacial disorder;
  - enlarged tonsils.
- Careful cardiac assessment will very occasionally identify evidence of pulmonary hypertension in children with severe longstanding OSA.

None of these findings may be present, and their absence does not exclude the possibility of OSA.

Consequences of untreated OSA

- Poor weight gain and growth is associated with OSA, probably due to a combination of increased work of breathing at night, poor feeding during the day, and possibly decreased nocturnal growth hormone secretion.
- Cognitive impairment (sometimes with poor school performance) and behavioural abnormalities are associated with OSA. There have been some studies suggesting that ADHD can be caused or exacerbated by OSA. Retrospective studies show improvement in school performance after treatment of OSA.
- There is increasing evidence that OSA can affect sympathetic tone with possible consequences for cardiovascular disease in adult life.
- Enuresis is more common in children with OSA. As many as 50% of 6–12 year olds with OSA will be enuretic with resolution or improvement in 75% after treatment of the OSA.
- Longstanding severe OSA with marked nocturnal desaturation and hypercarbia can cause cor pulmonale and right heart failure.
- Longstanding OSA may also be associated with decreased responsiveness to hypoxia and hypercarbia, giving rise to secondary alveolar hypoventilation. If these children are given oxygen therapy at night, the loss of any residual hypoxic drive can worsen the hypoventilation resulting in CO_2 narcosis. Hypoventilation is well described in adults and children with OSA associated with obesity. Normal ventilatory control usually returns once the obstruction has resolved.

Investigation

- Persistent snoring is the primary symptom of OSA but clinical symp toms alone are a poor guide to the presence of OSA. Overnight polysomnography (PSG) is the only reliable way to assess OSA. These studies can be done at home or in hospital. The complexity of the study and the number of channels recorded differs in different centres (see 📖 Appendix 3). There is a false negative rate for mild OSA and in this group the study may need to be repeated. Grading of OSA using PSG criteria also differs in different centres. One practical grading system is given in the box.
- Where severe OSA is suspected or proven, ECG and cardiac evaluation are sensible, particularly since anaesthesia and surgery will be the most likely intervention.

Grading of obstructive sleep apnoea

An obstructive event (apnoea or hypopnoea) is defined as paradoxical chest and abdominal movements for at least 2 respiratory cycles (with decreased or absent airflow if this is measured) resulting in either an arousal or an oxyhaemoglobin desaturation of at least 4%. There are a number of systems for grading severity of OSA. We use the following.

- *Upper airways resistance syndrome*
  - Chest and abdominal asynchrony without significant desaturation
- *Mild OSA*
  - An average of at least 5 obstructive events per hour
  - Lowest saturation never below 85%
- *Moderate OSA*
  - An average of at least 5 obstructive events per hour
  - Lowest saturation below 85% but never below 80%
- *Severe OSA*
  - An average of at least 5 obstructive events per hour
  - Lowest saturation below 80%

The number of obstructive events per hour is sometimes called the respiratory disturbance index (RDI). This can also be used, without saturation, to grade severity:

- RDI 5–10 is mild;
- RDI 10–15 is moderate;
- RDI > 15 is severe.

In most children the frequency of events correlates with the degree of desaturation. We prefer to incorporate the minimum saturation since there is some evidence that it is this that correlates best with neurobehavioural impairment.

Treatment

- In otherwise normal children with uncomplicated OSA, the first-line treatment is still adenotonsillectomy. Removing adenoids and tonsils is more effective than removing just one or the other. Whilst accepting an increased chance of residual obstruction, some surgeons prefer to do adenoidectomy alone in young children (< 15kg) since this minimizes the risk of bleeding.
- Adenotonsillectomy improves symptoms and PSG scores in most children (irrespective of the size of their tonsils and adenoids), although 15% of children will continue to show some evidence of obstruction. This is most likely in children with more severe OSA, and with comorbidity, including obesity (up to 50% of obese children will have some degree of persistent OSA after surgery).
- It is likely that surgery for OSA will improve many of its adverse effects on cognitive development, behaviour, enuresis, and sympathetic tone, but these outcomes have not been assessed by a prospective trial.
- Temperature-controlled radiofrequency treatment to reduce the bulk of the inferior turbinates can treat any coexisting nasal obstruction and can improve success of adenotonsillectomy.
- The presence of a narrow or contracted maxilla (recognized by the presence of nasal obstruction, often with a deviated septum, and a high-arched palate) can cause failure of adenotonsillectomy. This problem can be dealt with using orthodontic maxillary distraction devices.
- In otherwise normal children with mild to moderate OSA, a 6 week trial of nasal steroids can be expected to help 60–70% of children, and the benefits may be longlasting.
- When surgery is not appropriate or there is persistent residual obstruction following surgery, nasal mask CPAP is usually effective. Getting children of 2–5 years to tolerate a nasal mask can be quite a challenge, and requires skill and patience.
- Several oral drugs have been tried in adults with OSA, including respiratory stimulants and carbonic anhydrase inhibitors. None have shown convincing long-term benefits.

Postoperative respiratory complications

Respiratory problems after adenotonsillectomy are more common in those children with OSA (20%) compared to those without OSA (2%). Within the OSA group, the risk is higher in children:

- with more severe preoperative OSA—particularly those where the lowest recorded oxygen saturation was < 80%;
- under the age of 2 years;
- with comorbidities, especially craniofacial problems.

The majority (95%) of respiratory problems are characterized by desaturation and/or obstruction in the immediate postoperative period, whilst the child is still in the recovery room. These problems are presumed to be due to a combination of postoperative oedema and functional obstruction related to sedation. There may also be an element of right-to-left shunt caused by transiently elevated pulmonary pressures from a labile pulmonary circulation that has been sensitized by longstanding nocturnal hypoxia. In around 5% of children the problems persist for 24–48h postoperatively, requiring support with oxygen therapy and possibly nasal CPAP. Very occasionally an artificial airway will be needed. For these reasons, it is sensible to have a high-dependency bed available for the high-risk children undergoing adenotonsillectomy.

Long-term outcomes

There are very few long-term outcome studies in children and no RCTs of interventions. In the majority of children there is longlasting symptomatic improvement without evidence of morbidity. Thus it seems reasonable only to repeat sleep studies after adenotonsillectomy in high-risk children and in children whose symptoms have not improved. Much longer-term studies will be needed to assess the impact, if any, of childhood OSA on cardiovascular disease risk in later adult life.

Further information

Ali, N.J., Pitson, D., and Stradling, J.R. (1996). Sleep disordered breathing: effects of adenotonsillectomy on behaviour and psychological functioning. *Eur. J. Pediatr.* **155**, 56–62.

Brouillette, R.T., Manoukian, J.J., Ducharme, F.M., Oudjhane, K., Earle, L.G., *et al.* (2001). Efficacy of fluticasone nasal spray for pediatric obstructive sleep apnea. *J. Pediatr.* **138**, 838–44.

Carroll, J.L., McColley, S.A., Marcus, C.L., Curtis, S., and Loughlin, G.M. (1995). Inability of clinical history to distinguish primary snoring from obstructive sleep apnea syndrome in children. *Chest* **108**, 610–18.

Gozal, D. (1998). Sleep-disordered breathing and school performance in children. *Pediatrics* **102**, 616–20.

Lim, J. and McKean, M. (2003). Adenotonsillectomy for obstructive sleep apnoea in children. *Cochrane Database Syst. Rev.* **2003** (4), CD003136.

Mitchell, R.B. and Kelly, J. (2005). Child behavior after adenotonsillectomy for obstructive sleep apnea syndrome. *Laryngoscope* **115**, 2051–5.

O'Brien, L.M., Mervis, C.B., Holbrook, C.R., Bruner, J.L., Klaus, C.J., *et al.* (2004). Neurobehavioral implications of habitual snoring in children. *Pediatrics* **114**, 44–9.

Stradling, J.R., Thomas, G., Warley, A.R., Williams, P., and Freeland, A. (1990). Effect of adenotonsillectomy on nocturnal hypoxaemia, sleep disturbance, and symptoms in snoring children. *Lancet* **335**, 249–53.

Urschitz, M.S., Wolff, J., Sokollik, C., Eggebrecht, E., Urschitz-Duprat, P.M., Schlaud, M., and Poets, C.F. (2005). Nocturnal arterial oxygen saturation and academic performance in a community sample of children. *Pediatrics* **115**, 204–9.

Narcolepsy

Narcolepsy is characterized by periodic and often irresistible inappropriate daytime sleep. In addition there may be the following.

- Cataplexy. A sudden loss of muscle power, sometimes severe enough to cause a fall, but more usually enough to cause a head nod or the knees to buckle. Episodes may be brought on by emotion, such as laughter, or by being startled.
- Sleep paralysis. Paralysis of voluntary movement on waking from sleep.
- Hallucinations. Vivid hallucinations can occur at sleep onset (hypnagogus) or during wakening (hypnopompus) .

It is unusual for children to exhibit all 4 of these symptoms. Children may have apparent overactivity during the day.

- In half of affected adults, symptoms began between the ages of 10 and 20 years. In 5% onset occurs at < 10 years of age.
- Narcolepsy is rare with an incidence of around 1/10 000. It is poorly recognized by doctors and diagnosis is delayed on average by 10 years after the onset symptoms. Episodes of narcolepsy are frequently misdiagnosed as epilepsy or as hysterical.
- Narcolepsy–cataplexy is associated with specific damage to orexin (hypocretin)-containing neurons in the hypothalamus. Orexin (a class of neurotransmitter) levels are undetectable in the CSF of affected individuals.
- 90% of White European patients with narcolepsy–cataplexy carry HLA-DQB1*0602 (as do 20% of the general population). The orexin peptide fits the antigen presentation groove of the DQB1*0602 HLA protein and autoimmune-mediated damage of orexin neurons would be consistent with the strong HLA association. No autoimmune mediators (T cells or antibodies) have yet been identified in narcolepsy.
- There is an increased risk of narcolepsy in families and 5% of first-degree relatives have excessive daytime sleepiness.
- Rarely narcolepsy can occur after encephalitis or head injury.

Symptoms and signs

- Narcoleptic attacks are usually of sudden onset and last 15min or longer if the child is lying down. They occur more frequently during monotonous or boring situations, but may occur during eating and talking. The episode can be postponed by effort for minutes and sometimes hours.
- After an episode of sleep, the child will awaken refreshed following which there is a refractory period of 1–5h.
- Cataplexic episodes.
- Children can be woken from narcoleptic sleep episodes, and from episodes of sleep paralysis and cataplexy, by calling or shaking—an important difference from seizure activity.
- Children with narcolepsy may perform poorly at school and suffer ridicule from their peers. Cataplexy often takes the form of unexplained and abrupt falls or abrupt dropping of objects.
- Physical examination is normal.

Investigations

- Sleep studies show sleep-onset REM sleep. Outside infancy, REM sleep does not usually occur within 90min of sleep onset. A direct transition from wakefulness to REM sleep is suggestive of narcolepsy but may be seen following severe sleep deprivation or with severe OSA. The sleep study will otherwise be normal.
- Multiple sleep latency tests show that children with narcolepsy can readily fall asleep. In this test, which takes place after a sleep study showing at least 6h of sleep, the patient is given 5 opportunities where they are asked to lie quietly in bed and try to go to sleep. After 15min of sleep they are woken, and the cycle is repeated after 2h. Typically in narcolepsy sleep latency is less than 5min. Age-related normal values are not well-established in children.
- EEG is normal.
- CSF levels of orexin (hypocretin) can be assayed in specialist centres. Levels are low in narcolepsy–cataplexy, but less clear-cut in isolated narcolepsy.

Treatment and outcome

- A good sleep routine (sometimes called sleep hygiene) is important in controlling symptoms. This includes:
  - regular bedtimes with at least 8h sleep per night;
  - physical activity during the day, e.g. taking part in after school clubs;
  - scheduled daytime naps may help if necessary.
- Support at school will improve education and social achievement.
- Drug treatment, under the care of a specialist, may also help.
  - Stimulants such as methylphenidate or modafinil may improve daytime sleepiness.
  - Tricyclic antidepressants (clomipramine) and selective serotonin re-uptake inhibitors (fluoxetine) may help to prevent disabling cataplexy.
  - Recent evidence suggests that sodium oxybate may improve the symptoms of narcolepsy and cataplexy.
- Alcohol will exacerbate the condition.
- The condition is lifelong.

Dauvilliers, Y., Arnulf, I. and Mignot, E. (2007). Narcolepsy with cataplexy. *Lancet* **369**, 499–511.

Krahn, L.E. and Gonzalez-Arriaza, H.L. (2004). Narcolepsy with cataplexy. *Am. J. Psychiatry* **161**, 2181–4.

Weaver, T.E. and Cuellar, N. (2006). A randomized trial evaluating the effectiveness of sodium oxybate therapy on quality of life in narcolepsy. *Sleep* **29**, 1189–94

Respiratory control disorders

Congenital central hypoventilation syndrome

Definition and epidemiology

Congenital central hypoventilation syndrome (CCHS) is a condition in which there is blunted or absent respiratory response to hypoxia and hypercarbia in the absence of lung disease, neuromuscular disease, or an identifiable brainstem lesion. Most children with CCHS have adequate ventilation while awake but hypoventilate during sleep. More severely affected children hypoventilate both when awake and during sleep.

CCHS is thought to be a neurocristopathy, resulting from abnormal development of the neural crest, and this explains the observed association of CCHS with ganglioneuromas and Hirschsprung's disease. (See the box for other associations.) Over 90% of cases are associated with mutations in the transcription factor gene PHOX2b, which is expressed in the brainstem and in autonomic nerve cells. 5% of parents show somatic mosaicism for the mutation. In the remainder, the mutation arises de novo. CCHS is a very rare condition with a frequency of around 1/100 000 births.

Symptoms

- The majority of children are symptomatic from birth. In some there will be a history of abnormal fetal heart recordings—usually a lack of heart rate variability.
  - Affected infants usually make a good response to delivery and resuscitation is often not required.
  - Recurrent episodes of cyanosis or apnoea may become apparent in the first 1–12h after birth.
- If CCHS is not noticed in the neonatal period, it will usually present in the first 6 months of life. These infants are at risk of developing complications from prolonged episodes of hypoxia—either hypoxic brain injury or pulmonary hypertension, with cyanosis and signs of right heart failure.
- Occasionally a child with CCHS will present for the first time with an apparent life-threatening event (ALTE).
- A late presentation variant of CCHS is also recognized. These children present between 2 and 10 years of age. There is an association with hyperphagia, hypersomnolence, thermal dysregulation, emotional lability, and endocrinopathies.

Problems associated with CCHS

- Aganglionosis of the bowel (20%). This is usually in the form of long segment Hirschsprung's disease, but both short segment disease and total aganglionosis of the small and large bowel may occur.
- Autonomic dysfunction:
  - pupillary abnormalities (50%)—abnormal dilatation or unequal size with sluggish or absent response to light
  - oesophageal dysmotility (20%)
  - lack of heart rate variability
  - cardiac arrhythmias (20%)
  - episodes of pallor
  - episodes of profound sweating (40%)
  - fainting (25%)
- Ocular abnormalities:
  - 30% have strabismus (squint) and 10% have insufficient tears
- Tumours of the sympathetic nervous system (TSNS; 5–10%)
  - Neuroblastoma, ganglioneuroma. These tumours are more common in children with CCHS who have the frameshift type of mutations in PHOX2b with an incidence of up to 40% in this group. TSNS in CCHS tend to present after the first year of life
  - TSNS are more common in children with CCHS who have Hirschsprung's disease
  - Sporadic neuroblastoma without CCHS is also associated with mutations in PHOX2b
- Developmental delay (65%)
  - 50% have speech delay
  - 50% have motor delay, especially hypotonia
  - 30% diagnosed with cognitive impairment
  - 60% will have some learning problems
- Seizures (40%)—mainly in infancy
- Gastrointestinal problems:
  - gastro-oesophageal reflux (20%)
  - constipation (20%)
- Absence of fever in response to infections (20%)

Notes It is not clear whether the observed developmental delay and seizure activity are intrinsic parts of CCHS or whether they are secondary to periods of hypoxia and hypercarbia

Diagnosis

Diagnosis requires:

- evidence of hypoventilation that is unresponsive, or has a blunted response to both hypercapnia and hypoxia;
- absence of identifiable primary pulmonary or neuromuscular disease;
- absence of primary cardiac disease.

Demonstration of hypoventilation requires careful respiratory assessment. In infants who are self-ventilating, this can be done with polysomnography during wakefulness and sleep. In infants who are ventilated, recordings can be taken from the usual monitors and from the ventilator.

In the self-ventilating infant, the following is observed.

- Hypoventilation during sleep, and in the first 3 months of life during wakefulness as well, recognized by increases in CO_2 (> 8kPa), will be seen. This is characterized by hypopnoea and prolonged periods of apnoea. Infants with mild disease may sleep for up to 60min before showing evidence of hypoventilation.
- Hypoventilation is most severe in NREM sleep, during which breathing is primarily under chemical control. This distinguishes hypoventilation arising from disorders of central control from hypoventilation due to muscle weakness, which is more apparent during REM sleep.
- The infants fail to arouse in response to hypercarbia and often the expected increase in heart rate is also absent.
- Responses to hypoxia are more variable. In some infants there will be arousal and some respiratory effort.
- In mild cases, where there is doubt, more detailed chemoreceptor responses can be assessed using a re-breathing or steady-state challenge with 5% CO_2 administered via a head box.

In more severely affected neonates who are ventilator-dependent, it is important to ensure all sedative drugs are stopped for 24h prior to testing.

- Responses to hypercarbia can be assessed using the CPAP mode on the ventilator with a high FiO_2. Mixed responses to hypercarbia and hypoxia can be assessed using the CPAP mode with air.
- There may be a relatively prolonged period of apnoea before any ventilatory effort is apparent, and it is important to prevent unnecessary hypoxia during the assessment.
- By using a high FiO_2 in a hypoventilating infant it is usually possible to maintain normal oxygen saturation and yet induce an endogenous hypercarbia and respiratory acidosis. Lack of respiratory response (as assessed by measured minute volumes and respiratory effort), often combined with lack of heart rate response, is consistent with the diagnosis.

Investigations

Once the diagnosis has been suspected on the basis of blunted response to hypercarbia and hypoxia, additional investigations to exclude underlying causes include the following.

- Metabolic investigations. Plasma and urinary organic acids, plasma amino acids, carnitine levels. Tests of mitochondrial disorders, lactate, and possibly muscle biopsy.
- Imaging. MRI brain to exclude structural abnormality. The scan should include the chest and spine in children with associated Hirschsprung's disease to detect any potential TSNS.
- Echocardiography to exclude heart disease.

Additional investigations that increase the likelihood of a diagnosis of CCHS include the following.

- DNA analysis for PHOX2b mutations. Mutations are found in over 90% of affected infants.
- Rectal suction biopsy for Hirschsprung's disease. If this is positive, higher biopsies, including small bowel biopsies to determine the extent of the aganglionosis, will help in predicting long-term prognosis.

Management

- Most infants will initially be dependent on ventilatory support 24h per day. This will require insertion of a tracheostomy. There are a few case reports of infants being managed with face mask ventilation. This is generally impractical when continuous support is needed, not only because the skin may break down but also because pressure from the mask will cause mid-face hypoplasia.
- Respiratory stimulants such as doxapram are ineffective. Medroxyprogesterone has some effect but causes pituitary axis depression.
- Adequacy of ventilation will need to be assessed regularly using end-tidal CO_2 and oxygen saturation.
- As the infant becomes more active after 2–3 months of age, increasing periods of time off support when awake can be introduced as tolerated. Children who can apparently breathe during the day need careful daytime assessment to ensure they are adequately ventilated. The usual clinical signs of inadequate ventilation, such as distress, sweating, and pallor, will be absent.
- Intercurrent respiratory infection is common and may be difficult to diagnose in some children with CCHS who do not generate fever in response to infection. During infective episodes full-time ventilation may be needed in those usually only on night-time support.

- Associated medical problems, particularly in relation to feeding and Hirschsprung's disease, will need to be tackled.
- Discharge can be considered once the infant is stable, and the parents have become confident and capable in the care of their child and all the associated equipment. A fully ventilated child at home will need round-the clock nursing assistance, and the necessary funding and recruitment will need to be organized. This often takes several months.
- Daily assessment should include end-tidal CO_2 and saturation monitoring.
- Toddlers need careful assessment as they can develop daytime hypo-ventilation again for a period as their resting respiratory rate decreases.
- Older children will need assessment to determine their response to exercise. Since they do not perceive hypoxia and hypercarbia they can continue exercising to the point of collapse and need to be taught to take regular rests during sport.
- In children ≥ 6 years of age who have stable disease requiring night-time support only, conversion to face-mask ventilation and decannulation may be considered.
- In children who remain fully ventilator-dependent 24h per day, phrenic nerve pacing can be considered. This is only effective if there is normal lung compliance (i.e. no evidence of lung disease). It is expensive and associated with a number of complications including permanent phrenic nerve injury. If successfully implanted, pacing should only be used during the day to minimize nerve injury and diaphragm fatigue. Its use can lead to improved mobility and independence.
- Annual assessment of development.
- Annual ophthalmological review.
- Annual lung function testing when the child can cooperate with the required manoeuvres.
- Annual cardiac assessment. ECG and echo to look for evidence of pulmonary hypertension.
- Annual 24h ECG to detect periods of tachy- or bradyarrhythmia.
- Screening for TSNS for the 10% of children with CCHS who have frameshift or missense mutations in PHOX2B, and in whom there is a significant risk of neuroblastoma. There are no reports of successful screening, but 3 monthly urinary VMAs for the first 5 years seems reasonable. All reported TSNS have arisen within the first 5 years of life in this group of children.

Outcome
- All reported series describe a good quality of life in the majority of survivors. 65% attend mainstream school on a full-time basis.
- Overall mortality is 10–40%. Most deaths occur in the first 2 years of life, and include ethical decisions to withdraw care. Causes of death in older children include lung infection, cardiac arrhythmia, and accidental ventilator disconnection or dysfunction.

- Children with frameshift mutations (rather than the more common polyalanine repeats) are more likely to have extensive bowel aganglionosis, more severe respiratory involvement with a higher risk of needing daytime support, and a higher risk of developing invasive neuroblastoma.
- The average initial duration of hospital admission is 6–12 months.
- All infants presenting in the neonatal period will require 24h ventilatory support. The majority can be weaned off daytime support between 2 and 12 months of age as daytime activity increases.
- 5–10% will need chronic 24h ventilatory support.
- There is a lifetime risk of developing progressive pulmonary hypertension because of unrecognized hypoxia, which can only be avoided by scrupulous care with monitoring ventilation.
- Despite the challenges, there are now increasing numbers of children with this condition reaching adulthood. The majority do not require daytime ventilatory support and have normal or near-normal intelligence. Coexisting medical problems may significantly affect the quality of life of these children.

Further information

Maitraa, A., Shineb, J., Henderson, J., and Fleming, P. (2004). The investigation and care of children with congenital central hypoventilation syndrome. *Curr. Paediatr.* **14**, 354–60.

Katz, E.S., McGrath, S., and Marcus, C.L. (2000). Late-onset central hypoventilation with hypothalamic dysfunction: a distinct clinical syndrome. *Ped. Pulmonol* **29**, 62–8.

Amiel, J., Laudier, B., Attie-Bitach, T., Trang, H., de Pontual, L., Gener, B., Trochet, D., Etchevers, H., Ray, P., Simonneau, M., Vekemans, M., Munnich, A., Gaultier, C, and Lyonnet, S. (2003). Polyalanine expansion and frameshift mutations of the paired-like homeobox gene PHOX2B in congenital central hypoventilation syndrome. *Nat. Genet.* **33** 459–61.

Secondary central hypoventilation

Reduced respiratory drive may arise from blunting of chemoreceptor sensitivity or abnormalities of the respiratory centre in the brainstem (see boxes). Some of the conditions can be present at birth; others are acquired later.

Investigations and management

The clinical approach taken depends on the situation. A careful assessment will be needed to determine whether there are genuine problems of respiratory control. The possibility of weakness should be considered as a cause of inadequate ventilation.

When problems of respiratory control are identified, often there is a clear cause for the problem, and often there is no specific treatment. Decisions about long-term respiratory support are often difficult to make and require as much information as possible about likely outcomes. Where the cause is not known, extensive investigation may be required. These investigations may include the following.

- CNS imaging: usually MRI.
- Exclusion of CNS infection: may require lumbar puncture.
- Genetic tests. These may include:
  - *PHOX2B* analysis (congenital central hypoventilation);
  - tests for Prader–Willi (FISH or PCR or methylation analysis);
  - *IKBKAP* analysis (familial dysautonomia in Ashkenazi Jews).
- Tests for metabolic disease:
  - serum and urinary amino acids and organic acids;
  - serum and CSF lactate and pyruvate;
  - muscle biopsy for mitochondrial disease.

Treatment

Treatment will depend on the cause. Where there are potential reversible causes these should be addressed. Some of the secondary causes of hypoventilation are dealt with later in this chapter.

Respiratory centre abnormalities

These may arise from the following
- Asphyxia. These children usually have severe hypoxic encephalopathy
- CNS infection—usually viral encephalitis
- Head injury
- Brainstem tumour
- Brainstem stroke
- Metabolic disease. The mechanism by which most of these conditions affect respiratory drive is not well understood. The conditions include:
  - mitochondrial disease (especially Leigh disease)
  - pyruvate dehydrogenase deficiency
  - carnitine deficiency
- Congenital hypoplasia of brainstem nuclei (Mobius's syndrome) can be associated with central hypoventilation
- Arnold–Chiari malformation with brainstem compression
- Syndromic disorders, including Prader–Willi, may be associated with neonatal hypoventilation, sometimes requiring prolonged respiratory support
- Drugs. The use of respiratory depressants needs to be excluded
- Familial dysautonomia. Relatively common in Ashkenazi Jews and associated with decreased sensitivity to hypoxia and hypercarbia. See 📖 Chapter 54, p. 644

Blunted chemoreceptor sensitivity

- This is usually seen in the context of longstanding hypercarbia or hypoxia
- Some children with severe longstanding OSA may show central hypoventilation with insensitivity to episodes of hypoxia or hypercarbia. Once the obstruction is relieved periods of apnoea may worsen temporarily before chemoreceptor sensitivity returns. In extreme examples, usually associated with gross obesity, there may be daytime hypercarbia (Pickwickian syndrome)
- A similar situation may arise in children with longstanding hypercarbia who are dependent on hypoxic respiratory drive (type 2 respiratory failure). This most commonly arises now in the context of chronic lung disease of prematurity. Giving high concentrations of inspired oxygen to these infants may reduce their minute ventilation and lead to worsening hypercarbia

Arnold–Chiari malformation

- Chiari malformations are structural defects of the cerebellum. They are classified according to severity.
  - Chiari I. The cerebellar tonsils pass through the foramen magnum, but the brainstem is unaffected. There are usually no symptoms.
  - Chiari II. The cerebellar tonsils and the lower part of the brainstem herniate through the foramen magnum. The cerebellar vermis may be hypoplastic or absent.
  - Chiari III . More extensive herniation down into the cervical cord, often involving the 4th ventricle.
- The term Arnold–Chiari malformation (ACM) refers specifically to type 2 defects. ACM are usually associated with spina bifida, but may occur in otherwise normal children.
- The cause of Chiari defects is not known. They may arise because of a physically small posterior fossa or as a result of primary dysgenesis of the involved structures. The observation that early surgery can improve outcomes implies that, in at least some children, the brainstem dysfunction is acquired as a result of compression.
- ACM is associated with;
  - hydrocephalus;
  - tethered cord;
  - syringomyelia;
  - scoliosis.
- The incidence of ACM is not known precisely but is thought to be around 1/1000 births.

Symptoms and signs

- ACM may be asymptomatic. When symptoms occur, they do so most often in early infancy, and result from abnormal brainstem function. Possible symptoms include the following.
  - Stridor (from vocal cord dysfunction).
  - Weak or absent cry.
  - Difficulty swallowing (from bulbar dysfunction).
  - Aspiration lung disease.
  - Recurrent apnoea—often a combination of obstructive and central events. Obstruction may arise from vocal cord dysfunction or abnormal pharyngeal muscular tone. Central apnoeas are probably related to blunted responses to hypoxia and hypercapnia because of brainstem compression.
  - Upper limb weakness—from cervical cord compression.
- In later childhood, sometimes as late as adolescence, symptoms are likely to be less dramatic, but reflect disturbance of the same structures. There may be:
  - difficulty swallowing with aspiration events;
  - gastro-oesophageal reflux;
  - fainting episodes;
  - nystagmus;
  - ataxia.

- Breath-holding spells in toddlers with ACM can be associated with profound desaturation, possibly because of blunted central response to hypoxia. Typically these young children will cry, have prolonged expiration, and then fail to inspire and become cyanosed, sometimes resulting in loss of consciousness or seizures.
- Examination findings include the above, plus possible increased tone and brisk tendon reflexes and a diminished or absent gag reflex.
- Specialist respiratory opinion may be sought in infants or older children with apnoeas, stridor, or recurrent aspiration. It is in this group of children that ACM should be considered in the differential diagnosis.

Investigations and diagnosis

- The diagnosis is made by imaging, either with CT scan or MRI scan.
- There may be associated hydrocephalus and often areas of skull thinning, sometimes called a lacuna skull, a finding that persists up to around 6 months of age.
- Polysomnography is useful to document the presence and severity of any obstructive or central apnoea.

Management

- In infants with myelomeningocele, ACM and the associated brainstem dysfunction is a leading cause of mortality.
- Once the diagnosis is made, a decision as to whether foramen magnum decompression should be carried out needs to be made. This decision will be governed by the timing and severity of symptoms and MRI appearance of the ACM.
- Occasionally there is acute hydrocephalus and this will need urgent treatment.
- Foramen magnum decompression may not result in resolution of symptoms. There is some evidence to suggest that, in symptomatic infants, early intervention results in better outcomes. In one study, 10 of 13 children treated early recovered normal or near normal brainstem function.[1] Conversely, in a study of children with myelomeningocele and sleep-disordered breathing, of 8 children who had foramen magnum decompression, only 2 showed partial benefit.[2]
- Adenotonsillectomy may help obstructive symptoms, but residual obstruction is common.
- Respiratory stimulants such as theophylline can be tried. Anecdotal reports suggest that theophylline treatment can lead to improvement in frequency and severity of central apnoea.
- In children with persistent obstructive and central apnoeas, non-invasive support, usually with nasal BiPAP, will be required. The occurrence of central apnoea during wakefulness is a poor prognostic sign.
- There is no intervention that is known to help cyanosis with breath-holding.

1 Pollack, I.F., Kinnunen, D., and Albright, A.L. (1996). The effect of early craniocervical decompression on functional outcome in neonates and young infants with myelodysplasia and symptomatic Chiari II malformations: results from a prospective series. *Neurosurgery* **38**, 703–10.

2 Kirk, V.G., Morielli, A., Gozal, D., Marcus, C.L., Waters, K.A., D'Andrea, L.A. Rosen, C.L., Deray, M.J., and Brouillette, R.T. (2000). Treatment of sleep-disordered breathing in children with myelomeningocele. *Pediatr. Pulmonol.* **30**, 445–52.

Prader–Willi syndrome

- Prader–Willi syndrome (PWS) is a genetic hypothalamic obesity disorder characterized by the following.
  - Neonatal hypotonia, often with poor feeding. The hypotonia improves with age, but early motor milestones are usually delayed.
  - Hypogonadism. Small labia minora and clitoris in females and hypoplastic scrotum in males; incomplete and delayed puberty; and infertility.
  - Obesity secondary to overeating (hyperphagia).
  - Reduction in muscle mass is associated with diminished strength, physical function, and energy expenditure.
  - Cognitive impairment (mean IQ is 70) with some behavioural problems particularly related to social skills. Some children show surprising skill at solving jigsaw puzzles and simple word games.
  - Short stature.
  - Children with PWS may also have small hands and feet and characteristic facial features, including narrow bifrontal diameter, almond-shaped palpebral fissures, and down-turned mouth.
- The genetic defects in PWS arise early in embryonic life. In 75% of children with PWS, there is a deletion of 15q11–q13 derived from the father. In 22% there are 2 copies of the maternal chromosome 15 with no contribution from the father and in 3% there are imprinting errors because of either a sporadic or inherited microdeletion in the imprinting centre. There are a number of candidate genes in the affected regions and the precise genetic cause is not known. There is an equal sex incidence.
- Incidence is 1/25 000 births. Population prevalence is 1/50 000.
- In adults with PWS there is an increased risk of type 2 diabetes mellitus and osteoporosis.

Respiratory problems

- Sleep-disordered breathing occurs in 50–100% of children with PWS depending on the age and degree of obesity at the time of the study. Obstructive as well as central apnoeas can occur.
- Obstructive sleep apnoea (OSA) is thought to arise as a consequence of obesity leading to airway narrowing, combined with pharyngeal muscle hypotonia.
- Central apnoea arises because of blunted responses to both hypoxia and hypercapnia, probably because of reduced sensitivity of peripheral chemoreceptors. This is a primary defect in PWS. Further reductions in responsiveness can occur in children with longstanding OSA who have recurrent hypoxic events during sleep.
- The presence of obstructive events during sleep combined with lack of arousal to hypoxia can be life-threatening, and unexpected deaths during sleep are described.
- The presence of restrictive lung disease, caused by respiratory muscle weakness, scoliosis, and chest wall obesity, worsens the effects of obstructive and central events.

- Hypoventilation and hypotonia may be particularly troublesome in young children (< 4 years of age) with PWS and may be worsened by viral respiratory tract infection.

Growth hormone (GH)

- Some features of PWS (decreased total lean body mass, IGF-I levels, and poor linear growth) resemble those of GH deficiency, and children with PWS have demonstrably low levels of GH production. Treatment of children with GH improves linear growth, final height, physical strength, and agility. although some of the benefits wane once the treatment is stopped.
- Shortly after GH was introduced for the treatment of PWS, there were reports of unexpected deaths occurring within a few months of starting treatment.
- Treatment with GH actually improves central apnoea and responsiveness to hypoxia in children with PWS. However, it is possible that it worsens obstruction by causing increase in size of tonsillar and adenoidal tissue, or decreases lung compliance by temporarily causing fluid retention.
- In one study, polysomnography 6 weeks after GH was introduced in children with PWS showed 25% had worsening of apnoea hypopnoea index—nearly all obstructive events, whilst the remainder improved.[3]
- Children with PWS whose sleep-disturbed breathing is likely to worsen with GH treatment are those with gross obesity and those troubled by recurrent respiratory tract infection.

Management

- All children with PWS who have any symptoms of sleep apnoea or snoring should undergo polysomnography.
- All children with PWS who are going to be treated with GH should have polysomnography before and 6–8 weeks after starting treatment
- Where sleep-disturbed breathing is identified, there will nearly always be an obstructive element, which may be improved by adenotonsillectomy.
- The lack of response to hypoxia and hypercarbia, and reduced pharyngeal muscle tone are risk factors for general anaesthesia, and intensive care facilities may be needed postoperatively.
- Repeat polysomnography should be carried out after any surgical intervention as the likely success is reduced compared to that in the normal non-obese population.
- Where significant sleep-disturbed breathing remains after surgery, nasal CPAP or BIPAP may be needed, depending on the severity of events and the relative contributions of obstructive and central disturbance.
- Successful treatment of sleep-disturbed breathing in the children with PWS can significantly improve daytime sleepiness and behaviour.

3 Miller, J., Silverstein, J., Shuster, J., Driscoll, D.J., and Wagner, M (2006). Short-term effects of growth hormone on sleep abnormalities in Prader–Willi syndrome. *J. Clin. Endocrinol. Metab.* **91**, 413–17.

Rett syndrome

- Rett syndrome is an X-linked genetic neurodegenerative disorder of girls characterized by the following.
  - Normal development until between 6 and 18 months of age, although in retrospect babies may be thought to be placid and hypotonic.
  - Onset of symptoms heralded by slowing of head growth followed by a period of developmental arrest (6–18 months) and then a period of regression (1–4 years).
  - Developmental regression is characterized by loss of purposeful hand movements, loss of oral language, and dyspraxia. Striking hand sterotypies develop between 1 and 4 years with clasping, wringing, and clapping movements. Seizures and vacant episodes are common.
  - Following the period of regression, the condition becomes stable with no further cognitive deterioration. There may be some improvement in communication and social skills. There may be further deterioration in later adult life.
- Most girls with Rett syndrome will be able to walk and undertake some activities and express a full range of emotions. They will generally always require assistance with most activities of daily living and will not be able to live independently.
- Rett syndrome is the most common genetic cause of profound combined intellectual and physical disability in Caucasian females. It has an incidence of 1/10 000 girls.
- The majority of Rett syndrome (80%) is caused by mutations in the X-linked gene encoding methyl-CpG-binding protein 2 (*MeCP2*). *MeCP2* mutations have also been identified in individuals with a variety of other neurological diseases. A proportion of atypical Rett syndrome cases may result from mutations in *CDKL5*, particularly the early onset seizure variant.
- Girls with Rett syndrome may survive to middle or old age. 70% reach the age of 35 years. There is an increased mortality, either related to seizure disorder or sudden death due to autonomic dysfunction. This results in either prolonged apnoea or possibly cardiac arrhythmia. About 25% of deaths in girls with Rett syndrome are sudden.
- In addition to the respiratory problems, girls with Rett syndrome may have scoliosis, gut motility problems (mainly reflux and constipation), autonomic dysfunction (cold extremities and risk of arrhythmia), and short stature.

Respiratory problems

- About 70% of girls with Rett syndrome show disorganized breathing during wakefulness.
- Many different patterns of abnormal breathing are described including:
  - periodic breathing;
  - hyperventilation followed by periods of apnoea (Biot's breathing) often associated with cyanosis;
  - runs of inspiratory breath-holding with Valsalva type manoeuvres.

- Breathing abnormalities, particularly hyperventilation and apnoea, tend to be more common and more severe in younger girls with Rett syndrome (those < 10 years of age) but are often observed in adults.
- Periods of hyperventilation can reduce partial pressure of CO_2, with levels down as low as 2kPa. This can be associated with tetany and may possibly trigger seizures.
- Apnoea following hyperventilation can last as long as 2min and can be associated with profound desaturation, which may contribute to further brain injury or lead to sudden death.
- Breathing during sleep is usually of normal frequency although the time spent in REM sleep is diminished.
- The cause of the breathing abnormalities is not understood but is thought to reflect neurotransmitter imbalances in the brain.

Management

- Girls with Rett syndrome who are having symptomatic daytime hyperventilation or apnoea should undergo awake polysomnography to document the severity and frequency of events. Those with hypocapnia or marked periods of hypoxia may benefit from a trial of treatment.
- Benzodiazepines seem to be effective (e.g. diazepam 1–2mg taken in the morning) in reducing frequency and severity of daytime apnoea and desaturatation, but can cause unacceptable sedation.
- Serotonin analogues or serotonin reuptake inhibitors (SSRIs) in theory may be beneficial by improving serotoninergic neurotransmission. There is a case report of improvements in breathing patterns after treatment with buspirone, a serotoninergic type 1A receptor agonist usually used as a short-term anxiolytic.[4] There are no reports on the use of SSRIs.
- There are also anecdotal reports of the use of clonidine and acetazolamide.
- There is little value in monitoring the events at home. It is unlikely that any form of monitoring would prevent sudden death.

4 Andaku, D.K., Mercadante M.T., and Schwartzmann, J.S. (2005). Buspirone in Rett syncrome respiratory dysfunction. *Brain Dev.* **27**, 437–8.

Further information

Julu, P.O., Kerr, A.M, Apartopoulos, F., Al-Rawas, S., Engerstrom, I.W. Engerstrom, L., Jamal, G.A., and Hansen, S. (2001). Characterisation of breathing and associated central autonomic dysfunction in the Rett disorder. *Arch. Dis. Child.* **85**, 29–37.

Joubert syndrome

- Joubert syndrome is a neurological condition characterized by the absence or underdevelopment of the cerebellar vermis.
- Joubert syndrome usually presents in early infancy with hypotonia and jerky eye movements (oculomotor apraxia). Abnormal respiratory movements are common in infancy (see below).
- As children get older ataxia develops and developmental delay becomes apparent. There is a wide range of severity depending on the extent of the cerebellar hypoplasia.
- Most cases of Joubert syndrome are sporadic but, in some families, Joubert syndrome appears to be inherited via a recessive gene that has yet to be identified.
- The combination of abnormal eye movements and respiration is also seen in Leigh disease and Pelizaeus–Merzbacher disease (in boys).

Respiratory problems

- Respiratory abnormalities are seen in 50–75% of infants with Joubert syndrome.
- Episodes of extreme tachypnoea (100–200 breaths per minute) are associated with alternating periods of central apnoea.
- Typically the episodes of tachypnoea start in the neonatal period, improve with time, and are often no longer observed after 6 months of age.
- Persistent tachypnoea is not seen.

Management

- No specific management for the respiratory abnormalities is required, and improvement is usually seen over a few months.
- It is useful for the respiratory specialist to be aware of Joubert syndrome to assist diagnosis when asked to consult on neonates with intermittent tachypnoea.

Leigh syndrome

- Leigh syndrome, also called subacute necrotizing encephalomyelopathy, is a heterogeneous group of rare inherited disorders characterized by degeneration of the central nervous system, particularly involving the brainstem or spinal cord.
- It is caused by both nuclear and mitochondrial gene mutations that affect respiratory chain production of ATP by mitochondria.
- Classically it presents between 3 months and 2 years of age with poor feeding, hypotonia, weakness, and loss of motor skills often with features of encephalopathy (irritability, persistent crying, vomiting, loss of appetite, seizures). Later onset forms affecting previously normal school-age children also occur.
- There is progressive brainstem involvement with opthalmoplegia, bulbar dysfunction, and problems of respiratory control—usually slow resting respiratory rate with prolonged apnoea. Periodic breathing (Cheyne–Stokes pattern) may also be seen.
- Elevated lactic acid, either in the blood or CSF, is frequent but not invariable.
- MRI imaging of the head shows lesions affecting the basal ganglia, brainstem, or spinal cord.

Respiratory problems

- Children with Leigh syndrome may present with apnoea before other features of neurodegeneration become apparent.
- Central hypoventilation in infants with Leigh syndrome may be misdiagnosed as congenital central hypoventilation syndrome (CCHS). Leigh syndrome is not found in the neonatal period (unlike CCHS).
- It is important for the respiratory physician to be aware of the condition and make prompt referral to a paediatric neurologist.
- There may be confusion with Guillain–Barré syndrome, where bulbar dysfunction and weakness, but not central apnoea also occur. Nerve conduction studies will be normal in Leigh syndrome.

Treatment and outcome

- Vitamin supplementation (thiamine and B_1) may help, but in most children there is rapidly progressive disease with death occurring 6 months to 4 years after onset. In later onset atypical disease seen in school-age children, there may be rapid deterioration followed by a prolonged plateau period lasting some years.
- Bulbar and brainstem dysfunction are the usual cause of death, which can occur suddenly probably as a combination of an obstructive and central apnoeic event.
- The provision of long-term ventilation via a nasal mask or via tracheostomy will depend on the severity and progression of neurological impairment. Often it will be inappropriate and pointlessly prolong suffering. Occasionally in older children there may a requirement for support during the initial deterioration phase following which there may be a prolonged period of stability.

Sudden infant death syndrome

Overview

Definition
The sudden death of an infant that is unexpected on the basis of history and unexplained by a thorough post-mortem examination and by examination of the scene of death.

Incidence
Incidence 1–2 per 1000 live births. It is the commonest cause of death in infants between 1 month and 1 year of age. 90% occur in the first 6 months of life.

Risk factors
- Sibling with SIDS.
- Maternal smoking.
- Maternal drug abuse.
- Maternal age <20 years.
- Prematurity.
- Low birth weight.
- Late or no prenatal care.
- Sleeping prone or on side.

Theories of causation
- Immature respiratory control fails to compensate for imposed physiological stresses.
- There may also be abnormal or immature control of temperature, chemoreceptor sensitivity, and heart rate responses.
- A deficit in sleep arousal in response to cardiorespiratory disturbance appears to be necessary for SIDS to occur.
- The imposed stresses may include URTI, overheating, and partial airways obstruction (by secretions or external material such as the infant's bedding).

Prevention
- Supine sleeping posture.
- Avoid maternal smoking pre- and postnatally.
- Avoid overheating during sleep. Use sheets and thin blankets, not duvets.
- Avoid the head becoming covered during sleep—arms outside sheets, feet at the bottom of the cot.
- Use a firm mattress and do not place soft toys in the cot.
- Avoid sleeping in same bed as parent.
- Safest environment for sleep seems to be in a cot in the parents' room.

Immediate management of SIDS

Most hospitals will have a written policy for the management of SIDS.

Resuscitation

- The vast majority of SIDS victims will be brought to hospital by ambulance.
- The paramedic crews will have started resuscitation.
- How long resuscitation is continued is a matter of judgement. On some occasions it will be obvious that this infant has been dead for some hours. In other cases it will be appropriate to continue for the standard 30min, after which, if there have been no signs of cardiac or respiratory activity, care should be withdrawn.
- It can be important for the parents to be present during resuscitation attempts so that they can see that everything that could be done was done. If parents are present they need to have a member of staff with them at all times to explain what is happening.

History

In addition to the standard history, additional information is needed. This will usually require a separate meeting with the parents, often the following day. If possible this meeting should be carried out in the parents' home.

- Any previous medical problems?
- Any recent change in health?
- When was the baby last seen alive? (Where and by whom?)
- Exactly how was he/she found (position, covers, clothing, room temperature)?
- Details of resuscitation carried out at home.
- Family structure.
- Family history of SIDS.
- Consanguineous parents?
- Description of usual sleeping arrangements.
- Bed sharing when found (with whom?).
- Smoking in pregnancy.
- Parental smokers (one or both).
- Parental alcohol (in last 24h). Who? How much?
- Parental drug use (in last 24h). Who? What?

Samples

Consent from the parents is required for the collection of samples. After death the body comes under the jurisdiction of the coroner, who has control over any subsequent measures that affect it. Advance agreement in principle with the local coroner for sample collection should be in place. It may be necessary to carry out a cardiac puncture to obtain sufficient blood.

- FBC
- Na, K, Ca, Mg.
- Urea and creatinine.
- Glucose.
- Albumin.

- ALT.
- AST.
- Alk. Phos.
- Plasma amino acids.
- acyl carnitine (collect a blood spot on a Guthrie card).
- Blood culture.
- Urine (SPA) for culture, amino and organic acids, and toxicology.
- Throat swab.
- Rectal swab.
- Nasal swab.
- Lumbar puncture.

Skin biopsy may be necessary, but can nearly always wait until the autopsy is performed.

Informing other parties

The following individuals will need to be informed.
- The coroner has a duty to investigate all sudden and unexpected deaths and must be informed. An autopsy will need to be performed. The responsible paediatrician will need to provide the coroner with a report based on their interview with the parents and any other relevant material (including information from the GP).
- The police will have to talk to the parents and the parents may have to identify the baby in their presence.
- The responsible consultant paediatrician.
- The GP.
- The health visitor (the infant will need to be removed from the immunization register).

Follow-up

A multidisciplinary meeting, involving the pathologist, the paediatrician, and the primary health care team, should be convened when the data from the autopsy are available. The purpose of the meeting will be to establish the likely cause of death and to identify any precipitating factors. The results of the meeting should be conveyed in a written report to the parents.

Further information

The Foundation for the Study of Infant Deaths (FSID): *www.sids.org.uk.*

'Sudden unexpected death in infancy'. The report of a working group convened by the Royal College of Pathologists and the Royal College of Paediatrics and Child Health. Chair: The Baroness Helena Kennedy QC. September 2004 *www.rcpath.org/resources/pdf/SUDI%20report%20for% 20web.pdf*

Chapter 28

Apparent life-threatening events

Definition

- Apparent life-threatening events (ALTEs) are those where:
  - the affected infant has a sudden change in behaviour, characterized by a combination of apnoea, choking, colour change, or change in tone;
  - the parent or carer is very alarmed and may think that the child is dying;
  - the parent or carer usually initiates some form of life support.
- Most infants will be 2–4 months of age. ALTE is commoner in babies born prematurely.
- The term 'near-miss cot death', which implies a causal link with SIDS, should be avoided.

For history, possible causes, and investigation, see 📖 Chapter 6.

Outcome and risk of sudden infant death syndrome (SIDS)

- In infants with idiopathic ALTE the outcome is not predictable.
- The link between ALTE and SIDS is unclear.
- Most infants dying of SIDS have not had previous ALTE.
- In follow-up studies of infants with ALTE there is a small increased risk of sudden death (about 1%), which appears to be highest in infants with recurrent episodes requiring resuscitation.
- Survivors of idiopathic ALTE have normal neurodevelopmental performance at follow-up.
- Parents of infants with ALTE should be taught basic life support.

Role of monitoring

- Where a cause for the ALTE is found and treated, the problem has usually been addressed and home monitoring is not indicated.
- Where no cause has been found, the use of home monitoring remains controversial. The following points should be borne in mind.
  - Deaths have been reported despite the use of monitors.
  - Most monitors are simple movement detectors and will not detect obstructive events.
  - Monitors can cause heightened anxiety as a result of repeated false alarms.
  - Parents using monitors need regular follow-up and technical support.
- Where monitors are used, they need to combine respiratory and cardiac surveillance. Repeated false alarms will be detected for nearly all infants.

Cerebral palsy

Introduction

Cerebral palsy is a chronic non-progressive neurological disorder predominantly affecting motor function. Children with cerebral palsy frequently have respiratory problems.

It is important to remember that the aim of respiratory management is to improve the child's quality of life and that of his/her family. It is not to prolong suffering.

Aspiration pneumonia

Children with cerebral palsy are at increased risk of aspiration and LRTI as a consequence of:
- immobility;
- bulbar dysfunction;
- gastro-oesophageal reflux (GOR).

Clinical features
- The child may drool and may be unable to swallow saliva.
- There may be a frequent loose rattle from the back of the throat.
- The swallow may be unsafe (i.e. the child is likely to aspirate oral contents), particularly at times of URTI.
- GOR, indicated clinically by frequent effortless vomiting or finding milk in the mouth after feeds, increases the risk of significant aspiration events, particularly in children fed via gastrostomy.
- An aspiration event usually gives rise to an acute or acute on chronic cough, associated with fever and breathing difficulties (tachypnoea, chest wall retractions, with or without hypoxia).

Management
Treat the acute episode with oxygen, antibiotics, and chest physiotherapy as needed. Preventive management includes the following.
- Good positioning and regular chest physiotherapy to avoid problems of secretion retention related to immobility.
- Bulbar dysfunction can be difficult to manage. The swallow should be assessed by videofluoroscopy while the child is challenged with fluids or solids of different consistency. In some children the swallow is unsafe and gastrostomy feeding is needed. Hyoscine patches or glycopyrronium may be used to decrease oral secretions. In rare cases botulinum toxin injection of the salivary glands or surgical diversion of the salivary ducts may be needed to prevent recurrent aspiration.
- GOR is treated first by medical means but this may not be adequate and anti-reflux surgery is often required. Gastrostomy may make existing GORD worse and it is particularly important to consider anti-reflux surgery before a gastrostomy is inserted so that both procedures can be carried out under the same anaesthetic.
- Children with cerebral palsy are candidates for pneumococcal vaccination and annual flu vaccine. Children with recurrent chest infection may benefit from prophylactic antibiotic therapy once daily during the winter months. Second generation cephalosporins such as cefaclor have an appropriate spectrum of activity and are well tolerated.

Restrictive lung disease

This can be secondary to muscle weakness, to discoordinate muscle activity, or to the development of scoliosis (see 📖 Chapter 40).

Upper airway obstruction

Obstruction during wakefulness

Some children with cerebral palsy develop significant stridor and/or stertor. There are three main contributing factors:
- muscle spasm;
- muscle weakness;
- GOR.

GOR to laryngeal level results in irritation, oedema, and hypertrophy of aryepiglottic structures. Some children have poor laryngeal muscle tone and aryepiglottic folds that are sucked inwards on inspiration.

Management
- Effective control of GOR as a first step.
- An aryepiglottoplasty may be useful and may be combined with trimming of bulky aryepiglottic folds.
- Stridor related to spasm alone may be partly positional and may show some response to agents such as baclofen.

Obstruction during sleep

Upper airway obstruction, particularly during sleep, is common in cerebral palsy as one or more of the factors involved in airway patency are abnormal. Factors involved in airway patency are:
- anatomical size and resistance of upper airway;
- upper airway neuromuscular tone;
- effects of sleep state and arousal;
- central ventilatory responses to hypoxia, hypercapnia, and airway occlusion.

Assessment of upper airway obstruction
- Watch the child breathing.
- Is the obstruction positional?
- Monitor oxygen saturation overnight with chest and abdominal movement or airflow recordings (see 📖 Chapter 25).

Possible solutions to airway obstruction
- Positioning, including prone positioning or using a sleep system to hold the child in a comfortable position.
- Removal of tonsils and adenoids if they are thought to be contributing.
- Nasopharyngeal tube—to bypass the upper airway obstruction.
- Nasal CPAP.
- Tracheostomy.

Abnormal breathing during seizure activity

Seizures are common in children with cerebral palsy. Seizure activity can result in:

- disorganized breathing;
- obstructive apnoea;
- central apnoea;
- combination of above.

Seizure activity can result in oxygen desaturation, which can be profound. Polysomnography can be useful in investigating desaturation episodes where the cause is not clear.

Management

- Control of seizures.
- Oxygen therapy for episodes.
- Full resuscitation is rarely required.

Gastro-oesophageal reflux and aspiration lung disease

Overview

Gastro-oesophageal reflux (GOR) with or without aspiration and primary aspiration of material into the airway are relatively common mechanisms of lung disease in children (see box). Their presence should be actively sought in children who present with lung disease of unknown cause. Clinical decision-making is complicated because:

- lung disease may cause GOR, probably because of changes in intra-thoracic pressure consequent to less compliant lungs or increased airways resistance;
- GOR is common in asymptomatic children and may not be contributing to any lung disease that is present.

When there is doubt about the relative importance of GOR to respiratory symptoms a therapeutic trial of anti-reflux treatment can be useful.

Mechanisms of respiratory tract disease associated with GOR or aspiration

- Aspiration of material into upper trachea, especially acidic material, stimulates bronchospasm, coughing, and mucus secretion via irritant receptors in the trachea and upper airway. The aspirate remains in the trachea and is cleared by coughing and mucociliary clearance
- Aspiration of infected material from the sinuses or nasopharynx can result in tracheitis and bronchitis
- Recurrent aspiration of larger volumes can lead to aspirated material penetrating the lower airways, resulting in chronic airway irritation (bronchitis) and pneumonitis. This can progress to interstitial fibrosis and fixed airways obstruction (a combination restrictive and obstructive defect). These children may develop an absent or blunted cough reflex, so-called silent aspiration. Infants and neurologically impaired children may silently aspirate from the beginning
- Acid in the distal oesophagus may be able to trigger neurally mediated reflex bronchospasm. The evidence for this phenomenon is conflicting
- Small amounts of liquid reaching the top of the larynx can induce laryngospasm—this is most common in young infants. The liquid may be a milk feed or refluxed gastric contents
- In neonates and preterm infants, small amounts of liquid at the top of the larynx can stimulate laryngeal receptors and result in reflex central apnoea and bradycardia

Definitions

Gastro-oesophageal reflux

- GOR refers to the retrograde movement of gastric contents into the oesophagus towards the oropharynx.
- GOR is very common in infants under 6 months and, for most, other than frequent small volume vomits (possetting) there are no noticeable consequences. The predilection of infants to reflux is thought to arise from their posture (often lying flat, especially after feeding), and the immaturity of the gastro-oesophageal junction.
- These features improve with time and, in the vast majority, GOR is a self-limiting condition and resolves in the second year of life.
- Predisposing factors for GOR include:
  - respiratory distress (more negative intrathoracic pressure);
  - coughing (increased abdominal pressure);
  - feeding via gastrostomy or NG tube;
  - hiatus hernia;
  - oesophageal dysmotility, e.g. previous tracheo-oesophageal fistula.

Aspiration

- Aspiration can be divided into 2 types:
  - primary aspiration: via the larynx or more rarely directly into the trachea via an H-type tracheo-oesophageal fistula or laryngeal cleft;
  - aspiration following GOR.
- Normal infants and children aspirate small amounts of saliva and mucus, mostly during sleep. These small volumes are rapidly cleared by mucociliary mechanisms and usually do not cause symptoms.
- Normal infants can also aspirate milk during feeds when stressed or tired. This either occurs in the context of a respiratory illness with tachypnoea or as a consequence of fatigue, usually caused by some other intercurrent illness. These events are usually obvious with immediate symptoms of coughing and choking, with or without apnoea.
- Normal children can also aspirate small amounts of acidic material, consequent to GOR, or small amounts of infected material from the nasopharynx. Aspiration of either of these substances will often cause symptoms, but will not usually cause severe aspiration pneumonitis.
- Aspiration associated with GOR is more likely when there is oesophageal dysfunction (e.g. after tracheo-oesophageal fistula repair). Normally, when acid refluxes into the oesophagus, swallowing and peristalsis of the oesophagus are triggered and this rapidly clears the acid. When these protective mechanisms are defective, aspiration is more likely.
- Aspiration of larger volumes, sufficient to penetrate the lower airways and cause chronic pneumonitis, usually requires additional abnormalities to be present. These are listed in the box. Normal infants can also aspirate sufficient material to cause aspiration pneumonia, probably because of immature swallowing reflexes.

- Children with neurological impairment and some normal infants may have no immediate symptoms (coughing or choking) associated with the aspiration event. This is sometimes called silent aspiration and these children may first be referred to a respiratory specialist with symptoms of the resulting lung disease. It is therefore important to actively consider and investigate the possibility of aspiration in children with unexplained wheeze and/or pneumonia.

Conditions predisposing to large volume aspiration

- Structural abnormalities:
  - cleft palate
  - H-type tracheo-oesphageal fistula
  - laryngeal cleft
  - choanal stenosis
  - craniofacial disorders with upper airway obstruction
- Abnormal coordination or weakness of pharyngeal and or laryngeal muscles:
  - cerebral palsy
  - vocal cord palsy
  - neuromuscular weakness, e.g. SMA, myotonic dystrophy
  - bulbar palsy, including Mobius syndrome
- Loss of protective reflexes:
  - cerebral palsy
  - any cause of decreased level of consciousness, including sedation
  - some syndromes (e.g. Cornelia de Lange)
- Artificial airway:
  - endotracheal tube
  - tracheostomy

Notes

Cleft palate often causes reflux of milk into the nasopharynx where it is more likely to be aspirated in the feeding infant. Feeding any infant with upper airways obstruction increases the risk of aspiration. Children with cerebral palsy are amongst those with the highest risk for aspiration lung disease. They may have a blunted cough reflex, disordered swallowing, and loss of protective laryngeal reflexes

Symptoms

Symptoms suggestive of GOR

- Abdominal or retrosternal pain.
- Irritability in infants, which may lead to abnormal posturing, such as back-arching.
- Gagging after feeding in infants, especially if preceded by cough.
- Refusal to feed.
- Vomiting.
- Waterbrash (foul-tasting material brought up to the mouth).
- Dysphagia.

Symptoms suggestive of primary aspiration

- There may be immediate coughing and choking.
- In young infants there may be signs of distress, with body extension and eye widening during feeding.
- In some infants and children aspiration may occur without any obvious signs at the time of aspiration.

Respiratory symptoms

Caused by micro-aspiration or reflex responses
- Cough: sometimes associated with feeding. Cough may be dry or productive. Presence of a productive-sounding cough may have led to the diagnosis of recurrent chest infections. The cough may also be nocturnal, possibly because of reflux occurring whilst child is lying flat.
- Wheeze. This may occur without coughing, and may coexist with wheeze caused by asthma.
- In young infants, especially those born prematurely, there may be:
  - obstructive apnoea;
  - reflex central apnoea and bradycardia;
  - apparent life-threatening episodes.

Caused by larger volume aspiration Recurrent episodes of respiratory distress with CXR changes and requirement for oxygen therapy. There may be no symptoms of coughing or choking to suggest aspiration as the cause.

Caused by aspirating small amounts of infected secretions
- Chronic nasal discharge.
- Night-time productive-sounding cough, sometimes associated with post-tussive vomiting. The symptoms usually occur at night when the child lies flat. The infected secretions from the nasopharynx pool at the back of the throat stimulating cough. This is a problem mainly in the under 6-year-olds who cannot yet effectively clear their nasal secretions by blowing their nose.

Investigations

To demonstrate GOR

- Contrast swallow may show gross reflux, but its main purpose is to demonstrate normal structure and position of oesophagus and stomach and to exclude hiatus hernia.
- 24h pH monitoring. The pH probe is positioned in the lower oesophagus. Total time with pH < 4 exceeding 8% is usually taken to indicate significant acid reflux. Anything reducing gastric acidity, e.g. proton pump inhibitors, H_2-receptor antagonists, or antacids, should be stopped prior to the study. Studies on children being given milk-containing feeds may miss reflux episodes. To increase the sensitivity of the test, the milk can be acidified or additional feeds with acidic liquids, such as apple juice, can be given.
- pH monitoring can be combined with multichannel oesophageal impedance measurements. This technique measures electrical activity in the oesophagus and can distinguish between air and solid or liquid boluses. By having multiple sensors it can quantify the level of reflux. It has the advantage of being sensitive to non-acid reflux. It is only available in specialist centres and interpretation of the data is not standardized.
- Gastric scintigraphy. The child is given a feed containing a radiolabel and then monitored continuously using a scintillation camera for 1–2h. A column of increased activity re-appearing above the diaphragm indicates reflux.
- Oesophagoscopy may show oesophagitis, consistent with GOR.

To demonstrate aspiration

There are no gold-standard tests for aspiration and the diagnosis of aspiration lung disease requires a combination of factors—likely symptoms and signs as well as suggestive findings on investigation.
- CXR changes are non-specific (Fig. 30.1).
  - Air-trapping and hyperinflation.
  - Bronchial wall thickening.
  - Patchy atelectasis and streaky consolidation—in ambulant children with significant aspiration, CXR changes may be more severe in the lower, dependent lobes.
  - CXR may be normal in children with micro-aspiration.
- Gastric scintigraphy may show activity appearing in the peripheries of the lung after an oral feed, but the signal is often close to background making interpretation difficult.
- Radionuclide salivagrams use small amounts of radioactivity placed in the mouth. A series of images is then collected until the tracer has left the mouth. Presence of tracer in the trachea indicates aspiration. The test is simple and uses very small doses of radioactivity. There have been no studies to evaluate the diagnostic accuracy of this test.
- Videofluoroscopy is a useful method of demonstrating swallowing abnormalities and will show aspiration of contrast material into the trachea (Fig. 30.1).

- Fibreoptic-endoscopic evaluation of swallowing (FEES). This can be carried out by skilled operators in children of any age without sedation. A small flexible endoscope is passed through the nose and positioned between the soft palate and epiglottis. The image can be shown on a monitor and the ability of the child to swallow foods of different textures can be observed by a multidisciplinary team including speech and language therapists.

- Prone oesophagram can show an H-type fistula. In infants with respiratory distress, this investigation may precipitate an episode of reflux and apnoea. Personnel experienced in paediatric resuscitation should be present in the radiology department during this investigation. It should be noted that a simple contrast swallow does not exclude an H-type fistula.

- Bronchoscopy may show reddened mucosa around the larynx in patients with GOR. It may also show evidence of tracheal and bronchial irritation. Bronchoalveolar lavage may show the presence of inflammatory cells and lipid-laden macrophages. The cells can be stained for fat (using oil red-o) and the amount of intracellular lipid in alveolar macrophages assessed semi-quantitatively to give a lipid-laden macrophage index. Macrophages scavenge lipid from any source, including the membranes of cells shed into the lumen. The lipid-laden macrophage index, even when quantified, has a high false positive rate in children with other respiratory disease. A low score indicates that gross aspiration is not occurring, but does not exclude microaspiration.

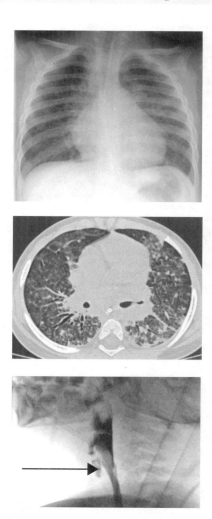

Fig. 30.1 CXR, CT scan, and videofluoroscopy of a 14-month-old girl who developed progressive respiratory distress over a 3-month period. The CXR shows bilateral streaky changes. The CT scan shows extensive airspace disease and bronchiectasis. The video swallow shows free aspiration into the trachea (black arrow), which did not cause coughing. This girl had also developed brisk tendon reflexes and a mild facial nerve palsy and was subsequently shown to have a brainstem glioma.

- There are some data to suggest that BAL levels of salivary amylase and gastric pepsin may help to identify primary aspiration and aspiration after GOR, respectively. These tests require further evaluation before their clinical usefulness is established.
- In children with tracheostomies or endotracheal tubes it may be possible to demonstrate GOR and aspiration by using dye (e.g. methylene blue) added to feeds and later identifying it in tracheal aspirates.

It is often impossible to demonstrate with certainty that aspiration is taking place, or that there is a direct link between demonstrated GOR and respiratory symptoms. Sometimes the history given, and the context of the history, e.g. a child with severe cerebral palsy, is highly suggestive of aspiration lung disease and the investigations, whilst not definitive, are consistent with diagnosis. In other children, e.g. those with poorly controlled asthma and symptoms of GOR, it may be appropriate to start a trial of antacid and anti-reflux treatment rather than pursue investigations that may be unhelpful.

Treatment and outcome

Treatment

Gastro-oesophageal reflux

- Feed thickeners may help symptoms associated with mild GOR, e.g. in infants who have had brief episodes of choking or apnoea. Smaller more frequent feeds can also reduce GOR. In severe cases, continuous nasogastric feeds can allow growth.
- Antacids, H_2 antagonists, and proton pump inhibitors will reduce symptoms mediated by gastric acid. If omeprazole is used it may need to be given twice daily to provide control over a 24h period.
- Agents to increase gastric emptying and lower oesophageal tone, such as metoclopramide or domperidone, are often also tried. Domperidone is usually preferred in children as it has fewer CNS side-effects.
- If medical therapy is ineffective, and there is good evidence that GOR is responsible for, or contributing to, the respiratory symptoms, then surgical correction should be considered. This is usually a Nissen or Thal fundoplication, now both commonly performed laproscopically.

Aspiration

- The most important priority is to identify the cause. If there is structural abnormality, this should be repaired where possible. If there is GOR, this should be treated. If the child has chronic sinusitis, a long course of antibiotics may be helpful. Teaching the child to effectively blow their nose will also help where this is possible.
- In cases where there is no useful intervention, the aim will then be to reduce the amount and nature of the aspirated material. Videofluoro-scopy can confirm that oral feeds are being aspirated. Speech and language therapists may be able to improve the effectiveness of swallowing and reduce any tendency to aspirate. Stopping oral feeds may lead to an improvement in symptoms.
- Aspiration of oral secretions, even in the absence of food, can cause symptoms. This is particularly true in children with problems swallowing, and in whom oral secretions tend to pool in the back of the throat. These children may be helped by the following.
  - Positioning the head so that secretions can drain out of the mouth.
  - Reducing the volume of secretions with hyoscine, scopolamine, or glycopyrollate. Hyoscine and scopolamine are available as patches. In some children these medications make their secretions thicker with mucus plugging, areas of atelectasis, and worsening of symptoms. There is also a risk of constipation and urinary retention.
- When oral secretions are thought to be a major contributor, e.g. in a child with persistent significant respiratory problems despite gastro-stomy and fundoplication, reduction in the volume of saliva can be achieved either by:
  - salivary ablation—this involves surgical removal of the submandibular glands and parotid duct ligation. This does not appear to have a significant impact on digestion (the pancreas produces lots of amylase); or

- injections of botulinum toxin. Ultrasound is needed to guide the injections—sometimes the glands cannot be clearly identified making injection impossible. Care must be taken not to leave the child with a dry mouth.
- Some children with recurrent aspiration, particularly if it leads to episodes of respiratory failure and chronic lung disease, may be managed with a tracheostomy. The tracheostomy will not reduce the likelihood of aspiration; it may actually make it worse. It does have the advantage of allowing suction of the trachea to remove aspirated material and provides a safe airway. Use of cuffed tubes may help if the material above the cuff can be effectively suctioned before the cuff deflated.
- If aspiration is intractable and causing severe respiratory distress, e.g. with multiple admissions to ICUs, more radical surgical options should be considered. Supraglottic laryngeal closure, leaving a small opening for phonation (but not enough for breathing) combined with a tracheostomy, can reduce aspiration. However, in 50% the closure breaks down and aspiration recurs. Laryngotracheal separation forming a blind-ending upper trachea and an end tracheostomy is more successful. Several centres have reported their experience, and nearly all children have immediate symptomatic improvement. The procedure deprives the child of speech and should not be undertaken without wide consultation. In a small number, the procedure has been successfully reversed with a return to normal phonation and laryngeal function.

Outcome

Aspiration is often unrecognized or misdiagnosed. Untreated, chronic aspiration may result in recurrent and intractable pneumonitis and bronchiectasis. As a consequence the child may fail to thrive and have frequent and prolonged admissions to hospital. There may be permanent loss of lung function. It is important to have a high index of suspicion for aspiration and GOR in all children with chronic lung disease and to have a low threshold to investigate. Aggressive treatment can prevent much of the morbidity.

Further information

Boesch, R.P., Daines, C., Willging, J.P., Kaul, A., Cohen, A.P., Wood, R.E., and Amin, R.S. (2006). Advances in the diagnosis and management of chronic pulmonary aspiration in children. *Eur. Respir. J.* **4**, 847–51.

Foreign body aspiration

Epidemiology

- Foreign body aspiration is a significant cause of morbidity and mortality in childhood and accounts for 5–10% of lethal accidents in the 1–3 year olds.
- Incidence is around 1/15 000 children per year,
- Mobile toddlers between 18 months and 3 years are most at risk, but foreign body aspiration has been reported in infants as young as 6 weeks of age,
- Older children can also aspirate objects but are more likely to give a clear history of the event.
- Younger children tend to aspirate foodstuffs—especially nuts, seeds, and pieces of vegetable.
- Older children are more likely to aspirate non-organic objects such as small pieces of plastic (pen tops, bits of toys).
- Objects small enough to get through the vocal cords are usually small enough to fit within the main bronchi. 65% of inhaled foreign bodies will lodge in the right main bronchus and 35% in the left main bronchus.

History

- A clear history of a choking event is given by most families. The child will usually have violent coughing for several minutes to hours afterwards. The cough often then becomes less impressive and more intermittent. Wheeze may be reported.
- It is important to get a detailed account of what might have been aspirated, e.g. if a piece of carrot, what size were the pieces and how well were they cooked, i.e. were they mushy or al dente?
- A clear history of choking should always be investigated, even if the child has apparently recovered.
- In around 15% of cases, no clear history of choking is obtained. These children present with recurrent or persistent coughs with or without wheeze or fever. Focal changes are usually seen on CXR.
- Rarely, children may be referred with 'atypical asthma' or chronic productive cough.

Examination

- Most children will not have any evidence of respiratory distress.
- There may be unequal chest expansion or unequal breath sounds.
- There may be monophonic expiratory wheeze.
- Examination may be normal.

Investigation

- CXR will be abnormal in 80% and may show the following.
  - Hyperinflation of the affected side. This is most effectively shown by comparing inspiratory and expiratory films. If the child is too young to cooperate with inspiratory and expiratory manoeuvres, they can be placed on the side with the suspected abnormal side dependent. CXR taken in this position should normally show some reduction in lung volume of the dependent side. If this fails to occur it implies air-trapping consistent with a foreign body.

- Collapse/consolidation (Fig. 31.1). This may be relatively subtle. It may be missed, particularly in the left lower lobe behind the heart.
- A radio-opaque foreign body (only in 10% of cases).
- A normal CXR does not exclude aspirated foreign body.
- Bronchoscopy is the definitive investigation.
  - Where the presence of a foreign body is very likely, rigid bronchoscopy is the examination of choice, since the object may be removed using optical forceps.
  - When there is more uncertainty, flexible bronchoscopy can allow an easier and more detailed inspection of the lower airways. The small instrument channel on flexible bronchoscopes makes them unsuitable for removing foreign bodies in most circumstances.

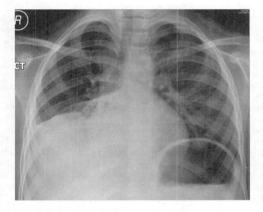

Fig. 31.1 CXR of a 6-year-old girl who gave a 7-week history of recurrent cough and fever that had persisted despite 2 courses of antibiotics. The CXR shows collapse and consolidation of the right middle and lower lobes. Only after direct questioning did the family give an account of an episode 8 weeks earlier when a pen top had disappeared from the child's mouth with an inspiratory gasp. Although she coughed and choked for a minute or so, the incident was soon forgotten. At bronchoscopy the pen top was found tightly wedged in the right main bronchus, just below the origin of the right middle lobe. After removal large volumes of foul-smelling pus were aspirated from the lower airways.

Management

- Prevention is the most effective management. Parents must be warned not to give nuts to young children. The increase in food allergy, particularly to nuts, has helped to get this message across.
- A high index of suspicion is needed to prevent delay in diagnosis. Aspirated foreign body should be considered in all children with persistent or unusual respiratory symptoms.
- If there is a clear history of a choking episode and the possibility that a discrete foreign body has been aspirated, bronchoscopy should be performed even if examination and CXR are normal.
- If the episode of choking involved liquids or very soft solids (such as pureed food) and the child has made a full recovery, no immediate action is necessary. These children can be reviewed after 5–7 days. If no symptoms have developed and examination remains normal, the likelihood of aspiration is remote.
- Where the history of choking is not as clear and both examination and CXR are normal, review after 7 days can also be helpful. If a repeat CXR remains normal, without symptoms and in the presence of a normal examination, aspiration is very unlikely.
- If in doubt, do the bronchoscopy.
- Flexible bronchoscopy can be carried out under sedation. Although the flexible bronchoscope can be used to remove foreign objects (using a device such as a Dormier basket) it is not safe to do so in a sedated child when there will be less than complete control of the airway.
- Where a foreign body that is wedged tightly into an airway has been in place for a number of weeks there may be a significant volume of pus distal to the obstruction. When the foreign body is removed, suction should be immediately available to deal with the pus.
- Nuts often elicit a rapid and marked inflammatory reaction. It is much easier to take them out before this has become established. Broncho-scopic removal should take place as soon as possible.

Outcome

- Delay in diagnosis is associated with significant morbidity, often recurrent pneumonia and bronchiectasis.
- After removal, some symptoms may persist in up to 30%, usually a combination of cough and wheeze. The symptoms may respond to inhaled bronchodilators and inhaled steroids.
- 30–50% of children will have either abnormal CXRs or abnormal ventilation perfusion scans 5 years after removal of the foreign body. Aspiration of nut fragments in particular can cause long-term problems. These fragments cannot be retrieved by bronchoscopy and may predispose to recurrent infection in the distal lung segments. Great care must be taken not to crush nut fragments during removal at rigid bronchoscopy.

- Persistence of symptoms and radiological abnormality is most likely:
  - in children who aspirated organic material—presumably because of the associated granuloma formation;
  - where the diagnosis was delayed;
  - where the foreign body was in the left main bronchus.
- If a CT scan is performed shortly before or after removal of a long-standing airway foreign body, bronchiectasis may be seen. Once the foreign body is removed, the bronchiectasis may resolve.
- Outpatient follow-up of all children who have aspirated foreign bodies should be arranged.

Further information

Karakoc, F., Karadag, B., Akbenlioglu, C., Ersu, R., Yildizeli, B., Yuksel, M., and Dagli, E. (2002). Foreign body aspiration: what is the outcome? *Pediatr. Pulmonol.* **34**, 30–6.

Mansour, Y., Beck, R., Danino, J., and Bentur, L. (1998). Resolution of severe bronchiectasis after removal of long-standing retained foreign body. *Pediatr. Pulmonol.* **25**, 130–2.

Inhalational lung disease

Overview

- Inhalational lung disease refers to damage to the lungs and airways through direct contact from toxic substances.
- Accidental ingestion of toxic domestic chemicals is common in childhood. The lungs may be exposed through aspiration of gastric contents after accidental ingestion, or directly by inhalation of fumes from volatile chemicals, e.g. petrol, petroleum products, and some concentrated bleaches.
- Smoke inhalation from fires involves both thermal and chemical damage to the airway.
- The possibility of CO poisoning should be considered in all cases of inhalational lung disease.

Presentation

The pattern of damage is common to many toxic substances and includes:
- tracheobronchitis;
- pulmonary oedema;
- mucosal oedema, sloughing of mucosa and airway debris leading to airway obstruction.

General principles of management

- Supportive care is the mainstay of treatment.
- Humidified oxygen to maintain oxygen saturations.
- Deliver 100% oxygen via reservoir mask if CO poisoning suspected.
- Respiratory failure may occur many hours after exposure and CXR may appear normal in early stages.
- Mechanical ventilation may be necessary in children with:
  - severe burns to the face or mouth because of the risk of airway oedema;
  - stridor and laryngeal oedema;
  - difficulty handling secretions;
  - respiratory failure;
  - altered mental status.
- Tracheostomy may be necessary in cases of severe upper airway oedema and mucosal sloughing.
- Extracorporeal membrane oxygenation (ECMO) may be needed if conventional ventilation fails.
- Bronchodilators may be useful for reflex bronchoconstriction.
- IV antibiotics are used to cover secondary bacterial infection.
- Careful fluid replacement to prevent pulmonary oedema.
- Corticosteroids show no documented benefit.

Specific substances

Household bleach (sodium hypochlorite)

- Commercial bleach products contain 5–10% sodium hypochlorite. Sodium hypochlorite itself is corrosive at concentrations > 10% but intoxication from inhalation is very rare as volatile gases are not released under normal conditions.
- When mixed with acid, sodium hypochlorite produces chlorine and, when mixed with ammonia-based products, it releases chloramines. Both products are highly irritant gases.
- Burning of the eyes, nose, throat, and lungs with chest tightness, coughing, wheezing, and dyspnoea may occur, but such a reaction is unusual with bleach at household concentrations.
- Very rarely, pneumonitis, airway oedema, and ARDS may occur.
- Reactive airways dysfunction syndrome (RADS), a chemical irritant-induced type of asthma, has been described after repeated exposures.
- Ingestion of sodium hypochlorite at household bleach concentration does not usually cause significant ulceration but large volumes or concentrated products may cause a corrosive oesophagitis.
- Aspiration of sodium hypochlorite together with gastric contents is more likely to cause severe disease and ARDS.

Highly volatile hydrocarbons

- Highly volatile liquids such as petrol, paraffin (or kerosene), naphthalene lighter fluid, and mineral spirits are more easily aspirated because of their low viscosity and low surface tension.
- Low surface tension also results in more widespread deposition within the tracheobronchial tree.
- Solvent hydrocarbons are directly destructive, causing desquamation, accumulation of airway fluid, and airway obstruction. Interstitial exposure causes an intense inflammatory reaction.
- Pulmonary oedema, haemoptysis, and respiratory failure may develop quickly.
- CXR may show pneumonitis, atelectasis, or air trapping, with the development of pneumatoceles in the recovery phase.
- Long-term follow-up of patients with hydrocarbon pneumonitis shows persistent obstructive lung disease in the majority.

Lipid-containing liquids

- Aspiration of lipid-containing liquids, such as polyethylene glycol or aromatic oils, often results in a combination of airway obstruction and intense inflammatory pneumonitis with progressive deterioration.
- Treatment is supportive. Flexible bronchoscopy and BAL have been advocated to clear the aspirated liquid from the airways. Corticosteroid therapy may be beneficial.

Smoke inhalation

- The pulmonary manifestations of smoke inhalation account for much of the mortality and morbidity seen in accidental fires.
- Thermal damage, which accounts for the majority of smoke injury, is primarily seen in the supraglottic airway and rarely below the carina. Exposure to steam causes more extensive thermal injury.
- Chemical injury is produced by the many noxious gases that are released.
  - Sulphur dioxide and nitrous oxide are corrosive acidic gases.
  - Acetaldehydes induce protein denaturation and pulmonary oedema.
  - Chlorine and hydrochloric acid are generated from burning PVC, hydrocarbons from polyethylene, and hydrogen cyanide from polyurethrane.
  - Wood generates high levels of CO.
  - Soot itself is benign but acts to carry noxious chemicals into the lungs and may induce bronchoconstriction.
- In fire survivors, suspect smoke injury to the airway if there is evidence of peri-oral burns, black or speckled sputum, respiratory distress, altered voice, or stridor.
- CO levels should be checked immediately.

Carbon monoxide poisoning

- CO is a product of incomplete combustion.
- Accidental poisoning is mainly due to faulty heating systems in the home and is more common in the winter.
- CO is a colourless, odourless, non-irritant gas. Exposure is usually occult.
- Non-accidental exposure is mainly from car exhaust fumes. It is an uncommon mode of suicide or attempted suicide in children and adolescents.

Pathophysiology

- CO combines with haemoglobin (Hb) in the blood to form carboxyhaemoglobin (COHb).
- The affinity of Hb for CO is 240 times its affinity for oxygen. A small amount of CO can therefore occupy a large amount of Hb, making it unavailable for oxygen transport. In this situation, Hb concentration and PaO_2 are normal, but there may be profound hypoxia.
- Pulse oximetry may show normal saturations as COHb and oxyHb have comparable absorption spectra.
- CO also alters the oxygen binding properties of Hb, by shifting the oxygen dissociation curve left. This reduces the capacity for oxygen release in the tissues and increases tissue hypoxia.
- CO dissolved in the plasma may react with other haem proteins such myoglobin or mitochondrial cytochromes, thereby disrupting metabolism.

Clinical features
- Clinical features depend on the COHb level.
  - Up to 20% COHb: headaches and nausea.
  - 20–40% COHb: fatigue and confusion.
  - > 40% COHb: ataxia, collapse, and coma; cardiac arrhythmias, cerebral oedema, acidosis.
- Classic healthy look with 'cherry red' lips and nail-beds is unusual.
- Suspect CO poisoning if other family members have similar symptoms.
- Suspect in fire survivors. Manage airway for smoke inhalation and treat associated injuries. Consider cyanide poisoning as CO levels correlate with cyanide levels in this group.

Investigations
- Pulse oximetry and arterial PaO_2 may be normal even if hypoxic.
- COHb levels can be measured using a CO-Oximeter. *or*
- Breath CO can be measured in end tidal expired air.

Management
- Oxygen displaces CO when administered at high concentrations.
- The half-life of COHb is 6h when breathing air. This is reduced to 1h when breathing 100% oxygen.
- To administer 100% oxygen, a reservoir mask with oxygen at flow rates exceeding the child's minute volume is necessary. Intubation and ventilation may be necessary in older children and adolescents.
- Hyperbaric oxygen given at 2–3 atm reduces the COHb half-life to 20min thereby accelerating removal of CO. Risks of treatment include oxygen toxicity and the need for tympanotomy. Long-term cognitive deficit is reduced in adults given hyperbaric oxygen for acute CO poisoning. No data exist for children and the use of hyperbaric oxygen remains controversial.

Non-cystic fibrosis bronchiectasis

Introduction

Bronchiectasis is defined as dilatation of the airway accompanied by inflammatory destruction of the bronchial and peribronchial tissue. It was previously thought to be irreversible but there is now clear evidence that early bronchiectasis in children can resolve. The pathogenesis is thought to be bronchial obstruction with retention of secretions and infection.

Prevalence

There have been a number of recent attempts at estimating prevalence.
- Northeast England: 172/million children aged < 15 years.
- New Zealand: 335/million children aged < 15 years
- Aboriginal population of Alice Springs, Australia: 10 000/million.

Aetiology

Careful investigation can reveal an underlying aetiology in 60–70% of cases. In most populations, post-infectious cause is most common followed by immunodeficiency. See box.

Aetiology of non-CF bronchiectasis

Post-infectious

Any severe LRTI can lead to bronchiectasis. In children the following are the most likely causative organisms

- *Streptococcus pneumoniae, Staphylococcus aureus*
- Adenovirus
- Measles virus
- Influenza virus
- *Bordetella pertussis*
- *Mycobacterium tuberculosis*

Immunodeficiency

Particularly the following

- Antibody defects:
  - agammaglobulinaemia
  - common variable immune deficiency
  - IgA and IgG subclass deficiency
- Following chemotherapy
- Acquired secondary to HIV infection
- Ataxia telangiectasia

Primary ciliary dyskinesia

Post-obstructive

- Foreign body aspiration
- Bronchial compression, e.g. by lymph nodes or tumour

Chronic aspiration

Congenital abnormality of the airways

- Williams–Campbell syndrome (congenital cartilage deficiency)
- Mounier–Kuhn syndrome (tracheo-bronchomegaly)

Syndromic

- Yellow-nail syndrome (abnormal nails, lymphoedema, bronchial infection, pleural effusion)
- Young syndrome (azoospermia and sinobronchial infection)

Allergic bronchopulmonary aspergillosis

Associated with bronchiolitis obliterans

- Post-infectious
- Following lung transplantation

Traction bronchiectasis associated with pulmonary fibrosis

Clinical features

The presenting clinical feature is chronic productive cough with or without:
- purulent sputum (young children rarely expectorate);
- chest pain during exacerbation;
- wheezing;
- breathlessnes on exertion;
- haemoptysis.

Physical examination may be normal or may reveal:
- clubbing;
- inspiratory crepitations.

A chronic productive-sounding cough that persists or recurs after initial treatment with physiotherapy and antibiotics warrants further investigation (see 📖 Chapter 4).

Investigations and diagnosis

Imaging

- CXR. May show evidence of bronchial wall thickening or airway dilatation and/or areas of volume loss. However, it may be normal.
- HRCT. Required for diagnosis. Features of bronchiectasis are:
  - bronchial wall thickening;
  - internal diameter of bronchus cut in cross-section being larger than accompanying artery (the signet ring sign);
  - poorly tapering bronchi as move to periphery of the lung;
  - bronchi clearly seen near periphery of lung.
- Bronchiectasis occurs in lower lobes > middle lobe > upper lobes.
- Bilateral upper lobe bronchiectasis is more common in CF than other causes of bronchiectasis. Unilateral upper lobe bronchiectais can be seen after TB. Focal bronchiectasis, particularly of the lower lobes, makes foreign body more likely. Multiple lobe involvement can be seen after viral pneumonia, aspiration (particularly bilateral lower lobe disease), or associated with a systemic disorder such as immune deficiency or primary ciliary dyskinesia.

Bronchoscopy

Bronchoscopy is not always required, e.g. in children with known immuno-deficiency or primary ciliary dyskinesia, bronchoscopy will add little (unless samples are needed for microscopy or culture).

Thresholds for carrying out bronchoscopy vary in different centres. We suggest that bronchoscopy should be carried out:
- when there is focal bronchiectasis (to exclude airway narrowing);
- when the HRCT suggests the possibility of airway abnormality;
- to assist the investigation of possible aspiration lung disease.

Other investigations looking for aetiology

- Sweat test—always worth repeating.
- FBC for lymphocyte and neutrophil counts.
- Immunoglobulin levels including IgE and IgG subclasses. Low levels of subclasses of IgG are especially important if IgA levels are also low (see 📖 Chapter 35).

- Specific antibody levels to vaccinations and response to booster doses if initial response is poor.
- Ciliary brush biopsy of nose or trachea (if bronchoscopy performed).
- Contrast swallow and pH study (evidence of GOR makes aspiration more likely).
- Videofluoroscopy if aspiration is suspected.
- HIV test if high risk or other evidence of immunodeficiency.

Microbiology
Airway culture may suggest aetiology, e.g. the presence of *Pseudomonas* species makes CF likely. Close attention to airway infection is an essential part of the management of bronchiectasis to limit any progressive damage. Samples can be obtained by:
- sputum including induced sputum;
- cough swab;
- BAL.

Lung function testing
Many children with mild bronchiectasis will have normal lung function. In more severe disease, airways obstruction and a degree of restriction can occur.

Management
The aim of treatment is to clear secretions from the dilated bronchial tree and prevent further infection thus halting disease progression and, in early cases, providing an environment for healing. Apart from replacement immunoglobulin in children with antibody deficiency, treatment is supportive.

Physiotherapy
There are no trials of physiotherapy in this condition but plenty of anecdotal evidence that it is beneficial.

Antibiotics
The most commonly found organisms are:
- non-encapsulated *Haemophilus influenzae*;
- *Streptococcus pneumoniae*;
- *Moraxella catarrhalis*.

Some children respond to antibiotics such as amoxicillin given only at times of exacerbation and, between exacerbations, produce only small amounts of clear secretions. Other children benefit from a continuous antibiotic such as cefixime.

Infection with *Pseudomonas aeruginosa* does sometimes occur in children with non-CF bronchiectasis and both treatment and eradication regimes similar to that used in CF have been used, although there is no evidence whether they are beneficial or not. In a trial in adults with non-CF bronchiectasis the addition of regular nebulized antibiotics did not affect clinical outcome.

Other agents
- DNase was not helpful in adult trials of non-CF bronchiectasis,[1] and probably isn't helpful in children with this condition.
- Bronchodilators may be helpful in children where wheeze is a prominent feature.
- Two recent studies of inhaled steroids in adults with bronchiectasis have shown a decrease in 24 hour sputum volume, exacerbation frequency and dyspnoea and an improvement in quality of life scores.[2,3]
- Azithromycin. Pilot and non-controlled studies have suggested that the regular use of azithromycin decreases exacerbations in adults.

Surgery
Surgery is an option for localized bronchiectasis if:
- there are significant symptoms not responding to medical treatment;
- there is resectable disease causing persistent focal infection;
- there is life-threatening haemoptysis.

Outcome
Children with bronchiectasis should be followed regularly in the outpatient clinic with monitoring of their symptoms, growth, and lung function. It can be helpful to repeat the HRCT to determine if there is disease progression or improvement.

The long-term outcome is dependent on the underlying condition. In most cases treatment should halt progression. There are well recorded cases of improvement and reversal of bronchiectasis in children.

Further information

Fall, A. and Spencer, D. (2006). Paediatric bronchiectasis in Europe: what now and where next? *Paediatr. Respir. Rev.* **7**, 268–74.

Gaillard, E.A., Carty, H., Heaf, D., and Smyth, R.L. (2003). Reversible bronchial dilatation in children: comparison of serial high-resolution computer tomography scans of the lungs. *Eur. J. Radiol.* **47** (3), 215–20.

1 O'Donnell, A.E., Barker, A.F., Ilowite, J.S., and Fick, R.B. (1998). Treatment of idiopathic bronchiectasis with aerosolized recombinant human DNase I. rhDNase Study Group. *Chest* **113**, 1329–34.

2 Martinez-Garcia, M.A., Perpina-Tordera, M., Roman-Sanchez, P., and Soler-Cataluna, J.J. (2006). Inhaled steroids improve quality of life in patients with steady-state bronchiectasis. *Respir. Med.* **100**, 1623–32.

3 Tsang, K.W., Tan, K.C., Ho, P.L., Ooi, G.C., Ho, J.C., Mak, J., Tipoe, G.L., Ko, C., Yan, C., Lam, W.K., and Chan-Yeung, M. (2005). Inhaled fluticasone in bronchiectasis: a 12 month study. *Thorax* **60**, 239–43.

Primary ciliary dyskinesia

Background and epidemiology

Cilia are fine tubular structures present on the apical surface of epithelial cells of several tissues (see Fig. 34.1). Each cilium contains a core of microtubules that allows it to flex actively. Ciliary activity on epithelial surfaces is coordinated to allow propulsion of overlying fluid. The normal ciliary beat frequency is > 11 beats/second.

- In the airway ciliary activity propels surface mucus towards the larynx and provides one of the major methods by which the lung clears inhaled particles and pathogens. Ciliary activity also appears to be one mechanism by which fetal lung liquid is cleared immediately after birth.
- In the Eustachian tube ciliary activity is an important mechanism keeping the middle ear clear of fluid.
- In the Fallopian tubes, ciliary activity assists the passage of the oocyte towards the uterus.
- In the developing embryo, ciliary activity controls the movement of fluid that is critical in determining laterality. In the absence of ciliary activity, laterality is random.
- In the spermatozoa, a specialized cilium is used for propulsion.
- There are also cilia lining the ventricles of the brain where they may be important in directing the flow of CSF, although loss of function does not seem to result in disease. In the fetus there may be mild ventriculomegaly, which can be a clue when primary ciliary dyskinesia is suspected in a fetus with situs inversus.

Primary ciliary dyskinesia (PCD) is a condition in which the efficient action of cilia is diminished or absent. PCD is caused by genetic defects of ciliary proteins, usually with autosomal recessive inheritance. It has been detected in all major ethnic groups worldwide. Over 250 different genes are involved in ciliary assembly and function. In most families the gene defect has not been identified. PCD has an estimated incidence of 1 in 15 000.

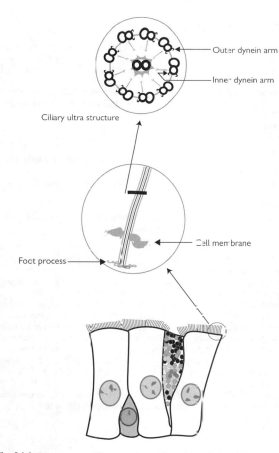

Fig. 34.1 Cilia structure. The nose, sinuses, Eustachian tubes, and lower airways, as far as the terminal bronchioles, are lined with ciliated respiratory epithelium. The cilia propel overlying airway mucous and particulate matter towards the mouth. Each cilium has a foot process beneath the apical membrane that fixes its position within the cell. The ultrastructure of the cilium shows a ring of microtubules around the edge of the cilium surrounding a pair of central microtubules—the so-called 9 + 2 arrangement. Each of the peripheral microtubules has inner and outer dynein arms that are critical in generating ciliary movement.

Clinical features

There is a wide variation in clinical severity in individuals with PCD, and symptoms may become apparent at any time in life from the newborn period to adulthood. Clinical problems that may be caused by PCD include the following.

- Unexpected neonatal respiratory distress in a term baby, either with a condition resembling prolonged transient tachypnoea of the newborn (TTN) or pneumonia.
- Persistent nasal discharge.
- Recurrent sinus infection.
- Persistent or recurrent otitis media.
- Persistent productive-sounding cough, including children with 'idiopathic' bronchiectasis.
- Severe or atypical asthma, particularly if there is an associated productive-sounding cough.
- Diminished fertility in men or women.
- Rarely, PCD can be associated with disorders of non-motile cilia including cystic kidney disease and retinal degeneration.

PCD and situs inversus

- PCD is associated with situs inversus totalis (Kartagener syndrome).
- The association arises from the presence of ciliated cells in early embryological development whose activity is important in determining situs, where there is no cilial activity, situs is random.
- Overall, about 40% of children with PCD have situs inversus, presumably because residual cilial activity in some is sufficient to determine situs.
- It also turns out that around 50% of individuals with situs inversus have PCD (the other reasons for having situs inversus are not understood). This information is useful when counselling families in which dextrocardia and situs inversus have been detected by antenatal ultrasound. As noted above, if ventriculomegaly is also present, the likelihood of PCD is increased.
- There is a smaller increased risk (1–5%) of PCD in isolated dextrocardia with situs solitus, and in infants with heterotaxia (right or left atrial isomerism).

Diagnosis

Diagnosis

Diagnosis of PCD usually requires a combination of tests. CXR is often normal, but may show situs inversus or isolated dextrocardia. Bronchus angle will be symmetrical in heterotaxia. The position of the abdominal viscera should be noted. There may be evidence of bronchial wall thickening. CT scan is not usually indicated as part of the assessment of a child with PCD unless bronchiectasis is suspected.

Saccharine test

The saccharine test is unreliable in children and should not be used for diagnostic purposes. It is described here so that the reader is aware of what is involved and, as a consequence, why it is not going to work in children.

A particle of saccharine is placed on the inferior turbinate. The subject is then asked to sit still for up to 60min with head tilted slightly forwards. Sniffing, sneezing, coughing, eating, or drinking is not permitted during the test. If saccharine is not tasted after 60min, a particle is placed on the tongue to check that the subject can recognize the taste. If they can, the test is positive. If saccharine is tasted within 60min the test is negative.

Ciliary brush biopsy

- Brush biopsies from the nasal turbinates are straightforward to perform in children (see 📖 Chapter 67).
- Ciliary activity in nasal samples correlates very well with that found in the lower airways.
- Secondary ciliary dyskinesia (including ultrastructural abnormalities detected by electron microscopy) is almost inevitable during and after respiratory viral infections, so it is important that the child has been free from URTI for at least 6 weeks prior to the biopsy. This can be difficult to assess in children with chronic nasal discharge.
- If children are undergoing bronchoscopy as part of their clinical evaluation, tracheal brushings can be obtained. They are usually of better quality than those obtained from the nose in children with purulent nasal discharge.
- Full evaluation of the ciliary biopsy sample requires measurement of the ciliary beat frequency (CBF; should be over 11Hz) and assessment of the nature and coordination of the ciliary activity by using high-speed digital video. This type of analysis is only available at a small number of centres (only 3 in the UK: Leicester, Southampton, and The Brompton Hospital, London). The sample is stable for several hours in tissue culture media. It can be transported to reference laboratories if necessary.
- Where this service is not available, estimation of the beat pattern and frequency by an experienced observer will detect most abnormalities (80–90%), particularly if combined with nasal nitric oxide assessment. Assessment of the ability of the cilia to propel particles along the epithelial surface is a reasonable proxy for coordinate function.
- Observed abnormalities of function include:
  - absent or nearly absent ciliary activity (65%);
  - stiff cilial movements with decreased amplitude, but near normal CBF (25%);

- rotary cilial activity (10%), which can only be appreciated by using an overhead high speed video.
- The sample should also be analysed using electron microscopy (EM) for evidence of ultrastructural abnormalities including the following.
  - Absent outer dynein arms alone or combined with inner dynein arm defects (65%). These are all associated with immobile or barely flickering cilial activity.
  - Absent inner dynein arms alone (15%). Of these 10% are immotile and the rest have stiff reduced amplitude motion with near normal CBF.
  - Absent radial spokes (15%). Of these, 30% are immotile and the rest have the stiff movement seen in the inner dynein arm defect.
  - Absent central pair microtubules (10%), also called transposition defect since one of the peripheral microtubules moves the core to replace the missing central pair. These defects cause the rotary motion with a normal CBF.
  - Random ciliary orientation. This was once thought to be relatively common but repeat biopsies are usually normal and in most cases this pattern represents a form of secondary dyskinesia.
- Samples showing abnormal ciliary activity may have no apparent ultrastructural abnormalities. Abnormal ultrastructure can also be secondary to viral infection and a repeat sample is always required.
- Repeat biopsies should be taken after 4–6 weeks to confirm the diagnosis.

Nasal nitric oxide

- For reasons that are not understood, nasal NO is low in children and adults with PCD. Exhaled NO is also low, but the range is greater and more likely to overlap with normal values.
- At present only exhaled NO analysers are widely available and nasal NO measurements are only available at specialist centres.
- To obtain a nasal sample, a sampling tube is placed in 1 nostril and samples the air at around 0.5L/min. The child must be able to take and hold a deep breath and to close their soft palate to prevent contamination from the pharynx. This restricts the measurement to cooperative children over the age of 3–5 years. If a large inspiration is taken and held, the soft palate will usually close. Some studies suggest gentle exhalation pressure to make sure this happens, e.g. by blowing into a suitable fixed volume toy. **No** measurements are made until a plateau is reached—usually in 15–20s. Normal values range between 150 and 1000ppb. Values in PCD are usually less than 100ppb. Low values are also seen in children with blocked noses, sinus disease, or CF.

Genetic testing

Mutations in 2 genes (DNAI1 and DNAH5) are found in about 40% of families with PCD. Clinical genetic tests are being developed for these genes and may in future provide part of a useful additional diagnostic test. Some interesting genotype–phenotype observations have been made, e.g. around 50% of families with outer dynein arm defects have mutations in DNAH5.

Management and outcome

Management

Chest disease

- The lungs are effectively normal at birth and become damaged as a consequence of repeated low grade bronchial infections. The impact of these infections can be minimized by daily airway secretion clearance combined with prolonged courses of antibiotics for respiratory exacerbations.
- Children should be seen 2–3 monthly with a cough swab or sputum sample obtained on each occasion. All positive cultures should be treated in an analogous way to the management of a child with CF. The main infecting organism is *Haemophilus influenzae*, but infections with *Staphylococcus aureus* and *Streptococcus pneumoniae* also occur. *Pseudomonas aeruginosa* infection may be a problem in older adolescents.
- Children with PCD should receive an annual influenza vaccination and immunization with the conjugate pneumococcal vaccine. Children over the age of 2 years should also receive the 23-valent Pneumovax.

Middle ear disease

- Recurrent acute otitis media and secretory otitis media are common in children with PCD.
- Reduction in hearing may result, with associated delay in language skills.
- Regular (6–12 monthly) hearing assessments should be performed in young children. Hearing loss is best treated with hearing aids.
- Grommet insertion leads almost inevitably to chronic discharge from the ear.
- Hearing aids can usually be discarded in later childhood.

Outcome

- The outcome for children with PCD is good with a normal life expectancy, provided that their lung disease is actively managed.
- Lung disease tends to stabilize after treatment is started. If treatment is suboptimal or diagnosis is delayed, outcomes are less good and in some published series the majority of adult patients had established bronchiectasis, some with significant loss of lung function ($FEV_1 < 50\%$).
- Around 50% of men with PCD will be infertile, and women will have decreased fertility. It is impossible to predict which men will be infertile from the severity of their lung disease or airway ciliary defect. Seminal fluid analysis is recommended to allow accurate assessment of reproductive capability. *In vitro* fertilization with intracystoplasmic sperm injection is possible.

Further information

Bush, A., Cole, P., Hariri, M., Mackay, I., Phillips, G., et al. (1998). Primary ciliary dyskinesia: diagnosis and standards of care. *Eur. Respir. J.* **12**, 982–8.

Chilvers, M.A., Rutman, A., and O'Callaghan, C. (2003). Ciliary beat pattern is associated with specific ultrastructural defects in primary ciliary dyskinesia. *J. Allergy Clin. Immunol.* **112**, 518–24.

Hornef, N., Olbrich, H., Horvath, J., Zariwala, M.A., Fliegauf, M. et al. (2006). DNAH5 mutations are a common cause of primary ciliary dyskinesia with outer dynein arm defects. *Am. J. Respir. Crit. Care Med.* **174**, 120–6.

Van Der Baan, S., Veerman, A., Wulffraat, N., Bezemer, P., and Feenstra, L. (1986). Primary ciliary dyskinesia: ciliary activity. *Acta Otolaryngol.* **102**, 274–81.

Zariwala, M.A., Leigh, M.W., Ceppa, F., Kennedy, M.P., Noone P.G., et al. (2006). Mutations of DNAI1 in primary ciliary dyskinesia: evidence of founder effect in a common mutation. *Am. J. Respir. Crit. Care Med.* **174**, 858–66.

Primary immuno-deficiency

Introduction

Children with immunodeficiency frequently present with respiratory problems. These include dramatic severe infections causing respiratory failure, as well as lower grade chronic or recurrent infections of the sinuses or lung. Children with the latter may have a chronic productive cough but seem otherwise well.

The range of possible underlying primary immune diseases is large. Over 80 different diseases have been described. Fortunately, most can be detected with a relatively straightforward battery of tests. The diseases can be characterized by deficiency of the different components of the immune system.

- Severe combined B- and T-cell deficiencies:
  - various forms of SCID;
  - hyper-IgM syndrome.
- Other T- and/or B-cell dysfunction:
  - DiGeorge syndrome;
  - Wiskott–Aldrich syndrome.
- Predominant antibody deficiency:
  - agammaglobulinaemia;
  - IgA and IgG subclass deficiency;
  - common variable immunodeficiency;
  - transient hypogammaglobulinaemia of infancy.
- Phagocyte/neutrophil defects:
  - chronic granulomatous disease;
  - congenital and cyclical neutropenia;
  - leucocyte adhesion defects;
  - Chediak–Higashi syndrome.
- Complement disorders.
- Interferon-gamma associated immunodeficiency.

The defect underlying hyper-IgE (Job) syndrome, which may present with respiratory infections in early or late childhood, has not been characterized. There is altered T-cell function and abnormal neutrophil chemotaxis. T- and B-cell numbers are usually normal. IgE and eosinophil count are both elevated. Respiratory involvement is usually in the form of recurrent bacterial bronchitis and/or repeated *Staphylococcal* and *Haemophilus* pneumonias often with pneumatocele formation.

When to consider immuno-deficiency

Underlying immune deficiency should be considered in all children whose respiratory infections are prolonged, recurrent, or unusually severe. Other factors that increase the likelihood of immune deficiency are:

- chronic diarrhoea;
- poor growth;
- eczematous rash (seen in Omenn's, hyper-IgE, and Wiskott–Aldrich syndromes);
- previous significant infections;

- parental consanguinity;
- family history of SCID;
- previous infant deaths;
- any autoimmune disease.

None of these risk factors may be present, and an apparently otherwise well and well-grown infant can present with an opportunistic lung infection. Clues on examination that may indicate immunodeficiency include:
- absence of any palpable lymph nodes;
- absent tonsils;
- thymus may not be visible on the CXR.

These findings are variable, depending on the form of immune disease.

Investigations

Suggested investigations in children with lung infection
and suspected immune deficiency

To investigate the infection

- CXR.
- Blood culture.
- Blood for CMV PCR.
- BAL for:
  - bacterial, mycobacterial, and viral culture;
  - immunofluorescence and/or PCR for RSV, influenza A and B,
    parainfluenza, human metapneumovirus, adenovirus, Epstein–Barr
    virus, CMV, HSV, and enterovirus.
  - cytology, including silver stain for *Pneumocystis* and evidence of
    fungal infection.
- Urine for culture (including *Candida*) and CMV PCR.

To investigate the possible immune defect (see Table 35.1)

Initial tests

- FBC and film.
- IgA, IgM, IgG, and IgE levels.
- Functional antibody responses to vaccinations and pneumococcal
  antigens.
- HIV test.

Subsequent tests

- Lymphocyte subsets:
  - total T-cell count (CD3) and T-cell subsets (CD4 and CD8 cells);
  - B-cell count (CD19);
  - NK-cell count (CD56);
- Lymphocyte stimulation assays.
- IgG subclasses.
- Neutrophil function tests.
- Complement tests (C3, C4, CH50, AP50) if there is invasive disease
  with *Streptococcus pneumoniae*.

Table 35.1 Commonly measured markers of immune function.

Primary immune deficiency	Lympho-cyte count	Eosinophil count	Neutro-phil count	Specific antibodies responses to vaccination	IgG	IgA	IgM	IgE	B cells (CD19)	CD4 T cells	CD 8 cells	other test
X-linked SCID	Low	Normal*	Normal	Always low	Low	Low	Low	Low	May be normal	Low	Low	NK (CD56) cells low
Bare lymphocyte syndrome	May be normal	Normal*	Normal	Always low	Low	Low	May be low	Low	May be normal or high	Low	May be normal	Low % cells carrying MHC II
Omenn's syndrome	May be normal	High	Normal	Always normal	May be normal	Low	Low	High	Low	May be normal	May be normal	Abnormal mitogen responses
PNP deficiency	Low	May be normal	Normal	Always low	May be normal	May be normal	May be normal	May be normal	Normal	Low	Low	Abnormal mitogen responses
ADA deficiency	Low	May be high	Normal	Always low	Low	Low	Low	May be high	usually low	Low	Low	Abnormal mitogen responses
Hyper IgM (X linked)	May be normal	Normal*	Often low	Always low	Low	Low	Usually high	Low	Usually normal	Usually normal	Usually normal	CD40 Ligand low. Response to mitogen normal

Table 35.1 (Contd.)

Primary immuno defiency	Lympho-cyte count	Eosinophil count	Neutro-phil count	Specific antibodies responses to vaccination	IgG	IgA	IgM	IgE	B cellsl (CD19)	CD4 T cells	CD 8 cells	other test
Hyper IgE	Normal	High	Normal	Usually normal	Normal	Normal	Normal	High	Usually normal	Usually normal	Usually normal	Abnormal neutrophil chemotaxis
Di George	Usually normal	Normal*	Normal	May be low	Normal	Normal	Normal	Normal	Normal	May be low	May be low	Abnoraml mitogen responses
Wiskott Alrich (X linked)	May be low in later childhood	Normal*	Normal	Low	Usually low	May be high	Usually low	May be high	Usually normal	Usually normal	Usually normal	Low platlets T cell mitogen responses derpressed.
Alaxia te langiectasia	May be low	Normal	Normal	Often low	May be low	May be low	May be high	May be low	Usually normal	May be low	May be low	Mat have T cell mitogen responses.
Common variable	Usually normal	Normal	Normal	Always low	Low and falls with age	Low and falls with age	May be normal	Normal	Usually normal	Usually normal	Usually normal	CD 40 ligand expression may be diminished
XLA	Usually normal	Normal	Normal	Always low	Low	Low	Low	Low	Low	Normal	Normal	

* Eosinophil count can be elevated during infection with *Pneumocytis carinii*.

Severe combined immune deficiency

Definition, types, and epidemiology

Severe combined immune deficiency (SCID) refers to a group of genetic conditions that result in impaired T- and B-cell immunity. The overall incidence of these disorders is approximately 1 in 100 000 births.

- The commonest form is X-linked disruption of the common gamma chain of the interleukin receptor for IL-2, IL-4, IL-5, IL-9, and IL-15. This deficiency disrupts normal activation and proliferation of T and B cells after antigenic stimulation. It accounts for around 50% of all children with SCID.
- The other 50% comprises a large number of autosomal recessive defects that either:
  - cause lymphopenia due to abnormalities leading to lymphocyte cell death (e.g. deficiencies of adenosine deaminase (ADA) and purine nucleoside phosphorylase (PNP)) or due to defects in lymphocyte production in the bone marrow (e.g. reticular dysgenesis);
  - disturb T- or B-cell function (e.g. loss of HLA class II molecules required for antigen presentation—the 'bare lymphocyte syndrome') or cause deficiency of IL-2, which is required for T- and B-cell proliferation;
  - or a combination, such as disruption of production of the B- and T-cell antigen receptors, which disrupts function but also leads to absence of B cells—Omenn's syndrome.
- Hyper-IgM also disrupts T- and B-cell function and causes similar problems to other forms of SCID. It is an X-linked disease caused by deficiency of CD40 ligand on T cells, which prevents the normal signalling for B cells to switch production from IgM to IgG and IgA. As a consequence IgM is usually (but not invariably) elevated and IgG and IgA are low. T-cell function is also affected. T- and B-cell numbers are often normal. Neutropenia is found in 50%; the cause is unknown. Most boys present in the first year of life with recurrent chest infection (40% get *Pneumocystis*), and nearly all will have presented by the age of 3 years.

Presentation

Children with SCID usually present as young infants with opportunistic, persistent, or overwhelming viral, bacterial, or fungal infection, often affecting the lungs. ADA and PNP deficiency may have phenotypes presenting later in childhood with recurrent bacterial infection, particularly sinus or lung disease, or with severe forms of chickenpox, herpes, or candida infections. Children with ADA and PNP deficiencies may also have neurological impairment, and PNP deficiency and hyper-IgM can be associated with autoimmune diseases.

Investigations

- Full investigation of possible infection is required (see 📖 p. 428 and Table 35.1).
- FBC and film, Ig levels, and lymphocyte subsets are usually sufficient to make a diagnosis.

- One or more class of lymphocyte will be reduced usually combined with reduction in one or more class of immunoglobulin. In this context a high eosinophil count suggests Omenn's syndrome, hyper-IgE syndrome, or *Pneumocystis* infection.

Treatment

Treatment of SCID requires expert immunological input and urgent referral to such a team should be made. Many forms require bone marrow transplantation. ADA deficiency may be managed with replacement therapy. X-linked forms can be treated by interleukin receptor gamma-chain gene therapy. The following treatments may be required urgently:

- co-trimoxazole prophylaxis for PCP (if not already started);
- fungal prophylaxis with fluconazole, or treatment with amphotericin B (usually as AmBisome®);
- ganciclovir if there is any evidence of CMV infection;
- ribavirin if there is any evidence of RSV infection;
- IV immunoglobulin infusions if there is hypogammaglobulinaemia.

Antibody deficiency

Antibody deficiency accounts for around 70% of children with primary immune deficiencies. The deficiencies predispose to recurrent bacterial infection, particularly of the upper and lower respiratory tract, and can present for the first time in children of all ages, depending on the severity of the defect. Untreated disease can progress to bronchiectasis.

X-linked agammaglobulinaemia

This is the most severe form of antibody deficiency. Most boys will present in the first 2 years of life with recurrent bacterial infection—often recurrent or severe pneumonia. More rarely, children are not diagnosed until later in childhood, although symptoms will usually have been present from early life. Usual pathogens are *Streptococcus pneumoniae*, *Haemophilus influenzae*, *Staphylococcus aureus*, and *Pseudomonas* species. Severe entero-viral infections (including encephalitis) can also occur. 20% of children develop large joint arthritis, and there is an increased risk of leukaemia and other malignancies. Examination shows absent or minimal lymph nodes and tonsillar tissue.

Investigations
- Low B-cell numbers.
- Very low or absent IgG, IgM, and IgA.
- Very poor or absent responses to vaccinations.

Treatment
IVIg replacement therapy plus long-term broad-spectrum antibiotics. If there is chronic productive-sounding cough, chest physiotherapy will be helpful.

Transient hypogammaglobulinaemia of infancy

Starts at about 6 months of age, when maternal Ig is diminishing. It usually comes to light because of investigation for recurrent otitis media or respira-tory infection. Examination is normal, with normal lymph nodes and tonsils.

Investigations
- IgG and IgA are low; IgM often normal.
- B-cell count is normal.
- Specific antibody responses to vaccinations may be normal or low. If vac-cine response is below protective level, vaccination should be repeated.

Treatment
Prompt use of antibiotics for coughs combined with chest physiotherapy is all that is required. Frequency of infections diminishes around the age of 3 years, although it may take a little longer for Ig levels to reach normal age-adjusted ranges.

IgA and IgG2 deficiency

Isolated IgA deficiency is common, around 1/750 people in most Western countries. In the majority it is asymptomatic. When combined with IgG2 deficiency there does appear to be an excess of URTIs and LRTIs. These are usually mild bronchitis-like infections, but may cause lung damage if not treated. The IgG2 defect may improve with age.

Investigations

- Total IgG s often normal. A low IgA in a symptomatic child should prompt testing for IgG subclasses.
- B-cell count is normal.
- Specific antibody responses to vaccinations may be normal or low. If vaccine response is below protective level, vaccination should be repeated.

Treatment

Treatment is symptomatic: chest physiotherapy and broad-spectrum antibiotics for exacerbations.

Note IgA deficiency is important to consider when using IVIg to treat other conditions such as Kawasaki disease, since there may be circulating IgE antibodies to IgA, which can trigger anaphylactic responses to IVIg. Prior to infusion, IgA levels should be checked, and IgA deficient children given IgA depleted IVIg.

Common variable immune deficiency (CVID)

- CVID is a group of poorly understood primary immune disorders whose predominant effect is antibody deficiency.
- Most are sporadic, but all forms of genetic inheritance have been described. CVID is one of the commonest forms of immune deficiency with an incidence of around 1/10 000.
- CVID usually presents between the 2nd and 4th decades of life and is the most common diagnosis in adults on long-term IVIg replacement therapy.
- Respiratory infections with *Streptococcus pneumoniae Haemophilus influenzae, and Staphylococcus aureus* are common, usually as recurrent bronchitis. They can progress to bronchiectasis if not treated.
- T-cell function may be affected and some children will present with infections caused by *Pneumocystis*, atypical mycobacteria, or *Herpes simplex*.
- Unlike IgG2 subclass deficiency, CVID tends to get worse with age. It is therefore important to follow up children with recurrent respiratory infections and *to re-test their immune responses* (particularly Ig levels, IgG subclasses, and specific antibody responses) on an annual basis if symptoms persist.
- Up to 50% of patients with CVID will develop autoimmune disease: haemolytic anaemia; thrombocytopenia; neutropenia; thyroid disease; rheumatoid arthritis; hepatitis. There is an increased risk of lymphoma.

Investigations

- IgG and IgA low. IgM may be normal. Ig levels may fall with age.
- Specific antibody responses to vaccinations will be low or absent.
- B-cell numbers usually normal, but may be low.
- T-cell numbers usually normal, but may be low.
- Expression of CD40 ligand may be diminished.

Treatment

IVIg replacement therapy is usually required. Prompt use of antibiotics for suspected infection. Chest physiotherapy is helpful for children with chronic productive-sounding cough.

Neutrophil defects

Neutrophil defects predispose to recurrent bacterial infections of the following types:
- pneumonia, especially with abscess formation or empyema;
- otitis media;
- sinusitis;
- osteomyelitis;
- bacteraemia;
- skin infection, especially abscesses.

Usual bacteria are *Staphylococci*, *Escherichia coli*, and *Serratia maracascens*. Infection with fungi (*Aspergillus* and *Candida*) can also cause severe disease.

Possible disorders

These include the following.
- Chronic granulomatous disease—a genetic defect of NADPH oxidase which prevents effective intracellular killing of phagocytosed micro-organisms. 70% is X-linked (*CYBB* gene); 30% is autosomal recessive (*NCF1*, *NCF2* and *CYBA* genes). Incidence is around 1 in 200 000. Usually presents in the first 5 years of life, but occasionally not until the 2nd decade. It should be considered in children presenting with severe pneumonias, even if they have apparently been previously well. 30% have an associated granulomatous colitis.
- Neutropenia.
  - Cyclic neutropenia. Neutrophil counts vary with a 21 day cycle. At the nadir there is a 3–4 day period where there is a high risk of infection.
  - Severe congenital neutropenia. Due to maturational arrest in the bone marrow. It is associated with early and severe infection. Delayed umbilical cord separation is common.
  - Shwachman–Diamond syndrome. Pancreatic insufficiency, bone marrow dysfunction, and short stature. Neutropenia is variable and may be cyclical. Neutrophil migration is always abnormal.
  - Hyper-IgM can be associated with neutropenia.
  - Milder chronic neutropenias are also described.
- Leucocyte adhesion defects. Very rare genetic defects of leucocyte surface molecules required for migration of neutrophils out of the blood and into the tissues. There is delayed umbilical cord separation and high resting white cell counts that become very high (> 40×10^9/L) during infection. Severe pneumonias can occur.
- Chediak–Higashi syndrome is a severe autosomal recessive multisystem disease that includes hypopigmentation of the skin, eyes, and hair, easy bruising, and recurrent infections, predominantly because of neutrophil dysfunction. Diagnosis usually follows identification of albinism rather than because of recurrent respiratory infection.
- Hyper-IgE syndrome is associated with abnormalities of neutrophil chemotaxis.

Investigations
- FBC for neutropenia.
- Bone marrow aspirate may be required.
- Nitroblue tetrazolium (NBT) dye test. The patient's neutrophils are stimulated with phorbol myristate acetate in the presence of NBT. In these circumstances, more than 95% of normal neutrophils will reduce NBT and become stained with a blue-black precipitate. In patients with chronic granulomatous disease (CGD), there is usually no NBT reduction. Carriers will show a mosaic pattern with 20–80% of neutrophils showing normal activity. More specific tests of neutrophil oxidase activity are available. Mutation analysis for the faulty gene (one of the phagocyte oxidase (phox) genes) is also possible.
- Neutrophil migration assays can be performed in specialized centres.

Treatment
Treatment depends on the underlying defect. Prompt use of antibiotics or antifungal treatment may be required. Granulocyte transfusion may be helpful during severe infection. For the neutropenic diseases, treatment with granulocyte colony-stimulating factor is usually effective.

Complement disorders

The complement system is part of the innate host response to infection. It can be activated by micro-organisms through the alternative pathway (activates C3 directly), and by the adaptive immune response (antigen–antibody complexes) via the classical pathway (C1–C4). Both pathways feed into a common final pathway via C3 that leads to activation of the terminal sequences (C5–C9). Activated complement promotes opsonization and direct killing of micro-organisms by lysis. It is also chemotactic for leucocytes and augments antibody production by B cells. Mannose-binding lectin is also considered to be part of the complement system and is one of the collectin group of proteins that promote opsonization of micro-organisms.

Complement deficiency is relatively rare, and deficiency is not always associated with disease. Deficiencies of factors in the classical pathway and of C5–C9 increase the risk of invasive bacterial infection, particularly with the encapsulated bacteria *Neisseria meningitides* and *Streptococcus pneumoniae*. It is possible that these children may present with severe pneumonia, but more likely that they will have a septicaemic illness. Recurrent bronchitis and bronchiectasis have not been described in these disorders. If complement deficiency is suspected, the following tests can be performed.

- CH50 test. Total serum classic haemolytic complement. Measures the ability of the patient's serum to lyse antibody-coated sheep red blood cells. Inability to do so indicates deficiency in the classical pathway.
- AP50 test. Alternative haemolytic complement. Measures the ability of the patient's serum to lyse uncoated rabbit red blood cells. Inability to do so indicates deficiency in the alternative pathway.
- Levels of C3 and C4.

DiGeorge syndrome

- DiGeorge syndrome comprises the triad of cardiac defects, thymic aplasia or hypoplasia with T-cell immunodeficiency, and hypoparathyroidism. It has an incidence of around 1/30 000. Microdeletions on chromosome 22q11 are found in 90% of affected children. Most arise *de novo*.
- The vast majority of children will present as a consequence of their cardiac defects, rather than with infections.
- Cardiac defects are principally the conotruncal lesions. The commonest are aortic arch anomalies, Fallot's tetralogy, ventricular septal defects, and truncus arteriosus.
- 60% have hypoparathyroidism. Hypocalcaemic tetany or seizures may occur in the neonatal period. Hypocalcaemia usually improves with time, but may require treatment with calcium supplements and vitamin D.
- In 80% of children with DiGeorge syndrome, immunodeficiency is mild. The small group of children with profound T-cell immunodeficiency (sometimes called complete DiGeorge syndrome) is similar to those with SCID. They are predisposed to *Pneumocystis jiroveci* pneumonia and disseminated viral infections. T-cell function tends to improve with time.
- Recurrent respiratory tract infections (upper and lower) are common, affecting up to 80% of children with DiGeorge, and sometimes result in bronchiectasis. These appear to result from defective humoral immunity, particularly to polysaccharide antigens.
- Dysmorphic features are common—hypertelorism, micrognathia, short philtrum with fish-mouth appearance, widely spaced eyes with short palpebral fissures, low-set ears, cleft palate.
- Behaviour problems, developmental delay, and poor growth may occur.

Investigations

- Lymphocyte count may be normal.
- T-cell responses to mitogens are low even when T-cell counts are normal. Infants with low T-cell counts tend to have more severe functional immune defects.
- Serum immunoglobulin levels are usually normal, but specific antibody responses to vaccinations may be low, particularly to pneumococcal polysaccharide antigens.
- Genetic test for 22q11 deletion. This is usually done by fluorescent *in situ* hybridization (FISH).
- Serum calcium and PTH level.

Treatment
- No specific treatment for the immune defect is usually required and it tends to improve with time.
- For children with severe recurrent pneumonias or bronchiectasis who have low levels of serum immunoglobulin, IV g replacement can be beneficial.
- For the small proportion of children with severe immunodeficiency bone marrow transplantation may be required.
- Where DiGeorge is suspected, usually because of the presence of cardiac defects, CMV-negative irradiated blood must be used to prevent CMV infection and graft versus host disease. As with all T-cell deficiency syndromes, live immunization should be avoided.

Wiskott–Aldrich syndrome

- Wiskott–Aldrich syndrome is an X-linked defect of T- and B-cell immunity caused by mutations in the WASP (Wiskott–Aldrich syndrome protein) gene seen predominantly in boys.
- The severity of immune disease in WAS patients correlates in many cases with specific mutations and with the level of WASP in blood cells.
- Female carriers of WASP mutations are usually asymptomatic. Rarely disease will occur in girls due to altered X chromosome inactivation.
- Thrombocytopenia, often with small platelets, is invariably present. Most children present with bleeding, often bloody diarrhoea in infancy. Severe eczema is common.
- Children are at risk of recurrent viral and bacterial infection, including pneumonia. Infection with *Pneumocystis jiroveci* can also occur.
- The immune defect gets worse with time.
- There is an increased risk of lymphoproliferative malignancy and autoimmune disorders.

Investigations

- FBC and film: low platelet count with small platelets. Lymphopenia is apparent in later childhood.
- IgM is usually low. IgA and IgE may be elevated.
- T-cell responses to mitogens may be depressed
- Specific antibody responses to vaccinations are usually low or absent.

Treatment and outcome

Treatment is supportive. Monthly IVIg may help. Platelet transfusions are needed to control severe bleeding.

Children with Wiskott–Aldrich syndrome often die in their teenage years from a combination of bleeding, infection, and lymphoproliferative malignancy. Bone marrow transplantation can reverse many features of the disease.

Ataxia telangiectasia

- Ataxia telangiectasia (AT) is an autosomal recessive disease caused by mutations in the ATM gene, a DNA-dependent protein kinase required for efficient DNA repair. Mutations of the ATM gene result in sensitivity to DNA damage including increased sensitivity to radiation. Chromosome breaks are particularly likely to affect genes related to the T-cell receptor and immunoglobulin heavy chains.
- AT is recognized clinically by the triad of ataxia, telangiectasia of the eyes and skin, and recurrent bronchopulmonary infections.
- The ataxia occurs early, is usually evident as the child begins to walk, and usually progresses so that the child will require a wheelchair by 10 years of age. The telangiectasiae develop between 3 and 6 years of age.
- Bronchopulmonary infections are common and affect over 80% of children with AT often resulting in bronchiectasis. The infections are usually first noticed between 5 and 7 years of age.
- Immunodeficiency worsens with age.
- 10–30% of children with AT develop solid or lymphoproliferative malignancies.
- 30% of children have mild cognitive impairment.

Investigations

- CXR shows bronchial wall thickening. CT scan may show bronchiectasis. Careful use of X-rays is particularly important in this group of children because of the increased radiosensitivity.
- IgA is often low; IgG and IgE may also be low. IgM may be elevated.
- Total lymphocyte count may be low and T-cell responses to mitogens are often low.
- Serum alpha-feto protein levels are usually elevated.
- DNA analysis of the ATM gene will identify mutations in 20–70% of patients depending on the population being studied.
- Chromosomal radiosensitivity tests and assays of the level of ATM protein in lymphocytes can also be carried out.

Treatment and outcome

- Antibiotics and chest physiotherapy for bronchial infection.
- Regular IVIg may be helpful.
- Children with AT usually die in their teenage years from a combination of respiratory failure related to chronic bronchopulmonary infection and malignancy. Occasionally, with milder phenotypes, survival into the 20–30s is possible.

Further information

Gennery, A.R., Barge, D., O'Sullivan, J.J., Flood, T.J., Abinun, M., and Cant, A.J. (2002). Antibody deficiency and autoimmunity in 22q11.2 deletion syndrome. *Arch. Dis. Child.* **86**, 422–5.

Taylor, A.M. and Byrd, P.J. (2005). Molecular pathology of ataxia telangiectasia. *J. Clin. Pathol.* **58**, 1009–15.

Swift, M., Morrell, D., Massey, R.B., and Chase, C.L. (1991). Incidence of cancer in 161 families affected by ataxia-telangiectasia. *N. Engl. J. Med.* **325** (26), 1831–6.

Post-infectious bronchiolitis obliterans

Introduction

Bronchiolitis obliterans (BO) is defined histologically by the presence of granulation tissue within small airways and/or destruction of the small airways by fibrous tissue. The distinction from organizing pneumonia (OP), in which alveolar spaces are also affected, is subtle, particularly since causes of BO and OP are similar. Histologically BO can be separated into constrictive bronchiolitis where there is inflammation and fibrosis around the bronchiolar wall and proliferative bronchiolitis where there is intra luminal fibrosis. Post-infectious BO is predominantly constrictive, often with accompanying bronchiectasis. Although BO can be caused by inhalation of noxious gases, and may be associated with connective tissue disease, by far the most likely cause in children is severe LRTI. BO syndrome associated with lung transplantation is dealt with in 📖 Chapter 55. BO is relatively rare in most parts of the world, and most centres would expect to see only 1 or 2 cases per year. There is a much higher incidence in some regions of Asia and South America, for reasons that are not yet understood.

Causative organisms

- Adenovirus is the most common infectious agent, accounting for around half of cases. Some serotypes, particularly serotype 7, appear to be more likely to result in BO than others. Co-infection with measles virus seems to be particularly damaging.
- *Mycoplasma pneumoniae* is responsible for 10–30% of cases in children.
- Several other infectious agents have also been implicated, including:
  - measles virus;
  - influenza virus;
  - parainfluenza virus;
  - respiratory syncytial virus;
  - *Bordetella pertussis*;
  - *Chlamydophilia pneumoniae*.

Symptoms and signs

- In most affected children the acute infection occurs before the age of 6 years, with an average at around 3 years of age.
- The acute illness is usually severe, with fever and respiratory distress requiring hospital treatment for oxygen therapy and sometimes mechanical ventilation.
- Following the acute illness there is persistence of symptoms:
  - wheeze—in about 50%;
  - breathlessness—universal;
  - exercise intolerance—universal;
  - cough, which may be productive-sounding.
- Examination findings include:
  - tachypnoea;
  - chest wall deformity—usually hyperinflation, but occasionally scoliosis;
  - crepitations—focal or diffuse;
  - digital clubbing;
  - desaturation—sometimes the requirement for supplemental oxygen can persist for several months or years.

Differential diagnosis

The usual clinical picture of a previously well child who develops a severe acute illness that is slow to resolve will suggest the diagnosis. Important differential diagnoses to consider:

- cystic fibrosis;
- atypical infection associated with immunodeficiency;
- tuberculosis;
- pulmonary venous obstruction;
- cardiac disease, including pulmonary arterial hypertension;
- aspiration pneumonitis (including that due to H-type TOF);
- hypersensitivity pneumonitis;
- idiopathic pulmonary haemosiderosis;
- pulmonary alveolar proteinosis;
- interstitial lung disease, including that associated with connective tissue disease (see 📖 Chapter 46);
- eosinophilic pneumonia;
- Langerhan's cell histiocytosis;
- lymphocytic interstitial pneumonitis with HIV infection;
- lymphangioleiomyomatosis;
- congenital lymphangiectasis.

Some of these diagnoses can be excluded clinically on the basis of a clear history of the onset of the illness, and the absence of symptoms before the acute illness occurred. This may be more difficult to establish in infants. Several chronic illnesses can present with an apparently acute onset (e.g. atypical infection with immunodeficiency, aspiration lung disease, TB, and CF). These need to be excluded by careful investigation.

Investigations

- NPA for viral culture and PCR for adenovirus, influenza viruses, human metapneumovirus, parainfluenza viruses, RSV.
- Serology for *M. pneumoniae* and *C. pneumoniae*. Elevated IgM or 4-fold rise of IgG over 2–3 weeks.
- Sweat test.
- Blood tests:
  - FBC;
  - total immunoglobulins;
  - specific antibody responses to immunizations;
  - HIV test.
- Mantoux test.
- CXR. Findings are non-specific and may be normal. Abnormalities include atelectasis, confluent densities, hyperlucent lung, and bilateral peribronchial thickening. The commonest abnormality is hyperlucency. This may affect one or both lungs. Where the affected lung is normal size or small, with air trapping on expiration, the radiological appearance is sometimes called Swyer–James or Macleod syndrome.

- CT scan. An HRCT scan of the chest is likely to be the most informative investigation. The most usual findings are areas of hyperinflation giving a mosaic pattern of attenuation. This is best demonstrated by inspiratory and expiratory scans. Air-trapping becomes apparent on the expiratory film. There may also be bronchial dilatation, bronchial wall thickening, areas of collapse, and bronchiectasis.
- Lung function tests. These can be difficult to obtain in young children but, when they can be obtained, an obstructive pattern is seen, with little or no response to bronchodilators.
- Bronchoscopy to exclude tracheomalacia or other structural airway abnormality and to obtain samples for microscopy and culture.
- Contrast swallow, videofluoroscopy, and pH study to look for evidence of gastro-oesophageal reflux and aspiration.
- Lung biopsy. This investigation should be reserved for children in whom there is significant difficulty in making the diagnosis. If the clinical picture and CT scan are consistent with a diagnosis of post-infectious BO and other likely causes have been excluded, lung biopsy is not usually necessary. Furthermore, the disease can be patchy and a normal lung biopsy does not exclude the diagnosis.
- Bronchography. This investigation is not available in most centres and is not usually required. If performed, it will show a relatively sharp cut-off at medium-sized airways, the so-called 'tree in bud' appearance, in parts of the lungs affected by BO.

Diagnosis

The diagnosis is reached on the basis of a compatible history combined with clinical evidence of fixed airways obstruction, CT chest findings suggestive of small airways disease, and the absence of evidence suggesting an alternative diagnosis. In the small number of children where there is still uncertainty about the diagnosis, a lung biopsy is required.

Treatment

- No treatments have been shown to work well and, by definition, the airway obstruction is not reversible. However, children with BO may have exacerbations, often with viral infections, during which courses of steroids and bronchodilators may help.
- There is anecdotal evidence that pulsed methyl prednisolone given 3 consecutive days per month may benefit children with severe oxygen-dependent disease.
- Recurrent infection is also common in children with BO, and usually reflects underlying bronchiectasis. It may therefore be appropriate to use courses of antibiotics for exacerbations, and to consider prophylactic antibiotics during the winter months. As with all children with chronic respiratory disease, annual influenza vaccination and pneumococcal vaccination should be given.

Outcome

Most children with post-infectious BO will show improvement with age, and most will be oxygen-free 3–5 years after diagnosis. However, there is an ongoing risk of exacerbation and most will be left with varying degrees of chronic respiratory impairment.

Further information

Chang, A.B., Masel, J.P., and Masters, B. (1998). Post-infectious bronchiolitis obliterans: clinical, radiological and pulmonary function sequelae. *Pediatr. Radiol.* **28**, 23–9.

Smith, K.J. and Fan, L.L. (2006). Insights into post-infectious bronchiolitis obliterans in children. *Thorax* **61**, 462–3.

Pleural effusion

Introduction

In most children with pleural fluid collections there is an obvious cause. Occasionally, the pleural fluid will be the primary problem and investigations will be needed to determine the nature of the underlying disease.

The normal pleura

- The pleural membranes are separated by a small volume of fluid (0.3mL/kg of body weight) with few cells.
- There is a continuous pleural circulation with secretion from apically placed lymphatic channels and absorption through lymphatic pores at the base of the thorax.
- The circulation can cope with greatly increased fluid production.
- The pressure in the normal pleural space is around −4 to −8cmH$_2$O during tidal breathing, increasing to > −100cmH$_2$O during maximal inspiration against resistance.
- Normal pleural fluid has the following characteristics:
  - pH 7.60–7.64;
  - protein content < 1–2g/dL;
  - fewer than 1000 white cells/mL;
  - glucose content similar to that of plasma;
  - lactate dehydrogenase (LDH) level less than 50% that of plasma;
  - electrolyte content similar to that plasma.

Increased fluid in the pleural space

- This can occur for several reasons.
  - There is a low serum protein level. This affects the physical forces encouraging tissue fluid to return to the capillaries. Fluid collects in body cavities, particularly the peritoneum and pleural space. The low pressure in the pleural space may be an additional reason for fluid collection here.
  - There is high systemic venous pressure. This has an end result on oncotic pressure similar to that of low serum protein, reducing the ability of the venous system to effectively collect tissue fluid.
  - There is an inflammatory process within the pleura that both increases pleural capillary permeability leading to plasma leak into the pleural space and reduces pleural fluid reabsorption by blocking the basal pleural lymphatic pores. Inflammation is most commonly caused by infection, but other inflammatory conditions may also result in pleural effusion (see box).
  - There is malignancy in the pleural space. Malignant deposits are often highly vascular and may have low capillary permeability.
  - There is an abnormality within the pleural lymphatic system or thoracic duct. This can result in alterations in lymphatic permeability within the thorax with increased formation of pleural fluid with a high protein and triglyceride content and a high lymphocyte count.
  - The fluid is blood, usually from trauma affecting an intercostal vessel.

- The lung cannot expand into the normal space within the thorax, e.g. this can be seen after diaphragmatic hernia repair with associated pulmonary hypoplasia.
- The fluid is coming from a misplaced central line.
- Low serum protein or high venous pressure cause transudates.
- Processes affecting capillary permeability cause exudates.

Causes of pleural effusions

Transudates
- High systemic venous pressure:
  - heart failure
  - superior vena cava obstruction
- Low oncotic pressure:
  - liver disease
  - malabsorption
  - protein-losing enteropathy
  - renal protein loss (e.g. nephrotic syndrome)

Exudates
- Pulmonary infection with parapneumonic effusion:
  - any bacterial lobar pneumonia
- Pleural infections:
  - tuberculosis
  - empyema
- Inflammatory disorders:
  - connective tissue disease (e.g. SLE, systemic juvenile arthritis)
  - sarcoidosis
- Adjacent inflamed structure:
  - pancreatitis
  - hepatic abscess
- Malignancy:
  - lymphoma
  - chest wall or pleural sarcoma

Chylothorax (see p. 456)
- High systemic venous pressure
- High pulmonary venous pressure
- Damage or compression of thoracic duct
- Abnormal pulmonary and pleural lymphatics
- Idiopathic, either isolated, or associated with Turner's syndrome or other chromosomal anomaly

Iatrogenic
- Misplaced central line

Symptoms and signs

- Symptoms caused by pleural effusions depend on the size of the fluid collection and the presence of inflammation. There may be no symptoms until collections are large. When symptoms occur they are usually a combination of:
  - breathlessness;
  - chest pain.
- Physical signs present also depend on the cause. There may be:
  - scoliosis towards the affected side;
  - dull percussion note;
  - a pleural rub;
  - decreased breath sounds.

Investigations and management

Investigations

Where the cause is not apparent, consider the following.
- Protein count. Levels over 50% of serum protein level suggest the fluid is an exudate. LDH can also be measured. Values above 2/3 that in plasma are also consistent with an exudate.
- Cytology for cell count and types of cell present, including possible malignant cells. High lymphocyte count is consistent with TB and chylothorax. High neutrophil count suggests bacterial infection.
- Gram stain. Presence of bacteria is consistent with empyema.
- Culture. May need to specifically ask for mycobacterial culture. Recovery of M. tuberculosis from tuberculous pleural effusions is poor, and diagnosis may require pleural biopsy.
- Triglyceride level. > 1.1mmol/L suggests the presence of chyle.
- High levels (> 40U/L) of the enzyme adenosine deaminase (ADA) in pleural fluid are suggestive of TB.

Management

- Treatment depends on cause.
- There is little value in draining transudates unless there is significant respiratory distress since they will persist until the cause is addressed.
- 📖 Chapter 18 deals with empyema.
- Chylothorax is discussed in more detail on 📖 p. 456.

Chylothorax

Background

- Fatty acids and monoglycerides released by intestinal lipases are absorbed by epithelial cells of the intestinal brush border where they are re-assembled into triglycerides and combined with carrier proteins to form chylomicrons. The chylomicrons then pass via the lacteal in the centre of the intestinal villus into the lymphatic system and eventually reach the thoracic duct where they join the systemic circulation and pass to sites of metabolism in the liver and adipose tissue.

- Lymph is fluid derived from plasma, which passes out from the capillary bed to bathe all tissues in the body. A proportion of the fluid re-enters the venous capillary bed and the remainder is collected in the lymphatic system. Lymph contains high numbers of lymphocytes and, like plasma, has a high protein content.

- Chyle is the term used for fluid containing lymph and chylomicrons draining from the small intestine.

- Most of the fat we eat is in the form of triglycerides containing long chain fatty acids (LCFA). Medium chain fatty acids differ from LCFA in that they are liquid at room temperature and much more soluble in water. Medium chain triglycerides (MCTs) are readily hydrolysed in the intestinal lumen by lipase and, unlike LCTs, can also be absorbed directly and hydrolysed within the intestinal epithelial cell. MCFA released from MCTs are largely transported via the portal venous system rather than the lymphatic system because of their higher water solubility. Thus MCTs can provide a source of fat nutrition independent of chyle formation, with the added benefit of reducing the volume of chyle produced.

- The thoracic duct carries all the lymph from the body except the right side of the head and neck, the right lung and right side of the thorax, and the right arm. This includes chyle from the small intestine and lymph from the lungs and pleura. The thoracic duct enters the thorax through the aortic hiatus of the diaphragm and ascends just to the right of midline as far as the 5th thoracic vertebra where it moves across to the left side. It joins the systemic circulation at the junction between the left internal jugular and left subclavian vein. Note that the thoracic duct loops above the clavicle into the base of the neck before joining the venous system. The lymph not collected by the thoracic duct passes via the *right* thoracic duct and joins the systemic circulation at the junction between the right internal jugular and subclavian veins.

How does chyle get into the pleural space?

- A true chylothorax requires that chylomicrons are found in the pleural space.

- This can occur because of disruption of the thoracic duct within the thorax caused either by shearing trauma such a motor vehicle accident or damage during surgery.

- Compression of the thoracic duct, most often by lymphoma, can result in chylothorax because of back-pressure and seepage.

- Increased systemic venous pressure can result in chylothorax, probably by increased thoracic duct pressure and subsequent seepage. This is most usually seen after cardiac surgery where the systemic venous circulation is anastomosed to the pulmonary arteries. e.g. the Fontan procedure.
- Chyle can also enter the pleural space when there is increased pressure within the pulmonary lymphatic bed, either because of abnormal lymphatics (e.g. pulmonary lymphangiectasia) or because of high pulmonary venous pressure. Presumably this reflects some transmission of the increased pressure to the thoracic duct with subsequent seepage of its contents into the pleural space.
- The pleural space seems to be particularly at risk as a site of lymph and chylous effusion because of the low pressures within the space generated by respiratory movements.

Causes of chylothorax

- Thoracic duct-related:
  - tear—caused by surgery or, more rarely, shearing forces from external trauma
  - compression—usually caused by lymphoma
- Abnormal pulmonary lymphatics:
  - pulmonary lymphangiectasia (see 📖 Chapter 54)
  - pulmonary lymphangiomatosis (see 📖 Chapter 54)
  - Turner's syndrome
- Increased systemic venous pressure:
  - usually following surgery—bidirectional cavopulmonary shunt, Fontan-type procedures, and right ventricular dysfunction after repair of tetralogy of Fallot
- Increased pulmonary venous pressure:
  - pulmonary vein stenosis
  - mitral valve stenosis
- Idiopathic neonatal:
  - associated with chromosome abnormality
  - no cause identified

Symptoms and signs

- True chylothorax is usually left-sided. Bilateral lymphatic effusions may be seen when there is increased lymphatic or pulmonary venous pressure or systemic venous pressure. Chylothorax can be right-sided and can be bilateral. Since true chylothoraces contain chylomicrons and must therefore include chyle draining from the intestine via the left thoracic duct, the presence of chyle in the right hemithorax presumably means that there is some communication between lymphatic drainage of the right hemithorax and the left thoracic duct or anatomical variation of the left duct allowing leakage of the left duct into the right hemithorax.

- Chylothorax may be part of neonatal hydrops, usually due to pulmonary lymphangiectasia. Other forms of neonatal hydrops may have pleural effusions, but these are non-chylous. Chylothorax in the neonatal period may also be seen with Turner's and Noonan's syndromes.
- Symptoms will depend on the underlying cause. There may be no direct symptoms attributable to the chylothorax. Large collections may cause respiratory distress.

Investigations

- The diagnosis of a chylothorax requires the identification of high levels of triglyceride (> 1.1mmol/L) in the pleural fluid. A cell count and differential is also helpful. Lymphocytes should account for more than 80% of the cells present.
- Not all chylous effusions look milky-white.
- Not all pale white effusions are chylous. Some will be lymphatic fluid without chyle.
- Traumatic and post-surgical chylothoraces usually require no further investigation.

Management and outcome

- There are 2 main objectives in the management of chylothorax:
  - to reduce and eventually stop the production of chylous fluid;
  - to maintain nutrition.
- Reduced volumes of chyle can be achieved by decreasing the fat content in the diet.
- Maintenance of adequate nutrition can be achieved by replacing normal fat content with MCT or, less commonly, with total parenteral nutrition.
- Octreotide, a long-acting synthetic analogue of somatostatin, may also have a role in reducing lymph production. It can be given as a daily SC injection.
- When effusions persist, surgery may be considered. The most successful procedure is pleurectomy. Depending on the cause of the chylothorax, ligating the thoracic duct may make the situation worse and induce a protein losing enteropathy.
- Longstanding chylothorax will have detrimental effects on nutrition and immune competence.
- Outcome depends on the cause. Damage to the thoracic duct will usually resolve with time and nutritional management. Octreotide therapy may play an increasing role in chylothoraces that persist for more than 7–10 days. When the chylothorax is due to increased venous pressure, improvement is related to reduction of venous pressures as well as approaches to reduce chyle and lymph production.

Further information

Chan, S.Y., Lau, W., Wong, W.H., Cheng, L.C., Chau, A.K., and Cheung, Y.F. (2006). Chylothorax in children after congenital heart surgery. *Ann. Thorac. Surg.* **82**, 1650–6.

Paget-Brown, A., Kattwinkel, J., Rodgers, B.M., and Michalsky, M.P. (2006). The use of octreotide to treat congenital chylothorax. *J. Pediatr. Surg.* **41** (4), 845–7.

Pneumothorax

Clinical features and investigations

Definitions

- The term pneumothorax refers to a condition in which there is air in the pleural space with associated lung collapse.
- Spontaneous pneumothorax, not directly caused by an immediately preceding event such as trauma, can be divided into primary and secondary according to whether there is apparent underlying lung disease. It is an important distinction since it influences management.
- Management outlined here is based on the BTS guidelines, with some adaptation.in[1] The BTS guidelines define pneumothorax size in terms of centimetres. This is not appropriate for children and can be confusing when using re-scaled digital X-rays.

Primary spontaneous pneumothorax

Annual incidence in children is not well reported but is around 2–3/100 000. It occurs almost exclusively in adolescents and in boys more frequently than girls. The affected children are usually tall and thin. The cause of the air leak is thought to be an area of weakness in the surface of the lung, sometimes identified as a bleb. These are usually in the apex of the lung. Cigarette smoking is an important risk factor.

Secondary pneumothoraces

These occur in the presence of underlying lung disease, usually asthma or CF. Occasionally they will complicate pneumonia and empyema. They can also occur in children with Marfan's syndrome where there may be inherent weakness in the lung parenchyma (emphysema can occur in adult life and in the severe neonatal form of Marfan's syndrome) and in children with congenital cystic lung disease (e.g. cystic adenomatoid malformation).

Clinical presentation

Spontaneous pneumothoraces usually come on at rest. Symptoms include:
- sharp chest pain, often pleuritic (worse on inspiration);
- breathlessness—may be minimal;
- cough.

Examination findings include:
- increased respiratory rate;
- decreased expansion on affected side;
- hyperresonant percussion note;
- decreased or absent breath sounds on the affected side.

Investigation

CXR is diagnostic (Figs 38.1 and 38.2). There is clear delineation of the edge of the lung, with a black featureless rim of air between the lung and chest wall. Pneumothoraces can be more difficult to spot on supine films, when the air can collect anteriorly. This situation is most likely to occur

---

1 Henry, M., Arnold, T., and Harvey, J. (2003). BTS guidelines for the management of spontaneous pneumothorax. *Thorax* **58**, 39–52.

in a ventilated patient, where there is a high index of suspicion and one lung field looks darker than the other. In children with significant underlying lung disease, such as CF, a small amount of air in the pleural space can have a disproportionately large impact on their lung function.

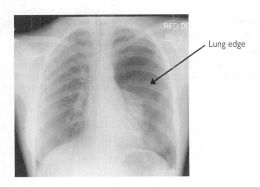

Fig. 38.1 Primary spontaneous pneumothorax in a 15-year-old girl.

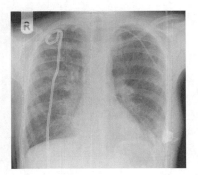

Fig. 38.2 Secondary spontaneous pneumothorax in a 14-year-old boy with cystic fibrosis. The lung re-inflated after an apical chest drain was inserted.

Role of CT scans

Blebs may be identified on CT scan, including blebs on the contralateral lung. Identifying blebs does not influence management and, for most patients, CT scan is unnecessary. CT scans can be helpful if symptoms or signs are suggestive of underlying disease. If surgery is subsequently required, many surgeons will request a CT scan pre-operatively, although direct inspection of the lung surface at operation is likely to provide more information.

Recurrence of pneumothorax

The recurrence rate of primary spontaneous pneumothorax is around 40%. Half of the recurrences will occur within 30 days of the first event. There is also an increased risk of pneumothorax in the contralateral lung. In some series this carries as lifetime risk as high as 25%.

Management

Primary spontaneous pneumothorax

Small pneumothorax, no respiratory distress

- Small means < 20% of the distance from the hilum to the chest wall on erect CXR is occupied by pneumothorax.
- In this instance, the patient should be observed for 4h and re-X-rayed.
- If the pneumothorax is the same size or smaller, patient can be discharged and reviewed after 48h.
- If symptoms are improving and pneumothorax has resolved at 48h, patient can be discharged, with appropriate advice about recurrence.
- If the pneumothorax is still present, patient needs to be seen every 3–4 days until resolution.

Large pneumothorax or pneumothorax with respiratory distress

- Large means > 20% of the distance from the hilum to the chest wall is occupied by pneumothorax on erect CXR.
- Large pneumothoraces should be aspirated.
- Smaller pneumothoraces with respiratory distress should also be aspirated. This can be done using a 16 gauge IV cannula. The same cannula can be used to pass the guide wire for a chest drain, if one is needed.
- The 2nd intercostal space in the mid-clavicular line is easiest site to use. The site for aspiration should be anaesthetized with lignocaine.
- The needle from the cannula should be removed after insertion, and IV tubing and a 3-way tap connected.
- Air should be aspirated using a 50mL syringe. If 1500mL of air is aspirated, with no evidence of a slow down, the procedure should be stopped and a drain inserted.
- If a point is reached where no more air can be aspirated, the cannula is removed and a repeat CXR should be performed. If this shows a nearly fully expanded lung, the patient should be observed for a further 4h and the CXR repeated. If there is no re-accumulation of air, no further action is required. In practice these patients would normally be admitted to hospital overnight.

Secondary spontaneous pneumothorax

- In children with underlying lung disease, pneumothorax is always potentially dangerous. Always admit these children to hospital.
- The threshold for draining secondary pneumothoraces is much lower, and there is a higher expectation of a persistent air leak.
- After a single event, consideration should be given to a pleurodesis procedure or excision of any cysts.

Indications for inserting a chest drain

A chest drain should be inserted:
- simple aspiration fails to re-inflate the lung;
- the pneumothorax recurs within 7 days;
- for all patients with underlying lung disease except those who are not breathless and have a very small pneumothorax.

Small-bore pig-tail drains are usually adequate. They cause less pain than large bore tubes, both on insertion and once *in situ*.

- A 10F drain is large enough for all simple pneumothoraces. The procedure for inserting the drain is given in 🕮 Chapter 65.
- We would recommend using the 2nd intercostal space in the mid-clavicular line as the site for the drain (the same site used for aspiration) with the aim of positioning the drain into the apex of the chest cavity. This site gives the best chance of allowing full re-inflation of the lung. The incision needed for a pig-tail drain is tiny, and will not leave any significant scarring.
- Suction is not required for the first 24h. If the lung has failed to re-inflate after 24h, suction can be applied at $-20cmH_2O$
- The drain should be left in until the lung has been fully re-inflated for 24h without bubbling of the underwater seal.
- Re-expansion pulmonary oedema (RPO) may occur, particularly in complete pneumothoraces where the lung has been down for a few days. Overly rapid re-inflation by early use of suction may increase the likelihood of this complication. Clinically the patient will complain of cough, breathlessness, or chest tightness. The symptoms usually resolve spontaneously. If they progress, intervention, including positive pressure ventilation may be required.
- In children with persistent air leaks, particularly those who are ventilated, larger chest drains (14–20F) on suction may be needed to allow the lung to re-expand.
- A bubbling chest drain should never be clamped. If a drain appears to have stopped bubbling, but there is uncertainty, it can be clamped for a few hours and then released whilst closely observing the underwater seal. If bubbles are seen, a small leak remains. This procedure should only be undertaken by experienced personnel.

High flow oxygen

Giving high flow oxygen (10L/min) can increase the rate at which air is reabsorbed by the pleura. It works by increasing the partial pressure of oxygen in the blood and thereby decreasing the partial pressure of nitrogen. This increases the diffusion rate of nitrogen from the pleural space into the blood. In practice high flow oxygen is unpleasant and, once a drain has been inserted, it adds little to the management of these patients.

Pleurodesis

Pleurodesis refers to the process of sticking together of the parietal and visceral pleural surfaces and obliterating the pleural space. Successful pleurodesis will prevent pneumothorax. It should be offered to any patient who has:
- first pneumothorax where there is underlying lung disease;
- a second ipsilateral primary pneumothorax;
- first contralateral primary pneumothorax;
- bilateral spontaneous primary pneumothorax;
- persistent air leak for more than 5–7 days or failure to re-expand the lung.

Surgical pleurodesis is the method of choice and should be used in all suitable patients. Two approaches are possible. Video-assisted thorascopic blebectomy together with either pleural abrasion or parietal pleurectomy. This procedure has a recurrence rate of around 5% and is preferred by most centres. The alternative is extensive open pleurectomy. This is the most effective procedure with a very low recurrence rate (1%), but requires a thoracotomy, results in increased blood loss, and has a longer recovery time.

For pleurodesis to be successful the pleural surfaces must be adherent after the procedure. This is most likely to be achieved if the drain placed at surgery has its tip at the apex of the chest cavity.

Closed chemical pleurodesis is an alternative for occasional patients who are not suitable for surgery. This can be carried out with doxycyline or with talc. Doxycycline (500mg doxycycline in 50mL saline) is painful (premedication with pethidine and midazolam is needed). Recurrence rate is 25%. Talc is more effective, but can be associated with acute respiratory distress syndrome, and the long-term effects of talc are not known.

Specific situations

Tension pneumothorax

- Tension pneumothorax occurs when air accumulates in the pleural space through a leak with a one-way valve.
- Air enters the pleural space with each inspiration and the pressure in the pleural space increases.
- The increased pressure compresses the lungs and mediastinal structures and impedes venous return, causing hypotension and the potential for cardiac arrest.
- It will normally occur with a complete pneumothorax and mediastinal shift away from the pneumothorax.
- In patients with significant lung disease, such as CF, the lungs can be very stiff allowing significant increases in intrapleural pressure with a relatively small-looking pneumothorax.

If tension pneumothorax is suspected it should be treated before getting a CXR.

- Give high flow oxygen and insert a 14 gauge cannula in the second intercostal space in the mid-clavicular line on the side of the pneumothorax.
- A hiss of escaping gas through the cannula and immediate clinical improvement confirm the diagnosis. Leave the cannula in place and insert a chest drain anteriorly in the 2nd intercostal space, mid-clavicular line.

Spontaneous pneumothorax in newborn infants

Spontaneous pneumothorax is more common in the neonatal period than at any other time in childhood. It presents with respiratory distress shortly after delivery and probably occurs as a result of the high pressures generated with onset of breathing. It is more common in large babies requiring instrumental delivery. There is usually no underlying lung disease, and most will settle without intervention. A small proportion will have pulmonary hypoplasia or cystic lung disease.

Pneumothorax in children with cystic fibrosis

See also ☐ Chapter 15.

- Pneumothorax occurs in around 3% of patients with CF.
- Most will have severe lung disease, with an FEV_1 of < 40%.
- All children with this complication should be admitted to hospital. The underlying lung disease should be treated vigorously with antibiotics and physiotherapy.
- A chest drain will be needed if the pneumothorax is large (> 20%) and for all symptomatic pneumothoraces. Most air leaks arise from the upper lobes and the drain should be sited with this in mind.
- Chest drains hurt, and often the pneumothorax itself will cause pain. Chest pain will impair sputum clearance manoeuvres and for this reason antibiotics should be started.

- Pleurodesis will be required when the air leak is persistent (> 3–5 days). The method of choice is VATS with partial pleurectomy or pleural abrasion.
- In 40% there will be recurrence on the ipsilateral or contralateral side.
- Pleurodesis will make lung transplantation more difficult but does not preclude it. Discussion with the local transplant team is advisable.
- Following pneumothorax in children and adults with CF there is an increased morbidity (increased number of days in hospital) and increased mortality compared to that in similar patients without pneumothorax.

Flying and diving

Children who have had a pneumothorax should not fly for at least 2 weeks after the pneumothorax has resolved. The family must be aware that there is a risk of recurrence, even after a pleurodesis procedure, which can affect the opposite lung. Children who have had pneumothoraces should never undertake any scuba diving activity.

Further information

Flume, P.A., Strange, C., Ye, X., et al. (2005). Pneumothorax in cystic fibrosis. Chest **128**, 720–8.
Baumann, M.H., Strange, C., Heffner, J.E., et al. (2001). Management of spontaneous pneumothorax: an American College of Chest Physicians Delphi consensus statement. Chest **119**, 590–602.

Chronic lung disease of prematurity

Definition and aetiology

Chronic lung disease (CLD) of prematurity is defined as the need for supplemental oxygen at or beyond 36 weeks postmenstrual age (PMA). This definition is a better predictor of pulmonary outcome than the previously used definition of an oxygen requirement at 28 days of age. Whilst there is some variability between different neonatal ICUs, most will use supplemental oxygen to keep saturations between 88% and 94%.

The cause of CLD following premature birth is multifactorial, and depends on the gestation of the infant.

- In the past, the majority of survivors were above 28 weeks gestation, and their CLD was related to the severity of their initial respiratory distress syndrome (RDS) and the amount of ventilator support required. Likely causes for the observed lung damage in this group are volutrauma, barotrauma, pulmonary infection, and aspiration. This form of CLD is called bronchopulmonary dysplasia (BPD). CLD is now unusual in infants over 30 weeks gestation, probably as a result of the use of antenatal steroids, pulmonary surfactant, and gentler modes of ventilation.

- In more recent years, an increasing number of extremely preterm infants have survived without significant RDS and without long periods of ventilator support. Despite this apparently trouble-free early neonatal course, some of these infants develop or retain an oxygen requirement by the time they reach term, have persistent CXR changes, and suffer longer-term respiratory morbidity similar to that of those with classic BPD. This form of CLD, which has been called the 'new BPD', is thought to arise because of poor postnatal alveolar growth with impaired remodelling, and is worsened by infection (including chorioamnionitis) and increased pulmonary blood flow caused by a patent ductus arteriosus.

CLD of prematurity can be complicated by the presence of tracheo-bronchomalacia, gastro-oesophageal reflux, and aspiration lung disease. Some infants with BPD have pulmonary hypertension as a consequence of abnormal development of the pulmonary vascular bed. Others may develop pulmonary hypertension as a result of unrecognized hypoxia and hypercarbia.

Symptoms and signs

Symptoms will vary according the severity of the CLD. They include:

- breathlessness;
- difficulty feeding, sometimes combined with gastro-oesophageal reflux and vomiting;
- cough;
- wheeze;
- poor growth;
- episodes of profound desaturation suggesting coexisting tracheo-bronchomalacia and/or pulmonary hypertension.

Examination findings include the following.
- Hyperinflated chest.
- Increased work of breathing with tachypnoea and chest wall retractions.
- Abnormal breath sounds:
  - scattered crackles;
  - wheeze.
- Evidence of pulmonary hypertension should be sought:
  - loud second heart sound;
  - enlarged liver.

Investigations
- CXR appearance can include:
  - hyperinflation;
  - faint, poorly defined opacities, giving a hazy appearance to the lungs;
  - coarse linear–reticular opacities extending out to the periphery of the lungs possibly with coalescence around the hila;
  - cystic areas.

Infants with 'new BPD' tend to have hyperinflation with fewer opacities and fewer cystic areas.
- CT scan is not usually required. If performed, findings include areas of hyperinflation, linear opacities, and bronchovascular bundle distortion or thickening.
- If there are symptoms suggestive of tracheobronchomalacia, further investigation may include bronchoscopy, bronchogram, or CT scan (for further details on tracheobronchomalacia, see 📖 Chapter 24).
- If there are symptoms suggestive of gastro-oesophageal reflux (GOR) or aspiration, further investigations may include contrast swallow, pH study, and videofluoroscopy (see 📖 Chapter 30).

Management
Regular and frequent assessment is essential, not only to assess oxygen requirements but also to review growth and developmental progress and to screen for the presence of complications, most importantly, pulmonary hypertension.
- Optimize nutrition. Initially this may need to include NG feeds.
- Early use of dexamethasone (< 14 days of age) has been associated with poor neurological outcome. Its routine use is no longer recommended.
- Pulmonary interstitial oedema may contribute to chronic lung disease. Diuretics, such as furosemide and thiazides and spironolactone, may be useful for exacerbations of disease in the neonatal period. They may be considered for longer-term use, although there is no evidence showing improved outcomes. Long-term use of diuretics (particularly furosemide) is associated with nephrocalcinosis and renal stones.
- Wheeze can be treated with inhaled bronchodilators. Careful assessment of benefit is required since there may be coexisting tracheo-bronchomalacia, which can be made worse by bronchodilators.
- Methylxanthines such as theophylline or caffeine may also be helpful in treating reactive airways disease. Their use can exacerbate GOR.

- The role of inhaled steroids is not clear. A trial of treatment may be justified.
- Exacerbations of lung disease are common, particularly in association with viral infections. Short courses of oral steroids may have benefit in this situation.
- Infants with CLD should, in addition to regular scheduled vaccinations, be given the conjugate pneumococcal vaccine and annual influenza vaccination. The risk of hospitalization in association with RSV infection can be halved by passive immunization during the RSV season.

Home oxygen therapy

- Home oxygen therapy for infants with CLD is provided to prevent hypoxic pulmonary vasoconstriction and the development of cor pulmonale. Giving oxygen may also reduce the work of breathing, thereby allowing calories to be used for growth. Oxygen therapy is provided for infants with evidence of day- or night-time desaturation.
- The amount of oxygen required needs to be assessed before discharge, and can then be continued at home in stable infants.
- Two large studies have shown that supplementing oxygen to keep saturations to 89–94% gives the same outcomes in terms of growth and neurodevelopment as that obtained by supplementing to 94–99%. Benefits of using the lower targets are shorter stay in hospital and shorter time on oxygen.[1, 2]
- Oxygen saturation as measured by Ohmeda pulse oximeters is 2 points lower than that measured by other commercial oximeters (e.g. the Nellcor), to correct for assumed carboxyhaemoglobin and methaemoglobin levels.
- An infant's oxygen requirements will vary according to their degree of alertness and whether or not they are feeding.
- A pragmatic approach is needed to select the level of oxygen that will keep the saturations at a safe level at all times. The risk of retinopathy of prematurity after 32 weeks gestation is negligible.

Weaning home oxygen

There is little evidence to guide the method by which home oxygen is weaned. One suggested approach is as follows.

- Arrange a clinic visit for 1 month after discharge home. If the infant has made good progress, stop the oxygen therapy and carry out a spot-check oxygen saturation measurement during wakefulness 30min later. If the infant's saturation is above 94%, introduce periods of 2h per day at home when the infant is off oxygen. Continuous oxygen saturation monitoring is not required. Spot oxygen saturations at the end of a 2h period off oxygen should be performed twice per week.

1 Askie LM., Henderson-Smart DJ., Irwig L. *et al.* Oxygen-saturation targets and outcomes in extremely preterm infants (BOOST I). *N Engl J Med* 2003; **349**: 959–67.

2 The STOP-ROP Multicenter Study Group. Supplemental therapeutic oxygen for prethreshold retinopathy of prematurity (STOP-ROP), a randomized, controlled trial, I: primary outcomes. Pediatrics 2000; **105**: 295–310

- If the infant remains well (no increase in breathlessness, feeding well, alert) after 1 week on this regime, with saturation spot checks > 94% at the end of the 2h period off oxygen, then the period of time off oxygen can be increased by 1h every week. This process can be repeated weekly to sequentially extend the time off oxygen.
- Continue to see the infant monthly in clinic and check saturations during visits. Additional saturation checks can be made at home. After 2–3 months, the infant will be using night-time oxygen only.
- At this stage an overnight oximetry study, with the infant off oxygen can be performed. If this study is satisfactory, all oxygen therapy can stop.
- Leave oxygen equipment in the home for a further 2 months in case oxygen is needed for intercurrent illnesses.

Outcome

Short-term outcomes
- The median duration of oxygen therapy for infants with CLD of prematurity is 4–6 months.
- Two-thirds of these infants will be re-admitted to hospital with respiratory exacerbations, usually associated with viral respiratory tract infection.
- Common symptoms are cough and/or wheeze. Some infants will have stridor from subglottic stenosis.

Longer term outcomes
- Children who had CLD of prematurity as infants have diminished lung function at school age.
- One study of extremely low birth weight infants (mean weight 700g, mean gestation 26 weeks) born in the 1980s and assessed at 11 years of age showed the following.
  - Infants with CLD in infancy had FEV_1 values 55–85% predicted.
  - Children with a history of CLD were also more likely to have cough and/or wheeze.
  - Infants who did not have an oxygen requirement at 36 weeks gestation (the usual definition for CLD of prematurity) had lung function that was not different from that of normal birth weight controls. The long-term outcome of infants with new BPD is not known but is likely to be similar.
- Children with fixed airways obstruction as a consequence of CLD of prematurity will be at increased risk of developing symptomatic chronic obstructive lung disease as adults.

Further information
Kilbride, H.W., Gelatt. M.C., and Sabath, R.J. (2003). Pulmonary function and exercise capacity for ELBW survivors in preadolescence: effect of neonatal chronic lung disease. *J. Pediatr.* **143**, 488–93.

Chapter 40

Chest wall deformity and scoliosis

Pectus excavatum

- Pectus excavatum (PE) is a chest wall deformity in which body of sternum is displaced posteriorly to produce funnel-shaped depression.
- It accounts for 90% of congenital chest wall deformities in children. Incidence of PE is between 1/400 and 1/1000 live births, with a male-to-female ratio of 5:1.
- There is a familial effect. 40% of families have > 1 affected member. Nature of inheritance is not resolved: likely to be multifactorial.
- The pathogenesis of PE is not understood. It is possible that abnormal growth in the costochondral regions results in the sternal depression. In some children it may occur because of underlying pulmonary hypoplasia or other lung disease.
- PE is associated with collagen disorders such as Marfan's and Ehlers–Danlos syndromes. Even in non-syndromic forms of PE, abnormalities of type 2 collagen have been detected and there may be hypermobility of joints.
- PE may be unilateral or asymmetrical.

Physiological effects of PE

- The major complaint of children and adults with PE is the cosmetic appearance of their chest rather than any physiological impairment.
- As a group, children with PE have decreased exercise ability and cardiovascular function and lower lung volumes than age- and size-matched controls. Effects often mild and may fall within normal range.
- Effects on cardiopulmonary function are real and not secondary to poor conditioning as was suggested in the past. This suggestion was made on the basis that children and adults with PE deformity avoid exercise because of embarrassment about their chest shape.
- The physiological effects arise because of restrictive movement of the chest wall and compression of the mediastinum such that the heart is displaced to the left with the apex beat in the mid-axillary line. This can result in restrictive lung function and a limited cardiac output response to exercise.

Symptoms

- Reduced exercise ability.
- Chest discomfort during exercise.

Signs

- Look for evidence of Marfan's syndrome (long limbs and fingers, high arched palate, visual problems, ligamentous laxity, aortic regurgitation).
- Listen for murmurs—mitral valve prolapse is occasionally present. Aortic regurgitation may occur in Marfan's syndrome.
- Look to see if the PE deformity is symmetrical or asymmetrical. Latter is associated with less favourable cosmetic results after surgery.
- Look to see if there is scoliosis.

Investigations

- Pulmonary function testing.
- Exercise testing.
- Echocardiography if there is a murmur or if surgery is contemplated.
- CT chest if surgery is contemplated. The severity of the PE can be quantified by dividing the inner width of the chest at the widest point, by the distance between the posterior surface of the sternum and anterior surface of the spine. The normal mean index is 2.5.

Treatment

- No treatment is a reasonable option.
- Whether or not the family opts for surgical intervention is largely dependent on how much the child is bothered by the deformity.
- Procedure most widely used now is correction, usually called a Nuss procedure, in which the sternum is elevated by a shaped metal bar. The bar is left in place for 2–4 years so that permanent correction of the anterior chest wall contour can be obtained. This procedure has largely superseded the Ravitch procedure, which involved anterior chest incision, resection of costal cartilages, and sternal osteotomy.
- Immediate complications of the Nuss procedure occur in about 10%: mainly small pneumothoraces. 1–5% develop wound infections; rarely, these require bar removal. Bar displacement (including bar flipping over) may occur at any time and affects 5–10% of patients. Significant bar displacement will require re-do surgery.
- There are several case reports of near-fatal bleeding; there have been rare deaths. Hard to quantify risk of severe bleeding but it is probably around 1/500, usually caused by the bar eroding into adjacent arteries.
- Following closed correction there is immediate good or excellent cosmetic result in 80–90% of children. In 5% there is recurrence of the deformity when the bar is removed.
- The procedure is effective in adults so there is no immediate pressure on an adolescent to have the surgery before growth is completed. There is a slightly higher risk of bar displacement in adult patients.
- Benefits on cardiopulmonary function are modest. there appears to be:
  - genuine improvement of exercise ability—probably around a 10% improvement in most children;
  - genuine improvement in cardiovascular function—between 5% and 25% improvement;
  - a possible effect on improvement in lung function. This has been more difficult to demonstrate. Most children with PE have lung function within the normal range and any possible benefit is going to be small. In children with an FVC < 70% there may an increase of 5–10%. Improvement in lung function should not be used as justification for surgery.

- In infants with severe PE not associated with underlying lung disease, increasing the size of the chest cavity can potentially allow lung growth. Alveolar development continues until 8 years of age. Benefit of PE surgery on final lung function in these young children has not been evaluated but it would not be unreasonable to expect benefit. Most centres do not offer surgery in the under-sixes and outcomes of any surgery in younger children would need to be evaluated carefully. Bar displacement may be an important consideration since enforcing restricted activity (most surgeons advise no vigorous physical activity for 6 weeks after surgery) in children < 6 years of age is likely to be difficult.

Further information

Aronson, D.C., Bosgraaf, R.P., van der Horst, C., and Ekkelkamp, S. (2007). Nuss procedure: pediatric surgical solution for adults with pectus excavatum. *World J. Surg.* **31**, 26–9.

Lawson, M.L., Mellins, R.B., Tabangin, M., Kelly, R.E. Jr, Croitoru, D.P., Goretsky, M.J., and Nuss, D. (2005). Impact of pectus excavatum on pulmonary function before and after repair with the Nuss procedure. *J. Pediatr. Surg.* **40** (1), 174–80.

Malek, M.H., Berger, D.E., Marelich, W.D., Coburn, J.W., Beck, T.W., and Housh, T.J. (2006). Pulmonary function following surgical repair of pectus excavatum: a meta-analysis. *Eur. J. Cardio-thorac. Surg.* **30**, 637–43.

Malek, M.H., Berger, D.E., Housh, T.J., Marelich, W.D., Coburn, J.W., and Beck, T.W. (2006). Cardiovascular function following surgical repair of pectus excavatum: a metaanalysis. *Chest* **130**, 506–16.

Rowland, T., Moriarty, K., and Banever, G. (2005). Effect of pectus excavatum deformity on cardiorespiratory fitness in adolescent boys. *Arch. Pediatr. Adolesc. Med.* **159**, 1069–73.

Cahill, J.L., Lees, G.M., and Robertson, H.T. (1984). A summary of preoperative and postoperative cardiorespiratory performance in patients undergoing pectus excavatum and carinatum repair. *J. Pediatr. Surg.* **19**, 430–3.

Kravarusic, D., Dicken, B.J., Dewar, R., Harder, J., Poncet, P., Schneider, M., and Sigalet, D.L. (2006). The Calgary protocol for bracing of pectus carinatum: a preliminary report. *J. Pediatr. Surg.* **41**, 923–6.

Pectus carinatum

- Pectus carinatum (PC) describes a chest wall shape where the sternum and anterior chest wall are unusually prominent. Overgrowth of the costal cartilage has been proposed as a mechanism, but the reason for the overgrowth is not known.
- PC is less common than PE with an incidence estimated at just under 1%. It is commoner in boys.
- As with PE there is an increased incidence in first-degree relatives.
- PC deformity is asymmetrical in 1/3 of children.
- PC is usually apparent from birth, but may worsen with the growth spurt in adolescence.
- The effects of isolated PC on lung function and exercise ability are less well studied that those for PE. What data are available suggest that there is little if any effect on lung volumes, except in the most severe cases. Children may complain of chest pain and apparent increased respiratory effort compared to their peers, but there is no evidence of decreased exercise-related cardiac output. There does appear to be an association with mitral valve prolapse, although the functional significance of this is uncertain.
- Occasionally PC-like deformity is seen in children with underlying lung disease, usually those with air-trapping and hyperinflation, such as children with asthma or CF. In these children respiratory symptoms are due to the underlying lung disease rather than the chest wall deformity.
- PC can also be seen in children with neuromuscular weakness, thoracic dystrophies, scoliosis, and collagen disorders such as Ehlers–Danlos and Marfan syndromes.
- Isolated PC can have adverse psychological effects on children, particularly adolescents. This may deter them from situations, like sport, where they may have to undress. This in turn can contribute to lack of fitness and apparent decreased exercise ability.
- Surgery is possible for PC, generally a modification of the Ravitch technique that uses resection of the deformed costal cartilages along with sternal osteotomy. There are potentially serious complications from this surgery and long-term results are variable.
- Non-surgical approach using external bracing is a safe alternative to surgery and has been reported to have good cosmetic results in small numbers of children. The brace is worn for an initial period of 24h, during which time the defect usually flattens, and thereafter every night until axial growth is complete.

Scoliosis

Adolescent scoliosis (AS)

- AS is defined as a structural lateral curvature of the spine that occurs at or near the onset of puberty, for which no cause is apparent.
- AS is the commonest form of scoliosis with a prevalence of around 2%.
- Overall there is an equal sex incidence, but the severe forms are much more common in girls.
- The lateral curve may be in a single direction or S-shaped.
- Scoliosis is often most apparent on inspection of the back as the child bends forward and, where possible, this should be done. When scoliosis is present, lateral curvature of the spine with or without asymmetry of the posterior chest wall will be seen.
- Severity of scoliosis is assessed by the Cobb angle. Lines are drawn parallel to the end plates of the vertebral bodies at the beginning and the end of the curve. A second set of lines perpendicular to each of the first lines are then drawn and the angle between these two perpendicular lines is measured
- Progression of scoliosis is variable but is more likely when the scoliosis:
  - is moderate or severe (Cobb angle > 30°);
  - is S-shaped or double scoliosis;
  - is associated with vertebral rotation;
  - affects girls;
  - affects the thoracic rather than the lumbar spine.
- Most progression occurs during the growth spurt. Scoliosis of > 30° at the end of growth can progress further in adult life.
- The degree of ossification of the iliac apophysis is a good guide to the stage of spinal growth (Risser sign). Once the apophysis is fully ossified, spinal growth has ceased.
- Most AS is asymptomatic. Back pain can occur during adolescence or later in adult life. Adolescents and adults may feel self-conscious and embarrassed by their scoliosis.
- Mild scoliosis (Cobb angle < 20°) requires no active treatment. The child should be watched until growth has ceased.
- Bracing is effective for moderate scoliosis (Cobb angle 20–40°). The brace must be worn day and night, usually for 2–3y, to be effective.
- Surgery is required for severe scoliosis. Benefits usually limited to reduced back pain in adult life and a better cosmetic result. The effects on lung function are discussed below.
- There are many different surgical techniques. Most use a combination of vertebral fusion with devices, usually spinal rods, to hold the spine straight whilst the fusion becomes secure.

Other forms of scoliosis

- There are other forms of idiopathic scoliosis that affect infants and young children that may be part of a thoracic dystrophy (see 📖 p. 502).
- Scoliosis may be secondary to muscular imbalance. This is seen in children with:
  - muscular weakness;
  - spasticity—usually children with cerebral palsy.

- Scoliosis is also seen in children with collagen disorders such as Marfan and Ehlers–Danlos syndromes.
- Where scoliosis is associated with an underlying problem, it is very likely to continue to progress when growth is complete.
- Bracing in children with neuromuscular weakness is likely to interfere with respiratory function, particularly at night. Braces fit from the iliac crest to the axillae and thus impede abdominal expansion on inspiration. Where there is evidence of night-time hypoventilation, braces should not be worn at night even though this may mean that the scoliosis will progress more rapidly.

Scoliosis and the lung

- Scoliosis has the potential to affect lung function by:
  - impeding the efficient action of the respiratory muscle;
  - reducing the thoracic volume;
  - decreasing the compliance of the chest wall.
- Lung function is only affected when the scoliosis affects the thoracic spine.
- In otherwise healthy adolescents, reduced lung volumes with a restrictive pattern are only seen when thoracic AS is severe (Cobb angles > 60°).
- The effects of scoliosis on lung function in children with muscle weakness are likely to be amplified.
- A mixed restrictive and obstructive picture may be seen in severe scoliosis. The airways obstruction is usually reversible and most likely represents airways irritation secondary to retained secretions.

Scoliosis surgery

- The effects of surgery on lung function remain controversial. The majority view is that surgery does not improve lung function in children with scoliosis. Successful scoliosis surgery will usually reduce the rate of decline of lung function in children with muscular weakness.
- Thoracic scoliosis surgery is a major undertaking. Most operations are performed using a posterior approach only. An anterior approach, traditionally via thoracotomy, may be required for more severe scoliosis to release anterior vertebral ligaments. The adverse impact of the anterior approach on lung function can be significantly reduced using thorascopic techniques.
- Postoperative respiratory failure is a significant risk in children with severe restrictive lung disease, particularly those with muscular weakness. Scoliosis surgery is associated with an acute fall in FVC of around 40% due to a combination of atelectasis and pain. Atelectasis occurs during the long operative period and immediately postoperatively because of poor secretion clearance.
- Postoperative recovery can be complicated by early heart failure and pleural effusions resulting from the massive volumes of fluid required to support these children during surgery. Blood loss can be very high: up to 30% of the circulating volume.

- Predicting which children are at risk of postoperative respiratory failure is not a precise science. Children at highest risk are those with neuromuscular weakness and severe scoliosis. All children undergoing scoliosis surgery should have their lung volumes assessed pre-operatively. If FVC < 40% we would recommend introducing the child to non-invasive mask support and cough-assist secretion clearance devices preoperatively. This makes their use in the postoperative period much more straightforward. Planned extubation on to mask ventilation is usually the best approach for this group of children. We also recommend that all children with neuromuscular weakness for whom scoliosis surgery is planned undergo a sleep study irrespective of their FVC. In a small number there may be unsuspected night-time hypoventilation, which is likely to put these children at high risk of postoperative respiratory failure.

Further information

Koumbourlis, A.C. (2006). Scoliosis and the respiratory system. *Paediatr. Respir. Rev.* **7**, 152–60.

Kishan, S., Bastrom, T., Betz, R.R., Lenke, L.G., Lowe, T.G., Clements, D., D'Andrea, L., Sucato, D.J., and Newton, P.O. (2007). Thoracoscopic scoliosis surgery affects pulmonary function less than thoracotomy at 2 years postsurgery. *Spine* **32**, 453–8.

Velasco, M.V., Colin, A.A., Zurakowski, D., Darras, B.T., and Shapiro, F. (2007). Posterior spinal fusion for scoliosis in Duchenne muscular dystrophy diminishes the rate of respiratory decline. *Spine* **32**, 459–65.

Thoracic insufficiency syndrome

- Thoracic insufficiency syndrome refers to a group of congenital and development disorders of the chest wall and spine that result in respiratory distress due to a combination of:
  - inadequate lung development *in utero* —pulmonary hypoplasia;
  - persisting small volume thorax;
  - poor chest expansion.
- Affected infants may have extensive and progressive congenital thoracic scoliosis, often associated with absent or fused ribs.
- Specific syndromic forms are recognized and include the following.
  - Jarcho–Levin syndrome (spondylothoracic dysplasia). This is usually autosomal recessive and characterized by dwarfism, short thorax with severe pulmonary hypoplasia, multiple vertebral and rib defects, posterior fusion and absence of ribs, lordosis, and kyphoscoliosis.
  - Jeune asphyxiating thoracic dystrophy. This autosomal recessive disease is associated with short-limbed dwarfism and microcystic renal disease.
  - VATER (vertebral anomalies, anal atresia, tracheo-oesophageal fistula with oesophageal atresia, and renal and radial abnormalities).
  - A number of different short rib syndromes.
- 80% of infants with congenital scoliosis will have other congenital malformations affecting 4 or more different organ systems, particularly genitourinary and cardiac anomalies.
- In many infants thoracic insufficiency is severe with hypoventilation, CO_2 retention, and hypoxia. Mechanical ventilation may be required from birth. There can be associated pulmonary hypertension and right heart failure.
- Other infants may develop respiratory failure as their thoracic scoliosis worsens.
- Congenital forms of scoliosis do not respond to bracing. In congenital scoliosis there are bony rather than the soft tissue abnormalities seen in adolescent scoliosis and scoliosis associated with neuromuscular conditions.
- Early surgery has the potential of allowing thoracic cage and therefore lung growth, although this has yet to be demonstrated. Isolated spinal surgery on scoliosis can have unsatisfactory results with progressive downward collapse of the ribs like a folding umbrella. This leads to progressive loss in lung volume. Early spinal fusion will result in reduced thoracic spine growth and decreased lung volumes in the longer term. Since 2000, a new approach based on supporting and expanding the rib cage has been developed. The vertical expandable prosthetic titanium rib (VEPTR) attaches to superior and inferior ribs or the spine and can be used unilaterally or bilaterally to increase the spacing between the ribs and increase the thoracic volume. The devices can be expanded sequentially (under general anaesthetic) to allow for the child's growth.

- The VEPTR method is successful in improving spinal curvature and increasing thoracic volume. There are very limited data on whether it improves functional lung volumes and whether the devices on the chest wall improve or impair chest wall compliance. There are significant technical challenges in measuring infant lung function in children with chest wall devices *in situ*. The 'pump-up and squeeze' method cannot be used.
- VEPTR surgery does appear to reduce respiratory rates and to improve saturations in some but not all children who were de-saturated preoperatively, which suggests better lung function. In some children respiratory failure has been worse after surgery.
- By reducing the progression of the scoliosis whilst allowing linear growth, subsequent spinal surgery in later years may be more straightforward.
- VEPTR surgery is only carried out a specialist centres and children who might benefit from this treatment need to be carefully selected. There are risks, including wound infection and device displacement. A long chest wall incision is required and, once healed, this may affect chest wall expansion. Recovery from surgery is generally much quicker than from standard spinal fusion and blood loss is usually minimal. Good nutritional status is a requirement for surgery to prevent the devices eroding through the skin. This type of surgery is usually restricted to children at risk of progressive respiratory failure. The presence of other life-limiting conditions should also be taken into account when the possible benefits of surgery are considered.

Further information

Campbell, R.M. Jr, Smith, M.D., Mayes, T.C., Mangos, J.A., Willey-Courand, D.B., Kose, N., Pinero, R.F., Alder, M.E., Duong, H.L., and Surber, J.L. (2004). The effect of opening wedge thoracostomy on thoracic insufficiency syndrome associated with fused ribs and congenital scoliosis. *J. Bone Joint Surg. Am.* **86**, 1659–74.

Emans, J.B., Caubet, J.F., Ordonez, C.L., Lee, E.Y., and Ciarlo, M. (2005). The treatment of spine and chest wall deformities with fused ribs by expansion thoracostomy and insertion of vertical expandable prosthetic titanium rib: growth of thoracic spine and improvement of lung volumes. *Spine* **30**, S58–E8.

Waldhausen, J.H., Redding, G.J., and Song, K.M. (2007). Vertical expandable prosthetic titanium rib for thoracic insufficiency syndrome: a new method to treat an old problem. *J. Pediatr. Surg.* **42**, 76–80.

Congenital lung anomalies

Embryology

A basic understanding of the embryology of the lung is helpful when considering congenital lung anomalies. Lung development begins early—in the 4th week of gestation the laryngotracheal diverticulum appears in the foregut. This tube subsequently divides into 2 lung buds, which progressively branch to form the pulmonary tree eventually forming blind-ending terminal bronchioles. The airway epithelium is derived from the endoderm of laryngotracheal tube. The alveoli, blood vessels, and interstitial tissue are derived from the splanchnic mesoderm. At 24 weeks gestation the airway has 17 generations of subdivisions. At term there are 23 divisions.

There are 4 stages of lung maturation.
- Pseudoglandular period (5–17 weeks). All elements of the lungs are developed except those elements involved in gas exchange.
- Canalicular period (16–24 weeks). This period overlaps in different areas of the lung—cranial segments mature faster than caudal ones. Gas exchange units start to form, with the development of the blood supply, respiratory bronchioles, and alveolar ducts. By 20 weeks type II alveolar cells begin producing surfactant.
- Terminal sac period (24 weeks to birth). Many more alveoli develop and the alveolar membranes become thinner. The pulmonary capillary bed develops rapidly. Type 1 alveolar cells differentiate.
- Alveolar period (late fetal period to childhood). This is a period of further alveolar development. At term an infant will have one-sixth the adult number of alveoli. Alveolar numbers continue to increase until the 8th year of life.

Congenital cystic adenomatoid malformation (CCAM)

- This term describes an abnormality of lung development characterized by solid and cystic components.
- The incidence is around 1/25 000 births.
- CCAMs are usually unilateral and usually involve only one lobe of the lung; in 20% the CCAM will cross into an adjacent lobe. Any lobe can be affected. They apparently result from failure of the pulmonary mesenchyme to develop fully and contain disorganized and dilated distal components of the respiratory tract with varying cell types. The cause is not known.
- CCAM can be classified into 5 different types according to size and relative proportions of cystic and solid components. Classifications are histological and do not influence management. Usually CCAMs have a pulmonary arterial and venous supply and are connected to the tracheo-bronchial tree: a requirement for the cysts to become air-filled.
- Apparently large CCAMs seen on antenatal scan may regress during fetal development, but complete resolution is rare.

Presentation

- With improvements in the quality of antenatal scans most CCAMs are now detected *in utero*. More rarely they present in neonatal period with respiratory distress because of a mass effect, compression of main airways, and possible associated pulmonary hypoplasia. Large CCAMs may also be associated with polyhydramnios and hydrops fetalis.
- Outside the neonatal period symptomatic presentations include recurrent pneumonia, pneumothorax, or pulmonary bleeding.
- If CCAM presents with infection, the cystic appearance on CXR can suggest a necrotizing pneumonia. It can be difficult to differentiate between these conditions. In both cases, prolonged antibiotics will be needed. If the infection clears it is worth waiting 3–4 months before repeating the CXR since pneumatoceles associated with necrotizing pneumonias will usually heal completely. If there is persisting CXR abnormality after 3–4 months, a contrast CT scan should be carried out. If the findings are consistent with CCAM, surgery should be planned.
- Important differential diagnosis for CCAM, in addition to necrotizing pneumonia, is diaphragmatic hernia; loops of bowel can resemble cysts.
- There are case reports of malignant tumours (particularly pleuropulmonary blastoma) arising at site of CCAMs, although the attributable risk associated with CCAM is not known. Some tumours have arisen elsewhere in the lung in patients with CCAM and also after resection for CCAM, so it is not clear if surgery reduces risk of malignancy.

Management

- Following antenatal detection, presence of any congenital lung anomaly needs to be confirmed postnatally (Figs 41.1–41.3). In an asymptomatic infant, a CXR adds nothing (since the CCAM could be missed and a CT scan will be needed preoperatively in any case) and should be avoided.

A contrast-enhanced CT should be carried out at around 1 month of age. This will usually confirm the presence of a CCAM-like anomaly. It is important to identify the origin of the blood supply to the anomaly.

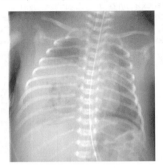

Fig. 41.1 This boy presented with respiratory distress in the neonatal period. His antenatal scan had shown a cystic mass in the chest. This CXR shows opacification of the majority of the lower half of the right hemithorax with some bubble-like radiolucencies projected over the region of the right lower lobe.

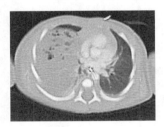

Fig. 41.2 CT scan of same child showing large non-enhancing mass with cystic lucent areas.

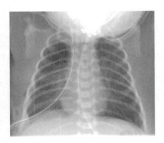

Fig. 41.3 CXR of the same child on first postoperative day. Histology was consistent with CCAM with some elements suggestive of pleuropulmonary blastoma.

- Occasionally what was thought to be a CCAM antenatally will turn out to be congenital lobar emphysema once the lung inflates.
- In children with respiratory distress, infection, pneumothorax, or bleeding, surgical excision of the CCAM is required. Large CCAMS may be associated with lung hypoplasia on the affected side.
- In asymptomatic children with a small CCAM, management is more controversial. Some units would do nothing, others would follow the children annually. Others, like our own unit, opt to remove the CCAM. This can be done safely between 3 and 6 months of age.

Bronchogenic cyst

Bronchogenic cysts arise during fetal development as abnormal budding from the foregut. They are more accurately called foregut duplication cysts. They are usually fluid-filled and most are found in the mediastinum (Fig. 41.4). More rarely they may communicate with the tracheobronchial tree and show an air–fluid level and are occasionally found outside the thoracic cavity. They are lined by respiratory epithelial cells.

Presentation

Most cause no symptoms and are incidental findings on imaging studies. They can:
- cause bronchial compression, resulting in recurrent LTRI;
- cause oesophageal compression, causing dysphagia;
- become infected. This is more likely if there is communication with the tracheobronchial tree and in these instances there may be expectoration of purulent material.

Management

CT scans will show a non-enhancing water-dense sharply demarcated cyst in the mediastinum. This appearance is diagnostic for bronchogenic cysts. Asymptomatic cysts should be left alone. Symptomatic cysts should be excised.

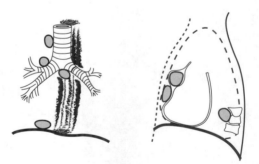

Fig. 41.4 Usual location of bronchogenic cysts.

Congenital lobar emphysema (CLE)

- This condition is thought to be caused either by a narrowed or malacic bronchus resulting in ball-valve obstruction during expiration or by a primary alveolar abnormality. Rarely there may be extrinsic compression of a bronchus by an anomalous vessel, teratoma, bronchogenic cyst, or other masses.
- Emphysema suggests that there is a reduction in alveolar number. This is not the case in CLE (in some affected lobes alveolar numbers are increased). The term congenital lobar overinflation is more accurate.
- In fetal life there is an overexpanded fluid-filled lobe that on antenatal ultrasound can look similar to a CCAM.
- The condition can affect more than one lobe, although this is unusual. The left upper lobe is most commonly affected (40%), followed by the right middle lobe (35%) and the right upper lobe (20%).
- After birth lung fluid clears more slowly from the affected lobe than the normal lung and can give a ground-glass appearance on CXR, before becoming more characteristically hyperexpanded and hyperlucent.

Presentation

- CLE may be detected by antenatal ultrasound. More usually it will present with neonatal respiratory distress, caused by compression of the ipsilateral and contralateral lungs and mediastinal structures by the affected lobe.
- The emphysematous lobes are not prone to infection.
- Occasionally CLE (or another congenital structural anomaly) will be identified unexpectedly on CXR performed as part of investigation of respiratory symptoms. Careful assessment of the nature, onset, and duration of symptoms will be required to determine whether they are related to the lung anomaly.
- CLE seen in older children needs to be distinguished from hyperinflation arising from acquired compression of a bronchus by a mass, such as lymphoma or TB lymphadenopathy, or intrinsic obstruction by a foreign body or carcinoid tumour.

Management

- Neonates with CLE may require support with mechanical ventilation. High inspiratory pressures can worsen the hyperinflation and should be avoided.
- A CXR is usually sufficient to make the diagnosis (Figs 41.5 and 41.6).
- CT scan (Fig. 41.5) can be helpful in determining the extent of the emphysema and identifying any cause of extrinsic compression.
- Bronchoscopy is not usually necessary if a CT scan has been performed. When presentation with lobar overinflation occurs outside the neonatal period, bronchoscopy is indicated to exclude intrinsic or extrinsic bronchial narrowing. In children with CLE, bronchoscopy findings are usually normal.
- Occasionally CLE can be mistaken for a pneumothorax (chest drains should be avoided!).

- 10% of infants with CLE will have other congenital anomalies, particularly heart disease. All infants with CLE should have a cardiac assessment.
- Infants with persistent respiratory distress will need to be treated by excision of the affected lobe. Less marked symptoms in infants who are thriving can be managed conservatively.

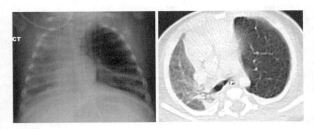

Fig. 41.5 CXR (left) and CT scan (right) of a 5-day-old infant who has a large CLE affecting the left upper lobe and who developed severe respiratory distress requiring mechanical ventilation. There is mediastinal shift, collapse of the left lower lobe, and partial collapse of the right lung. The CLE was resected.

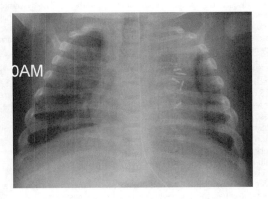

Fig. 41.6 Immediate postoperative CXR appearance of the same infant. His respiratory distress had resolved and he was self-ventilating in air.

Pulmonary sequestration

- This term refers to non-functioning lung tissue that does not have normal bronchial connections and receives its blood supply from one or more systemic arteries.
- Two forms are recognized: intralobar sequestration (ILS) and extralobar sequestration (ELS). (See Fig. 41.7) Both are usually around 3–6cm in diameter.
- ILS is more common (75% of cases), is contained within the lung parenchyma, and occurs almost exclusively in the lower lobes. Occasionally there may be a small communication to the bronchial tree or connections via the pores of Kohn. It is not usually associated with other anomalies. ILS may *not* be congenital in some instances, but acquired after necrotizing pneumonia. The pulmonary supply is lost and the systemic bronchial supply becomes hypertrophied. The tissue shows chronic inflammation and usually contains multiple fluid-filled cysts. Venous drainage is via the pulmonary veins.
- ELS lesions (25% of cases) lie outside the normal visceral pleura and have their own pleural covering. 80% are found between the lower lobes and the diaphragm. 5–10% are found below the diaphragm within the abdomen. ELS lesions probably arise as an accessory lung bud during embryological development. Other anomalies, such as bronchogenic cysts, CCAMs, diaphragmatic hernias, and congenital heart disease, occur in up to 50% of infants with ELS. The systemic arterial supply is usually from the descending aorta. Venous drainage is to the right heart via systemic veins in 85% and via pulmonary veins to the left atrium in 15%. Occasionally ELS lesions can have abnormal connections to the bronchial tree or GI tract.

Presentation

- Recurrent infection is the usual presentation for both ELS and ILS.
- ELS may also present in the neonatal period with respiratory distress or feeding problems, which may be caused by a connection to the oesophagus.
- ELS may also be found as part of the work-up for other congenital anomalies.
- Very large feeder vessels to sequestrated lobes can result in heart failure, usually in the first few weeks of life.
- ILS is a rare cause of haemoptysis.
- Contrast-enhanced CT will be diagnostic in most cases, showing a contrast-enhancing mass, which is occasionally cystic.

Management

- Infants with ELS should be investigated for other congenital anomalies. This usually means cardiac echocardiography in addition to the chest CT scan.
- Pulmonary sequestrations causing symptoms should be excised.
- The arterial and venous drainage may need to be carefully delineated before surgery, usually using a combination of contrast-enhanced CT scan (Fig. 41.8) and angiography.

- There is no broad agreement on the management of asymptomatic sequestration. The most usual situation is that of small sequestrations found at antenatal ultrasound.
  - A case for excision can be made because of the risk of infection.
  - An expectant approach can also be used, although surgery after an infective episode may be more difficult.
  - If the systemic supply is very large, this may mitigate in favour of surgery because of the increased cardiac work that can arise.
- ELS may be associated with adjacent CCAM and this may be used as an argument for surgical resection.

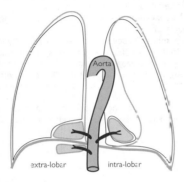

Fig. 41.7 Typical positions for extralobar and intralobar pulmonary sequestration.

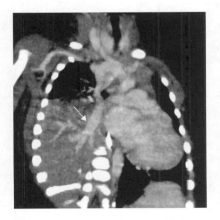

Fig. 41.8 Reconstructed CT image from a 4-week-old girl who presented in heart failure. The scan shows a very large artery (white arrow), probably arising from a remnant of the 4th brachial arch, feeding non-aerated lung tissue. Venous drainage was to the left atrium.

Scimitar syndrome

- This term, like many terms used to describe congenital lung anomalies, is often used imprecisely.
- The key feature is partial anomalous pulmonary venous drainage from a hypoplastic right lung. See Fig. 41.9, 41.10.
- The right upper pulmonary vein drains to the inferior vena cava (IVC) below the diaphragm. This vessel can be large and visible on a CXR giving the appearance of a scimitar.
- The right pulmonary artery is often hypoplastic, and the right lung may have an arterial supply from the aorta.
- The bronchial connections are usually normal and the right lung is usually ventilated effectively.
- Symptoms depend on the severity of the pulmonary hypoplasia. Simple partial anomalous venous drainage is often asymptomatic in childhood. The aberrant venous drainage is effectively a left to right shunt and, if it is large enough, it can eventually cause pulmonary hypertension.
- Treatment depends on the associated anatomy. It may be possible to correct the anomalous pulmonary venous drainage. Establishing normal arterial connections to the lung is more difficult and does not guarantee normal perfusion even if the surgery is technically successful.

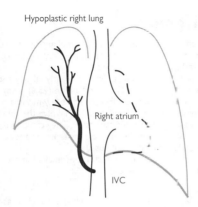

Fig. 41.9 Scimitar syndrome.

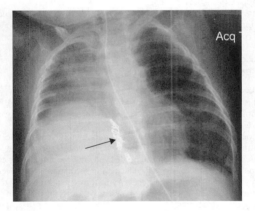

Fig. 41.10 CXR of a 4-month-old girl with scimitar syndrome The right lung is hypoplastic. Venous drainage was to the IVC; the scimitar vein cannot be seen on this film. The right pulmonary artery was hypoplastic and a large systemic artery supplied most of the right lung. This resulted in a significant left to right shunt, which was reduced by occluding the systemic supply with coils (arrow).

Cystic hygroma

- Cystic hygromas, also called cavernous lymphangiomas, are benign cystic lesions that occur deep in the dermis, forming painless swellings of the skin and subcutaneous tissue.
- They are usually first noticed at birth or in early infancy and are most frequently found in the neck (75%) and axillae (25%). They can be massive at birth and grow rapidly in the first few months of life.
- Cystic hygromas in the head and neck can involve the tongue, pharynx, and larynx resulting in airway obstruction. They can also extend down into the mediastinum and the thoracic cavity where they can compress the trachea and surrounding lung tissue.
- Cystic hygroma is associated with chromosomal anomalies, including Turner and Down's syndromes.

Presentation

- Large cystic hygromas may be detected by antenatal ultrasound. Otherwise, most will be obvious as a painless swelling of the head, neck, or axilla at birth.
- Occasionally the swelling may not be obvious until the second year of life. Rarely they may present as thoracic or airway lesions without any obvious external component.
- At any stage they can cause respiratory distress by airway obstruction or compression or, in the case of an intrathoracic lesion, by compressing and collapsing the lung. Cystic hygromas can become infected or bleed into the cysts.
- A sudden bleed can result in cyst expansion and acute airways obstruction.

Management

- MRI is needed to identify the extent of the hygroma (Fig. 41.11). The lesions often surround neurovascular structures including the facial nerve and brachial plexus.
- Although sclerosing agents have been tried, the primary mode of treatment is surgical excision. If the airway is unaffected and the infant can feed normally, excision can be delayed until around 2 years of age.
- Complete removal can be very difficult and recurrence is relatively common (> 10%). It may be necessary to form a tracheostomy to protect the airway in children with cystic hygromas affecting the supraglottic structures.
- Infection with cystic hygromas can occur and may lead to involution of the cysts.
- Recurrent hygromas are not usually treated surgically because of the technical difficulties that result from scarring and fibrosis at the original operation site.
- Blood should be sent for chromosome analysis in all infants with cystic hygroma.

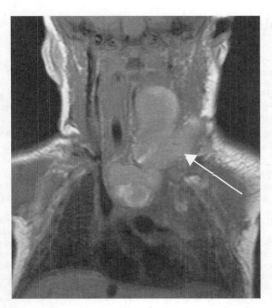

Fig. 41.11 MRI scan of a 6-month-old who presented with stridor requiring intubation following a bleed into a previously undetected cystic hygroma (white arrow). The extrathoracic component was resected with complete resolution of symptoms.

Pulmonary hypoplasia and agenesis

Pulmonary hypoplasia

Pulmonary hypoplasia can arise either because:
- there is insufficient space for the lung to grow,
- there is inadequate blood supply
- there are inadequate breathing movements in utero. (It is thought that breathing movements are an important stimulus to lung growth both *in utero* and in early life.)

The likely causes depend on whether the pulmonary hypoplasia is unilateral or bilateral: see boxes.

Management depends on the cause

- BIPAP may stimulate lung growth in infants with limited lung expansion, particularly those with neuromuscular weakness who have normal lung and chest wall compliance. These possible effects of BIPAP are unproven.
- For conditions where there is active lung compression, allowing space for lung growth should result in some improvement, as there may be compensatory increased expansion of alveolar numbers. The extent of recovery depends on the timing and nature of the underlying mechanism. Space effects present from early development will permanently affect lung size since airway branching is complete by 16 weeks gestation. Draining large effusions *in utero* may be helpful. The benefits of *in utero* surgery for diaphragmatic hernia, including trying to increase lung volume by temporary tracheal occlusion, remain unproven.
- Where there is no reversible cause, treatment is supportive. Severity ranges from mild tachypnoea to severe respiratory distress, and support needed may include long-term oxygen therapy or long term ventilation. Some infants cannot be successfully supported.

Pulmonary agenesis

- Pulmonary agenesis is a developmental defect in which there is unilateral or bilateral complete absence of the lung, bronchus, and vascular supply.
- It is a rare anomaly with an incidence of 1/20 000. The cause is not known.
- Bilateral agenesis results in stillbirth.
- Unilateral agenesis affects right and left lungs equally. Right-sided aplasia is associated with a higher mortality, possibly because of greater shift of mediastinal structures.
- There may be a residual stump of bronchial tissue at the carina, which can be a site of mucus collection and predispose to recurrent infection.
- The remaining lung is generally larger than usual with greater numbers of alveoli.
- There may be ipsilateral hypoplasia of the face and forearm and ipsilateral renal agenesis.
- Bronchial or tracheal compression can occur, often from vascular structures, because of anatomical distortion, which can be improved surgically.

- Children are often symptomatic, presenting with recurrent infection with respiratory distress.
- Outcome is variable and may depend on the presence of associated anomalies. Long-term survival has been reported.

Causes of bilateral pulmonary hypoplasia

Space
- Ascites usually with large pleural effusions, often with hydrops fetalis
- Large abdominal tumours such as teratomas
- Abnormal chest wall: large and tight amniotic bands or abnormal ribs such as in Jeune's asphyxiating thoracic dystrophy
- Oligohydramnios: usually caused either by premature rupture of membranes (< 26 weeks gestation) or urinary tract obstruction

Blood supply
- Conditions associated with decreased lung perfusion, such as Fallot's tetralogy are associated with decreased alveolar number. The pulmonary hypoplasia is usually mild and asymptomatic.

Breathing movements
- Neuromuscular weakness, particularly spinal muscular atrophy and myotonic dystrophy, can reduce fetal breathing movements, which are required for normal lung growth

Causes of unilateral pulmonary hypoplasia

Space
- Diaphragmatic hernia
- Congenital cystic adenomatoid malformation
- Congenital lobar emphysema

Blood supply
- Pulmonary artery branch stenosis, systemic arterial supply, Fallot's tetralogy, and anomalous venous drainage can all be associated with pulmonary hypoplasia. Whether the hypoplasia results from the abnormal blood supply or is part of a more global defect is not known. Scimitar syndrome is an example of systemic supply with anomalous drainage and unilateral lung hypoplasia.

Breathing movements
Effects are always bilateral.

Diaphragmatic hernia

- In this condition abdominal contents are present in the thoracic cavity as a result of a defect in the diaphragm. Most will occur as a congenital abnormality. More rarely they can be traumatic.
- The congenital form is most usually a defect in the posterolateral diaphragm (so-called Bochdalek hernia), more commonly on the left than the right. The anterior Morgagni hernia is found in only 5% of cases.
- The presence of the abdominal contents in the chest cavity during fetal development leads to variable degrees of pulmonary hypoplasia. In its severest form this will affect both the ipsilateral and contralateral lungs.
- 40% of infants with congenital diaphragmatic hernia will have another congenital abnormality, usually cardiac, renal, or chromosomal anomalies (especially trisomies).
- Traumatic diaphragmatic hernia is a rare consequence of blunt trauma, usually as a result of a road traffic accident. There is nearly always associated liver or spleen injury.

Presentation

- The majority of congenital diaphragmatic hernias will either be detected by antenatal ultrasound scan or present with respiratory distress immediately after delivery.
- Smaller diaphragmatic defects may not present until later in childhood. In these cases, it is possible for increasing amounts of small bowel to move into the chest cavity through a relatively small defect. These children can present with abdominal pain, recurrent 'pneumonia', or, occasionally, acutely with small bowel volvulus.
- Diaphragmatic hernias detected early and resulting in significant pulmonary hypoplasia are usually left-sided (right-sided defects are partially plugged by the liver).

Management

- The definitive management of diaphragmatic hernia is surgical.
- In the late-presenting child, the CXR appearances can be confused with a staphylococcal pneumonia with pneumatoceles or a congenital cystic lung abnormality. If there is doubt, an ultrasound can show peristaltic movements of the bowel in the chest, and an upper GI contrast study will show bowel above the diaphragm. If there is any suggestion of volvulus, urgent surgery is life-saving.
- Following surgery for neonatal diaphragmatic hernia, outcome is dependent on the severity of pulmonary hypoplasia. This can be complicated by pulmonary hypertension and dysfunctional diaphragm function.
- On occasions where there is difficulty weaning infants from the ventilator or when, once extubated, infants struggle with respiratory distress and poor growth, non-invasive ventilatory support can be very useful. Used intermittently during the day and for overnight support, non-invasive ventilation can provide periods of respiratory rest, which allow the infant to grow and any parenchymal lung damage to improve.

This type of support, along with oxygen therapy, may be needed for several months in the more severely affected infants. Progress can be complicated by recurrent herniation, a particular risk with large original defects closed with an artificial patch, patch infection, and incidental LRTI. Feeding problems are also common, including severe gastro-oesophageal reflux.

Further information

Bush, A. (2001). Congenital lung disease: a plea for clear thinking and clear nomenclature. *Pediatr. Pulmonol.* **32**, 328–37.

Calvert, J.K. and Lakhoo, K. (2007). Antenatally suspected congenital cystic adenomatoid malformation of the lung: postnatal investigation and timing of surgery. *J. Pediatr. Surg.* **42**, 411–14.

Craniofacial abnormalities

Introduction

The craniofacial abnormalities can be divided into two main groups:
- children with micrognathia but normal midface anatomy;
- children with midface hypoplasia.

Within these groups there are children with asymmetrical problems and children with a combination of problems. Many of the craniofacial abnormalities are syndromic and the responsible genetic mutations are increasingly being defined. Airway problems are generally of obstruction and sometimes obstruction occurs at more than one site. There are significant changes with growth and many of these children need long-term respiratory assessment. Less commonly children with craniosynostosis may develop central hypoventilation as a result of brainstem compression usually associated with raised intracranial pressure.

Syndromes with micrognathia

Children with syndromes that involve micrognathia, such as Pierre Robin sequence, Treacher–Collins syndrome, and Goldenhar syndrome, become obstructed at the hypopharyngeal level. The hypopharynx, sometimes called the laryngopharynx, is the lower part of the pharynx that connects the throat to the oesophagus.

Robin sequence

This sequence was described in 1923 by Pierre Robin as airway obstruction associated with glossoptosis and hypoplasia of the mandible. Pierre Robin sequence has 3 essential components: micrognathia and/or retrognathia; central cleft palate; and relative glossoptosis. Approximately 30% of children with this combination of problems have Stickler syndrome and a further 15% have velocardiofacial syndrome. Others are sporadic and may be related to intrauterine problems restricting mandibular growth. The sporadic forms have better mandible growth postnatally and associated airways obstruction is more likely to improve without surgical intervention.

Stickler syndrome

Stickler syndrome is a multisystem connective tissue disorder that can affect the eye, craniofacies, inner ear, heart, and joints. Incidence is 1 in 7500–9000. Inheritance is autosomal dominant or sporadic. Mutations affecting one of three genes (COL2A1, COL11A1, and COL11A2) have been associated with Stickler syndrome.

- Eye problems include:
  - congenital or early-onset cataract;
  - vitreous anomaly, retinal detachment;
  - myopia greater than −3 diopters.
- Craniofacial problems include:
  - midface hypoplasia, depressed nasal bridge, anteverted nares;
  - bifid uvula, cleft hard palate;
  - micrognathia;
  - Robin sequence (micrognathia, cleft palate, glossoptosis).
- Ear problems include sensorineural or conductive hearing loss;
- Joint problems include:
  - joint hypermobility;
  - mild spondyloepiphyseal dysplasia;
  - early onset osteoarthritis.
- Heart problems include:
  - mitral valve prolapse.

Velocardiofacial syndrome

- 22q11.2 deletion syndrome and, less commonly, 10p13–p14 deletion syndrome are both associated with velocardiofacial syndrome and the same mutations can also result in DiGeorge syndrome. The incidence of velocardiofacial syndrome is around 1 in 15 000–18 000.
- Individuals with the 22q11.2 deletion syndrome (del 22q11.2) have a range of abnormalities that include:

- characteristic facial features (present in the majority of Caucasian individuals);
- learning difficulties (70–90%);
- congenital heart disease (74%; tetralogy of Fallot, interrupted aortic arch, ventricular septal defect, and truncus arteriosus);
- immune deficiency (abnormal T-cell function; 77%);
- hypocacaemia (hypoparathyroidism; 50%)
- palatal abnormalities (69%), particularly velopharyngeal incompetence (VPI), submucosal cleft palate, and cleft palate;
- significant feeding problems (30%);
- hearing loss (both conductive and sensorineural);
- laryngotracheo-oesophageal anomalies, e.g. vascular ring and laryngeal web;
- renal anomalies (37%).

Goldenhar syndrome (oculo-auricular vertebral syndrome)

- The features of Goldenhar syndrome include
  - asymmetrical skull with unilateral micrognathia;
  - vision defects, including unilateral vestigial eye;
  - conjunctival dermoid cysts;
  - auricular appendices with pretragal blind fistula;
  - conductive hearing defect of variable degree sometimes with absence of the middle ear cavity;
  - skeletal abnormalities, e.g. accessory ribs and abnormal vertebrae;
  - moderate mental retardation in approximately 10% of cases.
- When the vertebral defects and eye anomalies are present the condition is designated as the Goldenhar syndrome. When one side of a child's face is smaller or underdeveloped in comparison with the other side without other abnormalities, it is known as hemifacial microsomia.
- The aetiology is unknown.
- Male-female ratio 2:1.
- The incidence is 1 in every 3000–5000 live births.

Treacher–Collins syndrome

- Treacher–Collins syndrome (TCS) is characterized by;
  - hypoplasia of the zygomatic bones (midface. 89%);
  - hypoplasia of the mandible (78%);
  - external ear abnormalities (77%);
  - coloboma of the lower eyelid (45%);
  - absence of the lower eyelid cilia (50%);
  - conductive hearing loss (40–50%) most commonly due to malformation of the ossicles and hypoplasia of the middle ear cavities;
  - cleft palate (28%) with or without cleft lip;
  - unilateral or bilateral choanal stenosis or atresia;
  - normal intellect.
- Aetiology. Mutations in TCOF1 are found in 90–95% of individuals.
- Inheritance: autosomal dominant (40%) or sporadic.

Airway problems associated with micrognathia

- The airway problems in micrognathia are caused by the posteriorly sited tongue falling back on to the posterior wall of the pharynx (particularly where there is a cleft palate) and causing airway obstruction. As the infant attempts to breathe and generates a negative pressure below the site of obstruction this simply 'sucks' the tongue on to the pharyngeal wall exacerbating the airway obstruction.
- The airway difficulties range from minimal to severe and are related to the extent of the mandibular hypoplasia.
- Mild problems are managed by positioning alone with side or prone lying and careful positioning during feeding.
- Infants with moderate or severe problems can almost always be managed with a nasopharyngeal airway. The airway acts both as a physical restraint to the tongue falling on to the posterior palate but more importantly maintains equal pressure along the airway. Ventilation may occur through mouth or the opposite nostril as well as the naso-pharyngeal tube. See 📖 Chapter 63 for advice on passing and securing a nasopharyngeal airway.
- Polysomnography can be used to determine if the nasopharyngeal tube is in the correct position to relieve obstruction. Occasionally small adjustments (0.5cm) need to be made to tube length to obtain optimum position.
- Once parents have learned to look after the tube in position and to replace a tube and can cope with feeding (many children will have some of their feed by NGT) the child can go home. Arrangements are made for review sleep studies. The usual pattern, e.g. with an infant with Robin sequence, is for the nasopharyngeal tube to be in day and night for 4–6 months, then nocturnal only until 9–12 months of age dependent on initial severity, growth, and progress.
- In Goldenhar syndrome and Treacher–Collins syndrome the facial asymmetry may make the problem more severe and interventions other than a nasopharyngeal tube are more likely than in Robin sequence.
- Other techniques that are occasionally used include tongue–lip adhesion, where the tongue is pulled forward and the undersurface of the tongue stitched to the lower lip. Another surgical technique is glossopexy where the tongue is held by a stitch through the tongue to a button under the mandible. The tongue is thus prevented from falling backwards.
- Early distraction osteogenesis is favoured by some surgeons. This technique for progressive elongation of the mandible carries risks of damage to nerves and tooth eruption.
- In the most severe cases tracheostomy is the only way to secure a safe airway.
- In an infant with airway compromise the repair of cleft palate is delayed until the obstruction has resolved with growth. In non-syndromic Robin sequence this generally means that the palate is not repaired until 12–18 months.

Syndromic craniosynostosis

Fibroblast growth factor receptor (FGFR)-related craniosynostosis syndromes

- There are eight disorders considered to be part of the FGFR-related craniosynostosis spectrum. These are:
  - Pfeiffer syndrome;
  - Apert syndrome;
  - Crouzon syndrome;
  - Crouzon syndrome with acanthosis nigricans;
  - Beare–Stevenson syndrome;
  - FGFR2-related isolated coronal synostosis;
  - Jackson–Weiss syndrome;
  - Muenke syndrome (FGFR3-related isolated coronal synostosis).
- Incidence: Crouzon syndrome, 1.6/100 000; Apert syndrome, 1/100 000; all Pfeiffer syndromes, 1/100 000. The other syndromes are even rarer.
- Mutations in FGFR2 gene cause 100% of Crouzon, Apert, and Pfeiffer types 2 and 3 and 95% of Pfeiffer type 1 (the remaining 5% being caused by a mutation in FGFR1). Crouzon with acanthosis nigricans is caused by a mutation in FGFR3.

Crouzon syndrome

- Craniofacial: significant proptosis; external strabismus; mandibular prognathism.
- Hands and feet: normal.
- Intellect: normal.
- Other: high risk of intracranial hypertension; progressive hydrocephalus (30%), with tonsillar herniation.
- Cutaneous: 5% of individuals with Crouzon syndrome have acanthosis nigricans. Acanthosis nigricans can be present in the neonatal period or appear later.

Apert syndrome

- Craniofacial: turribrachycephalic (tower-shaped) skull shape; moderate-to-severe midface hypoplasia.
- Hands and feet: soft tissue and bony ('mitten glove') syndactyly of fingers and toes involving variable number of digits; occasional rhizomelic shortening; elbow ankylosis.
- Intellect: varying degrees of developmental delay/mental retardation (50%), possibly related to the timing of craniofacial surgery.
- Other: fused cervical vertebrae (68%), usually C5–C6; hydrocephalus (2%); occasional internal organ anomalies.

Pfeiffer syndrome

Pfeiffer syndrome is subdivided into 3 types; types 2 and 3 are more common than type 1.

Pfeiffer syndrome type 1

- Craniofacial: moderate-to-severe midface hypoplasia.
- Hands and feet: broad and medially deviated thumbs and great toes; variable degree of brachydactyly.

- Intellect: usually normal.
- Other: hearing loss, hydrocephalus can be seen. A better prognosis than Pfeiffer syndrome types 2 and 3

Pfeiffer syndrome type 2

- Craniofacial: cloverleaf skull (a trilobar skull deformity caused by synostosis of coronal, lambdoidal, metopic, and sagittal sutures); severe proptosis (often unable to close eyelids).
- Hands and feet: broad and medially deviated thumbs and great toes; ankylosis of elbows, knees; variable degree of brachydactyly.
- Intellect: developmental delay/mental retardation common.
- Other: choanal stenosis/atresia; laryngotracheal abnormalities; hydrocephalus; seizures; increased risk of early death.

Pfeiffer syndrome type 3

- Craniofacial: turribrachycephalic skull shape; severe proptosis (often unable to close eyelids).
- Hands and feet: broad and medially deviated thumbs and great toes; ankylosis of elbows, knees; variable degree of brachydactyly.
- Intellect: developmental delay/mental retardation common.
- Other: choanal stenosis/atresia; laryngotracheal abnormalities; hydrocephalus; seizures; increased risk of early death.

Other craniosynostosis syndromes

There are other craniosynostosis syndromes associated with other genetic mutations but in general these are less likely to be associated with significant airway problems.

Saethre–Chotzen syndrome (also known as acrocephalosyndactyly type 3)

- Craniofacial: coronal synostosis; ptosis; facial asymmetry; small ears.
- Hands and feet: finger syndactyly second and third digits.
- Intellect: normal.
- Genetics : mutation in TWIST transcription gene, which maps to 7p21–p22.
- Inheritance : autosomal dominant.

Airway problems associated with syndromic craniosynostosis

- The characteristic facial features related to airway obstruction are:
  - midfacial hypoplasia with proptosis;
  - choanal stenosis or atresia;
  - high-arched palate (frequent); cleft palate (rarely).
- There is usually generalized narrowing of the nasal passages with a very shallow nasopharynx. Breathing problems can occur in the first few weeks or months of life because of upper airway obstruction. They may present anywhere on the spectrum from life-threatening respiratory failure to failure to thrive resulting from poor feeding.
- Investigations include airway imaging and polysomnography.
- Most often the choanal stenosis is such that a nasopharyngeal airway cannot be passed. Rarely choanal stents can be used. For infants who have obstruction only during sleep then nasal CPAP can be very effective. In some infants a full face mask needs to be used and in others custom-made nasal masks are needed. Careful mask fitting is essential to avoid damage to prominent eyes. For infants with severe obstruction (and almost universally in Pfeiffer syndrome) a tracheostomy is necessary.
- Lower airway abnormalities. There are a number of associated lower airway abnormalities. Subglottic stenosis is particularly associated with Crouzon syndrome. Complete tracheal cartilage rings, existing either as a short segment or a complete vertically fused trachea of nonsegmented cartilage, have been described in Apert, Crouzon, and Pfeiffer syndromes. These children commonly present with episodes of recurrent LRTIs and reactive airway disease and can have chronically retained secretions.
- Variation with growth. The variety of potential causes of airway obstruction means that there may be significant changes with growth. A child with primarily nasal obstruction in infancy can develop oropharyngeal problems later in childhood as anatomy changes, the palate thickens, and tonsils grow.
- Regular assessment should include consideration of sleep-disordered breathing. There is interaction between sleep-disordered breathing and intracranial hypertension, which is a common result of craniosynostosis. Both conditions can cause failure to thrive, somnolence, vomiting, and behavioural problems. CO_2 retention may contribute to raised intracranial pressure and raised intracranial pressure can cause cerebellar tonsillar herniation with central disturbance of control of breathing.

Down's syndrome

- There are a number of craniofacial abnormalities in Down's syndrome, which are variable between individuals but which predispose to upper airway obstruction. These include:
  - midface hypoplasia;
  - micrognathia;
  - a small nasopharynx;
  - large tongue.
- These anatomical problems are exacerbated by:
  - muscle hypotonia;
  - recurrent URTI and chronic rhinitis consequent to relatively decreased cell-mediated immunity.
- Many children with Down's syndrome are mouth-breathers and noisy breathing during sleep is almost universal. There is a high incidence (60%) of obstructive sleep apnoea (OSA).
- Tonsillectomy and adenoidectomy result in improvement but some children remain obstructed. MRI in children with OSA after palatine tonsillectomy has revealed a higher incidence of lingular tonsils in Down's syndrome.
- There is an increased incidence of pulmonary hypertension in Down syndrome even in those with structurally normal hearts and no evidence of OSA. The pulmonary circulation is more labile and pulmonary pressures may not ever have fallen to normal levels in the transition from fetal to newborn life.
- Lung histology from children with Down's syndrome shows changes consistent with a primary abnormality of the pulmonary bed. The peripheral pulmonary arteries are small with medial hyperplasia combined with tortuous dilatated pulmonary veins. There are associated parenchymal changes, often with reduced numbers of enlarged alveoli and subpleural cysts.
- The pulmonary capillary bed abnormalities predispose children with Down's syndrome to low grade alveolar haemorrhage.

Further information
Perkins, J.A., Sie, K.C., Milczuk, H., and Richardson, M.A. (1997). Airway management in children with craniofacial anomalies. *Cleft Palate Craniofac. J.* **34**, 135–40.

Atopic eczema and allergic rhinitis

Atopic eczema (atopic dermatitis)

Epidemiology and definitions

- Atopy (allergic sensitization) is a manifestation of altered T-cell function and is characterized by raised IgE levels and eosinophilia. It can be defined as the inherited tendency to develop one or more of the following conditions:
  - atopic asthma;
  - allergic rhinitis;
  - atopic dermatitis;
  - acute allergic urticaria.
- Atopic eczema normally appears in the first year of life but is uncommon under 2 months of age.
- Common initial sites in infancy are the face and hands, then extensor surfaces of the limbs. In older children the pattern changes to principally affect flexural aspects of limbs and other sites of friction.
- Atopic eczema appears as papules and vesicles with background erythema. Chronic excoriation may lead to lichenification and superinfection.
- *Staphylococcus aureus* colonization is highly prevalent in affected patients. Immunostimulatory superantigen toxins produced by both staphylococci and streptococci contribute to exacerbations of eczema.
- Prevalence approximately 20% under age 12 years. In 60% of individuals eczema clears by age 12 years and in 75% it has resolved by age 16 years. Up to 10% will recur in adult life.

Management

- Treatment is aimed at reducing itchiness, inflammation, and infection.
- The mainstay of treatment is with liberal use of emollients, bath oils, topical corticosteroids, oral antihistamines, antibiotics, and wet wraps to break an intractable itch–scratch–itch cycle (wet wraps are emollient with or without diluted steroid applied to the skin and covered with a moist elastic tubular bandage).
- For severe disease, immunomodulatory drugs such as tacrolimus or pimecrolimus in topical preparation or systemic azathioprine or ciclosporin may be used. These drugs should be administered under the supervision of a paediatric dermatologist.
- Breastfeeding may delay the onset of atopic eczema.
- In cases of severe atopic eczema, where cow's milk protein intolerance is suspected, a trial of hydrolysed formula feed (such as Nutramigen) with exclusion of dairy products and egg may be warranted, and should be supervised by a paediatric dietician. Other dietary manipulations are generally unsuccessful.

Allergic rhinitis

Allergic rhinitis is a symptomatic disorder of the nose induced after allergen exposure by an IgE-mediated inflammation of the nasal membranes.

Epidemiology

- Allergic rhinitis affects 10–25% of the population.
- It is most common during school-age years and is unusual before the age of 2 years.
- Symptoms of allergic rhinitis may impair school performance. This may be exacerbated by sedating antihistamine treatment.
- Asthma and allergic rhinitis are common comorbidities.
- Conjunctivitis and sinusitis are commonly seen in association with allergic rhinitis, but the reported links with nasal polyposis and otitis media are less clear.
- Classification is by chronicity and severity of symptoms.
  - Persistent rhinitis is present > 4 days/week and for > 4 weeks duration. Less frequent disease is called intermittent rhinitis.
  - Moderate–severe disease causes one or more of: abnormal sleep; impairment of daily activities; problems at school; troublesome symptoms. Less severe symptoms are classified as mild rhinitis.
- Triggers for allergic rhinitis are:
  - domestic allergens including house dust mites, domestic animals, and insects;
  - common outdoor allergens including pollens and moulds—these are responsible for seasonal allergic rhinitis (hay fever);
  - pollutants such as tobacco smoke, domestic aerosols, and traffic exhaust may exacerbate symptoms.

Symptoms

- Symptoms may vary from sneezing, itching, and rhinorrhoea to nasal blockage.
- 'Sneezers and runners' are worse in the day, improve at night, and are more likely to have associated conjunctivitis.
- 'Nasal blockers' have continuous symptoms that may worsen at night.

Examination

- The nasal mucosa in children can be easily inspected with an otoscope.
- The mucosa in allergic rhinitis is usually a pale greyish colour, with turbinate oedema.
- In infective rhinitis, the mucosa will be red.
- Nasal secretions in rhinitis are typically thin and clear, but thicker yellow secretions can be found in allergic rhinitis. Purulent secretions with fever and facial pain suggest sinusitis.

Differential diagnosis

- Simple infective rhinitis. Troublesome rhinitis in young children is usually infective in origin. Rhinitis associated with URTI will last 7–10 days; recurrent infections can give the appearance of persistence.

- Primary ciliary dyskinesia. Suggested by persistent purulent discharge, especially with recurrent otitis media.
- Cystic fibrosis. Suggested by the presence of nasal polyps (and usually chest or GI symptoms).
- Nasal foreign body. Often offensive discharge of relatively short duration.
- The diagnosis of allergic rhinitis is usually made clinically. Skin prick testing and allergen-specific IgE testing may be useful in identifying responsible allergens. Nasal cytology and nasal imaging can also be performed, but usually add little to history and examination findings.

Treatment options

Intranasal preparations

- Corticosteroids reduce nasal reactivity and inflammation and are the most effective treatment for all symptoms of allergic rhinitis including nasal obstruction.
- H1-antihistamines provide rapidly effective treatment for nasal symptoms except nasal congestion. Consider as add-on treatment if itch/sneeze symptoms are prominent.
- Anticholinergics are particularly effective for rhinorrhoea.
- Cromoglicate provides short-acting and moderately effective treatment for nasal symptoms. Eye drops are more effective for ocular symptoms.
- Decongestants are effective for nasal congestion but recommended for short-term treatment only. Prolonged use can cause rebound symptoms on discontinuation, leading to a repetitive cycle of decongestant use and persistent symptoms—rhinitis medicamentosa.
- Sympathomimetics may affect sleep.

Oral therapy

- H1-antihistamines have a rapid effect on nasal and ocular symptoms and are a good first-line treatment for intermittent symptoms but work poorly for nasal congestion. Second generation drugs such as cetirizine, loratidine are non-sedative.
- Montelukast is well tolerated drug with good effect on most symptoms of allergic rhinitis including nasal obstruction. A sensible choice in children with concomitant asthma symptoms.
- Oral corticosteroids are reserved for severe symptoms refractory to intranasal treatment.

Specific immunotherapy

- Specific immunotherapy (SIT) has been documented to be effective in children for symptoms of allergic rhinitis. Immunotherapy results in a decrease in antigen-specific IgE, an increase in antigen-specific IgG, and modification of the cytokine profile.
- SIT is used widely in Europe and some parts of the US. It is used infrequently in the UK.
- SIT is usually reserved for children with debilitating symptoms.
- Subcutaneous immunotherapy carries a remote risk of severe adverse reaction, particularly in asthmatics or during an exacerbation. Compliance is particularly difficult during the induction phase.

- Induction phase subcutaneous injections of escalating dose are administered weekly. Maintenance phase maintenance dose is given on a monthly basis for several years.
- Symptom remission following SIT may last for up to 3 years after discontinuation of treatment.
- High dose sublingual-swallow and nasal-specific immunotherapy (SLIT) has a good safety profile and has been shown to be effective in children with allergic rhinitis. Long-term benefits after discontinuation not fully clarified
- Administration is by trained practitioners only.
- SIT is not recommended in children < 5 years of age.

Further information

Bachert, C. and van Cauwenberge, P. (2003). The WHO ARIA (allergic rhinitis and its impact on asthma) initiative. *Chem. Immunol. Allergy* **82**, 119–26.
ARIA website: *www.whiar.org*.

Food allergy

Definitions and epidemiology

Food allergy is common in children, particularly in the pre-school age group in whom it has an incidence of 5–8%. Symptoms are generally mild and can include any of the following:
- skin—flushing, rashes, and itching;
- nose—with sneezing, nasal congestion, and itching;
- eyes—tearing and itching;
- gut—vomiting, cramps and diarrhoea, colic;
- mouth—swelling of the lips and tongue, oral tingling.

A small proportion (much less than 1% of those with food allergy) suffers from more severe reactions. A practical definition of *anaphylaxis* includes one or both of:
- respiratory difficulties caused by laryngeal oedema and/or bronchospasm;
- hypotension (light-headedness or dizziness) caused by loss of vasomotor tone.

Fatal anaphylaxis is very uncommon in the UK; a survey identified only 8 paediatric deaths over the 10-year period 1990–2000. Risk factors for anaphylaxis are:
- the presence of asthma, especially poorly controlled asthma;
- previous episodes of anaphylaxis;
- allergy to peanuts, tree nuts (walnuts and pecan nuts), and shellfish.

The contribution of food allergy to asthma symptoms is controversial, but up to 10% of children with asthma may have food-associated triggers to their usual wheeze.

History

A good history is the key to making a diagnosis of food allergy. Important features include the following.
- Timing: symptoms should occur within 2h of ingestion.
- Amount: small amounts of food are usually sufficient to cause the reaction.
- Repetition: symptoms should occur on each occasion the food is consumed.
- Other atopic illness: eczema, hay fever, asthma. Most children with significant allergic reactions will be atopic.
- The severity and nature of the reactions should be documented.

Investigation

Skin prick tests

Where there is history suggesting an allergic reaction, skin prick tests (SPT) can be helpful. Commercially extracts are available for most of the likely foods. Extracts from fruit and vegetables are less reliable because the proteins in these foods are readily degraded. Although SPT are generally very safe, even in those with a history of severe allergy, systemic reactions can occur and resuscitation equipment and trained personnel should be available on site. Oral antihistamines need to be stopped at least 48h prior to the test, and any topical emollients at the test site should be omitted on the day of the test.

- A negative SPT means that the child is very unlikely to react to that food.
- A positive SPT has a predictive value of around 60%.
- The severity of the reaction to a SPT does not correlate with the severity of clinical symptoms.

Serum-specific IgE

These blood tests (RAST and ELISA) are not superior to SPT but may be helpful when skin tests cannot be performed, either because of severe eczema or because antihistamines cannot be stopped. The interpretation of positive and negative results is the same as for SPTs. There is no added value in carrying out serum-specific IgE tests in children who have had SPTs.

Food challenge

- This remains the gold-standard test.
- For most immediate allergic reactions it is not required, particularly where the history is clear and there is a positive SPT.
- Where there is doubt, usually where the symptoms are more chronic and persistent (often gut symptoms), food challenge can be the best way to identify the causative food.
- The suspected foods need to be excluded from the diet for at least 2 weeks and the associated symptoms must have abated. A double-blind challenge can then be used to test individual foods.

Treatment

- Once a food has been identified as being very likely to be or definitely associated with allergy, avoidance is the main aim of management. This is best achieved by discussion with a dietician.
- Simple treatment with oral antihistamines will reduce the duration of symptoms from mild allergic reactions.
- Children with a history of severe reactions (difficulty breathing, light-headedness, or dizziness) should be provided with an adrenaline auto-injector. These devices deliver an IM injection of adrenaline. Two strengths are available, 0.3mg for those > 30kg and 0.15mg for those < 30kg. The dose should be repeated after 5min if there has been no improvement.
- The consequences of prescribing an adrenaline auto-injector should not be underestimated. The child and family must be told exactly how and when to administer the dose. The school will also need to be informed, and a member of staff identified who would be able to give the injection. The child will need to carry the adrenaline at all times when it is possible they will be exposed to the allergen. The auto-injector will need to be replaced every 6 months. The need to carry the auto-injector should be reviewed on an annual basis.

Emergency treatment of anaphylaxis

- A severe reaction in the hospital setting should be treated with IM adrenaline (10mcg/kg of 1 in 1000), repeated if necessary
- This should be followed by chlorpheniramine by slow IV or IM injection and hydrocortisone IV
- If there is evidence of shock, a bolus of 20mL/kg of normal saline may be necessary
- If there is marked stridor a nebulized dose of adrenaline (5mL of 1 in 1000) can be given
- Wheeze should be treated with nebulized salbutamol

Outcome

Food allergies tend to become less severe as children get older. 85% of children with milk allergy will no longer react by the age of 3 years. Allergies to peanut, tree nuts, and shellfish are more likely to persist. Subsequent exposures do not tend to result in increasingly severe reactions.

Heart disease

Introduction

Neither the heart nor the lungs exists in isolation. Respiratory complications frequently accompany cardiac disorders. The disorders fall into 3 main groups:
- high pulmonary blood flow secondary to large volume left to right shunts;
- high pulmonary venous pressure;
- large airway compression secondary to vascular abnormalities.

High pulmonary blood flow

Cardiac abnormalities that cause significant left to right shunts are common. Less common abnormalities such as atrioventricular canal defects, single ventricle, or truncus arteriosus are associated with bidirectional blood flow.

Pathophysiology

High pulmonary blood flow distends the small pulmonary arteries and increases pulmonary arterial pressure. It also increases pulmonary venous pressure resulting in peribronchial and interstitial oedema. The distended small pulmonary arteries cause some extrinsic compression of the small airways and the peribronchial and interstitial oedema can result in muco-sal oedema of the small airways. In combination this results in narrowed airways and high airways resistance. In addition the high pulmonary blood flow decreases lung compliance. The combination of increased airways resistance and decreased lung compliance results in increased work of breathing.

Clinical features

The clinical features are those of tachypnoea with recession accompanied by high-pitched auscultatory wheeze (cardiac asthma) and fine crackles. There will usually be a cardiac murmur, cardiomegaly, and hepatomegaly.

Investigation

- CXR: usually shows cardiomegaly and increased interstitial markings consistent with cardiac failure.
- Echocardiography: will show evidence of ventricular dilatation and underlying structural defects.

Management

- The management is that of the cardiac failure.
- Respiratory failure may occur, often during an intercurrent respiratory illness. Mechanical ventilation may be needed. See 🕮 p. 538.

High pulmonary venous pressure

This can occur because of the following.
- Pulmonary venous obstruction:
  - usually as part of more complicated congenital heart disease, especially total anomalous pulmonary venous drainage (TAPVD);
  - stenosis of pulmonary veins after surgery, e.g. after repair of TAPVD.
- Obstruction within the left atrium:
  - cor triatriatum;
  - mitral stenosis.

- High left atrial pressures:
  - mitral regurgitation;
  - cardiomyopathy;
  - poor left ventricular emptying—severe aortic stenosis or co-arctation.

Pathophysiology

High pulmonary venous pressure results in increased pulmonary blood volume and interstitial and peribronchial oedema. This causes small airway obstruction and decreases the compliance of the lungs resulting in increased work of breathing.

Clinical features

The clinical features are those of tachypnoea with recession accompanied by high-pitched auscultatory wheeze and fine crackles.

Investigation

- CXR: depending on the cardiac lesion the CXR may show a normal cardiac shadow, or the shadow of a large left atrium or cardiomegaly with, in each case, increased venous or interstitial markings. Asymmetry of lung markings may suggest unilateral venous obstruction.
- Echocardiography: to define the cardiac lesion.

Management

Medical management is directed towards reducing pulmonary venous pressure under the direction of a cardiologist. Definitive management is usually surgical.

Compression of the airways

There are three main groups of cardiac conditions that may result in airway compression.

- Congenital variation in the position of major blood vessels resulting in vascular rings. These are discussed in 📖 Chapter 24.
- Large vessel dilatation and compression of adjacent airways, e.g. that caused by absent pulmonary valve.
- Atrial enlargement causing compression of adjacent airways.

Pathophysiology

- In absent pulmonary valve syndrome the pulmonary arteries become hugely distended and compress both main bronchi and the lower trachea.
- Enlargement of the left atrium usually results in compression of the left main stem bronchus but can with continuing enlargement also cause compression of right main bronchus and carina.

Clinical features

- The features are those of airway obstruction with a prolonged expiratory phase and recurrent or persistent wheezing.
- Sometimes the airways obstruction is absent at rest but appears with increased cardiac output during exercise.
- In severe cases there may be air-trapping and hyperinflation.

Investigation
- CXR: depending on the cardiac lesion, the CXR may show variable cardiac shadows. The lungs may be bilaterally or unilaterally hyperinflated.
- Echocardiography: used to define the cardiac lesion.

Management
The management strategy is to relieve the airway obstruction primarily by addressing the underlying lesion. Although airway stenting has been used in selected circumstances the potential risks generally outweigh any short-term benefit. Even after the compression has been relieved, residual tracheobronchomalacia may continue to cause significant problems.

Respiratory support
- Children with cardiac disease can develop respiratory failure, often during intercurrent respiratory tract infection. Decompensated respiratory function results in hypoxia and hypercapnia, which may worsen both cardiac function and adversely affect pulmonary blood flow.
- These children will require respiratory support for the duration of the intercurrent illness and until any worsening heart failure or pulmonary hypertension is controlled.
- In the acute situation respiratory support will nearly always be provided using intubation and mechanical ventilation.
- Some children with cardiac disease can be difficult to wean from mechanical support (see box).
- For some children, where weaning from mechanical ventilation is difficult, non-invasive support can be helpful. This can be delivered using bilevel positive airway pressure via a nasal mask or, less commonly, using the Hayek RTX negative pressure ventilator. This form of support allows the child to leave the ICU whilst medical management is optimized and any future surgery is planned.
- In children with both chronic lung disease and cardiac disease it can be difficult to determine the cause of acute deterioration. There will usually be worsening of both conditions, most often triggered by a viral respiratory tract infection.

Possible reasons for failure to wean from mechanical ventilation

- Associated tracheo-bronchomalacia
- Chronic lung disease: either associated pulmonary hypoplasia or acquired, usually as a combination of recurrent infection, aspiration, and ventilator-associated injury
- Worsening pulmonary hypertension
- Muscular weakness, including diaphragm palsy caused by operative phrenic nerve injury
- Upper airway obstruction: caused by vocal cord palsy, which may result from laryngeal nerve injury during surgery or from direct compression of the nerve by enlarged vascular structures

Interstitial lung disease

Introduction

Most children who present with symptoms and signs of interstitial lung disease (ILD) will have a relatively easily identified aetiology, the commonest being either post-infectious disease or that related to aspiration. In the remainder the cause of the disease requires more detailed investigation and, in some cases, although a pathological diagnosis is reached, the aetiology remains unknown. Despite a wide range of underlying causes, the symptoms and signs of children with interstitial lung disease are similar and often non-specific. Here we will adopt the concept of the children's interstitial lung disease syndrome (chILD) proposed by the chILD cooperative group of the US NIH-sponsored Rare Lung Disease Consortium (http://www.childfoundation.info/chILD_Cooperative.htm). This group considers ILD in children as a syndrome defined by a specific constellation of symptoms, signs, and investigation findings. The advantage of this approach, rather than the traditional classification by histological findings, is that it is directly applicable to clinical problems, rather than starting with a histological diagnostic category. By identifying these children as a group, planned systematic investigations can then be carried out to identify likely causes.

Once a cause for ILD-like symptoms has been identified, these children are often no longer classified as having ILD; this has been part of the confusion in the literature. For example, if the cause of the chILD syndrome is aspiration, the final diagnosis is usually aspiration pneumonitis, rather than ILD secondary to aspiration. The same should probably be true for other identified aetiologies such as surfactant protein mutations, idiopathic pulmonary haemosiderosis, and hypersensitivity pneumonitis. True differential diagnoses should be those conditions that mimic ILD but do not cause it, such as cystic fibrosis and cardiac disease.

Some further points are also worth making.

- The interstitium of the lung is the connective tissue between the alveoli, between alveolar epithelium and capillary endothelium, and around the blood vessels and airways, and which provides the fibrous structure to the lung. Children who present with chILD syndromes and many diagnosed in the past with ILD have pathology that predominantly affects the airspaces and small airways rather than the interstitial tissue itself. The blood vessels in the lung may also be affected. This means that, although there may be restrictive lung disease classically seen in adult ILD, obstructive disease is also common and may be the predominant abnormality.
- Inflammation and fibrosis, often thought to be required elements of ILD, are not universally found in chILD syndromes.
- Usual interstitial pneumonitis (UIP), the histological pattern associated with idiopathic pulmonary fibrosis, the commonest ILD in adults, is rarely if ever, seen in children.
- Some forms of ILD, such as neuroendocrine hyperplasia (NEHI) and pulmonary interstitial glycogenesis (PIG), are only seen in children.
- All forms of ILD are rare in childhood; accurate incidence data are not available. A large respiratory centre might see 2 or 3 such children each year.

ChILD syndrome

About 30% of children with ILD will develop symptoms in the first year of life. The chILD Cooperative suggests that ILD be considered in children without known pre-existing condition who have 3 of the 4 following abnormalities.

- Symptoms of impaired respiratory function (cough, breathlessness, exercise intolerance).
- Evidence of impaired gas exchange (hypoxia or hypercarbia either at rest or induced by exercise).
- Diffuse abnormality on CXR or CT scan.
- Adventitious sounds on auscultation (crepitations or wheeze).

Typical presentations in infancy will be as an infant who has either had respiratory distress from birth, or who apparently has a respiratory infection from which they fail to make a full recovery. Older children will be seen with what is thought to be poorly controlled asthma, or unexplained breathlessness and poor growth.

History

Specific history that may assist in the diagnosis includes the following.
- Age at onset of symptoms.
- Rate of progression of symptoms.
- Gestation.
- History of choking or regurgitation or heartburn may be consistent with aspiration. Developmental delay makes this more likely. An H-type tracheo-oesophageal fistula may give symptoms that are worse at mealtimes.
- Family history of:
  - neonatal deaths;
  - lung disease requiring oxygen therapy (about 10% of children with ILD will have an affected relative).
- Previous episodes of lung infection may suggest infective cause or immunodeficiency.
- Exposure to organic dusts, in particular exposure to birds, suggests hypersensitivity pneumonitis.
- Involvement of other systems, e.g. skin, joints, eyes, suggests connective tissue disease or sarcoidosis.
- Haemoptysis suggests pulmonary haemosiderosis.
- Abnormal bowel habit may suggest CF.
- A history of wheeze is common in ILD and may have led to an erroneous diagnosis of asthma.

Examination

Examination findings in children with ILD include:
- tachypnoea;
- chest wall recession;
- inspiratory crepitations;
- wheeze;
- clubbing;
- desaturation.

Differential diagnosis and causes of ILD

Differential diagnosis There are many relatively common conditions that can present with symptoms and signs similar to those of ILD, and these must be excluded as part of the initial assessment. These conditions are shown in the box.

Conditions that may mimic ILD

- Cystic fibrosis
- Primary ciliary dyskinesia
- Cardiac disease, especially pulmonary vein obstruction and primary pulmonary hypertension
- Asthma
- Recurrent infection, including that secondary to immunodeficiency
- Tuberculosis
- Neuromuscular disease
- Scoliosis
- Thoracic cage abnormality
- Pulmonary hypoplasia
- Bronchopulmonary dyplasia
- Respiratory distress syndrome
- Alveolar capillary dysplasia
- Langerhan's cell histiocytosis
- Lymphangioleiomyomatosis
- Congenital lymphangiectasis
- Pulmonary infiltrates with eosinophilia
- Bronchiolitis obliterans

Causes of ILD

The likely causes of ILD depend on the age of the child (see box opposite). Please be careful to note that the box refers to causes of ILD not to the histological appearance of lung biopsies.

In a significant number of children no underlying cause will be found. The best classification will then be based on histological findings at lung biopsy.

Causes of ILD

Children under 2 years
- Aspiration lung disease
- Idiopathic pulmonary haemosiderosis
- Surfactant dysfunction mutations (SPB and SPC and ABCA3)
- Infectious or post-infectious: usually related to either viral infection (adenovirus, CMV, EBV, or influenza) or atypical bacterial infection (*Chlamydia trachomatis, Mycoplasma pneumoniae*)

Older children
- Aspiration lung disease
- Infectious or post-infectious: organisms as for the under-twos, plus *Chlamydophila pneumoniae* and *Legionella pneumophilia*
- Hypersensitivity pneumonitis
- Sarcoidosis
- Lymphocytic interstitial pneumonitis with HIV infection
- Idiopathic pulmonary haemosiderosis and Goodpasture's syndrome
- Connective tissue disease and vasculitis:
  - SLE
  - Juvenile chronic arthritis
  - Wegener's granulomatosis
  - Churg–Strauss syndrome
  - Dermatomyositis
  - Polyarteritis nodosa and microscopic polyangiitis
  - Mixed connective tissue disease
- Surfactant dysfunction mutations (SPC and ABCA3 mutations can present later in childhood; SPB invariably presents in early infancy)
- Pulmonary alveolar proteinosis

Investigations

Investigations should be directed at excluding other forms of lung disease and to determining the cause, nature, and severity of the ILD. Imaging is an important part of diagnosing ILD. CXR appearances may be normal even with active disease. More usually there is a combination of increased reticular or reticulonodular markings and generalized hazy shadowing (ground-glass appearance). HRCT scans will nearly always be abnormal with reticular markings and ground-glass attenuation. To get good information about the nature of ground-glass changes (e.g. are they the normal or abnormal parts of the lung) careful controlled ventilation inspiratory and expiratory scans are needed. It will usually be necessary to sedate or anaesthetize children < 4 years of age. Poor quality images will only confuse the clinical picture. It may be possible to combine sedation or anaesthesia used for CT scan with a subsequent BAL (don't do the BAL first: the subsequent CT scan will cause some alarm!). The CT may also show architectural distortion and traction bronchiectasis. Increased interstitial markings can give a honeycomb appearance to the lung.

First round investigations

- Lung function tests including DLCO if old enough.
- Oxygen saturation at rest and on exercise.
- Blood tests.
  - FBC and film.
  - Immunoglobulins.
  - Specific antibody responses to vaccination.
  - Serological tests for adenovirus, EBV, CMV, influenza.
  - CMV PCR.
  - HIV ELISA or PCR.
  - ESR.
  - Auto-antibody panel (anti-nuclear, anti-basement membrane, antineutrophil cystoplasmic).
  - RAST test to any suspected organic dusts.
  - Angiotensin-converting enzyme (elevated in sarcoidosis).
- Airway secretions for viral culture and PCR.
- Sweat test.
- Ciliary brush biopsy.
- pH study: may show evidence of GOR.
- Contrast swallow: may show evidence of GOR.
- CXR.
- ECG and echocardiogram.
- Urine for CMV PCR.

Second round investigations

- High resolution controlled ventilation inspiratory and expiratory CT scan.
- Bronchoscopy and BAL: send for cytology (Langerhan's cells; iron-laden macrophages, alveolar proteinosis) as well as culture.
- Prone oesophagram looking for H-type fistula.
- Consider videofluroscopy looking for evidence of aspiration.

- Consider cardiac catheterization to check pulmonary venous drainage and pulmonary arterial pressure.
- Consider assessing lymphocyte subsets and lymphocyte function tests.
- Consider tuberculin skin test or TB-Elispot test.

Third round investigations

- Lung biopsy.
  - Almost all children with ILD will require a lung biopsy as part of definitive investigation.
  - The biopsy may be diagnostic, e.g. showing evidence of vasculitis or interstitial fibrosis, but this is not always the case.
  - Although lung biopsy can be performed using transbronchial and percutaneous approaches the amount of tissue obtained may be too small to make an accurate histological diagnosis. Thorascopic or open lung biopsy is preferred by most centres.
  - The site for biopsy should be guided by the CT scan. In general, the right middle lobe and the lingular (which are the surgeon's favourites) should be *avoided* as they are often spared in patchy disease. Ideally 2 sites should be biopsied: one site thought to be affected, and one site thought to be normal.
  - Since ILD is often patchy a negative biopsy does not exclude the diagnosis.
- DNA for mutations in SPB, SPC, and ABCA3 (only available at specialist centres). The ABCA3 gene is massive and mutation analysis is only possible as part of research projects. It is possible that a significant proportion of younger children with idiopathic ILD will turn out to have mutations in genes related to surfactant function.

Histological classification

This is where some confusion can arise. The histological classification is often *not* the diagnosis; rather it is the pattern of disease that the pathologist describes on the lung biopsy. For example, desquamative interstitial pneumonitis (DIP), chronic interstitial pneumonitis of infancy (CIP), and non-specific interstitial pneumonitis (NSIP) can all be seen in children with surfactant dysfunction mutations (SPB, SPC, and ABCA3 genes). Histological classification depends on the:

- presence and severity of any interstitial fibrosis;
- presence of alveolar thickening;
- degree of desquamation of material into the alveolar spaces, and the presence of inflammatory cells (lymphocytes, neutrophils, plasma cells, or macrophages);
- presence or increase in specific cell types (such as pulmonary neuroendocrine cells and interstitial spindle cells).

Two specific histological appearances require special mention. These are those of NEHI and PIG.

Neuroendocrine hyperplasia of infancy (NEHI)

Pulmonary neuroendocrine cells, PNECs, also known as Kulschitzky cells, are granulated epithelial cells found in normal airway epithelium and occasionally as small clusters within the lung parenchyma as neuroepithelial bodies (NEB). They are thought to be oxygen-sensing cells that secrete several bioactive products (bombesin-like peptide, serotonin, and calcitonin) capable of bronchoconstriction, vasoactivity, epithelial differentiation, and smooth muscle alteration. PNECs are abundant in fetal life and may play a role in pulmonary development. They are also increased in several lung diseases in children, including diaphragmatic hernia, CF, and bronchopulmonary dysplasia. In the normal infant they account for around 2% of airway cells. This drops in the adult lung to around 0.5% of the cells.

An increase in this cell type has been described in a group of children with a relatively well-defined ILD phenotype. These children present in the first year of life with tachypnoea and hypoxia, usually having had no problems in the neonatal period. Most have impressive inspiratory crepitations. Full investigation finds no cause for the symptoms. CXR shows hyperinflation. BAL is normal. CT scan shows some segmental ground-glass opacity. Lung biopsy is remarkably normal, without significant inflammation or fibrosis. Immunostaining for bombesin and serotonin shows an excess of PNECs (increased to around 6%) and an increase in the numbers and size of NEBs.

The diagnosis is a useful one to make because these children have a good prognosis. They do not respond to steroids or hydroxychloroquine, although a trial of steroids will nearly always be given. There is a plateau period where the clinical condition remains unchanged, followed by slow improvement, without significant relapses. Most children require daytime oxygen for several months and night-time oxygen for 2–3 years. In older childhood lung function may be normal or may show mild obstruction. There may be minor exercise limitation. Whether the increased number of PNECs is the primary abnormality that causes the lung disease, through increased production of bioactive molecules, or whether they have increased in response to other stimuli is not known.

Pulmonary interstitial glycogenesis (PIG)

Children with PIG present either at birth or within the first 4 weeks of life with tachypnoea, hypoxia, and crepitations. The CXR shows increased interstitial markings and hyperinflation, both of which are also seen on CT scans. Lung histology shows thickened interstitium due to the presence of immature oval to spindle-shaped interstitial cells containing abundant cytoplasmic glycogen with little evidence of inflammation and no fibrosis. The condition is thought to represent dysmaturity of the interstitial cells, with expectation of improvement with time. The clinical course is similar to that of NEHI with near normal function by 6 years of age, but often with persistent crackles and radiographic abnormality. There may be some benefit in steroid treatment, but it does not seem to affect longer-term outcome.

Other histological classifications

The following may also be mentioned in pathology reports.

- *Desquamative interstitial pneumonitis* (DIP). In DIP there is diffuse involvement of the lung with macrophage accumulation within most of the distal airspaces. The alveolar septa are thickened by a sparse inflammatory infiltrate. Lymphoid aggregates may be present. A familial form has been described.
- *Chronic interstitial pneumonitis of infancy* (CIP), characterized by marked alveolar septal thickening, alveolar type 2 cell hyperplasia, and an alveolar exudate containing numerous macrophages and foci of eosinophilic debris. Primitive mesenchymal cells predominate within the widened alveolar septa and inflammatory cells are scant.
- *Non-specific interstitial pneumonitis* (NSIP), a term used to describe histological findings that do not fit into the descriptions of UIP, DIP, or CIP. There is evidence of mild to moderate interstitial inflammation and evidence of fibrosis.
- *Lymphoid interstitial pneumonitis or follicular bronchiolitis*. These are thought to be part of the same spectrum of disorders causing lymphoid hyperplasia. There is a heavy lymphoid interstitial infiltrate that may contain germinal centres. If these affect the airway walls the term follicular bronchiolitis is often used. There is a strong association with immunodeficiency (including that caused by HIV infection), possibly combined with EBV infection. In others there may be underlying connective tissue disease.
- *Organizing pneumonia* (OP). OP is preferred to the previous terms, bronchiolitis obliterans and organizing pneumonia (BOOP), because it avoids confusion with conditions predominantly affecting the airways. OP is characterized by intraluminal organizing fibrosis or polypoid masses of granulation tissue in distal airspaces (bronchioles, alveolar ducts, and alveoli). OP in children is most often described after severe viral or *Mycoplasma pneumoniae*. It has also been associated with some connective tissue disorders. There are a few case reports where no cause has been identified, and these would now be called cryptogenic OP. The patchy involvement of airspaces (which can also be seen on CXR and CT scan) distinguishes OP from bronchiolitis obliterans.

Treatment and outcome

Treatment

Treatment depends on the cause. Where no cause has been identified, it is common practice to give a trial of systemic corticosteroids. Steroids may be of some help in children with SPC- and ABCA3-related lung disease. The dose and duration depend on the severity of the illness and the response. In most children an initial high dose (2mg/kg) course of 4 weeks can be used to assess response. If improvement is seen, a weaning course over a further 8 weeks, with or without a maintenance dose, can be tried. In children who do not respond, or who have severe oxygen-dependent disease, IV methylprednisolone (10–30mg/kg once daily for 3 days) is an alternative and can be repeated on a monthly basis for 6 months. There is also anecdotal response to hydroxychloroquine combined with prednisolone. Other immunosuppressive treatments, including azathioprine, cyclophosphamide, and methotrexate, have all been tried with varying success. Post-infectious organizing pneumonia usually responds to corticosteroids. In all forms of ILD, if medical therapy has failed, lung transplantation may be considered.

Outcome

Often the outcome will depend on the cause of the ILD or the specific ILD type. For example, ILD associated with genetic SPB deficiency is usually rapidly fatal, whereas PIG and NEHI have a very good outcome. Where the cause for the ILD is unknown, giving a prognosis is more difficult. Some series report up to 50% mortality; others none at all. An often quoted figure for overall childhood ILD mortality is 20%. The presence or absence of fibrosis does not correlate well with survival or respiratory morbidity. Some children seem to respond very well to first-line therapies with steroids and/or hydroxychloroquine whilst others make no response at all. There is a clear need to develop more information on this group of diseases. In the UK a database for ILD and other rare lung diseases has been established (http://www.bpold.co.uk) and in the US the chILD cooperative group is continuing to collect data on histology and clinical outcomes for children with these diseases.

Further information

American Thoracic Society/European Respiratory Society (2002). American Thoracic Society/European Respiratory Society International Multidisciplinary Consensus Classification of the Idiopathic Interstitial Pneumonias. *Am. J. Respir. Crit. Care Med.* **165**, 277–304.

Bullard, J., Wert, S., Whitsett, J., Dean, M., and Nogee, L. (2005). ABCA3 mutations associated with pediatric interstitial lung disease. *Am. J. Respir. Crit. Care Med.* **172**, 1026–31.

Canakis, A., Ernest Cutz, E., Manson, D., and O'Brodovich, H. (2002). Pulmonary interstitial glycogenosis—a new variant of neonatal interstitial lung disease. *Am. J. Respir. Crit. Care Med.* **165**, 1557–65.

Deterding, R., Pye, C., Fan, L., and Langston, C. (2005). Persistent tachypnea of infancy is associated with neuroendocrine cell hyperplasia. *Pediatr. Pulmonol.* **40**, 157–65.

Nicholson, A., Kim, H., Corrin, B., Bush, A., du Bois, R., Rosenthal, M., and Sheppard, M. (1998). The value in classifying interstitial pneumonitis in childhood according to histological patterns. *Histopathology* **33**, 203–11.

Hypersensitivity pneumonitis

Introduction

- Hypersensitivity pneumonitis (HP) is a rare disease in children. Incidence figures are not available, but a large respiratory centre might see fewer than 1 or 2 children each year.
- It can affect children of any age, including infants, although it most often affects school age children.
- HP is caused by a damaging host immune response to tiny (0.5–5µm in size) inhaled organic particles. The list of potential sources of the organic particles is long, particularly in adults. In children the most likely sources are bird proteins (especially pigeons) and fungi, particularly *Aspergillus* species and thermophilic *Actinomycetes* (from humidifiers and mouldy hay).
- About 50% of individuals exposed to large amounts of these types of organic dust will make an immune response, but only 5–15% will develop disease.
- The nature of the damaging response appears to involve both immune complex formation (type III hypersensitivity response) and T-cell mediated responses (type IV hypersensitivity response). It is not an IgE-mediated allergic response.
- Alveolar inflammation results in a diffusion defect that can lead to hypoxaemia.
- The condition can occur in acute, subacute, and chronic forms. The distinction between subacute and chronic is blurred. The major distinction is that with chronic disease there is only a partial recovery of lung function and respiratory symptoms when exposure to the cause ceases, whereas in the subacute form recovery is complete.
- HP is described in association with some drugs, such as bleomycin and methotrexate, and following radiation to the lungs. The mechanism behind these forms of HP is poorly understood, although peripheral and lung eosinophilia has been described. These conditions usually respond well to a combination of stopping the offending drug and a course of systemic corticosteroids.

Symptoms

The *acute form* of HP is unusual in children, although cases have been described. The episodes resemble 'flu-like' illnesses coming on 4–6h after exposure and lasting for 2–5 days. Typical symptoms include:
- dry cough;
- dyspnoea;
- fever (as high as 40°C);
- malaise.

Subacute or chronic HP, the common form of the disease in children, arises from more prolonged contact with smaller amounts of the antigen. Typical symptoms include:
- dry cough;
- exercise intolerance;
- weight loss;
- fever;
- wheezing episodes.

Signs

In acute disease the child may look unwell with respiratory distress and inspiratory crackles. In subacute and chronic disease findings include:
- inspiratory crackles;
- finger clubbing;
- hypoxia;
- tachypnoea;
- evidence of pulmonary hypertension in longstanding disease (RV heave, loud P2, enlarged liver).

Differential diagnosis

The differential diagnosis in a previously well child with a history of cough and exercise intolerance lasting for several weeks includes the following.
- Asthma.
- Atypical infection:
  - *Chlamydophila pneumoniae*;
  - *Chlamydia trachomatis* (in infants can be associated with eosinophilia);
  - *Mycoplasma pneumoniae*.
- Tuberculosis.
- Immunodeficiency, including HIV, either alone or combined with opportunistic infection (EBV, CMV, PCP).
- Cardiac disease, including cardiomyopathy.
- Pulmonary arterial hypertension, either primary or secondary (including secondary to chronic HP).
- Sarcoidosis.
- Other forms of interstitial lung disease.
- Pulmonary infiltrates with eosinophilia.

Investigations and diagnosis

The diagnosis is not straightforward. There is no simple diagnostic test. Immunological tests indicate exposure but do not indicate that the symptoms a child has are due to a hypersensitivity reaction. Careful investigation and consideration of other causes is usually necessary. Investigation of a child presenting with the symptoms described above will include the following.
- CXR: typically shows diffuse reticulo-nodular or micro-nodular infiltrate. However, early in the disease it is often normal.
- Lung function tests, including DLCO. There is usually evidence of restriction with a decreased DLCO. A mixed pattern including obstruction may also be seen. It is usually only possible to measure DLCO in children > 8–10 years of age.
- Resting and exercise oxygen saturation. In severe disease there may be resting hypoxia. In milder disease desaturation may become apparent only on exercise.
- Blood tests.
  - FBC and film: leucocyte count may be elevated. 10% have eosinophilia.
  - Total immunoglobulins, including IgE.

- Increased IgG (not IgE) antibodies directed against suspected antigens. The test used depends on the centre—either precipitation tests (such as Ouchterlony) or enzyme-linked (ELISA) or using radioisotopes (RAST). The term precipitating antibodies refers to the test method, not the activity of the antibodies *in vivo*.
- HIV test.
- EBV and CMV serology/culture/PCR.
- Serology of *Mycoplasma pneumoniae* and *Chlamydophila pneumoniae*.
- ECG and echocardiography.
- Bronchoscopy and BAL. Bronchoscopic appearances are usually normal. BAL should be sent for culture (viral, bacterial, and TB) and cytological analysis. Typically in HP there is a marked increase in T lymphocytes, up to 70% of the cells present, about half of which are CD8$^+$ cells (unlike sarcoidosis where the CD4$^+$:CD8$^+$ ratio is around 5:1).
- CT scan: may show nodular opacities with ground-glass attenuation, sometimes with a mosaic pattern. In more advanced disease there may be prominent interstitial markings, giving a honeycomb appearance.
- Lung biopsy: may be carried out in chronic disease when either the diagnosis is unsuspected or where there is clinical doubt. Typical findings are inflammatory nodules or granulomata containing lymphocytes, plasma cells, and foamy macrophages. Similar cells can be seen within the alveoli and interstitium. In severe disease there may be changes of interstitial fibrosis and/or obliterative bronchiolitis.

Diagnosis needs to be based on the presence of likely symptoms and signs, combined with CXR or CT scan appearance, plus a history of exposure and immunological evidence of exposure. If there is intermittent exposure, it may be possible to elicit a history of worsening symptoms during periods of exposure. The value of specific challenge tests in children has not been tested.

Treatment

The most important treatment is removal of the causative organic antigen. In most children this will be sufficient. 1–2mg/kg/day of prednisolone will speed recovery.

Outcome

In the vast majority of children full recovery will occur, with a return to normal lung function and normal chest imaging. Occasionally the disease is detected late, after irreversible interstitial fibrosis or bronchiolitis obliterans have become established. In these children there may be progressive hypoxia and pulmonary hypertension. Other immunosuppressant drugs can be tried in this group of children, although evidence of benefit is lacking.

Further information

Fan, L.L. (2002). Hypersensitivity pneumonitis in children. *Curr. Opin. Pediatr.* **14**, 323–6.

Chapter 48

Neuromuscular weakness

Introduction

Respiratory complications are a major cause of morbidity and mortality in children with neuromuscular diseases. Weakness of the muscles of respiration results in shallow breathing and ineffective cough, making these children vulnerable to hypoventilation, atelectasis, pneumonia, and tracheal obstruction from retained respiratory tract secretions. Children with respiratory complications fall into 2 broad groups:

- infants with severe weakness;
- older children who have progressive disease, most often boys with Duchenne muscular dystrophy, or those with weakness with progressive scoliosis.

In both groups of children, common problems that may occur are:

- rapid onset of respiratory failure, usually in association with a chest infection;
- gradual onset of respiratory failure, usually starting during sleep;
- failure to wean from ventilation after scoliosis surgery.

All these situations are much easier to manage if respiratory assessment and intervention occur before an acute deterioration. Effective management of respiratory problems has a major impact on quality of life and life expectancy for these children.

Management of respiratory problems

Assessment

Who should be assessed?

It is hard to predict which children with neuromuscular weakness will have impaired respiratory function. For many children, such as those with Duchenne muscular dystrophy and spinal muscular atrophy, respiratory problems are not a major problem whilst they are able to walk. Others, particularly those with structural myopathies or significant chest wall deformity, can retain the ability to walk and yet have significant night-time hypoventilation, with associated CO_2 retention and hypoxia. There are no established guidelines to identify those at risk. A reasonable approach would be the following.

- Assess all weak infants by polysomnography.
- Assess older children with a combination of history and spirometry. Those children who should undergo polysomnography are those:
  - with a history suggestive of night-time hypoventilation;
  - who are having recurrent respiratory exacerbations;
  - who have a vital capacity of less than 50% predicted;
  - who have conditions particularly affecting the chest wall, diaphragm, or intercostal or axial muscles. For example, some forms of congenital muscular dystrophy and structural myopathies are associated with a rigid spine and early respiratory compromise.

History

Specific information that is helpful in making a respiratory assessment includes the following.

- General well-being, growth, and global assessment of child's strength and ability: are they getting stronger or weaker?
- Number and nature of chest infections in the past: was hospital care required? Was oxygen needed?
- Nature and strength of cough and ability to clear respiratory secretions.
- Ability to feed and swallow: any choking?
- Any evidence of night-time hypoventilation, e.g.
  - disturbed sleep;
  - difficulty waking in the morning;
  - morning headache;
  - morning nausea (do they usually eat breakfast?);
  - daytime sleepiness;
  - difficulty concentrating during the day, including poor school performance.
- If there is established scoliosis, is this progressing and is any surgery planned?

Examination

- Assessment of child's strength: proximal, distal, facial, bulbar.
- Observation of respiratory movements:
  - chest expansion;
  - abdominal movement (is the movement of the diaphragm paradoxical?).

- Spine: is it straight? Assess with standing and bending forwards if scoliosis is not obvious.
- Nutritional status.
- If the child is able to cooperate, ask them to cough to assess its effectiveness.
- In an infant particularly, look for evidence of hypoventilation:
  - tachycardia;
  - desaturation;
  - sweating and pallor.

Investigations
- All children with weakness who are able to carry out the necessary manoeuvres should perform simple spirometry. Weak children may have trouble making a seal with their lips around a standard mouthpiece and special mouthpieces with a flange inside the lips may help. A slow vital capacity usually provides the most useful information. Measuring inspiratory and expiratory pressures and cough peak flow may also be helpful.
- Polysomnography, including CO_2 measurement, is often needed to assess evidence of night-time hypoventilation (see suggested criteria above). Some children with neuromuscular weakness also have abnormal respiratory control (e.g. those with myotonic dystrophy and mitochondrial disease), and this may also be demonstrated by polysomnography. A common pattern of abnormality is evidence of hypoventilation seen particularly during active (REM) sleep.
- Evaluation of swallowing (by videofluoroscopy) and gastro-oesophageal reflux are often required. Aspiration events are common and may precipitate respiratory failure.

Respiratory interventions
Physiotherapy
- Children with neuromuscular weakness have difficulty clearing respiratory secretions and have a tendency to develop atelectasis of the lung bases. Both problems predispose to respiratory infection, which in turn stimulates more mucus production.
- The main reason for both problems is the inability to take deep breaths to fully expand the lungs and to generate sufficient volume for an effective cough. Weakness of expiratory muscles and muscles of the glottis also contribute to ineffective coughing.
- Deep breathing or lung insufflation can be augmented either manually with a resuscitation bag or mechanically with either a ventilator or a cough-assist machine. Breath-stacking and glossopharyngeal or 'frog' breathing, in which the glossopharyngeal muscles are used to push air into the lungs, can also be used to augment lung volumes in motivated older children.
- Assistance with coughing can be achieved manually by compression of the upper abdomen or chest wall at the same time as the child tries to cough. Cough assistance can also be achieved mechanically using an increasing range of cough-assist devices.

- These devices use a face mask to deliver a relatively high pressure (+25 to +40cmH$_2$O) insufflation of 2–3s followed by a similar high pressure exsufflation of 1–2s as the child attempts to cough. Airway secretions are then either expelled into the mask or suctioned from the oropharynx. The timings of insufflation and exsufflation can be manual or automated. If these devices are used, it is important to finish the session with 2 or 3 good inflations to try and restore a good functional residual volume.
  - These devices have not been evaluated in RCTs but, at an anecdotal level, they appear to be a very useful addition to secretion clearance techniques, particularly during infective exacerbations.
- Assisted lung insufflation and exsufflation can be combined with standard chest physiotherapy to assist with secretion clearance.

Antibiotics and vaccination
- Early and aggressive use of antibiotics in children with neuromuscular weakness who develop respiratory signs seems sensible. In children with recurrent respiratory exacerbations, particularly during the winter, daily prophylactic antibiotics are sometimes used, although there is no objective evidence of benefit.
- As for all children at risk of respiratory infection, children with neuromuscular disease should be immunized against pneumococcus and annually against influenza.

Ventilatory support
- The aims of introducing non-invasive ventilation (NIV) are to:
  - improve quality of life by preventing night-time hypoventilation and reducing the impact of respiratory infections;
  - improve survival.
- Criteria for starting NIV are not well established. In infants with severe weakness and frank respiratory failure, respiratory support is clearly needed if the child is to survive. In older children who develop night-time hypoventilation the decision is less clear-cut.
- There is no evidence that 'prophylactic' NIV improves the quality of life or length of survival. Where there are no symptoms of hypoventilation and the child perceives no benefit of the NIV it is generally poorly tolerated and little used by the child.
- It is not known whether early use of NIV in younger children with neuromuscular weakness may have a beneficial effect on lung growth by promoting lung expansion, or whether, where there is mild asymptomatic night-time hypoventilation, NIV would improve cognitive development.
- When there is documented daytime hypercapnia, there is evidence of improved survival if NIV is introduced, at least in boys with Duchenne muscular dystrophy.
- When there is evidence of nocturnal hypoventilation, but daytime normocapnia, the decision to introduce NIV depends on:
  - the presence of symptoms of hypoventilation (but note that children with neuromuscular weakness may underestimate their symptoms, particularly those of daytime fatigue, and that these may only become recognized in retrospect after NIV has been started);

- the occurrence of troublesome recurrent respiratory infection;
- the nature of the neuromuscular weakness (for progressive conditions like Duchenne muscular dystrophy daytime hypercapnia will inevitably follow night-time hypoventilation, usually within 2–4y);
- whether scoliosis surgery is planned (children with neuromuscular weakness often require NIV support after extubation and this is much easier to provide if the NIV has been introduced preoperatively).
- When there is symptomatic daytime hypercapnia, a choice between NIV and ventilation via a tracheostomy tube also needs to be made. There are proponents of each approach.
  - NIV via nasal mask cannot usually be used continuously because pressure from the mask will result in breakdown of the facial skin. Other methods of augmenting daytime breathing can be introduced in older motivated children such as glossopharyngeal breathing and on-demand mouthpiece ventilators, which are usually attached to wheelchairs with a mouthpiece that the child can easily reach.
  - Tracheostomy is an alternative and has the advantage of being away from the face and, at least in theory, easier to use. Use of a speaking valve allows speech during ventilation, although speech will invariably be affected to some extent. Disadvantages include adverse effects on swallowing, increased risk of infection, and troublesome secretions requiring frequent suctioning. The cosmetic appearance of a tracheostomy is also distressing to many children and their families. There may also be more difficulty in getting a child placed at school if they have a tracheostomy.
- Daytime ventilation improves symptoms of dyspnoea, fatigue, and headaches, and probably improves survival.

Nutrition

- Good nutrition is essential to maximize muscle development.
- Weak children often have incoordinate swallowing movements and are prone to gastro-oesophageal reflux.
- Adequate nutrition may require the use of gastrostomy feeding. If a gastrostomy is needed, performing a fundoplication at the same time should be carefully considered.
- Excessive weight gain should be avoided to prevent unnecessary respiratory work.

Management in the ICU

Ventilation strategy

- Despite careful attention to physiotherapy and secretion clearance, some children with respiratory weakness will have exacerbations leading to respiratory failure that cannot be managed using non-invasive ventilation, usually because of increasing oxygen requirements associated with areas of lung collapse.
- Most experience of ventilating weak children with successful outcomes has been reported by Bach et al. who describe a successful protocol that has been evaluated in a retrospective study.[1] The protocol emphasizes the following points once a child is intubated and ventilated:

- aim for saturations of 95% (not higher);
- use a PEEP of 3–5cmH$_2$O;
- use a cough-assist device via the endotracheal tube to aid clearance of secretions;
- maintain inspiratory pressure to provide adequate minute volumes and only wean inspired oxygen as the child improves;
- do not attempt extubation until the child is ventilated in air, requirement of suction is not more than 6 hourly, any fever has resolved, and any nasal secretions have dried up;
- extubate to nasal ventilation, in air, using the cough-assist device to treat desaturations (typical ventilator settings would be 15–20cmH$_2$O peak and 3–5cmH$_2$O PEEP);
- repeated or prolonged desaturation is an indication for re-intubation.

Using this regime, Bach *et al.* report successful extubation (not requiring re-intubation during the same hospital admission) of around 80%. The likely duration of intubation is around 8–10 days.

- If a negative pressure jacket ventilator is available, this can be a useful adjunct after extubation, allowing time off NIV whilst still providing some respiratory support.
- A nasopharyngeal airway can be left *in situ* after extubation to allow suction catheters to be passed to the posterior nasopharynx with the minimum discomfort.

1 Bach, J. *et al.* (2000). Spinal muscular atrophy type 1: a noninvasive respiratory management approach. *Chest* **117**, 1100–5.

Ethical aspects of care

The approach to the care of children with severe muscle weakness, particularly those children requiring full-time ventilation, is controversial. The position of most UK units has been published[2] and can be summarized as follows.

- The family should be given all relevant information about likely outcome and possible interventions.
- Personal views of the medical team should not be used to judge the child's likely quality of life. Children with neuromuscular weakness rate their quality of life at a much higher level than some health care workers might imagine and in some cases no different from healthy age-matched children.
- If the family of a very weak child with respiratory failure opts for ventilatory support, a reasonable plan would be to:
  - use NIPPV overnight and also for daytime rescue periods during respiratory infections;
  - provide full physiotherapy support, including cough-assist manoeuvres;
  - provide short-term intensive care including periods of intubation for severe exacerbations;
  - if this is insufficient to support the child because they have daytime respiratory failure even when 'well', most units in the UK would recommend palliative care rather than tracheostomy and full-time ventilatory support in children with severe generalized weakness. Older children may manage without a tracheostomy using a regime of glossopharyngeal breathing or use of on-demand 'sip' ventilators.
- Placing a tracheostomy in a very weak child can result in complete ventilator dependence in a child who previously had some respiratory drive. This may reflect loss of ability to maintain residual volume, or difficulties in dealing with secretions from the tracheostomy.
- If the parents of very weak infants opt for palliative care from the outset, this position can be supported in good faith. To avoid undue distress because of CO_2 retention, NIPPV can be initiated and used during the night and for short periods during the day. Intensive physiotherapy regimes and intubation would not be appropriate in this setting.
- Families may alter their views about what they want for their child, and they must be allowed to do so.

2 Bush, A. *et al.* (2005). Respiratory management of the infant with type 1 spinal muscular atrophy. *Arch. Dis. Child.* **90**, 709–11.

Further information

Fauroux, B. and Lofaso, F. (2005). Non-invasive mechanical ventilation: when to start for what benefit? *Thorax* **60**, 979–80.

Bush, A. *et al.* (2005). Respiratory management of the infant with type 1 spinal muscular atrophy. *Arch. Dis. Child.* **90**, 709–11.

Spinal muscular atrophy (SMA)

- SMA is an autosomal recessive condition characterized by proximal muscle weakness caused by primary degeneration of anterior horn cells of the spinal cord and often of the bulbar motor nuclei without evidence of primary peripheral nerve or long-tract involvement.
- It has an incidence of 1/10 000 live births with a carrier frequency of approximately one in 50.
- Atypical forms of the disease have been described, including those with associated sensory deficits, hearing loss, arthrogryposis, and bone fractures. Some of these forms may be X-linked and unrelated to the SMN1 gene defect. SMA with respiratory distress (SMARD) is a distinct condition (see opposite).
- SMA is caused by mutation in SMN1 (survival of motor neuron) gene, nearly always a large deletion, usually of the entire gene. Rare point mutations are also described. The adjacent SMN2 genes are nearly identical to SMN1, but differ by 1 base in exon 7. This base change results in exon 7 being skipped in a high proportion of SMN2 transcripts with the formation of a truncated protein product. This means that, although some SMN protein is made from the SMN2 gene, this does not fully compensate for the loss of SMN1 function. Loss of both SMN1 and SMN2 genes causes embryonic death.
- Disease severity in SMA correlates with SMN2 copy number; this varies from 1 to 4 copies.
- SMN1 is expressed in all tissues, but appears to have effects only on motor neurons. SMN protein is involved in ribosome formation and in transporting mRNA in axons.
- SMA is divided into 3 types according to age of onset and clinical severity.
    - Type 1: muscle weakness (predominantly proximal) and hypotonia usually in the first few weeks of life and always before 6 months of age. These children are never strong enough to sit. Respiratory failure (at least during sleep) occurs before 2 years of age. Type 1 can be subdivided into 'true type 1' and intermediate type 1. True type 1s present in the first 3 months of life and, by the age of 18 months, they will be left with only residual finger, toe, and facial movements. The majority will have had one acute episode of respiratory failure requiring intubation. Intermediate type 1s present between 3 and 6 months of age and will be able to raise their heads off the bed, although they never sit. When these children are older they will be able to operate electric wheelchairs and to talk.
    - Type 2: onset of weakness before 18 months of age. Able to sit but not walk. May become weaker so that ability to sit is lost after 1–2 years.
    - Type 3: onset of weakness after the age of 2 years. Initially able to walk. May become weaker so that ability to walk is lost after a variable period.

- Usually the diagnosis will have already been made before a respiratory opinion is sought. Occasionally a weak infant with respiratory distress will be referred first to a respiratory paediatrician. The following signs suggest SMA type 1.
  - Hypotonia and proximal weakness lead to a frog-like posture.
  - Cry is often weak.
  - Tendon reflexes are absent.
  - Contractures are rare.
  - There may be fasciculation of the tongue.
  - The chest may be bell-shaped.
  - There is preservation of the diaphragm and weakness of the intercostal muscles. This means that, on inspiration, the abdomen moves out, but there is intercostal recession and limited chest expansion. Infants with weakness *in utero* may also have small volume lungs.
- Progression of weakness is inevitable, but the degree of progression is variable. Children who develop respiratory failure will usually have type 1 disease or the weaker end of type 2 who have lost the ability to sit. Most of the children with type 2 disease and intermediate type 1 disease are able operate an electronic wheelchair and to sit with special supports. Most are also able to talk and some will be able to feed orally. They have normal intellectual development.
- Some children with SMA will require intubation and ventilation during respiratory infections. These tend to become less frequent with age, and are relatively unusual after 5 years of age. Long-term survival in children with SMA type 1 supported either by non-invasive or tracheostomy support is now described.
- Children with SMA are prone to lactic acidosis during periods of illness or fasting. Whether there are metabolic abnormalities caused by an underlying defect associated with SMA is not known. Underweight patients with SMA with minimum muscle mass may be at risk for recurrent hypoglycaemia or ketosis, although patients typically recover in 2–4 days. The acidosis will make the child feel unwell and may induce vomiting. It will also drive respiration. It should be treated with NG feeds or IV dextrose depending on how unwell the child is at the time. Bicarbonate should be avoided as it will cause elevation of CO_2.

SMA with respiratory distress (SMARD)

- SMARD (also known as diaphragmatic spinal muscular atrophy, distal hereditary motor neuronopathy type VI, and severe infantile axonal neuropathy with respiratory failure) is an autosomal recessive condition caused by mutations in the immunoglobulin-binding protein 2 (IGHMBP2) gene.
- As with SMA, there is loss of α-motor neurons in the anterior horn of the spinal cord, leading to neurogenic muscular atrophy with subsequent symmetrical muscle weakness of trunk and limbs.

- In contrast to SMA, distal muscles rather than proximal muscles are more severely affected in SMARD, and diaphragm weakness is invariable and early (in SMA the intercostal muscles are weak with relative preservation of the diaphragm).
- All infants with SMARD will require full-time respiratory support to survive, almost always within the first year of life.
- There may be deformities of the feet and/or contractures of the fingers.
- Infants with SMARD may present at birth or as late as 6 months of age. In some infants, the first presentation may be with respiratory failure, before any limb weakness is noticed.
- Weakness rapidly progresses in the first year of life and becomes generalized, eventually affecting upper and lower limbs and trunk.
- After the first year, progression slows and any residual power tends to be preserved.
- Sensory and autonomic dysfunction can also occur.
- The inevitable requirement for full-time respiratory support—almost always via tracheostomy—needs to be explained to families when decisions are being made about the best course of management.

Treatment and outcome

- Management, as with all children with neuromuscular weakness, starts with fully informing the family of the problems the child has and is likely to face
- Attention to physiotherapy, nutrition, swallowing, gastro-oesophageal reflux, and respiratory support will be needed, as discussed above.
- The outcome depends to some extent on the level of intervention the family and medical team think is appropriate. Even with full support children with true type 1 SMA are at risk of death from sudden onset respiratory failure, usually associated with respiratory infection.

Further information

Bach, J. *et al.* (2000). Spinal muscular atrophy type 1: a noninvasive respiratory management approach. *Chest* **117**, 1100–5

Grohmann, K. *et al.* (2003). Infantile spinal muscular atrophy with respiratory distress type 1 (SMARD1). *Ann. Neurol.* **54**, 719–24.

Duchenne muscular dystrophy

Clinical features

- Inheritance is X-linked recessive. Mapping and molecular genetic studies indicate that Duchenne muscular dystrophy (DMD) and Becker muscular dystrophy (BMD) both result from mutations in the dystrophin gene, and may be considered together, using the term Xp21 dystrophy. Two-thirds of the mutations are deletions. Although there is no clear correlation found between the extent of the deletion and the severity of the disorder, in DMD 96% of deletions result in a shift in the amino-acid reading frame (frameshift mutations), which inevitably results in loss of protein function. In BMD, 70% of mutations are in-frame. 30% of mutations in DMD arise *de novo*.
- Onset is most commonly at age 3–5 years, manifest as symmetrical weakness more marked proximally and more marked in lower than upper limbs. Pseudohypertrophy, due to muscle fibrosis, is usually most marked in the calf muscles, and can be progressive.
- Motor function is reduced within 2–3 years of diagnosis, with a steady decline in strength beginning 6–11 years later. The ability to walk is usually lost by 9–13 years.
- Obesity, muscle contractures, dilated cardiomyopathy (after the age of 15), night blindness, and learning difficulties (mean IQ 88) are other common problems.
- Scoliosis usually follows the loss of ambulation. Onset may be delayed if walking and standing are prolonged. Surgical insertion of a spinal rod may be required. The timing of surgery is crucial. Where possible it should be undertaken when lung function is relatively preserved in order to lessen anaesthetic risk. A degree of correction by surgical means facilitates sitting and may lessen the degree of restrictive lung function that inevitably develops.

Diagnosis

Typical clinical picture plus:
- elevated creatine kinase;
- myopathic muscle biopsy.

Treatment and outcome

- Without respiratory support, death usually occurs between 15 and 25 years of age, usually from respiratory failure. With respiratory support, life can be prolonged by several years, although weakness continues to progress. Respiratory support is first needed at night-time only. With progressive weakness, daytime support will be required, either via a tracheostomy, or by using sip ventilation with or without glossopharyngeal breathing techniques.
- A regular chest physiotherapy regime is required to clear respiratory secretions. Cough-assist devices may be helpful.

• Oral corticosteroids taken on a continuous basis can prolong the ability to walk by 2–3 years, and delay the need for ventilatory support. Daily and alternate day regimes have been used. Side-effects, including weight gain, development of Cushingoid facies, short stature, hypertension, hyperglycaemia, cataracts, and osteoporosis, may prevent long-term use.

Further information

Troussaint, M. et al. (2006). Diurnal ventilation via mouthpiece: survival in end-stage Duchenne patients. *Eur. Respir. J.* **28**, 549–55.

Congenital muscular dystrophies

A group of at least 20 autosomal recessive disorders characterized by the following.

- Generalized weakness and hypotonia, usually from birth and always within the first year of life.
- Contractures—frequently present.
- Elevated serum creatinine kinase in most.
- Myopathic changes on muscle biopsy:
  - fibre size variation;
  - increased connective tissue or fat.
- CNS involvement with evidence of developmental delay may be present.
- Several different structural genes (e.g. merosin, fukutin) and enzymes (e.g. o-mannosyltransferase) are involved in these diseases. Severity varies. The more severe conditions are associated with progressive deterioration with eventual respiratory failure. In others weakness is mild and no progression is seen.
- Selenoprotein N1 (SEPN1) mutations are associated with the development of a rigid spine and axial weakness—congenital muscular dystrophy with early rigid spine. SEPN1 mutations are also found in children with minicore structural myopathy.
- *Rigid spine syndrome* (RSS) was first proposed by Dubowitz in the 1970s to describe a condition resembling muscular dystrophy, with onset in infancy but a relatively benign course of muscle weakness, associated with early and severe spinal and limb joint contractures. Nocturnal hypoventilation can be an early feature and a cause of mortality. Early spinal rigidity can also be found in some of the congenital myopathies (see 📖 p. 576). It is important to recognize that these children can develop severe night-time hypoventilation despite an FEV_1 > 50% and reasonable limb strength, including the ability to walk.

Further information

The Neuromuscular Disease Center at Washington University, St. Louis, USA website: *www.neuro.wustl.edu/neuromuscular*.

Myotonic dystrophy

- Inheritance is autosomal dominant.
- Incidence is around 14/100 000 live births.
- The disease is caused by a CTG expansion in the 3′ untranslated region of the dystrophia myotonica protein kinase gene. The mechanism by which the expansion leads to disease is poorly understood, but the abnormal mRNA derived from the expanded gene appears to affect the expression and splicing of several other genes, possibly by sequestering transcription factors.
- Disease severity depends upon the number of CTG repeats, which can vary within families, and is typically worse in offspring (genetic anticipation).
  - Mildly affected: 50–150 repeats.
  - Classic disease range: 100–1000 repeats.
  - Severely affected (usually congenital presentation): 1000–5000 repeats.

Clinical features

- Age at onset varies from birth to adulthood.
- Childhood forms are usually, but not always, associated with developmental delay.
- Myotonia is not usually detectable in young children.
- The severe neonatal form of the disease is most likely to be associated with respiratory impairment.
- Older children with myotonic dystrophy can develop hypoventilation, which may be exacerbated by a reduced response to hypoxia.
- Affected neonates usually have more mildly affected mothers in whom myotonia can be demonstrated (e.g. by delayed release of grip after a handshake). Neonates with myotonic dystrophy usually have:
  - marked hypotonia;
  - generalized weakness, including the face;
  - typical facial appearance with a triangular open mouth;
  - talipes and other contractures;
  - respiratory failure is common and respiratory support may be required.
- Other problems in later life include:
  - cataracts;
  - heart rhythm disturbance;
  - oesophageal dysfunction;
  - hypogonadism.

Investigations

- EMG in the mother (or more rarely the father) usually shows myotonia and the serum creatinine kinase is usually elevated.
- Serum creatinine kinase often normal.
- EMG may be normal.
- Muscle biopsy often normal.

- Head MRI may show enlarged ventricles with central white matter changes.
- Genetic tests show CTG expansion of the DMPK gene.

Treatment and outcome

- Treatment is supportive.
- In older childhood, myotonia can be troublesome and be helped by drug treatment, e.g. with procainamide.
- Although prolonged neonatal ventilation (>30 days) may be needed, most infants can be weaned on to night-time support by nasal mask, or off ventilation completely.
- There is apparent improvement over the first decade and most affected infants will be able to walk. There may be increased weakness in the second decade with the appearance of myotonia. Most children will have cognitive impairment requiring special schooling.
- Those already on ventilatory support as infants should have their need for support reviewed 6–12 monthly. Older children with worsening weakness should have annual assessment, usually by night-time polysomnography.

Further information

Campbell, C., Sherlock, R., Jacob, P., and Blayney, M. (2004). Congenital myotonic dystrophy: assisted ventilation duration and outcome. *Pediatrics* **113**, 811–16.

Roig, M. et al. (1994). Presentation, clinical course and outcome of the congenital form of myotonic dystrophy. *Pediatr. Neurol.* **11**, 289–93.

Congenital structural myopathies

- In children with congenital structural myopathies the serum creatinine kinase is often normal or only minimally elevated and the diagnosis is made on the striking structural abnormalities in the muscle fibres.
- These disorders are usually present at birth, but may not be noticed until later childhood.
- Most are mild and non-progressive; some are severe.
- Joint contractures and arthrogryposis can occur.
- Inheritance is usually autosomal dominant. Autosomal recessive forms are usually more severe.

Clinical features

- Generalized weakness.
- Muscle wasting.
- Delayed motor development.
- Joint contractures.

Investigations

- Creatinine kinase normal or marginally elevated.
- EMG: myopathic picture (brief, small amplitude, polyphasic potentials).
- Muscle biopsy appearance is diagnostic.

Specific conditions

- Central core:
  - non-progressive; usually mild, although can be severe; severity can vary within families;
  - normal intellect;
  - caused by mutations in ryanodine receptor gene;
  - can be associated with malignant hyperthermia.
- Minicore (multicore):
  - proximal moderate non-progressive weakness; occasionally severe;
  - normal intellect;
  - several possible genetic causes including tyanodine teceptor and selenoprotein N1 (SEPN1) gene mutations. SEPN1 mutations can be associated with rigid spine and early respiratory compromise.
- Nemaline:
  - can be autosomal dominant or recessive;
  - recessive form is severe and presents in early life with weakness, marked hypotonia, and respiratory failure;
  - usually due to mutations in alpha-actin; other proteins (nebulin, troponin) can be involved;
  - may be associated with pectus carinatum and pes cavus.
- Myotubular or centronuclear:
  - Dominant form (dynamin or MYF6 gene mutations) is usually mild;
  - X-linked recessive and autosomal recessive forms (myotubularin gene mutations) are severe.

- Congenital fibre-type disproportion:
  - usually type 1 and type 2 fibres are similar in size; variation is seen in several conditions, but where type 1 fibres are smaller than type 2, congenital fibre-type disproportion is likely;
  - non-progressive;
  - severity varies;
  - may be associated with short stature and foot deformities.

Treatment

Treatment is supportive. Respiratory support may be needed in the more severe forms.

Glycogen storage disease type II (Pompe disease)

- Although some weakness may be seen with type III and type V glycogen storage disease, marked weakness and associated respiratory failure are most frequent in Pompe disease.
- Pompe disease is a rare (incidence is 1/40 000) autosomal recessive disorder caused by mutations in the acid alpha-glucosidase gene. Acid alpha-glucosidase is a lysosomal enzyme required for the metabolism of a minor fraction (1–3%) of glycogen stores. Reduced activity does not lead to hypoglycaemia, but accumulation of glycogen in lysosomes and cytoplasm leads to cellular injury, particularly in muscle tissue.
- There are 3 forms of the disease depending on the level of residual acid alpha-glucosidase activity.
  - Infantile: severe, with cardiac involvement (hypertrophic cardiomyopathy).
  - Juvenile: presentation after the first year of life; no cardiac involvement.
  - Adult onset: presentation in the second decade or later. Often relatively mild proximal limb weakness, but at least 30% will develop respiratory failure.
- The infantile form presents in the first few months of life with hypotonia, weakness, and cardiac failure. It can resemble SMA type 1 and infants with Pompe never sit unaided. Without treatment death usually occurs in the first year of life from cardiorespiratory failure.
- Older children present with slowly progressive proximal muscle weakness following normal early motor development. The juvenile form progresses at a variable rate and, without treatment, children become confined to wheelchairs. Death usually occurs in the second or third decade from respiratory failure. The adult-onset form can be stable over a number of decades.
- Examination findings are those of hypotonia and muscle weakness. In the infantile form there is moderate hepatomegaly (in 80%) and macroglossia (in 60%). In older children these features are usually absent.
- Diagnosis is by EMG (myopathic pattern), muscle biopsy (myopathy with glycogen deposits), and leucocyte or fibroblast culture for acid alpha-glucosidase activity. Genetic analysis may help although rare mutations will not be detected. A blood film may show lymphocytes with glycogen containing cytoplasmic vacuoles.
- Enzyme replacement therapy has shown some dramatic beneficial effects and may become an established treatment. It is likely to be most effective when used early before extensive muscle damage has occurred.

Respiratory problems

- The diaphragm is weak in children with Pompe disease and the problems these children have are the same as those of any child with weakness of the respiratory muscles:
  - a weak cough and consequent risk both of recurrent and severe LRTIs and of aspiration;
  - night-time and daytime hypoventilation with associated symptoms.
- Infants with Pompe disease are at increased risk of left lower lobe collapse as a result of compression of the left lower lobe bronchus by the often massively enlarged heart.
- Polysomnography should be carried out to determine the presence and severity of any night-time hypoventilation.
- Respiratory support using non-invasive ventilation and cough-assist manoeuvres can reduce symptoms and improve quality of life in these children. In severely affected infants with daytime respiratory failure, the use of a tracheostomy for ventilation can be considered, although, until effective enzyme therapy is more generally available, it may not always be appropriate.

Further information

Van den Hout, J.M. et al. (2004). Long-term intravenous treatment of Pompe disease with recombinant human alpha-glucosidase from milk. *Pediatrics* **113**, 448–57.

Myasthenic syndromes

- The common adult form of autoimmune myasthenia gravis (MG) is defined by fluctuating muscle weakness as a result of antibodies directed against the acetylcholine (ACh) receptor of the neuromuscular junction synapses. This form of myasthenia can start in the second decade of life. Respiratory failure is rare, although it can occur during myasthenic crises.
- Respiratory problems as a result of myasthenia are more often associated with infants or young children who have severe generalized weakness. This group of children is likely to have one of a larger number of congenital or familial disorders of the neuromuscular junction rather than autoimmune disease. All of these disorders cause weakness, but not all are fluctuating or show fatiguability.
- Neonatal myasthenia, caused by transplacental transfer of anti-AChR antibodies, is seen in 10–30% of infants of mothers with autoimmune MG. Generalized weakness and respiratory failure are typical. The diagnosis is made by confirming MG in mother, detecting anti-AChR antibodies in the affected neonate, and demonstrating an objective improvement in symptoms when anticholinesterase inhibitors are administered. Treatment is with either pyridostigmine or neostigmine, with supportive management (including ventilation, adequate nutrition), as required until natural remission occurs. Symptoms usually subside over 1–4 weeks.

Congenital and familial myasthenic syndromes

These disorders can be classified as follows.
- Pre-synaptic— accounts for 10% of cases.
  - Defects in the synthesis of ACh, caused by mutations in the choline acetyl transferase (ChAT) enzyme and consequently insufficient ACh available in the synapse. This condition is sometimes called 'myasthenia gravis and episodic apnoea'.
  - Defects in the release of ACh.
- Synaptic—accounts for 15% of cases.
  - Defects in acetylcholinesterase (AChE). This prevents the rapid degradation of ACh resulting in depolarizing block. In these children, giving anti-cholinesterase inhibitors such as IV edrophonium chloride (Tensilon test) can cause deterioration and respiratory failure by further increasing synaptic ACh and worsening the depolarizing block.
- Post-synaptic—accounts for 75% of cases.
  - Most are caused by mutations in subunits of the ACh receptor.
  - Others are caused by mutations in other synaptic proteins such as rapsyn, dok-7, or plectin (which also causes epidermolysis).

Clinical features
- Myasthenic syndromes can present at any age from birth to adulthood, but usually there will be evidence of weakness at birth or in infancy.
- Weakness may be ocular, bulbar, or generalized.

- Typically there is fluctuation in severity but this is not always present. Fluctuation is particularly marked in ChAT deficiency. These infants may have severe deteriorations requiring ventilatory support, between which they can be apparently normal.
- Most forms can cause respiratory failure.
- Arthrogryposis (fixed flexion deformities of the limbs) may be present.

Investigations

- Anticholinesterase inhibitors (edrophonium V over 1min or neostigmine IM) will result in some improvement in pre-synaptic and most post-synaptic conditions, although the response is often incomplete. In AChE deficiency giving anticholinesterase inhibitors leads to deterioration. An increase in muscle strength after anticholinesterase inhibitors have been given is not specific for myasthenic conditions.
- Antibodies against ACh will be absent
- Electromyogram (EMG) may show suggestive abnormalities and
- typically will show decrement of the muscle action potential on repetitive testing as the pre-synaptic ACh is exhausted.
- Muscle biopsy with staining for ACh receptors may help with the diagnosis.
- Genetic tests looking for mutations in specific proteins may be diagnostic and provide some prognostic information.

Treatment and outcome

- Children with respiratory failure, even if intermittent, should be commenced on non-invasive BIPAP. This will typically be needed at night-time to prevent unforeseen respiratory compromise during the night. During the day when the child can be more easily observed, BIPAP may be used as needed. Weakness may become worse during intercurrent illness, and it is important that the child and family are familiar with a BIPAP system for use when needed.
- Anti-AChE medication is usually tried in all children. It will not be effective in AChE deficiency and often is only partially or ineffective in ACh receptor defects.
- 3,4-diaminopyridine or quinidine may be helpful in ACh receptor defects.
- Ephedrine may help in AChE deficiency.
- Prognosis is variable. Some children show improvement with age and even those with respiratory failure in infancy may become strong enough to walk. Other children show progression and some are severely disabled. The nature of the defect has some impact on severity but, even within each separate condition, wide variation in severity and disease progression is observed.

Guillain–Barré syndrome

- Guillain–Barré syndrome (GBS) is an immune-mediated acute demyelinating polyneuropathy that may occur at any age.
- Incidence in children is 0.5–1.5 in 100 000.

Clinical features

- There may be a prodromal viral illness followed 10–14 days later by generalized symmetrical weakness of acute onset, usually starting in the lower extremities and extending proximally.
- Respiratory muscles and those supplied by the cranial nerves may be affected. Bulbar dysfunction and difficulty swallowing may lead to aspiration and respiratory arrest.
- Pain and paraesthesiae in the lower limbs or back occur in up to 60% of affected children.
- Bladder dysfunction can occur.
- Headache, meningism (30%), and ataxia are not uncommon.
- Papilloedema occurs in < 5%.
- Mental clarity is usually fully preserved.
- Autonomic dysfunction (labile heart rate and blood pressure) occurs in up to 40% of affected children.

Diagnosis

The diagnosis is usually made on clinical grounds. Supportive laboratory investigations include:

- high CSF protein (elevated in 65% of cases in the 1st week, 80% in the 2nd week);
- CSF oligoclonal bands (10–30%);
- nerve conduction studies suggestive of demyelination.

Respiratory aspects of management

Approximately 15% of affected children develop respiratory failure. The likelihood of the need for mechanical ventilation is difficult to predict. It may be required in the following settings.

- Rapidly ascending weakness may affect respiratory muscle function (intercostal muscles, diaphragm) resulting in hypoventilation and, ultimately, respiratory failure. Sequential pulmonary function testing in children aged 5 years or more can be useful in indicating the degree of hypoventilation, and in tracking its severity. A slow vital capacity of < 20mL/kg or a decrease of > 30% from baseline are generally indicative of a need for invasive or non-invasive respiratory support.
- Bulbar dysfunction with a loss of the normal protective upper airway reflexes.
- The presence of bilateral facial weakness has been reported by some groups as a marker of impending respiratory failure.
- Severe dysautonomia (cardiac arrhythmias, blood pressure lability).

Although in adult studies, the duration of ventilator use and pulmonary morbidity are not increased in patients who required emergency intubation when compared with those intubated semi-electively, it is clearly preferable not to have an uncontrolled respiratory arrest on a general paediatric ward.

Prognosis

- Mortality is extremely low, with cardiac arrhythmias the commonest cause of death.
- Long-term neurological outcome is generally good, though minor residual deficits are relatively common.
- Outcome after mechanical ventilation is usually good, though a prolonged period of ventilation (with tracheostomy) may be required. The median duration of ventilation is around 21 days.
- Once extubated, a period of NIV may be required until sufficient strength has been regained. Once safely established this can be continued at home provided an adequate support network is in place.
- Gastrostomy feeding may be required in severe cases where length of recovery is protracted.
- The expectation is for full recovery with no requirement for long-term support.
- Lung function testing after recovery is normal.

Further information

Fauroux, B. and Lofaso, F. (2005). Non-invasive mechanical ventilation: when to start for what benefit? *Thorax* **60**, 979–80.

Bush, A. et al. (2005). Respiratory management of the infant with type 1 spinal muscular atrophy. *Arch. Dis. Child.* **90**, 709–11.

Bach, J. et al. (2000). Spinal muscular atrophy type 1: a noninvasive respiratory management approach. *Chest* **117**, 1100–5

Grohmann, K. et al. (2003). Infantile spinal muscular atrophy with respiratory distress type 1 (SMARD1). *Ann. Neurol.* **54**, 719–24

Troussaint, M. et al. (2006). Diurnal ventilation via mouthpiece survival in end-stage Duchenne patients. *Eur. Respir. J.* **28**, 549–55.

The Neuromuscular Disease Center at Washington University, St Louis, USA website: *www.neuro.wustl.edu/neuromuscular*.

Campbell, C., Sherlock, R., Jacob, P., and Blayney, M. (2004). Congenital myotonic dystrophy: assisted ventilation duration and outcome. *Pediatrics* **113**, 811–16.

Roig, M. et al. (1994). Presentation, clinical course and outcome of the congenital form of myotonic dystrophy. *Pediatr. Neurol* **11**, 289–93.

Van den Hout, J.M. et al. (2004). Long-term intravenous treatment of Pompe disease with recombinant human alpha-glucosidase from milk. *Pediatrics* **113**, 443–57.

Sladky, J.T. (2004). Guillain Barre syndrome in children. *J. Child Neurol.* **19**, 191–200.

Lawn, N.D. et al. (2001). Anticipating mechanical ventilation in GBS. *Arch. Neurol.* **58**, 893–8.

Wijdicks, E.M. et al. (2003). Emergency intubation for respiratory failure in GBS. *Arch. Neurol.* **60**, 947–8.

Freezer, N.J. and Robertson, C.F. (1990). Tracheostomy in children with Guillain Barre syndrome. *Crit. Care Med.* **18**, 1236–8.

Thoracic tumours

Presentation

- Primary tumours and metastases in the thorax are rare in children.
- Although the care of children with chest tumours will be coordinated by oncologists, the first presentation with respiratory symptoms is often to a general paediatrician or a respiratory specialist.
- Chest masses may be asymptomatic and detected either antenatally by fetal screening or coincidentally during assessment of an unrelated complaint.
- By the time respiratory symptoms occur thoracic tumours are often advanced. A space-occupying lesion within the chest may cause airway compression resulting in recurrent cough, dyspnoea, stridor, or wheeze. There have often been unsuccessful attempts to treat the symptoms with antibiotics or bronchodilator therapy.
- Refractory symptoms with persistent distal collapse or consolidation on CXR are common findings.
- Tumours impinging on the pleura may cause pleuritic pain.
- Compression of the recurrent laryngeal nerve may cause unilateral vocal cord palsy, change in character of the voice, hoarseness, and a brassy cough.
- Superior vena cava obstruction can be caused by mediastinal tumours.
- Neurogenic posterior mediastinal tumours may present with thoracic pain, Horner's syndrome, paraplegia, and other motor symptoms.
- Dysphagia does not usually occur even if the oesophagus is displaced, but may occur if peristalsis is affected by malignant progression, or organization secondary to local infection or haemorrhage.
- Metastatic disease in the chest may cause symptoms but is usually identified on radiological screening in those with a known diagnosis.

History and examination

- Assess for the presence of constitutional symptoms: fever; night sweats; pain; decreased growth velocity; cough; wheeze; stridor; and haemoptysis (rare).
- Tuberculosis is an important differential diagnosis, particularly for mediastinal masses and a history of TB exposure should be sought.
- Examination for respiratory distress and stridor and for evidence of tumour elsewhere—including signs of pallor and organomegaly.

Investigation and diagnosis

Blood investigations

- FBC and blood film (lymphoproliferative disease).
- Alpha-fetoprotein (teratoma).
- Beta-human chorionic gonadotrophin (teratoma).
- Carcinoembryonic antigen (bronchogenic carcinoma).
- Urinary VMA (tumours of sympathetic origin, e.g. neuroblastoma).

Radiology

- CXR may reveal a persistent infiltrate, collapse/consolidation, or abnormal mediastinal contour or chest wall abnormality, e.g. an osteolytic lesion.

- Lateral CXR may be useful in assessing the degree of tracheal compression.
- CT scan with contrast will highlight bronchial tumours and areas of calcification. Contrast is essential for discrimination of masses from vascular structures in the mediastinum.
- MRI. Most useful for assessment of spinal extension in posterior mediastinal masses. Superior to CT in the discrimination of masses from vascular structures in the mediastinum.

Biopsy

- Biopsy of palpable lymph nodes or pleural fluid may be diagnostic.
- Bronchoscopy may be used to visualize the airways and biopsy lesions within the airway and collect BAL samples for cytology looking for malignant cells.
- Thoracoscopy may be used to biopsy masses from the chest wall, the pleura, the diaphragm, the mediastinum, and lung parenchyma. It generally precludes the need for open thoracotomy for diagnosis.
- CT-guided fine-needle percutaneous biopsy may also be used for diagnosis but size of biopsy is limited.
- Open thoracotomy and biopsy may be necessary to produce a definitive diagnosis if all other approaches have failed.

Primary pulmonary tumours

Benign tumours

Plasma cell granuloma (other names: inflammatory psuedotumour; fibroxanthoma; histiocytoma)

- Accounts for 60% of all benign primary lung tumours and 20% of all primary lung tumours in children.
- A non-neoplastic reactive lesion. Positive antecedent history of infection is common.
- Lesion is a peripheral mass and may be large.
- Histology reveals multiple components (collagen, plasma cells, histiocytes, lymphocytes, foamy macrophages, and focal calcification).
- Mean age at presentation in childhood is 7 years.
- Tumour is slow growing with capacity for local invasion into neighbouring structures.
- Local recurrence after resection may occur.

Hamartoma

- Accounts for 25% of benign primary lung tumours.
- Developmental tumour consisting of normal tissue components in disorganized structure.
- Predominantly cartilage, with components of epithelium, fat, and muscle.
- Usually peripheral.
- Presentation in infancy is usually symptomatic with a large tumour and respiratory distress.
- Popcorn calcification on CT is pathognomonic.
- May occur in association with adrenal and GI tumours (Carney's triad).

Other very rare benign primary tumours include leimyoma, mucous gland adenoma, and myoblastoma. Papillomata and haemangiomata of the trachea are considered in Chapters 19 and 24 respectively.

Malignant tumours

Bronchial adenoma

- Bronchial adenomas are a group of heterogeneous tumours comprising 4 main types:
  - carcinoid;
  - cylindroma;
  - mucoepidermoid tumour (very rare);
  - mucous gland adenoma (benign and very rare).
- Together bronchial adenomas account for 80% of malignant primary tumours in childhood.

Bronchial carcinoid

- Account for 90% of bronchial adenomas in children.
- Arise from neural crest tissue with ability to secrete neuroendocrine peptides although carcinoid syndrome is extremely rare in children with primary bronchial carcinoid.
- Presentation usually in adolescence with history of cough, wheeze, haemoptysis, and recurrent pneumonia.

- Metastases are present in 10% at presentation.
- 85% of tumours arise in the mainstem or lobar bronchi. 15% arise in the lung periphery. Most common site is the right main bronchus. Bronchial obstruction with distal collapse is the typical finding.
- Tumour is often dumb-bell-shaped, with a small intrabronchial component that may be biopsied at bronchoscopy (caution needed as these tumours may be extremely vascular).
- Tumour is calcified in 25% of cases.
- Treatment is surgical.
- Overall survival 90%.

Cylindroma
- Most aggressive form of bronchial adenoma.
- Histology resembles mixed cell tumour of salivary gland.
- 40% incidence of metastasis.
- Treatment is early surgical excision.

Bronchogenic carcinoma
- Rare tumour in childhood. The most common form is undifferentiated small cell carcinoma.
- Presentation is late, usually with disseminated disease
- Prognosis is poor.
- Mortality, 90%.
- Mean survival, 7 months after diagnosis.

Pleuropulmonary blastoma
- Embryonic neoplasm arising from mesenchyme
- Classification:
  - type 1 (cystic);
  - type 2 (cystic and solid);
  - type 3 (solid).
- 5 year survival: type 1 (80%); types 2 and 3 (40%).
- May arise from within a congenital cystic adenomatoid malformation (CCAM).

CCAM-related malignant transformation
- The association between CCAM and malignancy remains controversial.
- Some series suggest that up to 8% of malignant tumours are associated with previously documented CCAM.
- Bronchogenic carcinoma is associated with type 1 CCAM,
- Pleuropulmonary blastoma is associated with type 4 CCAM.
- Sarcomas have also been documented in children with CCAM.
- Surgical removal may not prevent malignant transformation, which has been seen in the contralateral lung after surgery.
- Management of CCAM is discussed in 📖 Chapter 41.

Other malignant primary tumours
Other very rare primary malignant tumours include:
- fibrous sarcoma;
- rhabdomyosarcoma;
- leiomyosarcoma;
- synovial sarcoma.

Primary mediastinal tumours

- The mediastinum lies between the lungs, is bound laterally by the parietal pleura, anteriorly by the sternum, posteriorly by the vertebrae, superiorly by the suprasternal notch, and inferiorly by the diaphragm. It contains all the structures of the thoracic cavity except the lungs.
- Foregut duplication cysts (bronchogenic cysts, oesophageal cysts, and gastroenteric cysts) are benign congenital mediastinal cysts. Bronchogenic cysts are predominantly seen in the middle mediastinum; oesophageal and gastroenteric cysts in the posterior mediastinum.
- Bronchogenic cysts are considered further in 📖 Chapter 41.

Tumours of the anterior mediastinum

Teratoid tumours

Teratoid tumours are classified as benign cystic teratoma and solid teratoma.

Benign cystic teratoma
- Arises through abnormal embryogenesis of the thymus.
- Contains ectodermal tissue including hair, teeth, and sebaceous and sweat glands.
- Main symptoms arise from impingement on pulmonary structures causing cough, dyspnoea, and recurrent pneumonia.
- Rupture, haemorrhage, or infection may result in adherence to surrounding vital structures.
- CXR usually shows a well demarcated mass, commonly with patchy calcification.
- Evidence of teeth in a cystic mass is pathognomonic.
- Malignant transformation in cystic lesions is rare.
- Treatment is surgical excision.

Solid teratoma
- Solid tumours have greater chance of malignant transformation with an incidence at diagnosis of 10–25%.
- Serum alpha-fetoprotein, beta-HCG, and CEA levels are elevated.
- Benign solid teratomas are well differentiated with components similar to those of cystic teratoma.
- Connective tissue elements in malignant tumours are poorly assembled.
- Diagnosis is by excision biopsy.
- Malignant teratoma may be treated with chemotherapy and radiotherapy but outcome is poor.

Benign hyperplasia of the thymus
- An enlarged thymic mass is most likely to represent hyperplasia of the thymus, which tends to involute by 12 months of age.
- A large thymic shadow is present on CXR. Cervical extension of the thymus is common and tracheal compression may occur at the level of the cervical thoracic inlet. This may be managed with steroid therapy, irradiation therapy, or surgery.
- Malignant tumours of the thymus are rare.

Tumours of the anterior mediastinal lymph nodes

- Lymphoproliferative disease is one of the more common groups of childhood malignancy.
- Symptomatic compression of vital structures of the mediastinum is not an infrequent presentation of T-cell NHL/T-cell ALL disease.
- Other malignancies that can affect the anterior mediastinal lymph nodes include Hodgkin's lymphoma, lymphosarcoma, and reticulum cell sarcomas.
- Symptoms include SVC obstruction and biphasic or expiratory stridor.
- CXR (Fig. 49.1) shows a widened mediastinum with or without pleural effusion, and lateral CXR allows rapid assessment of the degree of tracheal compression.
- Other findings may include fever, anaemia, thrombocytopenia and bruising, bone pain, palpable lymphadenopathy, hepatosplenomegaly, and, rarely, CNS signs.
- Diagnosis is made from peripheral blood smear, lymph node biopsy, pleural fluid, or bone marrow examination.
- Surgical biopsy of the mediastinal lymphadenopathy may be necessary if all tests are normal.
- Children who present with an anterior mediastinal mass and stridor must be considered to have an *unsafe airway*. They should be monitored carefully and any sedation (e.g. that used to carry out a CT scan) may result in dangerous airway compromise. Assistance from a senior paediatric anaesthetist should be sought early.

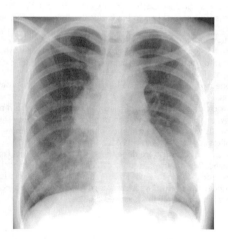

Fig. 49.1 CXR of a 13-year-old girl showing a mediastinal mass. Biopsy showed non-Hodgkin's lymphoma.

Tumours of the posterior mediastinum

Neurogenic tumours constitute the majority of posterior mediastinal masses and can be classified as:

- tumours of the sympathetic nervous system;
- neurofibromas;
- chemodectomas.

Tumours of the sympathetic nervous system (TSNS)

- TSNS are classified as:
  - neuroblastoma;
  - ganglioneuroma;
  - ganglioneuroblastoma;
  - phaeochromocytoma.
- TSNS arise from neural crest cells present in the adrenal medulla and in the ganglia along the cervico-lumbar sympathetic chain.
- The commonest presentation is with an abdominal mass.
- Most intrathoracic tumours arise in the upper two-thirds of the hemithorax and extend locally.
- Neuroblastoma is a malignant poorly differentiated tumour.
- Ganglioneuroma is a well differentiated benign tumour.
- Ganglioneuroblastoma is composed of elements from both tumours.
- Mediastinal phaeochromocytoma has not been reported in children.
- Neuroblastoma is likely to present before the age of 2 years; ganglioneuroma after 2 years. Radicular pain, paraplegia, Horner's syndrome, and respiratory symptoms are more likely to be present with neuroblastoma although often the initial presentation is with symptoms from metastases to bone, skin, lymph nodes, and bone marrow.
- Benign tumours are more likely to be asymptomatic.
- CXR findings for neuroblastoma are typically of a well demarcated oval mass located posteriorly in the paravertebral gutter. Calcification may be present. Thoracic bone metastases are not uncommon.
- Ganglioneuromas may be more elongated extending across several vertebrae.
- Unequivocal diagnosis of neuroblastoma is made either from tissue histology, or from the combination of bone marrow biopsy showing tumour cells together with evidence of urinary catecholamine metabolites (urinary VMA or HVA).
- Prognosis and treatment are dependent on many biological factors, e.g. amplification of n-myc, tumour cell chromosome number. Prognosis for local disease with favourable biological factors is good. Infants under the age of 1 year carry a good prognosis. Prognosis is poor in older children with advanced disease.

Vascular and lymphatic mediastinal masses

- Lymphangiomas (cystic hygroma) consist of tortuous ectatic lymphatic channels containing lymph. They are usually multilocular and are generally located in the anterior mediastinum, commonly with cervical extension. They can cause tracheal compression. They are considered in more detail in 📖 Chapter 41.
- Vascular tumours such as cavernous haemangiomas or angiosarcomas occur rarely and are generally located in the anterior mediastinum.

Primary tumours of the chest wall

Bone, cartilage, fat, skeletal muscle, vascular structures, and nervous tissue in the chest wall may all give rise to tumours. All chest wall tumours are rare.

Benign tumours

- Lipoma, lipoblastoma, fibroma, neurofibroma, lymphangioma, haemangioma, hamartoma, and chondroma may all occur in the chest wall.
- Chondroma of the rib is the most common benign chest wall tumour. The majority occur in the anterior tract of the ribs or the sternum. They are often asymptomatic. CXR shows a discrete expansion of bone with cortical thinning.
- Cavernous haemangioma may be very extensive and demonstrate intrathoracic extension. Similar lesions in other tissues including the oropharynx and tongue in the upper airway, and the trachea and bronchi in the lower airway should suggest a diagnosis of hereditary haemorrhagic telangiectasia. Kasabach–Merritt syndrome describes the combination of cavernous haemangioma, microangiopathic haemolytic anaemia, thrombocytopenia, and consumptive coagulopathy.

Malignant tumours

Sarcomas

- Sarcomas are the most common malignant chest wall tumours, and may be derived from bone, cartilage, or soft tissue.
- Bone-derived sarcomas often present with a mass, pain, and constitutional symptoms. Soft tissue sarcomas generally present with a palpable mass and few other symptoms until disease is advanced.
- Radiological assessment with CXR, CT, or MRI may reveal necrosis and bone destruction.
- Biopsy is required for definitive diagnosis.

Small cell tumours

- Small cell tumours of childhood comprise Ewing's sarcoma, primitive neuroectodermal tumours (PNET), and Askin's tumour.
- Presentation is usually in the second decade of life.
- 10% of Ewing's and 50% of PNETs originate in the chest wall. Askin's tumour is specifically of thoracopulmonary origin.
- All are aggressive bone-derived tumours with mixed prognosis, treated with a combination of chemotherapy, radiation, and surgery.

Solitary plasmacytoma

- A plasmacytoma is a discrete, solitary mass of neoplastic monoclonal plasma cells, with histology resembling that seen in multiple myeloma.
- The disease affects the axial skeleton, in particular, the thoracic vertebrae. The ribs, sternum, clavicles, or scapulae are involved in 20% of cases.
- Bone is thinned and may be greatly expanded.
- Presentation is usually with bone pain, pathological fracture, or spinal cord compression.

Langerhans cell histiocytosis (LCH)

- LCH is characterized by proliferation of bone marrow derived Langerhans cells. The pathogenesis is poorly understood and it is not known whether LCH is a neoplastic or reactive process.
- Disease is isolated to bones in 20% of cases but may also involve the brain, abdominal organs, and lungs.
- Localized bone disease (chronic eosinophilic granuloma) affects older children and adolescents. Bony lesions are lytic and may affect the ribs, vertebrae, and scapulae (as well as several other sites). Pathological fractures can occur.
- Multifocal bone disease (Hand–Schuller–Christian) is the classic form of LCH and includes the triad of diabetes insipidus, exophthalmos, and bony defects, particularly of the cranium.
- Disseminated disease (Letterer–Siwe and congenital LCH) affects children under 2 years of age, including neonates. It presents like systemic malignancy with skin eruptions, hepatosplenomegaly, and anaemia.
- Lung involvement can occur in any form of LCH and may be the first presenting feature. Symptoms of LCH lung disease include:
  - chest pain;
  - haemoptysis;
  - dyspnoea;
  - failure to thrive.
- CXR and/or chest CT scan may show micronodular interstitial infiltrate, which can give a honeycomb appearance. There may also be extensive cystic changes.
- Pneumothorax may occur.
- Extensive lung disease can result in a restrictive defect with decreased oxygen diffusion capacity.
- Diagnosis is usually established by biopsy of a bony lesion.
- Unifocal and mutifocal disease are often self-limiting, although young children do less well. Disseminated disease in infants is associated with 50% mortality. Systemic chemotherapy is often tried for this group of children.

Other malignant chest wall tumours Osteosarcoma, rhabdomyosarcoma, chondrosarcoma, and fibrosarcoma may all arise in the chest wall.

Metastatic chest disease

Pulmonary metastatic disease

- Pulmonary metastases may be identified because of symptoms or on screening, usually with chest CT scan, in a child with known primary malignancy.
- Most common lung metastases are from Wilms' tumour and osteosarcoma. Other malignancies that metastasize to the lung include Ewing's sarcoma, rhabdomyosarcoma, neuroblastoma, leukaemia, lymphoma, hepatoblastoma, hepatocellular carcinoma, and germ cell tumours.
- Haematological spread to the lungs commonly produces metastatic deposits in the lung periphery, particularly in the lower segments.
- Pulmonary metastases appear as single or multiple well demarcated nodules.
- Metastatic cavitation may occur with Wilms' tumour, osteosarcoma, and Hodgkin's disease.
- Metastatic ossification may occur in osteosarcoma.
- Lymphatic spread can occur in lymphoma, leukaemia, and neuroblastoma, and may produce a reticular or miliary type appearance on CXR (see Fig. 49.2). Cough, dyspnoea, fever, and pulmonary infiltrates due to leukaemic infiltration of the lung may mimic infection.
- The lungs may also be involved in Langerhans cell histiocytosis (see 🕮 p. 596).

Prognosis

- Outcome for patients with Wilms' tumour (Fig. 49.3) with pulmonary metastases is good with 75% survival at 4 years. Metastases are responsive to both irradiation and chemotherapy.
- 15% of children diagnosed with osteosarcoma have pulmonary metastases at diagnosis. >50% of patients are cured with resection of the primary tumour and adjuvant chemotherapy. Surgical resection should be considered for discrete relapse confined to the lung.

Chest wall metastatic disease

- Tumours in children that metastasize to bone include neuroblastoma, lymphoproliferative disease, Ewing's sarcoma, osteosarcoma, Langerhans cell histiocytosis, and, more rarely, rhabdomyosarcoma and primary renal tumours.
- MRI and isotope bone scans are most sensitive at detecting bone metastases. MIBG scan is indicated for the detection of bone metastases in patients with neuroblastoma.

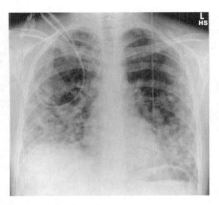

Fig. 49.2 CXR of a 14-year-old girl showing extensive infiltration of the lung parenchyma by a B-cell lymphoma.

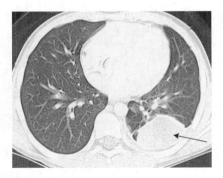

Fig. 49.3 Chest CT of a 12-year-old boy with a pulmonary recurrence of his Wilms' tumour (arrow) 12 months after completing treatment.

Pulmonary complications of cancer treatment

Introduction

In this chapter we will deal predominantly with non-infectious complications caused by radiation and drugs and associated with stem cell transplantation. Infections associated with immunosuppression are dealt with in 📖 Chapters 11 and 18–21.

Pulmonary complications of cancer treatment can cause both short- and long-term problems. Long-term sequelae of successful treatment regimes are becoming increasingly important as overall survival of childhood cancer improves and at least one chronic health condition is reported by > 60% of survivors of childhood malignancy. Chest-related sequelae include interstitial lung fibrosis, radiation-induced musculoskeletal deformity (less common now because of lower radiation doses and advances in technique), osteoporosis, secondary malignancy, and specific problems associated with stem cell transplantation.

Chemotherapeutic agents

- Multiple chemotherapeutic agents cause lung injury. The commonest manifestation is diffuse interstitial pneumonitis and the development of pulmonary fibrosis.
- Other syndromes include hypersensitivity lung disease, non-cardiogenic pulmonary oedema, alveolar haemorrhage, and bronchiolitis obliterans.
- Responses to drugs may be idiosyncratic but most are dose-dependent. Risk factors for lung disease include cumulative dose, use of multiple toxic drugs, concomitant use of radiotherapy, need for oxygen therapy, and patient age.
- Presentation of drug-induced lung injury is classically with non-productive cough, dyspnoea, hypoxaemia, malaise, and fever.
- Disease onset can be within a few hours of an IV infusion to up to 6 months after treatment has ended.
- Pulmonary function tests may be restrictive or obstructive.
- CXR and chest CT scans show diffuse interstitial or alveolar airspace disease (Fig. 50.1).
- Differential diagnosis includes:
  - malignant infiltration (e.g. leukaemia);
  - infective pneumonitis (e.g. CMV or PCP);
  - diffuse alveolar haemorrhage;
  - radiation-induced lung injury.
- Investigation should include BAL sent for microbiology, virology, and cytology assessment. BAL usually shows evidence of a chronic inflammatory infiltrate.
- Drug-induced lung disease may be diagnosed using the following criteria:
  - there is no other likely cause of disease;
  - symptoms are consistent with an administered drug;
  - time-course is appropriate;
  - BAL or tissue biopsy findings are compatible;
  - improvement is documented after drug withdrawal.
- Lung injury within the course of treatment is often difficult to ascribe to a single chemotherapeutic agent.
- Most drug-induced pneumonitis responds to systemic corticosteroid treatment. In acutely unwell children this can be given as a pulse of methylprednisolone.

Bleomycin

- Bleomycin is a DNA-damaging glycopeptide, used mostly in children in the treatment of Hodgkin's disease and other lymphomas.
- 5–10% of children treated will develop pulmonary disease.
- Two forms of lung disease are recognized.

Dose-dependent lung disease

- This is the usual form of bleomycin lung disease. It can minimized if the bleomycin is given by slow IV infusion and is exacerbated by concurrent oxygen therapy, radiotherapy, and possibly GCSF.
- Bleomycin-related lung disease starts within 1–6 months of therapy and onset is insidious.
- Fibrotic damage is irreversible. Steroid therapy may be effective in a subgroup of patients.
- Serial lung function monitoring of patients on bleomycin is mandatory. Bleomycin causes restrictive lung disease. Asymptomatic patients may show early decline in DLCO and withdrawal of the drug at onset of toxicity should be considered.

Dose independent lung disease

An acute hypersensitivity immune-mediated pneumonitis is also associated with bleomycin use and is not dose-dependent. This can rarely occur within a few hours of an infusion of bleomycin but more usually within 1–4 weeks. Hypersensitivity pneumonitis usually responds rapidly to systemic steroids, without long-term lung damage.

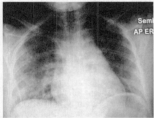 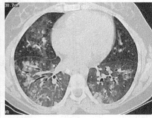

Fig 50.1 CXR (left) and chest CT (right) of a 12-year-old girl with Hodgkin's disease. She presented 1 month after receiving carmustine with a 4 day history of increasing breathlessness and worsening hypoxia. BAL was negative for *Pneumocystis* and bacterial culture and for viruses including CMV. The CXR shows diffuse interstitial changes. The CT scan shows patchy ground-glass airspace shadowing. A diagnosis of drug-induced pneumonitis was made and she was given a single IV dose of methylprednisolone. Within 48h her symptoms had resolved.

DNA alkylating agents

Cyclophosphamide

- Cyclophosphamide is used in children in the treatment of leukaemia, lymphomas, and autoimmune disease.
- Pulmonary toxicity is uncommon, but cyclophosphamide may have an important contribution when multiple chemotherapeutic agents are used. Atopy may predict risk.
- Presentation is usually subacute with onset of fever, dyspnoea, dry cough, diffuse bilateral infiltrates on CXR, sometimes with pleural thickening. Lung function testing shows restrictive lung disease.
- Biopsy demonstrates interstitial fibrosis with alveolar exudates.
- Treatment is withdrawal of the drug, corticosteroids, and supportive therapy but disease may be progressive despite intervention.

Chlorambucil

- Chlorambucil is also used in the treatment of leukaemia and lymphoma.
- Pulmonary complications occur rarely.
- Onset of symptoms is more insidious than for cyclophosphamide and may present up to 3 years after initiation of treatment.
- Disease may be progressive despite drug withdrawal and steroid therapy.

Busulfan

- Busulphan is principally used in the treatment of chronic myelogenous leukaemia, and with cyclophosphamide in preparation for bone marrow transplantation.
- Pulmonary manifestations are similar to those seen with chlorambucil.

Carmustine

Carmustine is a nitrosourea used in the treatment of lymphoma and gliomas. 30% of patients develop lung disease. Disease is similar to that seen with bleomycin. Disease is dose-dependent. Radiotherapy and cyclophosphamide may be synergistic.

Methotrexate

- Methotrexate is a folic acid antagonist used in the treatment of leukaemia, lymphoma, and osteosarcoma and in autoimmune disease.
- It is often administered with other drugs with toxic effects on the lung and in diseases that themselves cause lung disease.
- Methotrexate pneumonitis is a hypersensitivity reaction and is usually mild and often reversible.
- Presentation is with cough, dyspnoea, hypoxia, diffuse crackles on examination, and lymphocytosis with moderate eosinophilia on BAL.
- Lung function is relatively preserved.
- CXR shows mixed interstitial and alveolar infiltrates.
- Pulmonary infection may mimic these findings and needs to be excluded.
- Treatment is withdrawal of the drug, corticosteroids, and supportive care.
- Folinic acid rescue treatment does not prevent lung toxicity.

Others
6-mercaptopurine and cytosine arabinoside have been associated with pulmonary dysfunction in case reports. Rituximab, a monoclonal antibody directed against B cells used mainly in the treatment of lymphoma and B-cell mediated immune disease, is rarely (incidence < 1%) associated with interstitial lung disease.

Radiotherapy

- Children most commonly receive radiotherapy to the lung fields during the treatment of thoracic lymphoma or during total body irradiation as part of conditioning prior to stem cell transplantation.
- Classic radiation pneumonitis refers to predictable dose-dependent damage, which is avoided in modern regimes by fractionating the dose.
- Sporadic (acute) radiation pneumonitis occurs within 1–6 months of thoracic radiation and affects 5–15% of patients. It is thought to be an immune-mediated response to lung damage caused by irradiation and histologically resembles a lymphocytic alveolitis. Changes are most marked in the radiation field but need not be confined to these areas.
  - Symptoms include dry cough, fever, and dyspnoea and onset may be insidious.
  - The illness lasts 6–8 weeks and usually responds to systemic steroids. In most children there are no long-term effects.
  - There is an increased risk in children who have higher radiation doses, recent or concomitant chemotherapy, or oxygen.
- Pulmonary fibrosis is a late complication of radiation to the lungs and occurs within the radiation field. Pulmonary fibrosis may cause progressive respiratory impairment, traction bronchiectasis, and, occasionally, pneumothorax.
- Chest radiation is associated with a 3.5% incidence of lung fibrosis at 20 years post-diagnosis.

Musculoskeletal effects of radiotherapy

- The effect of radiation therapy on musculoskeletal development has historically been severe with depressed vertebral growth in the field of radiation leading to disproportionate body growth.
- Radiation of thoracic vertebrae may cause scoliosis and kyphosis, and failure of the thorax to grow may lead to restrictive lung disease.
- Advances in radiation dosing, schedule, and field selection have reduced the frequency of such severe complications.

Bone marrow transplantation

The term bone marrow transplantation has now been largely replaced by the more precise term stem cell transplantation (SCT). When the cells (usually derived from bone marrow, but occasionally from the umbilical cord) come from another individual, the transplant is said to be allogeneic. Where the cells have been harvested from the recipient earlier in their treatment, the transplant is said to be autologous.

Pre-transplant conditioning

- Bone marrow may fail because of underlying disease or because of treatment. Bone marrow transplant with prior obliteration of the host bone marrow space using high dose treatment may be curative in those who have not responded to conventional treatment. Pre-transplant conditioning using combination chemotherapy, often together with total body irradiation (TBI), serves to obliterate persisting bone marrow disease and host lymphocytes that will cause graft rejection.
- Combination chemotherapy used in pre-transplant conditioning often includes high dose busulfan and cyclophosphamide. This, in combination with high dose irradiation, puts these children at significant risk of the pulmonary complications outlined above. One series suggests that pre-transplant conditioning with chemotherapy and TBI results in restrictive lung disease in 50% of patients at 6 months after SCT, with persistent restrictive lung disease in 20% at 10 years post-SCT.

Graft-versus-host disease (GVHD)

- GVHD usually occurs after allogeneic SCT. More rarely it may follow solid organ transplants that contain immunocompetent cells (small bowel transplants are high risk for GVHD). The likelihood of GVHD depends on the HLA matching of the donor and recipient cells and ranges from 10% to 90%.
- Acute GVHD is an illness usually comprising hepatitis, enteritis, and dermatitis occurring within 100 days of transplantation.
- Chronic GVDH occurs after this time and affects the skin, eyes, lungs, mouth, liver, gut, and occasionally muscle.
- 35% of children will have lung function abnormality 5 years after SCT. Of these 2/3 will be asymptomatic. The causes of lung injury include the effects of conditioning, infection, and acute and chronic GVHD.
- GVHD can affect the lungs, usually as part of more generalized GVHD (e.g. affecting the eyes, hair, and tongue).
- Most chronic GVHD lung disease results in a bronchiolitis obliterans or constrictive bronchiolitis picture with predominantly obstructive changes on spirometry.
- More rarely an organizing pneumonitis may occur with restriction and decreased DLCO.
- CT scan shows a mosaic pattern consistent with patchy small airways disease.

- The diagnosis can usually be made on the basis of lung function, CT scan, and evidence of other GVHD. If there s doubt about the nature of the lung disease, a lung biopsy may be helpful. Lymphocytic inflammation would be consistent with active lung GVHD.
- Lung disease in GVHD is often progressive and may need aggressive immunosuppressant treatment. Initial therapy s usually an increase of existing treatment (often tacrolimus) combined with pulsed methylprednisolone.

Other pulmonary complications

- Infection (details can be found in 🕮 Chapters 18–21).
  - Bacteria: predominantly a problem in the early pre-engraftment period.
  - Fungi: delayed engraftment with prolonged neutropenia increases the risks of *Candida* infection. *Aspergillus* infection is more likely in the post-engraftment stage. *Pneumocystis* infection can also occur at this time.
  - Viruses: CMV reactivation occurs in the post-engraftment stage and can cause pneumonitis. Late CMV reactivation is associated with GVHD. Any respiratory viruses can cause troublesome infection after SCT.
- Pulmonary oedema can be seen in the first 2–3 weeks after transplantation. Several factors contribute, including drug-related cardiac and renal dysfunction and altered pulmonary capillary permeability. Treatment is usually with diuretics.
- Idiopathic pneumonia syndrome: seen in 5–10% of adults following SCT. Causes breathlessness and dry cough with restrictive lung function changes and non-specific infiltrates or CXR. Usually occurs within 2 months of transplantation although a similar interstitial type lung disease can been seen after 3 or more months. It can be severe enough to cause hypoxia and respiratory failure. Bronchoscopic lavage cultures are negative. Treatment is with systemic steroids.
- Diffuse alveolar haemorrhage can be seen within 4 weeks of transplantation. It is associated with the engraftment process and marrow recovery. The mechanism is not known. Treatment is supportive. Mortality is high and relapse is common.
- Pulmonary veno-occlusive disease can occasionally occur at any time after SCT resulting in pulmonary hypertension. The cause is not known.

Further information

Abrat, R.P. and Morgan, G.W. (2002). Lung toxicity following chest irradiation in patients with lung cancer. *Lung Cancer* **35**, 103–9.

Frisk, P., Arvidson, J., Bratteby, L.E., Hedenstrom, H., and Lonnerholm, G. (2004). Pulmonary function after autologous bone marrow transplantation in children: a long-term prospective study. *Bone Marrow Transplant* **33** (6), 645–50.

Michelson, P.H., Goyal, R., and Kurland, G. (2007). Pulmonary complications of haematopoietic cell transplantation in children. *Paediatr. Respir. Rev.* **8**, 46–61.

Uderzo, C., Pillon, M., Corti, P., Tridello, G., Tana, F., et al. (2007). Impact of cumulative anthracycline dose, preparative regimen and chronic graft-versus-host disease on pulmonary and cardiac function in children 5 years after allogeneic hematopoietic stem cell transplantation: a prospective evaluation on behalf of the EBMT Pediatric Diseases and Late Effects Working Parties. *Bone Marrow Transplant.* **39**, 667–75.

Pulmonary hypertension

Definition

Increased pressure in the pulmonary circulation can present as an isolated problem or can complicate the course of children with longstanding cardiac or lung disease. The high pulmonary pressure puts strain on the right ventricle and can increase right atrial pressure. Severe pulmonary hypertension will result in:

- poor forward flow through the lungs, which can lead to low cardiac output and systemic hypotension;
- systemic venous distension with associated hepatomegaly;
- right to left shunting at atrial level (if there is a patent foramen ovale) with subsequent desaturation.

Secondary pulmonary hypertension is often reversible initially. If the underlying cause is not treated, structural changes can occur in the pulmonary arterioles and the hypertension can become permanent and progressive.

Causes of pulmonary hypertension

Most children with pulmonary hypertension cared for by respiratory paediatricians will have underlying lung disease, often combined with heart disease, as the cause. Other causes and idiopathic pulmonary hypertension (see box) are less common, but important to consider in children who present with unusual or persistent breathlessness, cyanosis, or fainting episodes.

Respiratory patients at risk of pulmonary hypertension are those with persistent hypoxia

- Alveolar hypoxia leads to pulmonary arteriolar contraction, probably as a result of compensatory mechanisms to minimize ventilation perfusion mismatch. When alveolar hypoxia persists for months, pulmonary arterial resistance becomes elevated and this increase may become irreversible.
- Hypoxia from respiratory disease is often first apparent either on exercise or during sleep. Sleep-related hypoxia often represents a combination of reduced respiratory drive and upper airways obstruction. Both of these events are more common during active or REM sleep.
- The severity and duration of hypoxia necessary to cause pulmonary hypertension is not known and will almost certainly be different in each child.
- The relative contribution of hypercarbia is not known.
- Respiratory conditions most likely to be associated with alveolar hypoxia and subsequent pulmonary hypertension are:
  - chronic lung disease of prematurity;
  - chronic interstitial lung disease;
  - pulmonary hypoplasia, particularly associated with diaphragmatic hernia;
  - severe cystic fibrosis (usually with $FEV_1 < 30\%$);
  - neuromuscular disease with night-time hypoventilation;
  - untreated severe obstructive sleep apnoea.

Coexisting cardiac disease is a common contributor to pulmonary hypertension

- Infants with a combination of chronic lung disease and congenital structural heart disease are the largest group of children with pulmonary hypertension in many centres.
- The lung disease in these infants has usually arisen through a combination of long-term ventilation, recurrent infection, increased pulmonary blood flow, and possible aspiration.
- Infants with Down's syndrome, particularly those with heart or lung disease, are at increased risk of developing pulmonary hypertension.

WHO (1998) classification of pulmonary hypertension[1]

Pulmonary arterial hypertension (PAH)
This type of pulmonary hypertension includes:
- Idiopathic pulmonary hypertension
- Familial pulmonary hypertension
- PAH associated with:
  - increased pulmonary blood flow, usually caused by left to right shunts (such as PDA, VSD, ASD)
  - collagen vascular disease
  - portal hypertension
  - HIV infection
  - drugs including diet pills, fenfluramine and dexfenfluramine
  - thyroid disease, Gaucher disease, hereditary haemorrhagic telangiectasia, haemoglobinopathies
- Persistent pulmonary hypertension of the newborn
- Pulmonary veno-occlusive disease

Pulmonary venous hypertension
Caused by diseases of the left side of the heart, including:
- mitral valve disease and pulmonary vein stenosis
- left atrial or left ventricular disease

Pulmonary hypertension associated with disorders of the respiratory system or hypoxaemia
- Any chronic lung disease with hypoxia
- Alveolar hypoventilation, e.g. with neuromuscular weakness
- Obstructive sleep apnoea
- Chronic exposure to high altitude

Pulmonary hypertension caused by chronic thrombotic or embolic disease including large thrombi in proximal pulmonary arteries, pulmonary embolism, and in situ thrombosis as seen in sickle cell disease

Pulmonary hypertension caused by disorders directly affecting the pulmonary blood vessels
- Sarcoidosis
- Alveolar capillary dysplasia
- Schistosomiasis

---

1 Rich, S. (ed.) (1988). Primary pulmonary hypertension. The World Symposium—Primary Pulmonary Hypertension 1998. Available from the World Health Organization via the Internet (*www.who.int/ncd/cvd/pph.html*).

Symptoms and signs

- In children with pre-existing heart or lung disease, symptoms and signs of pulmonary hypertension may be masked by those of the underlying disease. Pulmonary hypertension should be suspected when there is unexpected deterioration in this group of children.
- More rarely, children who have apparently been previously well may present with pulmonary hypertension with any of the symptoms listed below.

Symptoms may include:
- shortness of breath with mild exertion;
- lethargy;
- chest pain or pressure;
- dizzy spells and fainting;
- palpitations;
- infants with a patent foramen ovale may have episodic cyanosis.

Unless the cause is obvious additional specific history should be obtained:
- use of diet pills;
- use of contraceptive pill;
- cocaine or metamphetamine use;
- family history of PAH.

Findings on examination

These include:
- right ventricular heave;
- loud pulmonary component of second heart sound;
- systolic murmur of tricuspid regurgitation;
- evidence of right ventricular failure—raised venous pressure, enlarged liver, peripheral oedema (older children).

Pulmonary hypertensive crises

Pulmonary hypertensive crises can occur in children with labile pulmonary circulations. They most often occur in children with increased pulmonary blood flow, but can occur in any patient with pulmonary hypertension. Episodes of hypoxia (e.g. caused by intercurrent infection and anaesthesia) result in sudden increases in pulmonary vascular resistance, which can dramatically reduce forward flow from the right side of the heart. This causes rapid falls in systemic BP, usually with cyanosis and acidosis. Unless reversed quickly, usually by intubation, paralysis, and hyperventilation with 100% oxygen, these events can be fatal.

Investigation

The most effective management of pulmonary hypertension is to identify a treatable cause. In children with complex combined heart and lung disease, the problem may be readily apparent—and may or may not be treatable. In other children who present symptomatically, a long list of investigations needs to be undertaken. Only when this list has been exhausted can a diagnosis of idiopathic primary pulmonary hypertension be made.
- CXR: cardiomegaly; evidence of lung disease.
- ECG: RV strain.

- Echocardiogram: structural heart disease, RV strain, estimate of RV pressure if there is tricuspid regurgitation, presence of normal pulmonary veins. If there is hypoxia, a bubble echo may demonstrate AV shunting more effectively than Doppler.
- Liver ultrasound: evidence of portal hypertension.
- Blood tests:
  - hypercoagulable states: D dimers or fibrin degradation products, fibrinogen levels, partial thromboplastin time, prothrombin time, factor V Leiden, prothrombin G20210A mutation, anticardiolipin antibodies, Russell viper venom time (for lupus anticoagulant), protein C, protein S and anti-thrombin III levels;
  - collagen vascular disease; antinuclear antibodies, RhF, complement, ESR;
  - thyroid function;
  - liver function tests;
  - HIV test;
  - FBC and haemoglobin electrophoresis for sickle-cell disease.
- Lung function testing:
  - simple spirometry;
  - transfer factor (minimum FVC of 1.0L needed for this measurement).
- Exercise testing with saturation monitoring.
- Sleep polysomnography: evidence of obstruction or hypoventilation.
- Chest CT scan: thromboembolic disease, or primary lung disease if lung function tests are abnormal. Ventilation–perfusion scan can also be used to investigate for thromboembolic disease.
- Lung biopsy may occasionally be needed, e.g. in neonates to diagnose alveolar capillary dysplasia. By inspecting pulmonary arterioles, lung biopsy can also give information about the severity and likely reversibility of the pulmonary hypertension.

If no cause has been found, or if the cause is not readily treatable, a *cardiac catheterization* should be performed to obtain more precise information about pulmonary artery pressures and pulmonary artery reactivity.

Management

The best management is prevention. Children with respiratory disease at risk of pulmonary hypertension should be assessed by overnight polysomnography and, where appropriate, by exercise testing. Cardiac evaluation by CXR and ECG may also be appropriate. Where night-time or daytime hypoxia is identified it should be treated—either with supplemental oxygen or with ventilatory support depending on the cause.

Treatment of the underlying cause for pulmonary hypertension is usually sufficient to bring the pulmonary pressures back into the normal range. For those children where this is not successful and for those children with primary idiopathic pulmonary hypertension, additional therapies need to be considered. Before these therapies are started, reversibility of the pulmonary hypertension should be evaluated at cardiac catheterization. Therapies include the following.

- Oxygen therapy: this is nearly always required.
- Diuretics and digoxin if there is right heart failure.

- Pulmonary vasodilators.
  - Nitric oxide: useful to assess vasoreactivity and for treatment of ventilated children.
  - Calcium channel blockers, e.g. nifedipine. Usually effective in children who have a vasodilator response to nitric oxide.
  - Prostacyclin—PGI2 (such as epoprostenol)—needs to be given as a 24h infusion via central line. Response to prostacyclin is not predicted by vasoreactivity to oxygen or nitric oxide in the cardiac catheterization laboratory. It can be used as chronic therapy. SC (treprostinil) and nebulizable (iloprost) forms are available, but there are little data on their use in children. The effects of iloprost last only 2h. Treprostinil injections are very painful.
  - Endothelin receptor antagonist, e.g. bosentan and sitaxentan. These are oral agents. Bosentan has the most data on use in children and appears to be the most effective long-term agent.
  - Phosphodiesterase-5 inhibitors, e.g. sildenafil, can also be given orally. Sildenafil may give good short-term results but the effects are often relatively short-lived.
- Anticoagulation with warfarin is usually recommended because forward blood flow in the pulmonary artery can be a little sluggish and lead to thrombus formation. It has been shown to prolong survival in adults.
- Atrial septostomy is a palliative procedure in uncontrolled pulmonary hypertens on to improve systemic BP and prevent syncope.
- Lung transplantation may be successful if medical therapy has failed.

The choice of therapy is determined by the cause and reversibility of the pulmonary hypertension. For example, pulmonary hypertension secondary to hypoxic lung disease may respond poorly to vasodilators since these can worsen V/Q mismatch. There is some evidence that combination therapy (e.g epoprostenol plus bosentan) can be more effective than monotherapy. Some oral medications have been tried in an uncontrolled manner in children with pulmonary hypertension secondary to bronchopulmonary dysplasia.

Outcome

The outcome for secondary pulmonary hypertension is largely dependent on the underlying cause. Idiopathic pulmonary hypertension was previously a rapidly fatal disease. Newer therapies now mean these children are surviving longer with a better quality of life. In a recent study the 2 year survival was over 90%.

Further reading

Rashid, A and Ivy, D. (2005). Severe paediatric pulmonary hypertension: new management strategies. *Arch. Dis. Child.* **90**, 92–8.

Rosenzweig, E.B. and Barst, R.J. (2005). Idiopathic pulmonary arterial hypertension in children. *Curr. Opin. Pediatr.* **3**, 372–80.

Rosenzweig, E.B. Ivy, D.D., Widlitz, A., et al. (2005). Effects of long-term bosentan in children with pulmonary arterial hypertension. *J. Am. Coll. Cardiol.* **46**, 697–704.

Pulmonary infiltrates
with eosinophilia

Introduction

- Pulmonary infiltrates with eosinophilia (PIE) is the agreed term for a collection of diseases with the common findings of lung disease and eosinophilia in the peripheral blood, BAL fluid, or pulmonary interstitium.
- The key observation is that there are infiltrates on the CXR. Simple atopic asthma is often associated with a mild blood eosinophilia (but < 8% of the total leucocyte count), but the CXR will either be normal or show hyperinflation only, and the condition readily responds to normal asthma therapy.
- The diseases causing PIE are all rare but form an important part of the differential of acute and chronic respiratory illness. When, after full investigation, no cause for the lung disease and eosinophilia can be found, a diagnosis of idiopathic acute or chronic PIE may be made, and a course of steroids given. Repeated investigation may be needed if the child fails to improve.
- Loeffler's syndrome, also called simple pulmonary eosinophilia, is a transient illness with migratory pulmonary infiltrates and peripheral blood eosinophilia. It represents a group of illnesses that overlap with those described below. Many of the original patients with Loeffler's syndrome had *Ascaris* infection, and would now be classified as chronic PIE.
- As with all components of the white cell count, it is best to refer to absolute cell counts rather than percentages. The normal range for peripheral blood eosinophils is $0.02–0.5 \times 10^9$/L.

Idiopathic acute PIE

This can affect children (but not infants; see 📖 p. 621) of any age, with durations from 1 to 7 days. The condition is also known as acute eosinophilic pneumonia. The cause is not known. Symptoms include:
- fever;
- myalgia;
- pleuritic chest pain;
- breathlessness;
- lethargy.

Findings include:
- hypoxia;
- tachypnoea;
- recession;
- breath sounds may be normal, or may have wheeze or crepitations.

The disease can progress rapidly to respiratory failure requiring intubation.
Investigations
- CXR/CT scan: diffuse bilateral infiltrates, sometimes with small bilateral pleural effusions.
- WBC: total count is usually normal or mildly elevated. Eosinophil count is elevated.
- IgE may be elevated.
- BAL may show increased numbers of eosinophils, but this is not invariable.
- Lung biopsy shows infiltration of interstitium, airways, and alveoli with eosinophils.

The diagnosis is one of exclusion. The differential will depend on the presentation, but may include the following.

- Other forms of interstitial lung disease.
- Immune defects and *Pneumocystis jiroveci* pneumonia. Some forms of SCID (adenosine deaminase deficiency and purine nucleoside phosphorylase deficiency) may present in later childhood, and can be associated with both raised IgE and eosinophilia.

Occasionally blood and BAL eosinophilia is absent and the diagnosis of acute eosinophilic pneumonia is only reached after lung biopsy.

Treatment

The condition usually responds quickly to corticosteroids. In acutely unwell children, this may be given as IV methylprednisolone. The total course is given for 4–8 weeks. Relapse is rare.

Infant disease

Infants may develop the acute or chronic forms of the disease, but are worth considering separately because of the increased possibility of underlying immune deficiency syndromes. There are several described forms of SCID, some of which are associated with peripheral blood eosinophilia, e.g. Omenn's syndrome (see 📖 Chapter 35). Hyper-IgM and hyper-IgE syndromes are also associated with eosinophilia as is eosinophilic leukaemia. BAL and peripheral blood eosinophilia may be seen in infants with *Chlamydophila trachomatis* pneumonia and in *Pneumocystis jiroveci* pneumonia associated with immune deficiency, including HIV infection.

Investigation

Searching for opportunistic infection is especially important.

- Nasopharyngeal aspirate for respiratory viruses and *Chlamydophila trachomatis* (culture or PCR).
- Blood, urine, and BAL fluid for CMV.
- BAL fluid for cytology, viral, and bacterial culture, and Grocott stain for *Pneumocystis jiroveci*.
- FBC and film.
- Serum immunoglobulins (including IgE).
- Lymphocyte subset counts.
- Lymphocyte stimulation tests.
- DNA for genetic tests for SCID variants.
- HIV test.
- CT chest.
- Consider lung biopsy if not improving.

Treatment

Treatment depends on the cause. If immune deficiency is excluded and there is no evidence of *Pneumocystis jiroveci* or CMV infection, a course of systemic corticosteroids may be tried. If the child is not critically ill, obtaining a lung biopsy should be strongly considered before starting the steroid treatment.

Chronic PIE

This includes a wide-range of conditions that develop over a variable period of time from 1–2 weeks to several months. In some conditions, although there are CXR infiltrates, there may be few or no respiratory symptoms. The following conditions are included in the category of chronic PIE.

- *Drug-induced disease*. The list of drugs is long, and includes oral medications like ampicillin and inhaled medications such as beclometasone and tobramycin. Symptoms include cough, breathlessness, and fever and usually occur within 4 weeks of starting the drug, although they may not arise for several months. Symptoms resolve on stopping the drug, a process that may be hastened by use of systemic corticosteroids.
- *Parasite-induced disease*. Many parasites can induce eosinophilia with lung involvement, including *Angcylostoma, Ascaris, Echinococcus, Schistosoma, Stronglyloides, and Toxocara*. Stool examination (for ova, cysts, and parasites) and/or serology are needed for the diagnosis.
- *Churg–Strauss vasculitis*. A systemic granulomatous small vessel vasculitis, usually preceded by a long history of asthma and allergic rhinitis. It can rarely occur in childhood. It can affect almost any system, including the peripheral nerves. ESR and serum IgE are elevated and in 70% (of adults) p-ANCA is positive.
- *Allergic bronchopulmonary aspergillosis*. This is rarely found in children with asthma, although it is much more likely if the child has cystic fibrosis (see 📖 Chapter 15). A child with asthma who develops ABPA should have a sweat test to exclude CF.
- *Idiopathic hypereosinophilic syndrome*. Only a few cases in children have been described. There is peripheral eosinophilia for more than 6 months combined with fever, night sweats, itchy papular rash, and cough. Complications can affect almost any organ system.
- *Chronic eosinophilic pneumonia*. This is an idiopathic condition that is well-described in adults. It has been occasionally reported in children. It causes chronic cough, fever, and diminished lung function, associated with infiltrates on CXR. It responds to high dose corticosteroids. Relapse may occur.
- *Hyper-IgE (Job) syndrome* may present in later childhood and can predispose to recurrent bronchitis as well as *Staphylococcal* and *Haemophilus* pneumonias with pneumatocele formation.
- *Sarcoidosis*. Although not usually included in this group of diseases, sarcoidosis is associated with eosinophilia in 50% of affected children. Sarcoidosis is described in more detail in 📖 Chapter 54.

Investigations

Investigations should follow the same lines as for acute disease and will usually include chest CT scan and bronchoscopy with lavage. Lung biopsy may be required. In addition it is worth checking immunoglobulin levels, lymphocyte subsets, and neutrophil chemotaxis, which is abnormal in hyper-IgE syndrome. Elevated serum angiotensin-converting enzyme would be consistent with sarcoidosis.

Treatment

Treatment will depend on the cause. Chronic eosinophilic pneumonia without any identified underlying cause usually responds to high dose systemic corticosteroids.

Further information

Oermann, C.M., Panesar, K.S., Langston C., Larsen, G.L., Menendez, A.A., Schofield, D.E., Cosio, C., and Fan, L.L. (2000). Pulmonary infiltrates with eosinophilia syndromes in children. *J. Pediatr.* **136**, 351–8.

Sickle cell disease

Acute chest syndrome (ACS)

ACS is defined as the appearance of a new pulmonary infiltrate on CXR accompanied by fever, cough, tachypnoea, and chest pain. Fever and cough are the most common symptoms in children. ACS is a common cause of hospitalization in children with SCD and, whilst it is frequently self-limited when the infiltrate is confined to a small area, it can progress rapidly into a acute respiratory distress syndrome (ARDS) and may be fatal. 30–40% of children with SCD will have ACS, and most of these will have recurrent episodes.

ACS may be precipitated by:
- infection (*Chlamydophila pneumoniae*, *Mycoplasma pneumoniae*, and respiratory syncytial virus are the commonest pathogens);
- painful crisis causing restricted breathing, typically caused by bone infarcts of the thorax;
- pulmonary oedema caused by overvigorous hydration;
- fat embolus from necrotic infarcted bone marrow.

Each of these processes, accompanied by local hypoxia, can lead to the inflammatory cascade associated with ACS.

Clinical features
- Fever.
- Cough (which can be productive).
- Tachypnoea.
- Wheezing.
- Hypoxia.
- Leucocytosis.
- New infiltrate on CXR. The CXR may be normal early in an episode of ACS.

Management
The best management is preventive.
- Although adequate hydration is important in sickle cell crises, fluid management should carefully monitored to prevent overloading the pulmonary circulation.
- Adequate analgesia, using a combination of opiates and NSAIDs, should be used to prevent hypoventilation because of pain.
- Taking 10 maximal inspirations every 2h has been shown to be effective in decreasing the risk of ACS during painful crises, presumably because this minimizes the risk of atelectasis resulting from decreased respiratory movements due to pain. The inspiratory manoeuvres can be optimized in children by using an incentive spirometer.
- Oxygen should be used to prevent hypoxia. Saturation monitors may not give an adequate indication of arterial saturation in children with SCD due to the presence of dyshaemoglobin and a shifted oxyhaemoglobin dissociation curve.

- Broad spectrum antibiotics such as macrolides should be given. Children with SCD are functionally asplenic and prophylaxis with penicillin can be helpful, as can immunization against *Pneumococcus* and *Haemophilus influenzae*.
- Simple or exchange transfusion should be considered in children with hypoxia to improve oxygen carriage and decrease the proportion of sickle haemoglobin. A haemoglobin level of 11g/dL should not be exceeded.
- In children with persistent or worsening hypoxia, consider using corticosteroids and nitric oxide.
- Hydroxyurea is effective at reducing the frequency of ACS in adults with SCD.

Chronic lung disease

- Older children with recurrent ACS can develop permanent reduction in lung function, associated with interstitial changes on CXR and CT scan. The lung function deficit is usually restrictive, but can include obstructive and diffusion defects.
- Children of any age can have recurrent small pulmonary infarcts without obvious acute chest syndrome. This can result in chronic hypoxia, often worse at night, which predisposes them to later pulmonary hypertension. The infarction is presumably of the bronchial supply leaving areas of perfused non-functional lung leading to V/Q mismatch.
- Pulmonary hypertension occurs in around 30% of adults with SCD, probably because of a combination of *in situ* thrombosis in the distal pulmonary arteries and chronic hypoxia. Symptoms include decreased exercise tolerance, right heart failure, and hypoxia. Pulmonary hypertension is responsible for around 20% of mortality associated with SCD.
- Reactive airways disease occurs in 40% of children with SCD, and in up to 80% of those with recurrent ACS. The wheeze is usually bronchodilator-responsive and prophylaxis with inhaled steroids is appropriate.

Nocturnal desaturation

- Nocturnal desaturation occurs in up to 40% of children with SCD and daytime hypoxia occurs in a smaller proportion.
- The mechanisms responsible for the desaturation are not clear. Some children will have obstructive sleep apnoea and others may have chronic parenchymal lung disease from previous infarction. However, the majority of children with night-time hypoxia will have normal lung function, no chronic chest disease, and no obstruction. In this group of children, the low saturations appear to be a combination of a right-shifted oxygen saturation curve (because of the sickle Hb) and increased levels of carboxyhaemoglobin and methaemoglobin, leading to lower saturations with normal or near-normal oxygen partial pressures.
- Nocturnal desaturation is associated with an increased risk of painful crisis and CNS morbidity (strokes, seizures, cranial nerve palsies, and coma). This suggests that even if the arterial PaO_2 is normal the reduction in oxygen carriage as a result of the low saturation, especially when combined with a low haemoglobin (often around 6–8g/dL) may lead to true tissue hypoxia, increased sickling, and increased micro-circulation occlusion and ischaemia.

Management

- Children with SCD should have annual spirometry and an annual CXR to monitor for the development of chronic lung disease. Assessment should be more frequent in those with recurrent ACS.
- Routine polysomnography to detect hypoxaemia is not part of most management plans, but should be considered in children with frequent ACS or painful crises, or those with daytime oxygen saturation of less than 94%.

- Where there is obstructive sleep apnoea this should be treated, usually by adenonsillectomy. It seems likely that using oxygen to treat nocturnal desaturation without obstruction will protect against sickle complications, although these benefits have not yet been demonstrated by a clinical trial.
- Annual ECGs may provide a method of early detection of pulmonary hypertension.

Further information

Hargrave, D.R., Wade, A., Evans, J.P.M., et al. (2003). Nocturnal oxygen saturation and painful sickle cell crises in children. *Blood* **101**, 846–8.

Kirkham, F.J., Hewes, D.K., Prengler, M., Wade, A., Lane, R., and Evans, J.P. (2001). Nocturnal hypoxaemia and central-nervous-system events in sickle-cell disease. *Lancet* **357**, 1656–9.

Needleman, J.P., Franco, M.E., Varlotta, L., Reber-Brodecki, D., Bauer, N., Dampier, C., and Allen, J.L. (1999). Mechanisms of nocturnal oxyhemoglobin desaturation in children and adolescents with sickle cell disease. *Pediatr. Pulmonol.* **28**, 418–22.

Siddiqui, A.K. and Ahmed, S. (2003). Pulmonary manifestations of sickle cell disease. *Postgrad. Med. J.* **79**, 384–90.

Spivey, J.F., Uong, E.C., Strunk, R., Bosaugh, S.E., and Debaun, M.R. (2006). Low daytime pulse oximetry reading is associated with nocturnal desaturation and obstructive sleep apnea in children with sickle cell anemia. *Pediatr. Blood Cancer* 2006 Oct 27 (Epub ahead of print).

Rare diseases affecting the lungs or airway

Alpha-1 antitrypsin deficiency

- Alpha-1 antitrypsin (AAT) is an enzyme produced by the liver that has activity against neutophil-derived proteases, and provides defence against protease-mediated tissue damage.
- AAT deficiency is common. About 1 in 5000 newborns of European descent will have the severe ZZ phenotype. This phenotype is associated with a marked (10-fold) reduction in enzyme activity.
- Between 60 and 80% of individuals with the ZZ phenotype will develop emphysema in adult life.
- Approximately 6% of affected babies will develop jaundice, of whom 1/3 will progress to cirrhosis. Up to 70% of affected babies have transient elevation of liver transaminases. AAT deficiency is the second commonest reason (after biliary atresia) for liver transplantation in childhood.
- Emphysema in individuals with the ZZ phenotype develops in adult life between the ages of 30 and 45 years and up to 10 years earlier if these individuals are regular cigarette smokers. Management is the same as for other forms of emphysema with the additional possibility of AAT replacement therapy for those with severe disease.
- One of the best studies of the effects on AAT deficiency on lung function in young people was carried out in Sweden. In 1972–1974 all newborns were screened for AAT deficiency and 129 infants with severe PiZZ deficiency were identified. The majority of these underwent lung function testing at 16, 18, and 22 years of age. Lung function was normal at all ages, although there did appear to be a more rapid decline than normally expected (-1.2% FEV_1/year).[1]
- AAT deficiency is not a risk factor for bronchiectasis. Since the ZZ phenotype is relatively common, the possibility of chance associations with bronchiectasis and other conditions is relatively high. Measuring AAT levels in children with bronchiectasis is not helpful since it may result in a false attribution of their lung disease to AAT deficiency.
- Occasionally, referrals are made to paediatric respiratory specialists to ask advice about children with the PiZZ AAT deficiency. On the basis of the available evidence, it is fair to say that lung disease in childhood is not significantly more likely than in the general population. There is an ongoing increased risk of liver disease. Smoking should be avoided.

1 Piitulainen, E. and Sveger, T. (2002). Respiratory symptoms and lung function in young adults with severe alpha(1)-antitrypsin deficiency (PiZZ). *Thorax* **57**, 705–8.

Alveolar capillary dysplasia

Alveolar capillary dysplasia (ACD) is a developmental abnormality of the pulmonary vasculature in which normal alveolar capillaries are absent and there is failure of the formation of the normal air–blood diffusion barrier. The cause is unknown. ACD usually affects term infants. There are often associated anomalies of the gastrointestinal, genitourinary, or cardiovascular systems. There may be a family history of neonatal death.

Histological examination of the lung shows:
- hypertrophy of the muscle coat of the small arteries;
- paucity of capillaries adjacent to alveolar epithelium;
- branches of the pulmonary vein running with branches of the pulmonary arteries rather than in the interlobular septa.

Presentation

Most infants present within 6h of birth with respiratory distress and cyanosis. Occasionally presentation is delayed, rarely for as long as 6 weeks. This is unlikely to represent any progression of the disease, but rather re-distribution of blood flow within the lung, changes in pulmonary shunting, and the development of right heart failure. Clinically, these infants are indistinguishable from those with persistent pulmonary hypertension of the newborn (PPHN). The initial CXR is often normal, but may show diffuse haziness or granularity.

Management

This is the same as for PPHN, often a combination of high frequency oscillatory ventilation and nitric oxide, or ECMO. Pneumothorax is common. In most cases, any improvement will be transient. It is very likely that those infants sick enough to need ECMO with ACD will die. A lung biopsy showing ACD could be considered as a contra-indication to ECMO since this treatment will be futile.

Outcome

In most infants the diagnosis is made at autopsy suggesting that the condition is uniformly fatal. However, it is possible that milder forms of the disease, which may have a patchy distribution within the lungs, may occur. At least one case of long-term survival has been reported.

Further information

Eulmesekian, P., Cutz, E., Parvez, B., Bohn, D., and Adatia, I. (2005). Alveolar capillary dysplasia: a six-year single center experience. *J. Perinat. Med.* **33**, 347–52.

Al-Hathlol, K., Phillips, S., Seshia, M.K., Casiro, O., Alvaro, R.E., and Rigatto, H. (2000). Alveolar capillary dysplasia. Report of a case of prolonged life without extracorporeal membrane oxygenation (ECMO) and review of the literature. *Early Hum. Dev.* **57**, 85–94.

Tibballs, J. and Chow, C.W. (2002). Incidence of alveolar capillary dysplasia in severe idiopathic persistent pulmonary hypertension of the newborn. *J. Paediatr. Child Health* **38**, 397–400.

Connective tissue disease

- Connective tissue diseases are rare in childhood and in most children the lungs are not involved.
- Children with connective tissue disease may present with respiratory symptoms, or may develop respiratory disease as part of their illness.
- Lung disease is usually of gradual onset and only slowly progressive and it can therefore be missed.
- Occasionally lung disease will present dramatically as an alveolar haemorrhage and acute respiratory failure.

Systemic lupus erythematosus

SLE is an autoimmune connective tissue disease with prevalence in children of around 1/10 000. It is commoner in African and Asian races than northern Europeans and is commoner in girls than boys (3:1), although this difference is less distinct in pre-pubertal children. In most individuals the cause is not known, although genetic and environmental factors have been proposed. A variant of SLE can be induced by drugs such as hydralazine, nitrofurantoin, and quinolones. SLE can affect children of any age, including infants.

Signs and symptoms
Usual initial symptoms, which may be intermittent or persistent, include:
- fever;
- fatigue;
- joint pain;
- malar rash (which may be photosensitive);
- painful or painless ulcers in the nose or mouth.

Signs may include:
- joint inflammation;
- hepatosplenomegaly;
- lymphadenopathy.

Respiratory problems
During the course of the disease, respiratory involvement is seen in 20–40% of children with SLE, and may be part of the presenting illness. Problems include the following.
- Pleuritis. Chest pain and breathlessness. Pleural effusion (exudates) may be present.
- Interstitial lung disease.
  - Gradual onset of breathlessness on exertion, with a dry cough and inspiratory crackles on auscultation. CXR usually shows reticulo-nodular shadowing. Chest HRCT scan may show ground-glass attenuation and increased interstitial markings, reflecting non-specific interstitial pneumonitis or patchy consolidation and bronchiectasis reflecting the presence of organizing pneumonia. Bronchiolitis obliterans may occur, but is uncommon.
  - Mild disease may be asymptomatic, and be picked up either by CT scan or by the presence of mild restriction on pulmonary function testing.

- Acute pneumonitis: fever, cough, breathlessness, chest pain with bilateral infiltrates on CXR. Illness can be severe, occasionally leading to respiratory failure.
- Pulmonary haemorrhage. Although this is relatively rare in childhood SLE (only 5% of cases), it may be the presenting symptom. Presents with breathlessness, fever, and cyanosis, and can progress to respiratory failure. Bilateral infiltrates on CXR. Haemoptysis is only seen in 50% of affected children with pulmonary haemorrhage.
- Increased risk of pulmonary infection, including *Pneumocystis* pneumonia, as a primary problem of the disease, but also as a consequence of immunosuppressive therapy.

Other organ involvement

- Renal tract The renal tract is affected in 50–60% of patients at presentation. Nephritis in children appears to be more severe than in adults, and usually requires aggressive treatment.
  - CNS. Neuropsychiatric manifestations occur in 30–60% of children with SLE during the course of disease. The commonest problems are headache, behaviour disorder, memory problems, lethargy, and dizziness. Encephalopathy, seizures (generalized and focal), depression, hallucinations, and transverse myelitis can also occur.
- Cardiac disease.
  - Myocarditis.
  - Pericarditis.
  - Endocarditis.
- Musculoskeletal disease.
  - Arthritis or arthralgia.
  - Myositis.
- Coagulopathy. There may be a pro-thrombotic tendency, associated with lupus anticoagulant or anti-cardiolipin antibodies. Although some of these anti-phospholipid antibodies prolong *in vitro* clotting tests (particularly the APTT) and are not corrected by adding normal plasma, they are associated with pro-thrombotic tendencies *in vivo*. They are associated with a number of collagen vascular diseases (also lymphomas and occasionally after viral infections), including SLE.

Investigations

The following investigations will help determine if a child has SLE.
- Blood tests:
  - anti-nuclear antibody: elevated in most children with SLE, but not specific;
  - anti-double-stranded DNA antibody: more specific and reflects disease activity;
  - Anti-Sm (Smith) antibody: very specific, not very sensitive;
  - FBC: haemolytic anaemia, leucopenia, and thrombocytopenia are all consistent with SLE;
  - complement levels: often reduced in SLE;
  - tests of clotting: prolonged APTT may suggest presence of lupus anticoagulant.
- Urine analysis: may indicate presence of glomerulonephritis.
- CXR: findings as described above.

- Chest HRCT scan: findings as described above.
- Lung function testing: in chronic respiratory involvement usually shows a restrictive pattern.

Diagnosis of SLE requires 4 out of 11 specific criteria (see box).

Diagnostic criteria of the American College of Rheumatology

A diagnosis of SLE requires 4 of the following to be present serially or simultaneously over any time period

- Malar rash
- Discoid rash
- Photosensitivity
- Oral ulcers
- Arthritis
- Serositis (pleuritis or pericarditis)
- Renal disorder—proteinuria or cellular casts
- Neurological disorder—seizures or psychosis
- Haematological disorder—haemolytic anaemia, leucopenia, lymphopenia
- Immunological disorder—raised anti-dsDNA or anti-SM or antiphospholipid antibodies
- Raised anti-nuclear antibody raised titre

Treatment

Treatment depends on the severity and pattern of organ involvement. Symptomatic lung disease would usually be treated with systemic corticosteroids. Severe disease may require addition of other immunosuppressants, usually either azathioprine or cyclophosphamide. Treatment duration is several months to years. Frequent re-evaluation for disease progression or development of new organ involvement is required. Serum markers such as anti-dsDNA, complement levels, and ESR can be used to monitor disease activity.

Outcome

Outcome 5-year survival is now > 90%, but long-term disease-free remission is rare and, in the majority of children, life span is limited by their disease. The possible role of biological agents such as anti-CD20 monoclonal antibodies (which target B cells) has not yet been established.

Dermatomyositis

- Juvenile dermatomyositis (JDM) is an inflammatory myopathy caused by a systemic vasculopathy.
- JDM typically presents with:
  - low grade fever;
  - weight loss;
  - arthralgia;
  - skin rash (typically in sun-exposed areas);
  - proximal muscle weakness.

- Diagnosis is suspected or the clinical findings plus elevated creatine kinase and often positive anti-nuclear antibody. MRI will show affected muscle, and EMG combined with muscle biopsy confirms the diagnosis.
- Treatment is with immunosuppressive agents—corticosteroids, cyclophosphamide, and methotrexate.

Respiratory problems

- Oropharyngeal muscles may be involved in the disease resulting in hoarseness, dysphagia, and difficulty handling secretions. Aspiration pneumonia may occur. Rarely, tracheostomy may be needed for adequate airway toilet. Dysfunction of the oropharynx is associated with a poor prognosis and requires aggressive treatment.
- Weakness of the respiratory muscles can also occur leading to a poor cough and increased risk of infection, as well as hypoventilation. As with other forms of muscle weakness, hypoventilation may first become apparent during sleep.
- Direct involvement of the lungs is unusual in JDM. Diffuse interstitial pulmonary fibrosis is well-documented in the adult form of dermatomyositis, but has been reported only occasionally in children with JDM.
- There are case reports of association between dermatomyositis and pulmonary alveolar proteinosis.

Scleroderma

- Scleroderma is a rare chronic systemic disorder of unknown aetiology characterized by:
  - Raynaud phenomenon;
  - skin fibrosis, ulceration, or atrophy, particularly affecting the face and hands;
  - organ involvement, especially lungs, kidneys, oesophagus, and heart.
- It is commonest in young adults but can affect teenagers and, rarely, children under the age of 10 years.
- Compared with adults, children are more likely to have localized scleroderma rather than systemic sclerosis.
- Nailfold video-capillaroscopy is a simple test to distinguish simple Raynaud phenomenon from that associated with underlying disease.
- Diagnosis is clinical, based on major and minor clinical criteria. Anti-nuclear antibody is often positive.
- There is no specific treatment, although immunosuppressant agents, such as pulsed IV cyclophosphamide and D-penicillamine have been tried with variable and limited success for lung disease.

Respiratory problems

- When scleroderma is part of systemic sclerosis, lung involvement is common (90% of patients) in both adults and children.
- Pulmonary fibrosis with a restrictive defect is the commonest abnormality. There is often a decreased carbon monoxide transfer factor.
- Aspiration lung disease, secondary to oesophageal dysmotility, can occur.

- Cardiac disease, such as cardiomyopathy, can present with respiratory symptoms or worsen pre-existing lung involvement.
- Pulmonary hypertension can occur and is usually a manifestation of the primary vasculopathy rather than occurring as a result of hypoxia. Children with systemic sclerosis and pulmonary hypertension may have relatively little parenchymal lung disease.
- Lung fibrosis is very slowly progressive. Pulmonary hypertension can be more aggressive resulting in right heart failure.
- There is an increased risk of lung malignancy in adults with systemic sclerosis.

Juvenile idiopathic arthritis

- Juvenile idiopathic arthritis (JIA) is defined as inflammation of one or more joints for at least 3 months in a child under the age of 16 years in whom other known causes of arthritis have been excluded.
- It has an incidence of 10–20/100 000 children.
- Pauciarticular disease (50% of cases) affects 4 or fewer joints, mainly knees and ankles. It is commoner in girls and usually presents at 1–3 years of age. Anti-nuclear antibody (ANA) may be positive, and is associated with chronic uveitis. A later onset form affects older boys and can be associated with acute uveitis.
- Polyarticular disease (30% of cases) affecting 5 or more small or large joints, is more common in girls than boys and, if rheumatoid factor (RhF) is positive, is the most likely form to cause joint deformity.
- Systemic onset disease (20% of cases) has an equal sex incidence and may affect a variable number of joints, although sometimes joint involvement is not apparent for several weeks after the start of the illness. Systemic-onset JIA typically presents with high spiking fevers, a faint rash that comes and goes with the fever, lymphadenopathy, and hepatosplenomegaly. ANA and RhF are usually negative.
- First-line treatment is high dose NSAID followed by disease-modifying drugs (such as methotrexate) for resistant disease. Corticosteroids are used for episodes of intense inflammation or systemic illness.

Respiratory problems

- Lung involvement in JIA is rare, and seen mainly in children with systemic onset disease.
- During the acute phase of systemic onset JIA, there may be pleural inflammation with effusion, sometimes with an interstitial pneumonitis. Concurrent pericarditis is common and may contribute to pain and breathlessness. These acute inflammatory conditions usually respond well to NSAID therapy or systemic corticosteroids.
- Longer-term respiratory problems that have been reported to be associated with JIA include:
  - bronchiolitis obliterans;
  - lymphoid interstitial pneumonia;
  - lymphoid bronchiolitis;
  - alveolar proteinosis;
  - primary pulmonary hypertension.

- There are no specific guidelines for the management of these rare lung diseases combined with JIA. It is possible that some may arise as a result of immunosuppressive therapies used for JIA. Each affected child needs to be investigated and treated according to the findings. Investigations are likely to include CT scan, bronchoscopy, and, where the diagnosis remains unclear, lung biopsy.
- Atypical infection, including *Pneumocystis* pneumonia, is an important differential in children with JIA on immunosuppressant therapy who develop lung disease.
- In asymptomatic children with JIA, lung function abnormalities may be found in up to 50%, including some with apparent small airways disease, and others with restriction and decreased transfer factor.

Sjögren's syndrome

- Sjögren's syndrome is an idiopathic systemic autoimmune disorder.
- It is relatively common in middle-aged adult women with usual symptoms of a dry mouth and dry eyes.
- It is rare in childhood. 75% of affected children are girls. Typical symptoms include:
  - recurrent parotid swelling, often with fever;
  - dry mouth (xerostomia), sometimes with oral ulcers;
  - recurrent conjunctivitis with dry eyes (keratoconjunctivitis sicca);
  - arthralgia.
- Investigation shows:
  - positive anti-nuclear antibody, anti-SSA, anti-SSB, or rheumatoid factor in 80% of affected children;
  - elevated amylase in 80%;
  - elevated ESR in 80%;
  - ocular examination may show keratoconjunctivitis and decreased tear production.

Respiratory problems

- Lung disease is reported in children with Sjögren's syndrome, often presenting as an interstitial lung disease, with breathlessness and dry cough.
  - Lung function shows a restrictive defect.
  - BAL can show increased numbers of neutrophils or lymphocytes.
  - Lung biopsies from affected adults show interstitial fibrosis with lymphocytic infiltration.
- Treatment is usually with a combination of systemic corticosteroids, hydroxychloroquine, or azathioprine.

Behçet disease

- Behçet disease (BD) is a multisystem vasculitis-like disorder characterized by the triad of recurrent:
  - mouth ulcers;
  - genital ulcers;
  - uveitis (less commonly seen in children).

- Other features include arthritis (large or small joints), erythema nodosum, and other skin rashes, CNS involvement (meningoencephalitis and psychiatric or behavioural disorders), vascular lesions including thrombosis (arterial and venous), and pulmonary arterial aneurysms.
- The cause is unknown but there does appear to be neutrophil hyperfunction. This can be demonstrated clinically using the pathergy test—a sterile 24 gauge needle is pricked under the skin. Neutrophil migration to the site results in the formation of a small nodule or pustule within 24–48h.
- BD is a rare disease (1/100 000) and very rare in children. It is thought to be commoner in the Middle East and Turkey. When it does occur in children it is nearly always in children > 10 years of age.
- Oral ulceration is the hallmark of the disease. The ulcers are painful, usually occur in crops, and resolve without leaving a scar.
- Blood tests are non-specific. Inflammatory markers (ESR, CRP) are usually raised. Anti-cardiolipin is elevated in 30% but other auto-antibodies (including ANA and ANCA) are negative.
- Diagnosis requires the presence of recurrent oral ulceration plus 2 of the following:
  - recurrent genital ulcerations;
  - anterior or posterior uveitis or retinal vasculitis;
  - erythema nodosum or other skin involvement, including pustular rash;
  - positive pathergy test.
- Differential diagnosis for recurrent oral ulceration includes SLE, sarcoidosis, and Crohn's disease or orofacial granulomatosis.
- Imaging of the head with MRI is indicated when there is CNS involvement. Vascular involvement (thrombosis or aneurysms) can be identified by angiography, CT with contrast, or MRA (magnetic resonance angiography). A history of haemoptysis should prompt this investigation to identify pulmonary artery aneurysm.
- Cardiac evaluation including echo may detect evidence of pulmonary hypertension associated with pulmonary thrombosis or emboli.
- Biopsy is often unhelpful and the diagnosis is made clinically. Histology of the mouth or genital ulcers may show lymphocytic and plasma cell infiltration. Occasionally there may be vasculitic necrosis.
- Treatment is usually a combination of colchicine (good for mouth ulcers), topical steroids, and systemic steroids. For more severe disease azathioprine, cyclophosphamide, ciclosporin, methotrexate, and TNF antagonists (e.g. infliximab) have all been tried.
- Overall mortality in adult series is 15–20% at 5 years. Death is usually related either to pulmonary haemorrhage, thrombosis, or CNS disease.

Respiratory problems

- Lung disease affects 10–20% of adults with BD. A smaller proportion of children with BD seems to have lung disease, but this reduced incidence seems likely to be related to the duration of the disease rather than any fundamental difference between adults and children.

- Most lung disease in BD is caused by either pulmonary artery aneurysms (PAA) or by pulmonary emboli. Symptoms include:
  - breathlessness;
  - cough;
  - pleuritic chest pain;
  - haemoptysis.
- Fatal pulmonary haemorrhage can occur, usually from rupture of a PAA. The aneurysms are often on peripheral pulmonary vessels and ulcerate into adjacent bronchi.
- Very rarely, PAA may be the only manifestation of BD.
- In one series of adults and children with BD, 80% of those with PAA had extrapulmonary thrombosis or thrombophlebitis. Nearly all has episodes of haemoptysis. This suggests that, in the absence of these problems, PAA are unlikely.
- Vascular inflammation can spread to the lung parenchyma and cause diffuse pulmonary haemorrhages, bronchiolitis, and organizing pneumonia.
- Pulmonary problems such as fibrosis and alveolitis that are not associated with vascular involvement are rare.
- Imaging usually reflects the consequences of thromboembolic disease or PAA. CXR may show pleural effusion, diffuse infiltrate, discrete densities, and hilar vessel prominence. HRCT may show pleural thickening, air-trapping (on expiratory scans), bronchiectasis and pulmonary nodules.
- Biopsy of involved lung tissue may show a predominant lymphocytic pulmonary vasculitis.

Further information

Uzun, O., Akpolat, T., and Erkan, L. (2005). Pulmonary vasculitis in Behcet disease: a cumulative analysis. *Chest* **127** (6), 2243–53.

Familial dysautonomia

- Familial dysautonomia, also known as Riley–Day syndrome, is an autosomal recessive disorder found almost exclusively in individuals of Ashkenazi Jewish descent. It occurs with an incidence of 1/4000 within the Ashkenazi Jewish population. It is caused by mutations in the *IKBKAP* gene.
- It is a progressive disease affecting autonomic and some sensory nerves. It usually presents in the first year of life with feeding difficulties, recurrent chestiness, lack of tears during crying, and autonomic crises (see below).
- Features of the autonomic dysfunction include:
  - decreased tears—which can cause corneal drying and significant eye problems;
  - abnormal sucking and swallowing;
  - gastro-oesophageal reflux;
  - unstable and variable blood pressure, including postural hypotension;
  - decreased sensitivity to hypoxia and hypercarbia, which can be associated with hypoventilation;
  - syncope during vigorous exercise.
- Autonomic crises are common. The frequency of crises varies from child to child—from several per day to 1 per month. They can be precipitated by infection, tiredness, or emotional stress and result in:
  - emotional lability;
  - increased secretions;
  - varying blood pressure (often hypertension);
  - tachycardia;
  - vomiting;
  - poor skin perfusion.
- Other neurological problems include:
  - decreased tendon reflexes;
  - hypotonia in infancy;
  - seizures in 10%;
  - ataxia;
  - decreased pain and temperature sensation;
  - altered taste sensation;
  - peripheral sensory neuropathy with consequent increased injury.
- Renal disease, particularly glomerulosclerosis, occurs in 20% and may result in renal failure.
- Scoliosis is common in mid-childhood and will worsen coexisting lung disease. Osteoporosis can also occur, which makes management of the scoliosis more difficult.
- Most individuals have normal intelligence. Behavioural problems, including breath-holding episodes, are common.

Respiratory problems

- The commonest problem is aspiration lung disease resulting in recurrent pneumonia, wheezing, and bronchiectasis.
- Night-time hypoventilation can also occur.

Investigation

- Diagnosis is based on clinical suspicion plus DNA test for *IKBKAP* mutations.
- Where there are persistent respiratory problems, CT chest may be helpful to determine extent of underlying lung disease.
- Polysomnography should be carried out annually to identify any problems of respiratory control, such as long respiratory pauses and blunted responses to hypoxia or hypercapnia.

Treatment and outcome

- Treatment is supportive. Eye care to maintain eye moisture is important.
- Most (80%) of affected children need gastrostomy and fundoplication to reduce aspiration events.
- Chest physiotherapy and prophylactic antibiotics can be helpful in children with chronic lung disease and bronchiectasis. Full vaccination is recommended, including annual influenza vaccination.
- Although significant night-time hypoventilation is unusual, affected children may benefit from non-invasive ventilation during sleep.
- Decreased responses to hypoxia and hypercarbia mean that children with familial dysautonomia should avoid underwater swimming and extra care should be taken with long-haul air travel, particularly in children with coexisting chronic aspiration lung disease.
- Respiratory disease is a major cause of morbidity and mortality. Median survival is 40 years of age. There is an undefined risk of sudden death.

Further information

Axelrod, F.B., Chelimsky, G.G., and Weese-Mayer, D.E. (2006). Pediatric autonomic disorders. *Pediatrics* **118**, 309–21.

Maayan, H.C. (2006). Respiratory aspects of Riley–Day syndrome familial dysautonomia. *Paediatr. Respir. Rev.* **7** (Suppl. 1), S258–9. http://www.thelamfoundation.org.

Hepato-pulmonary syndrome

Children with cirrhosis may develop a number of respiratory complications. These include hepato-pulmonary syndrome, pulmonary hypertension, breathlessness due to restriction (caused by compression usually from ascites), right basal pneumonia, and pleural effusions.

Hepato-pulmonary syndrome

- This condition is characterized by persistent hypoxia, the cause of which is not fully understood but which includes:
  - functional intrapulmonary right to left shunting—sometimes due to vasodilatation of the pulmonary arterioles leading to a rapid capillary transit time insufficient to allow full oxygenation. In other cases there may be true pulmonary arteriovenous malformations;
  - ventilation perfusion mismatch;
  - reduced diffusion capacity.
- Intrapulmonary shunting may be demonstrated by perfusion scans, which will show deposition of label in the brain and kidneys indicating bypass of the pulmonary capillary bed. It can also be demonstrated by bubble-contrast echocardiography.
- Clinically the circulation appears to be hyperdynamic because of the dilated pulmonary vascular bed.
- Cardiac catherization does not usually show true arteriovenous shunts. The shunting arises as a result of dilatation of pulmonary arterioles and capillaries.
- Occasionally hepato-pulmonary syndrome is caused by shunts that arise because of anastomoses between the pulmonary veins and systemic veins, usually either the portal or para-oesophageal veins.
- The severity of liver disease does not correlate with the likelihood of the presence of hepato-pulmonary syndrome.
- It has been reported in children of all ages, including infants.
- The frequency of hepato-pulmonary syndrome in children with cirrhosis ranges between 5% and 35% in different reported case series.
- Some children with hepato-pulmonary syndrome will have no symptoms. Other will have breathlessness and exercise intolerance. Breathlessness and the degree of hypoxia are worse in the upright position; the opposite is the case in most cardiac causes of these problems.
- Low-flow oxygen is usually sufficient to correct the hypoxia. Since the most likely cause is right to left shunting, the situation is analogous to that of cardiac disease and oxygen treatment need only be given for symptom relief.

Pulmonary hypertension
- This is occasionally seen in children with cirrhosis and may arise because of:
  - pulmonary thromboemboli arising in the portal system;
  - vasoactive substances bypassing liver metabolism.
- Symptoms are similar to those of other causes of pulmonary hypertension and are predominantly breathlessness and exercise intolerance. There will usually be hypoxia with evidence of right ventricular strain or hypertrophy.

Idiopathic pulmonary haemosiderosis

Idiopathic pulmonary haemosiderosis (IPH) is characterized by diffuse alveolar bleeding in the absence of vasculitis or cardiac disease. As the name implies, the cause is not known. Links with milk allergy (Heiner's syndrome) and fungal infection (with *Stachybotrys chartarum*) have been proposed but are not universally accepted and in any case only apply to a small proportion of children with IPH. The incidence of IPH is not known, but a large centre might see 1 case every 2 years. Minor epidemics of alveolar bleeding in infants have been described.

Symptoms and signs

- 70% are < 6 years of age at presentation.
- Recurrent haemoptysis (common but not invariable).
- Dry cough is common.
- During active bleeds there may be breathless and desaturation, either at rest or on exercise.
- Auscultation is often normal. There may be end-inspiratory crepitations.
- No signs of vascular disease (e.g. rash or arthritis). Although not well described in the literature, some patients with IPH have arthralgia.
- Children with Down's syndrome appear to have susceptible pulmonary capillary beds and are more likely to bleed. Diagnosis of IPH in this group requires particularly careful exclusion of any cardiac cause (high pulmonary blood flow or raised pulmonary venous pressure).

Differential diagnosis

The differential diagnosis for haemoptysis includes the following.

- Confusion with epistaxis or haematemesis.
- Inhaled foreign body.
- Bronchiectasis, including that caused by cystic fibrosis.
- Tuberculosis.
- Bleeding disorders, especially von Willebrand disease.
- Hereditary haemorrhagic telangiectasia—can be associated with tracheal telangiectasia.
- Pulmonary venous hypertension or high pulmonary blood flows.
- Pulmonary adenoma or carcinoid tumor.
- Goodpasture's syndrome.
- Pulmonary vasculitis:
  - Wegener's granulomatosis;
  - microscopic polyangiitis, a variant of polyarteritis nodosa.
- Connective tissue disease: systemic lupus erythematosus.

Where there is no observed haemoptysis, the differential will be the same as for other forms of interstitial lung disease (see 📖 Chapter 46).

Investigation
- Blood tests
  - FBC and film (iron-deficient anaemia and reticulocytosis);
  - ferritin, iron, and transferrin;
  - renal function: should be normal in IPH;
  - ESR: only mildly elevated in IPH;
  - autoimmune tests: ANA (SLE), ANCA (Wegener's granulomatosis and microscopic polyangiitis) should all be negative in IPH;
  - for completeness a RAST for milk protein should be done, at least in infants;
  - standard tests for clotting (prothrombin time and activated thromboplastin time) plus tests for von Willebrand disease (factor VIII and VWB antigen).
- Lung function tests will show a restrictive pattern. KCO will be increased because of the free Hb in the alveoli.
- Urine microscopy for red cells and white cells indicating renal involvement: negative in IPH.
- CXR: in IPH this may show diffuse alveolar shadowing indicating alveolar haemorrhage.
- Echocardiography and ECG may be needed to exclude evidence of pulmonary hypertension.
- CT scan: usually shows a ground-glass appearance with alveolar infiltrates. The appearance can be patchy or mosaic.
- Bronchoscopy and BAL. The airways will usually appear normal. BAL will show haemosiderin-laden macrophages, with mild increase in neutrophils. Culture is usually negative. Haemosiderin-laden macrophages may also be seen in gastric aspirates or induced sputum.
- The numbers of haemosiderin-laden macrophages are expressed as the number of positive cells out of 300 counted. Haemosiderin appears in macrophages 36–48h after alveolar bleeding and level of haemosiderin in macrophages peaks 6–8 days post-bleed. Levels fall below 50/300 by 6 weeks post-bleed.
- Lung biopsy is not usually necessary for the diagnosis providing clinical history and other investigations are typical for IPH. If performed it will show alveolar blood with haemosiderin-laden macrophages, but no evidence of vasculitis. Alveolar septae may contain mild focal infiltrate of neutrophils, which can be seen to be within capillary walls on electron microscopy. This may be reported as pulmonary capillaritis. It is not known whether the presence of pulmonary capillaritis affects the clinical course.

Diagnosis
Diagnosis usually based on history of recurrent haemoptysis or recurrent episodes of breathlessness, plus abnormal CXR and CT scan, plus iron deficiency anaemia, plus evidence (usually BAL) of pulmonary haemorrhage in absence of evidence (clinical or on investigation) of vasculitis.

Treatment

- Despite the absence of marked inflammation, the main treatment for IPH is immunosuppression with systemic steroids. Most regimes will use prednisolone 2mg/kg/day for 4 weeks followed by a slow wean over 6 months. Weaning too quickly seems to be associated with recurrence. If breakthrough bleeds occur on prednisolone, a second line agent should be added, either hydroxychloroquine or azathioprine, and prednisolone put back to 2mg/kg/day until bleeding has stopped. A slower wean should then be started. As for all children on long-term oral steroids, warnings about infection risk, particularly chicken pox, should be given.
- In children with severe hypoxic illness, a 3–5 day course of pulsed methylprednisolone can be used to try and control the bleeding. If no benefit is seen cyclophosphamide can be tried. Cyclophosphamide can take up to 2 weeks to be effective and supportive treatment should be maintained during this period, including mechanical ventilation if necessary.
- Iron deficiency should be treated with a 3 month course of iron.
- Children should be monitored monthly for the first 6 months. FBC and reticulocyte count are sensitive measures of bleeding. Some units like to carry out repeat BAL to demonstrate that bleeding has stopped. Others prefer to use clinical parameters only. The local tissue hypoxia that occurs during a lavage potentially increases the risk of re-bleeding.
- CXR should be repeated during exacerbations.
- Treatment can be withdrawn when there has been no evidence of bleeding on low dose therapy for 6 months.

Outcome

With relatively aggressive immunotherapy most children will now do well, and the disease will go into remission. Recurrence can occur, and may be precipitated by lung infection, exposure to irritants (including cigarette smoke), and hypoxia. Where treatment is less successful, or the diagnosis is made after some years, there is a risk of pulmonary fibrosis, significant restrictive lung disease, and respiratory failure.

Lymphangioleiomyomatosis

- Lymphangioleiomyomatosis (LAM) is a rare disorder occurring almost exclusively in women of child-bearing age, although it has been described in children (boys and girls) as young as 12 years of age.
- It is characterized by the progressive proliferation, migration, and differentiation of smooth muscle (SM)-like LAM cells in the lungs, kidneys, and lymphatic system. LAM cell proliferation is thought to obstruct small airways giving rise to cysts and pneumothoraces. Obstruction of lymphatics can cause pleural effusions and obstruction to pulmonary venules may cause haemosiderosis and haemoptysis.
- LAM occurs sporadically in association with mutations in the tuberose sclerosis complex genes TSC1 and TSC2 (sporadic LAM) and also in patients with tuberose sclerosis (TSC-LAM). TSC1/TSC2 complex functions as an integrator of signalling networks regulated by growth factors, insulin, and nutrients.

Clinical features
- Symptoms may include:
  - dyspnoea;
  - haemoptysis;
  - chest pain;
  - persistent cough;
  - fatigue.
- Pneumothorax is often the presenting problem and occurs in 65% of affected individuals at some time. Pleural effusions in 30% of affected individuals. The combination of a pneumothorax with pleural effusion in a young woman is suggestive of LAM.
- Physical findings are usually those of pneumothorax or pleural effusion. A search should be made for features of tuberose sclerosis:
  - facial or nail bed fibromata;
  - shagreen patch—rough discoloured skin near the sacrum;
  - café-au-lait spots;
  - retinal hamartomas—usually white spots around the disc.

Investigations
- CXR can be normal or can show:
  - cystic changes;
  - basilar reticulonodular changes;
  - pleural effusions;
  - hilar and mediastinal adenopathy;
  - pneumothoraces.
- HRCT scanning of the chest demonstrates profuse thin-walled cysts in all lung fields. Diffuse nodular changes may be present predominantly in patients with TSC LAM.
- Lung biopsy. Histopathologically the cysts are dilated distal airspaces and diffuse infiltration of atypical smooth muscle cells in the pulmonary interstitium , including spaces surrounding airways, vessels, and lymphatics.

- Renal ultrasound. Renal angiomyolipomas, unusual hamartomas containing fat, smooth muscle and blood vessels, are present in about 70–80% of patients with TSC-LAM and 50% of sporadic LAM.

Treatment

There is no treatment with proven effectiveness. Often anti-oestrogen therapies are tried. A trial of rapamycin is underway. The disease is progressive. Recurrence has been reported after lung transplantation.

Pelizaeus–Merzbacher disease

- Pelizaeus–Merzbacher disease (PMD) is a very rare neurodegenerative condition with an incidence of about 1/500 000.
- It is an X-linked condition seen only seen in boys. 70% have mutations in the proteolipid protein 1 (*PLP1*) gene.
- It is of relevance to the respiratory specialist because it is a cause of neonatal and infant stridor. Combined with hypotonia this often leads to recurrent respiratory infection, which is a frequent cause of death in these boys.
- Other characteristic features, usually present in the first few weeks or months of life, are:
  - striking nystagmoid eye movements present from birth or soon after;
  - neonatal hypotonia but subsequent severe spasticity;
  - ataxia and severe cognitive impairment.
- Affected boys do not walk or talk and have very limited purposeful movements.
- The stridor is caused by disco-ordinate laryngeal musculature.
- There is no effective treatment.

Pulmonary alveolar proteinosis

Pulmonary alveolar proteinosis (PAP) is characterized by the accumulation of surfactant-like material in the alveoli. The presence of this material reduces lung compliance and interferes with gas exchange. The incidence of PAP in children is not known, but it is rare and most paediatric respiratory centres would not expect to see more than one affected child every 2–3 years.

Types of disease

Neonatal disease due to surfactant protein B deficiency

Surfactant protein B deficiency is an autosomal recessive disorder caused by loss of function mutations in the SPB gene. It has an incidence of around 1/1.5 million in children of northern European descent. The usual clinical presentation is of a term infant who develops severe neonatal respiratory distress in the 1st day of life with CXR changes that resemble respiratory distress syndrome. Most infants require mechanical ventilation. Occasionally, initial presentation is with milder lung disease that progresses over the course of a few days. The disease is usually rapidly fatal. The only effective treatment is lung transplantation. Histological examination of lung tissue from infants with SPB deficiency shows large amounts of periodic acid Schiff (PAS)-positive lipoproteinaceous material in the alveoli much of which is precursor protein for surfactant protein C. This suggests that SPB is important in the turnover of other surfactant proteins.

Later onset disease

Outside the neonatal period PAP can present at any age from infancy to adolescence. Later-onset disease can either be primary and related to disturbance of the function of granulocyte–macrophage colony-stimulating factor (GM-CSF) or secondary and associated with a wide range of conditions, including the following.

- Infections (especially *Nocardia* and *Pneumocystis*).
- Haematological malignancy (especially myeloid leukaemia).
- Lysinuric protein intolerance. This is a systemic disorder caused by a defect of the transport of cationic amino acids (lysine, arginine, ornithine). Features of the disease include hyperammonaemia, GI symptoms, failure to thrive, hepatosplenomegaly, renal disease, osteoporosis, haematopoietic abnormalities, pancreatitis, and lung involvement. Lung problems include pulmonary haemorrhage, symptomatic and asymptomatic interstitial fibrosis as well as progressive and usually fatal alveolar proteinosis. Diagnosis is based on serum and urinary amino acid levels. Treatment with a low protein diet and oral citrulline has limited benefit.
- Sideroblastic anaemia.
- Dermatomyositis.

GM-CSF related PAP can be due either to a genetic defect in the GM-CSF receptor, which usually results in symptoms in the first few years of life, or the presence of acquired anti-GM-CSF auto-antibodies, which usually presents in adolescence or adult life.

Symptoms include:
- progressive breathlessness during feeding or on exercise;
- dry cough;
- poor growth or weight loss.

Less commonly there is:
- fever;
- chest pain;
- haemoptysis.

The rate of disease progression is very variable, ranging from symptoms that come on over several months, to those progressing to respiratory failure in a few weeks. Some children can have quite dramatic CT scan changes with little in the way of symptoms.

Investigations (for later onset disease)
- CXR shows bilateral diffuse airspace opacity.
- CT scan shows ground-glass opacification, often with interlobular septal thickening giving the appearance of crazy paving
- BAL returns creamy pinkish fluid containing PAS-positive material and foamy macrophages. BAL fluid should be sent for culture and microscopy looking for *Pneumocystis jiroveci*.
- Lung biopsy is the gold-standard diagnostic test.
- Other tests looking for aetiology include:
  - anti-GM-CSF antibodies;
  - DNA for GM-CSF receptor defects;
  - FBC and film;
  - immunoglobulin levels and specific antibody levels to check immune function;
  - serum and urinary amino acids for lysinuric protein intolerance (plus DNA for *SLC7A7* mutation analysis if high index of suspicion).
- Rarely, Niemann–Pick disease type B can present with similar CT and BAL findings. There is nearly always hepatosplenomegaly. See 📖 p. 674.

Treatment for later onset primary disease
When symptoms are mild, it is reasonable to watch and wait. In more severe disease, the treatment of choice is therapeutic lung lavage, using selective lung intubation and large volumes of pre-warmed saline to wash the lipo-proteinaceous material out of the alveoli. The procedure may need to be repeated on multiple occasions to keep the disease under control. In patients with severe disease who have anti-GM-CSF antibodies, daily SC GM-CSF may lead to improvement.

Outcome for later onset primary disease
The clinical course is variable. Some patients have mild to moderate stable disease, controlled with multiple lavage treatments, some have spontaneous remission, and some have disease with progression to respiratory failure.

Further information

de Blic, J. (2004). Pulmonary alveolar proteinosis. *Paediatr. Respir. Rev.* **5,** 310–2.

Trapnell, B.C., Whitsett, J.A., and Nakata, K. (2003). Pulmonary alveolar proteinosis. *N. Engl. J. Med.* **349,** 2527–39.

Santamaria, F., Brancaccio, G., Parenti, G., Francalanci, P., Squitieri, C., Sebastio, G., Dionisi-Vici, C., D'argenio, P., Andria, G., and Parisi, F. (2004). Recurrent fatal pulmonary alveolar proteinosis after heart–lung transplantation in a child with lysinuric protein intolerance. *J. Pediatr.* **145,** 268–72.

Pulmonary embolism

- Pulmonary embolism (PE) is the term used to describe arterial obstruction by thrombus that has either arisen at a distant location or that has formed and extended within the pulmonary artery.
- Large central or bilateral PEs are life-threatening.
- The incidence of PE in children is around 1/100 000. It is commonest in the first 2 years of life.
- As with many rare conditions, diagnosis is often delayed.
- Chronic recurrent small pulmonary emboli can cause pulmonary hypertension.

Risk factors

- Central venous lines.
- Congenital or acquired heart disease (risk of intracardiac clot formation).
- Obesity.
- Immobility.
- Inflammatory disease, including vasculitides.
- Malignancy.
- Prothrombotic disorder.
- Oral contraceptive pill.
- Smoking.
- Sickle cell disease.

Clinical features

Symptoms include:
- chest pain;
- haemoptysis;
- breathlessness;
- cardiovascular collapse.

Signs include:
- pleural rub;
- a loud P2 heart sound suggests right heart strain;
- evidence of a peripheral thrombus.

Investigation

- Measurement of serum D-dimers in adults is a highly sensitive test for excluding PE with an elevated level found in 97% of cases. It seems to be less sensitive in children. Normal levels were found in 5 of 14 children with PE in one case series.
- Chest CT with contrast (sometimes called CT-pulmonary angiogram) is usually the diagnostic test. Alternatives such as magnetic reasonance angiography (MRA), radionuclide perfusion scans, and standard angiography can be also be used but their availability may be limited, particularly outside of the normal working day.
- Echocardiography will identify any embolic foci in the heart or associated with central lines and indicate if there is any right ventricular dysfunction secondary to the PE.
- Blood investigations for pro-thrombotic risk factors:

- anti-thrombin III protein C and protein S levels;
- factor V Leiden;
- prothrombin gene mutations.
- When no cause is apparent investigation for occult malignancy or inflammatory disorders should be considered.

Treatment

- For most children treatment with standard doses of SC fractionated heparin is appropriate. Effectiveness is judged by clinical improvement. For infants, where absorption of fractionated heparin may be less reliable, IV heparin infusions with monitoring of clotting times may be required.
- Thrombolytic therapy with tissue plasminogen activator (TPA) can cause bleeding. It is reserved for children with haemodynamic compromise associated with large central or bilateral clots. Recent surgery is a contraindication.
- Long-term anticoagulation with warfarin may be indicated, depending on the cause of the thrombus.

Further information

Rajpurkar, M., Warrier, I., Chitlur, M., Sabo, C., Frey, M.J., Hollon, W., and Lusher, J. (2007). Pulmonary embolism—experience at a single children's hospital. Thromb. Res. **119**, 699–703.

Pulmonary lymphangiectasia

Pulmonary lymphangiectasia (PL) refers to a rare condition in which there is dilatation of the normal lymphatic channels. The incidence is not known. Increased fluid in the lymphatic channels decreases lung compliance and increases the work of breathing. Two forms of PL are recognized.

Primary PL is thought to be an intrinsic abnormality of the lymphatic channels, and may be associated with lymphoedema of other parts of the body, loss of intestinal lymph, and hemihypertrophy. Primary PL can be confined to the lung. The cause is not known. It may be found in association with genetic syndromes, including Down, Turner, and Noonan syndromes.

Secondary PL results from lymphatic obstruction (e.g. damage to the thoracic duct) or from increased lymph production because of raised pulmonary venous pressure, such as that caused by pulmonary vein stenosis or mitral valve stenosis.

Presentation

Primary PL will usually present in the neonatal period.

- Primary PL confined to the lung is particularly severe and may be fatal, despite intervention.
- More generalized lymphangiectasia can present pre-natally as non-immune hydrops.
- Rarely symptoms may not develop until later infancy or early childhood. Affected infants will have respiratory distress, usually with diffuse fine crackles.
- The diagnosis can be difficult. CXR will be abnormal but non-specific, with increased interstitial markings and hyperinflation. Similar changes will be seen on CT scan. 15% will have a pleural effusion that may be chylous.
- A lung biopsy is usually required to make a definitive diagnosis.

Secondary PL usually occurs where there is an easily recognized underlying condition.

Management

There is no specific treatment for PL. Management is supportive. Large pleural effusions may need to be drained and may continue to re-accumulate for several days or weeks. Resolution may be speeded by using a medium chain triglyceride diet or TPN to decrease the volume of chyle. Pleurodesis may be helpful.

Outcome

The outcome of primary PL is uncertain. With supportive care, the lung disease tends to improve with time. Lung function tests show a stable, predominantly obstructive pattern. There may be poor growth in the first 2 years and recurrent episodes of bacterial bronchitis. The presence of associated abnormalities may significantly affect outcome. The prognosis of secondary PL depends on the nature of the lymphatic obstruction or venous hypertension.

Pulmonary lymphangiomatosis

- Lymphangiomatosis is a rare disease characterized by diffuse or multifocal lymphangioma (abnormal proliferation of lymphatic vessels) that commonly affect the lung and mediastium and may also involve the liver, soft tissues, bones, and spleen.
- Lymphangiomatosis is differentiated from primary lymphangiectasia (see 📖 p. 660) by the increased number of complex anastomosing vessels with secondary dilatation rather than the simple dilatation of pre-existing lymphatic capillaries. Primary lymphangiectasia usually presents in the neonatal period or early infancy. Lymphangiomatosis presents at any time throughout childhood (including infancy) and early adult life. Most reported cases are in children.

Signs and symptoms

- Lung involvement is found in the majority (80%) of affected children and typically presents with breathlessness and exercise intolerance.
- Splenomegaly is found in 20% of affected children.
- Bony involvement is common (75% of children) and may be the reason for initial presentation because of either deformity or pain from a pathological fracture. The axial skeleton, including skull, ribs, shoulder girdle, spine, and pelvis, is most usually affected. After a fracture through an area of affected bone there is typically failure of healing followed by progressive reabsorption of bone around the fracture site. This condition is sometimes called Gorham's vanishing bone disease.

Investigations

- CXR may show unilateral or bilateral pleural effusions (chylothoraces), increased interstitial markings, and a widened mediastinum. Thickening of interlobular septa and the pleura is seen on CT scans.
- Typical radiographic appearance of the bony lesion is radiolucent cysts surrounded by a sclerotic rim.
- MRI will demonstrate mediastinal involvement.
- Biopsy of any masses present or thickened pleura will usually be necessary to make the diagnosis

Management

- Management of the pulmonary disease includes closed chest drainage of the chylothoraces; pleurodesis is often required. Involvement of the lung parenchyma can lead to progressive breathlessness and systemic therapies with interferon-alpha and etoposide have been tried.
- The natural history of lymphangiomas is progressive enlargement. Where there is compression of surrounding structures, or instability of bony structures such as the cervical spine, surgical excision may be necessary. Pathological fracture of the ribs can lead to a sudden worsening of respiratory status.
- Radiotherapy, electrical therapy, and bisphosphonates may be required to promote healing of fractures.

Outcome

The prognosis in children is poor, with a 40% 5-year mortality. Most children who die have extensive systemic disease, nearly always involving the lungs.

Further information

Alvarez, O.A., Kjellin, I., and Zuppan, C.W. (2004). Thoracic lymphangiomatosis in a child. *J. Pediatr. Hematol. Oncol.* **26**, 136–41.

Pfleger, A., Schwinger, W., Maier, A., Tauss, J., Popper, H.H., and Zach, M.S. (2006). Gorham–Stout syndrome in a male adolescent—case report and review of the literature. *J. Pediatr. Hematol. Oncol.* **28**, 231–3.

Pulmonary vasculitides

- The lungs may be involved in several systemic vasculitic disoders. All the diseases are rare in childhood. In most pulmonary involvement is unusual.
- Note that dermatomyositis (📖 p. 638) and Behçet disease (📖 p. 641) are both predominantly vasculitic diseases that can affect the lungs but are usually considered as connective tissue diseases.
- The clinical presentation depends on the size of vessel involved.
  - Medium to large arteritis can result in pulmonary infarction and necrosis. Granuloma formation may occur.
  - Small vessel disease can cause diffuse alveolar haemorrhage.
- Pulmonary symptoms and signs are non-specific. Alveolar haemorrhage can cause rapid onset respiratory failure with prominent hypoxia.
- CXR and CT scans will show diffuse alveolar shadowing when there is alveolar haemorrhage, and discrete abnormalities such as nodules and areas of consolidation, usually due to tissue necrosis, when larger vessels are involved.
- Biopsy of an affected site is usually required for diagnosis. This will show inflammation of affected vessels with associated tissue necrosis. There may be vessel thrombosis. Changes suggestive of diffuse interstitial pneumonitis are not associated with vasculitic conditions.

Pulmonary involvement in vasculitides

Common in
- Wegener's granulomatosis
- Kawasaki disease

Uncommon in
- Churg–Strauss vasculitis
- Polyartertis nodosa
- Henoch–Schönlein purpura
- Takayasu arteritis

Wegener's granulomatosis

Wegener's granulomatosis (WG) is an aggressive small vessel vasculitis characterized by the formation of necrotizing granulomata. It particularly affects the upper and lower respiratory tract and the kidneys. Although an accurate incidence is not known, WG is occasionally seen in childhood and frequently presents with disease involving the respiratory tract. WG can affect children of any age, from infancy to adolescence.

Symptoms and signs

Usual symptoms at initial presentation include:
- mouth ulcers;
- sinusitis and nasal discharge;
- nose bleeds;
- otitis and deafness;
- cough;

- wheezing;
- breathlessness;
- haemoptysis.

Other symptoms may include:
- weight loss;
- fever;
- malaise;
- myalgia;
- arthralgia;
- skin rashes.

Examination may reveal:
- tachypnoea with or without desaturation (suggesting alveolar haemorrhage);
- tender sinuses;
- oral or nasal granulomata, sometimes with nasal deformity;
- stridor (suggesting subglottic stenosis).

Possible organ involvement in WG
- Upper airway:
  - ulceration;
  - granuloma formation;
  - subglottic stenosis.
- Lower airway:
  - granulomata with airway compression;
  - alveolar haemorrhage;
  - parenchymal granulomata.
- Renal: glomerulonephritis (10–20% at presentation; 60–70% in later disease).
- Skin:
  - blanching or non-blanching macules and nodules in 50%;
  - more rarely massive necrotizing granulomata.
- Joints:
  - arthralgia of the knees, hips, wrists, or ankles in 50%;
  - objective evidence of arthritis is rare.
- Eyes:
  - conjunctival and corneal lesions;
  - uveitis;
  - proptosis from orbital granuloma.

Investigations and diagnosis
- Blood tests.
  - FBC and film: anaemia, leucocytosis, and thrombocytosis.
  - ESR: always elevated.
  - autoimmune tests: c-ANCA is elevated in 80% of children with WG and is reasonably specific, but may be increased in other conditions (such as CF and microscopic polyangiitis). p-ANCA is also elevated but less specific and is also elevated in Churg–Strauss disease. Diagnosis is made with tissue biopsy.
  - Renal function.
- Urine analysis for evidence of glomerulonephritis.

- CXR: may be abnormal in the absence of symptoms. Findings consistent with WG are focal opacities of varying size, up to 10cm, representing either nodules or atelectasis. Widespread diffuse infiltrates suggest alveolar haemorrhage. Hilar adenopathy and pleural effusion are less common.
- Chest CT scan: usually shows multiple focal opacities, sometimes with central necrosis. Diffuse opacity will be seen with bleeding. There may be evidence of airway stenosis or compression by granulomata.
- Sinus CT scan: may show sinus opacity with bone destruction.
- Biopsy. Histological examination of affected tissue, showing necrotizing granulomata, is the most certain method of diagnosis. Biopsy sites include sinuses, lungs, kidneys, and skin. Diagnosis is usually based on biopsy findings.

Treatment

Treatment usually involves a combination of high dose prednisolone and cyclophosphamide. Methotrexate has also been used.

Outcome

Outcome 5-year survival with treatment is 80%, but disease-free remission is rare and most children will have at least one relapse, usually 1–2 years after the original illness.

Kawasaki disease

- CXR changes, usually a reticulonodular appearance, are found in 15% of children with Kawasaki disease. Atelectasis and pleural effusion are also reported.
- At post-mortem evidence of pulmonary vasculitis has been seen in > 50% of children who died as a consequence of Kawasaki disease.
- Pulmonary involvement seldom causes symptoms and, when present, usually resolves after the usual treatment with IV immunoglobulin and salicylate.

Other vasculitides

Churg–Strauss syndrome

- Also called allergic granulomatous angiitis.
- Three phases of the disease are recognized:
  - a prodromal phase of allergic rhinitis and asthma that can last several years;
  - a period of peripheral eosinophilia and eosinophilic tissue infiltration;
  - a final phase of systemic vasculitis, which can be fatal if not treated.
- The vasculitis is predominantly small vessel including capillaries, and can involve the heart, kidneys, GI tract, brain, lungs, and eyes.
- Defined as one of the ANCA-associated vasculitides along with Wegener's and microscopic polyangiitis, although ANCA is frequently negative in children with biopsy-proven Churg–Strauss syndrome.
- The apparent association with leucotriene receptor antagonist use probably reflects unmasking of the disease as a consequence of decreased steroid use by these patients.

- Lung involvement may be associated with fever and breathlessness and occasionally haemoptysis. There is usually a diffuse reticulonodular infiltrate on CXR. More rarely, there may be pleural disease or cavitating eosinophilic abscess formation.
- Treatment is immunosuppression, usually with systemic corticosteroids.

Microscopic angiitis

- This is a form of polyarteritis nodosa.
- It is associated with a rapidly progressive glomerulonephritis
- Lung involvement, particularly alveolar haemorrhage, is common.
- ANCA is usually positive (unlike other forms of polyarteritis nodosa).
- Diagnosis is usually by renal biopsy.
- Treatment is immunosuppression.

Sarcoidosis

Sarcoidosis is an inflammatory granulomatous multisystem disease. It is found most often in young adults, particularly those of Irish, Scandinavian, or Afro-Caribbean descent. It is rare in children with an estimated incidence of 0.6/100 000. It can occur at all ages of children, including infants, but is commonest in those > 8 years of age. The cause is not known; clustering of cases can occur and suggests a combination of genetic and environmental factors, including viral infection and exposure to toxins. The following are the usual presenting symptoms and signs in children.

- General malaise.
- Weight loss.
- Fever.
- Skin involvement: painless nodules or plaques especially around the eyes and nose. More rarely erythema nodosum may occur.
- Eye involvement: redness, pain, photophobia caused by anterior uveitis. Conjunctival nodes and posterior uveitis may both be present.
- Oral mucosa: aphthous ulceration is reported.
- Arthritis: usually polyarticular, with large effusions and often painless.
- Lymphadenopathy: usually mobile and painless.
- Unilateral or bilateral parotid gland enlargement: non-tender, smooth.

Children < 5 years of age typically present with arthritis, uveitis, and skin involvement. Older children are more likely to have lung involvement, uveitis, and lymphadenopathy. Other tissues that may be affected include:

- nervous system: cranial nerve palsies (especially facial nerve), aseptic meningitis, hydrocephalus, peripheral neuropathy, spinal cord involvement;
- endocrine system: central diabetes insipidus;
- heart: cardiomyopathy, heart block.
- muscles: muscle nodules and weakness.

Lung involvement

In children > 5 years of age lung involvement is almost universal. Often the children are asymptomatic, but there may be a dry cough, chest pain, or breathlessness. Examination is usually normal, but wheeze and crepitations have been described. Lung involvement is graded:

- stage 0, no involvement;
- stage I, bilateral hilar lymphadenopathy (BHL) ± paratracheal lymphadenopathy;
- stage II, BHL plus parenchymal infiltrate;
- stage III, parenchymal infiltrate without BHL;
- stage IV, extensive fibrosis with bullae, cysts, and emphysema.

95% of those with lung involvement are stage I or II so the finding of an infiltrate without BHL makes sarcoidosis a possible but unlikely diagnosis.

Investigations

- CXR and chest CT scan: findings as per lung staging. Infiltrates are usually irregular discrete lesions surrounded by normal lung and range in size from a few mm to 2–3cm. Nodules are often seen along bronchovascular bundles. Pleural thickening may also be seen.
- Lung function testing: may be normal, or may show evidence of restriction. More rarely, there may be obstruction. KCO may be decreased.
- Bronchoscopy and BAL. Macroscopic appearances are usually normal; mucosal nodules with contact bleeding is described in adults. BAL reveals a moderate lymphocytosis (25–30% of cells present) with a 5:1 $CD4^+$ to $CD8^+$ ratio.
- Bloods:
  - FBC: leucocytes may be increased or decreased; eosinophils elevated in 50% of affected children;
  - electrolytes: serum calcium elevated in 30%;
  - urine electrolytes: hypercalciuria in up to 65% of children;
  - liver function tests: mild elevation of transaminases is common;
  - angiotensin converting enzyme (ACE) levels: elevated in 80%, but not specific for sarcoidosis (also increased in lymphoma and TB, both of which may cause BHL);
  - immunoglobulins: hypergammaglobulinaemia in 80%;
  - ESR: elevated in 60–80%.
- Liver ultrasound: may identify nodules or evidence of cholestasis.
- Renal ultrasound: may identify nephrocalcinosis or nodules.
- 12 lead ECG, 24h ECG, and echocardiography heart block may occur and nodules may be seen.
- Slit lamp examination needed to fully evaluate eye involvement.
- Biopsy: the most easily available involved tissue should be selected (conjunctiva, skin nodule, salivary gland). If no peripheral site is available, hilar lymph nodes may need to be selected; fine needle aspiration may be successful. Typical findings are well formed non-caseating granulomata with varying degrees of fibrosis.
- Tuberculin skin test or TB-Elispot to exclude TB.

Diagnosis

There is no single diagnostic test and making a firm diagnosis can be difficult. The ATS suggests a combination of:

- a compatible clinical picture;
- histological evidence of non-caesating granulomata;
- exclusion of other conditions, e.g. TB, neoplasm, hypersensitivity pneumonitis.

Treatment
- Asymptomatic children with hilar adenopathy caused by sarcoidosis do not need treatment.
- When there is loss of lung function, progressive radiological abnormality, or symptoms, treatment should be started.
- Other organ involvement, such as uveitis or CNS disease, may also be the trigger to start treatment.
- Standard treatment is immunosuppression with oral corticosteroids, usually at 1mg/kg/day for 4–8 weeks followed by a weaning regime over 3–6 months. Other immunosuppressants such as hydroxychloroquine and azathioprine have been tried in resistant disease.

Outcome

In older children, the prognosis is usually good, with spontaneous remission in 70%. 10–20% have long-term respiratory or other organ impairment. Younger children tend to fare less well.

Storage diseases

Storage diseases are a rare cause of lung disease in childhood and most usually occur after the storage disease has been diagnosed. Occasionally respiratory illness may be the first manifestation of the illness, e.g. in some cases of Niemann–Pick disease.

Gaucher's disease

- Gaucher's disease (GD) is a multisystem lysosomal storage disease caused by a genetic defect of the beta-glucosidase enzyme. This results in accumulation of glucosylceramide in macrophages.
- GD is an autosomal recessive condition, particularly common in the Ashkenazi Jewish population where it has an incidence of 1/1000.
- Three types are recognized. Type 1 (> 90% of cases) has no neurological involvement and can present in early childhood, but more often in adolescence. Type 2 disease is characterized by rapid neurodegeneration with death by 2 years of age. Type 3 is an intermediate form, with death usually by age 15 years.
- The diagnosis is made by identification of typical Gaucher cells (macrophages filled with glucocerebroside) in the bone marrow or spleen, and by demonstrating low beta-glucosidase enzyme activity in cultured fibroblasts or leucocytes.
- Typical presentation of type 1 GD includes:
  - bruising due to hypersplenism;
  - tiredness due to anaemia;
  - bone pain;
  - hepatosplenomegaly.

Respiratory problems

- 70% of children and adults with type 1 GD have abnormal lung function tests, showing variable degrees of airways obstruction, reduced lung volumes, and diffusion defects.
- Clinically apparent lung disease is much less common, affecting < 10% of patients. It is more common in children who present in early life and who have more severe systemic disease. It is also seen in children with type 2 disease.
- Lung disease can manifest as:
  - breathlessness;
  - exercise intolerance;
  - hypoxia (sometimes with pulmonary hypertension);
  - recurrent pneumonia.
- Respiratory problems may be due to direct lung involvement by GD, or due to hepatopulmonary syndrome, or due to mechanical compression of the lungs by massive hepatosplenomegaly.
- Direct lung involvement usually results in filling of the interstitial and alveolar spaces with Gaucher cells. CT scan of the chest shows diffuse ground-glass opacity with increased interstitial markings. BAL fluid will contain Gaucher cells.

- The visceral, but not neurological, effects of GD can be reversed by enzyme therapy (recombinant human beta-glucosidase) given by IV infusion 2–4 weekly. The dose of enzyme required to treat lung involvement is higher than that required for other organ systems.
- Bone marrow transplantation is also effective.
- There is one case report of a 10-year-old with type 1 GD who developed progressive lung involvement and underwent successful bilateral lung transplantation, with no recurrence of GD in the graft 5 years after transplantation.[2]

Mucopolysaccharidoses

- Mucopolysaccharidoses (MPSs) are characterized by the abnormal tissue deposition of the mucopolysaccharides (now called glucosaminoglycans, GAGs) heparin sulphate, keratin sulphate, and dermatan sulphate. They arise as a result of genetic mutations in lysosomal enzymes that normally metabolize these substrates.
- Nine forms of MPS (MPS-I to MPS-IX) have been described, dependent on the nature of the deposited material. A number of eponymous forms are also described according to the clinical picture.
- Hurler syndrome is a severe form of MPS-I. Scheie syndrome is a milder form of MPS-I. Characteristic features include:
  - normal appearance at birth; diagnosis between 6 and 24 months;
  - coarse facial features and coarse hair;
  - hepatosplenomegaly;
  - cardiomyopathy;
  - corneal clouding;
  - developmental delay;
  - enlarged tongue;
  - skeletal abnormalities: dysostosis mulitplex.
- Hunter syndrome is MPS-II and can be mild or severe. It is clinically similar to MPS-I with the exception of corneal clouding.
- MPS-III, also known as Sanfillipo syndrome, is characterized by progressive neurological involvement with relatively mild somatic features.
- MPS-IV, also known as Morquio syndrome, has predominant involvement of the skeleton. Patients are often very short but with normal intelligence. Instability of ondontoic process, which is found in most forms of MPS, is particularly severe in MPS-IV, and may require stabilizing surgery to prevent fatal atalanto-axial subluxation, which can, for example, occur as the neck is extended during intubation.
- MPS-V is no longer used. MPS-VI to IX are rare.

2 Rao, A.R., Parakininkas, D., Hintermeyer, M., Segura, A.D. and Rice, T.B. (2005). Bilateral lung transplant in Gauchers type-1 disease. *Pediatr. Transplant.* **9**, 239–43.

Further information

Goitein, O., Elstein, D., Abrahamov, A, Hadas-Halpern, I., Melzer, E. Kerem, E., and Zimran, A. (2001). Lung involvement and enzyme replacement therapy in Gaucher's disease. *Q. J. Med.* **94**:407–15.

Diagnosis is by spot urine analysis for GAGs, followed by lysosomal enzyme assay using fibroblasts or white cells. Clinical severity and life expectancy is variable in all forms of MPS. MPSs are autosomal recessive apart from MPS-II (Hunter), which is X-linked.

Respiratory problems

The respiratory consequences of MPS include the following.

- Upper airway obstruction secondary to deposition of GAGs in the upper airway and tongue. This is predominantly a problem in children with Hurler syndrome and may result in obstructive sleep apnoea (OSA). Polysomnography should be used to identify OSA in at-risk children.
- Restrictive lung deficit. Again this is most marked in children with Hurler, but can also be seen in severe Hunter syndrome. The restriction can be severe (FVC < 40%) and result in exercise intolerance. The cause of the restriction is multifactorial and includes:
  - hepatosplenomegaly, which affects diaphragmatic excursion;
  - restricted movement at costovertebral joints (GAGs are deposited in joints);
  - rib abnormalities;
  - deposition of GAGs in the lung interstitium reducing lung compliance.
- Recurrent respiratory infection. This is predominantly a problem in children with upper airways obstruction or restrictive lung disease or both. It probably represents secondary effects of these conditions on reduced ability to clear airway secretions. These problems will be compounded if there is significant neurodisability.
- Children with MPS-I and MPS-II frequently have a cardiomyopathy, which can present as acute cardiac failure. The presence of cardiac dysfunction can contribute further to decreased lung compliance and risk of respiratory infection.

Treatment

- Night-time nasal CPAP is usually effective in the treatment of OSA. Adenotonsillectomy may be helpful although great care should be taken to avoid atlanto-axial subluxation during intubation and surgery. Occasionally tracheostomy may be required when upper airway obstruction is severe.
- Cardiac disease should be screened for and treated appropriately.
- Children with recurrent respiratory infection may be helped by chest physiotherapy and prophylactic antibiotics, especially during the winter months. Pneumococcal and influenza vaccination should be used routinely.
- Bone marrow transplant can improve survival in severe Hurler syndrome, especially if carried out before the age of 2 years.
- Enzyme replacement (with laronidase) results in small improvements (10–15%) in the restrictive lung defect of children with MPS-I.

Niemann–Pick disease

- Niemann–Pick disease (NPD) is a rare autosomal recessive lysosomal storage disorder that results in the deposition of sphingomyelin and cholesterol in affected tissues, particularly affecting the brain and reticuloendothelial system.

- Six forms of NPD are recognized. Type A accounts for 85% of cases.
  - Type A, acute neuronopathic form.
  - Type B, visceral form.
  - Type C, chronic neuronopathic form.
  - Type D, Nova Scotia variant.
  - Type E, adult form.
  - Type F, sea-blue histiocyte disease.
- NPD arises because of decreased activity of the lysosomal enzyme sphingomyelinase, either directly because of mutations in the sphingomyelinase gene, *SMPD1* (NPD type A and B) or indirectly through effects on enzyme processing as a result of mutations in the *NPC1* gene (NPD type C).
- Neurological involvement is seen in types A and C, but not in type B.
- Infants with type A do not develop much beyond the skills of a 10-month-old and have progressive neurodegeneration and usually die within 5 years, often with bronchopneumonia.
- Children with type B disease have significant hepatosplenomegaly, like children with type A disease, but without neurological impairment.
- Type C disease often presents in school age children with ataxia and progressive intellectual impairment.
- The diagnosis of NPD types A and B is made by assaying sphingomyelinase activity in white blood cells or cultured fibroblasts. Type C disease is diagnosed by studying cholesterol metabolism in cultured fibroblasts.

Respiratory problems

- Pulmonary parenchymal involvement can be seen in all forms of NPD but is particularly prominent in type B disease.
- Lung disease usually occurs in the context of an older child or adult who has already been diagnosed with NPD, usually because of hepato-splenomegaly. Rarely, lung disease may occur earlier, sometimes in the first year of life before hepatosplenomegaly has developed. Thus NPD should be included in the differential for children who present with interstitial lung disease.
- Clinical presentation of lung involvement includes breathlessness, recurrent episodes of pneumonia, cough, and haemoptysis. Clinically, type B NPD disease is similar to type 1 Gaucher's disease. Lung disease in NPD can cause progressively worsening hypoxia and respiratory failure.
- Extensive bronchial casts have been described in NPD lung disease and, when these are combined with interstitial changes, NPD should be considered as a possible diagnosis.
- CT scan may show ground-glass opacities in the upper lung zones, possibly due to partial filling of the alveoli with 'Pick cells' and thickening of the interlobular septa.
- If lung function can be measured, it may be normal or more typically show a restrictive defect. There is usually a reduced transfer factor consistent with a diffusion defect.

- BAL will show foamy macrophages.
- Open lung biopsy will show foamy macrophages and thickened alveolar walls. The presence of foamy macrophages may raise the possibility of alveolar proteinosis.
- The main differential for type B NPD disease is type 1 Gaucher's disease, which can have a similar presentation and histological findings.

Treatment and outcome

- Pulmonary involvement in type B NPD is a significant cause of morbidity and mortality.
- Case reports in adults with severe pulmonary involvement suggest that whole-lung lavage may be of benefit in removing large numbers of lipid-laden cells. Bronchial casts may also be cleared by this process. Lung lavage may be less successful in children.
- Hypoxia can develop, requiring long-term supplemental oxygen therapy to prevent cor pulmonale.
- No specific therapy is available for NPD. Bone marrow and liver transplants have been tried for type B disease with little success.

Further information

Uyan, Z.S., Karadag, B., Ersu, R., Kiyan, G., Kotiloglu, E., Sirvanci, S., Ercan, F., Dagli, T., Karakoc, F., and Dagli, E. (2005). Early pulmonary involvement in Niemann–Pick type B disease: lung lavage is not useful. *Pediatr. Pulmonol.* **40**, 169–72.

Nicholson, A.G., Florio, R., Hansell, D.M., Bois, R.M., Wells, A.U., Hughes, P., Ramadan, H.K., Mackinlay, C.I., Brambilla, E., Ferretti, G.R., Erichsen, A., Malone, M., and Lantuejoul, S. (2006). Pulmonary involvement by Niemann–Pick disease. A report of six cases. *Histopathology* **48**, 596–603.

Nicholson, A.G., Wells, A.U., Hooper, J., Hansell, D.M., Kelleher, A., and Morgan, C. (2002). Successful treatment of endogenous lipoid pneumonia due to Niemann–Pick type B disease with whole-lung lavage. *Am. J. Respir. Crit. Care Med.* **165**, 128–31.

Transfusion-related acute lung injury

- Transfusion-related acute lung injury (TRALI) has a reported incidence of 1 in every 2000 transfusions. It occurs in adults and children.
- The serious hazards of transfusion (SHOT) data from the UK and Ireland identified only five cases of TRALI reported in children from 1996 to 2003, out of a total of 145 cases.
- TRALI is characterized by an acute respiratory distress syndrome (ARDS)-like illness. There is rapid onset of respiratory distress, hypoxia, and non-cardiogenic pulmonary oedema during or soon after (within 6h) blood transfusion. The diagnosis requires the absence of fluid overload or other identifiable cause of acute lung injury.
- TRALI is probably immune-mediated, possibly related to anti-HLA or anti-granulocyte antibodies in the donor blood. These antibodies are thought to activate host neutrophils within the lung capillaries leading to capillary leak.
- Donor blood associated with TRALI is usually derived from multiparous women who will have had several exposures to paternal HLA and leucocyte antigens. This group makes up 30% of the donor population. There has been a reduction of immune-mediated TRALI in the UK following implementation by the UK Blood Services of a policy of using male donors, as far as possible, for fresh frozen plasma (FFP) and the plasma contribution to platelet pools.

Investigations

- CXR shows bilateral pulmonary infiltrates.
- Pulmonary oedema fluid has high protein content (almost the same as plasma); this test can be used to demonstrate that fluid arises as capillary leak, not because of high left atrial pressure (cardiogenic oedema).
- Cardiac echo can be used to identify evidence of left atrial overload and hence distinguish cardiogenic from non-cardiogenic oedema.
- There may be transient leucopenia, perhaps reflecting sequestration of white cells in the lung. The WBC count recovers within 24h of onset.

Treatment and outcome

- Treatment is supportive, including the use of mechanical ventilation.
- It is important to recognize early that the cause is non-cardiogenic. Inappropriate use of diuretics can worsen associated hypotension.
- Systemic steroids are sometimes used, but there is no evidence of benefit and their use is controversial.
- TRALI usually resolves after 3–4 days.
- Mortality ca. 1–5% in adults. No mortality data available for children.

Further information

Bux, J. and Sachs, U.J. (2007). The pathogenesis of transfusion-related acute lung injury (TRALI). *Br. J. Haematol.* **136**, 788–99.

Church, G.D., Price, C., Sanchez, R., and Looney, M.R. (2006). Transfusion-related acute lung injury in the paediatric patient: two case reports and a review of the literature. *Transfus. Med.* **16**, 343–8.

Serious Hazards of Transfusion website: *www.shotuk.orgs*

Lung transplantation

Patient selection

- An estimated 60 lung transplant procedures are carried out in children worldwide per year.
- Lung donors are currently found for only around 50% of children who require a lung transplant. This means that half of all children listed for lung transplant will die before a suitable organ is found.
- The general paucity of donated organs is compounded for paediatric lung transplant candidates for 2 reasons. First, only an estimated 25% of multiorgan cadaveric donors provide suitable lungs for transplantation. Second, the donor organ needs to be of suitable size. Matching is based on major blood groups and organ size only.
- The most common indication for lung transplantation is respiratory failure secondary to cystic fibrosis, accounting for one-third of all transplants, and two-thirds of lung transplants in adolescents.

Underlying conditions leading to lung transplantation

- Cystic fibrosis
- Primary pulmonary hypertension
- Congenital heart disease
- Bronchiolitis obliterans
- Idiopathic pulmonary fibrosis
- Idiopathic pulmonary haemosiderosis
- Pulmonary veno-occlusive disease
- Surfactant B deficiency
- Alveolar capillary dysplasia
- Pulmonary AV malformations

Timing of referral

- Discussion with child and family regarding referral for transplantation should be initiated before the child has end-stage disease so that there can be a period of reflection and decision.
- Consideration of referral for transplantation involves frank discussion within the family unit and an open acceptance of life limitation for the patient.
- This may be the first time the family has broached this subject and it will be difficult for many families.
- A substantial proportion of children and families will decline referral for transplantation.

Disease-specific guidelines for timing of referral
Cystic fibrosis

- FEV_1 < 30% predicted or FEV_1 > 30% with rapid fall in FEV_1 or clinical deterioration.
- Hypoxia (PaO_2 < 7.7kPa); hypercapnia ($PaCO_2$ > 6.7kPa).
- Poor exercise tolerance.
- Severe haemoptysis despite embolization.
- Female patients with rapid deterioration should be considered for early referral.

Primary pulmonary hypertension
- Symptomatic progressive disease.
- Right atrial pressure > 15mmHg.
- Cardiac index > 2.1L/min/m².
- Mean pulmonary artery pressure > 55mmHg.
- Pulmonary artery saturation < 63%.
- 6 minute walk test < 400m.
- Consider referral at time of starting epoprostenol as some will be unresponsive to this therapy.

Eisenmenger's syndrome Severe and progressive symptoms despite maximal medical therapy.

Indications for referral for lung transplantation

- Predicted life expectancy < 2 years
- Severely impaired quality of life
- On maximal medical treatment
- Child and family committed to the transplant process

Contraindications to lung transplantation

These may vary between centres

Absolute
- Severe failure of other organ systems
- Ventilation dependence
- Acute tuberculosis,
- Hepatitis B, hepatitis C, HIV
- Psychiatric illness
- Active malignancy

Relative
- Long-term high dose steroid treatment (> 5mg/day)
- Previous pleurodesis/thoracic surgery
- Osteoporosis
- The presence of multiresistant organisms, e.g. some genomovars of *Burkholderia cepacia* complex (especially *B. cenocepacia*), MRSA, panresistant *Pseudomonas aeruginosa*; NTM infections, invasive pulmonary aspergillosis
- Psychosocial issues/lack of family support
- Non-adherence to current treatment
- Minor dysfunction of other organ systems

Pre-transplantation investigations and management

Consult the transplant centre for details of required investigations prior to referral. Some investigations may otherwise be repeated at transplant assessment.

Important investigations
- Full spirometry and lung volumes.
- Exercise performance (e.g. 6 minute walk).
- Liver function, viral serology (hepatitis B,C, CMV, HIV).
- Renal function with 24h creatinine clearance.
- Sputum microbiology including *Pseudomonas* resistance patterns; *B. cepacia*, MRSA, or NTM infection/colonization; history of allergic bronchopulmonary aspergillosis.
- CXR.
- HRCT.
- ECG.
- Echocardiography and, in some children, cardiac catheter.

Important information for the transplant service
- Detailed past medical and surgical history.
- Rate of decline in respiratory function.
- Detailed microbiology.
- Possible contraindications.
- Compliance history.
- Psychosocial assessment of patient and family.

Ongoing medical care at referring hospital
- Monitor disease.
- Optimize nutrition.
- Maintain mobility and exercise.
- Treat chest exacerbations aggressively.
- Consider early non-invasive ventilatory support.
- Avoid intubation if possible.
- Avoid high dose steroid treatment if possible.

Surgical techniques in lung transplantation

Evaluation of donor lungs
- Potential donor lungs are assessed using arterial blood gases, CXR, airway cultures, and laryngobronchoscopy.
- The donor is screened for hepatitis A, B, and C, HIV, VZV, CMV, EBV, and herpes viruses.
- Ischaemic time is limited to 4h.

Surgical approaches for lung transplant
- Heart–lung transplant. Historically, lung transplantation involved total heart–lung transplantation or domino surgery where the recipient received a donor heart–lung transplant and donated his/her healthy heart to a patient awaiting heart transplant. This avoided the need for tracheal anastomosis and the consequent complications associated with tracheal stenosis.
- Bilateral sequential lung transplantation is now performed in the majority of cases in children. The procedure is performed through a bilateral transsternal 'clamshell' incision, and utilizes mainstem bronchial anastomoses, therefore eliminating the complications of tracheal anastomosis. This approach avoids unnecessary post-transplant cardiac complications and is performed in some centres without the need for by-pass surgery as the patient may be managed using selective lung ventilation.
- Single lung transplant is performed much more rarely in children than in adults and is never performed in CF.
- Living donor lower lobe (or complete lung) transplantation is available in a few centres worldwide, principally for transplant candidates who are unlikely to survive to receive an organ from a deceased donor. These organs are in good condition and are HLA-matched. This procedure is currently on clinical trial for adults only in the UK.

Post-transplant management
- Induction immunotherapy. Anti-lymphocyte or anti-thymocyte globulin, or a monoclonal IL-2 receptor antagonist (basiliximab or daclizumab) may be given at the time of transplantation.
- Post-transplant triple-drug immunosuppression:
  - calcineurin inhibitor (tacrolimus, ciclosporin);
  - azathioprine or mycophenolate mofetil;
  - corticosteroids.
- The majority of patients continue to take corticosteroids at 5 years post-transplant.
- Antimicrobial treatment.
  - IV antibiotics pre- and post-transplant. Donor and recipient sputum cultures are used to determine the specific regimen.
  - Trimethoprim–sulfamethoxazole (TMP-SMZ) 3 times weekly as prophylaxis for *Pneumocystis jiroveci* for 1 year (oral dapsone is an alternative).

- CF patients who have isolated *Aspergillus* sp in the past receive IV amphotericin or voriconazole peri-operatively, with transition to oral itraconazole or voriconazole thereafter.
- Oral nystatin for prevention of candidal disease
- CMV prophylaxis if either the donor or recipient is seropositive. Ganciclovir or valganciclovir are generally given for 1–3 months post-transplant.

Complications

Immediate surgical

- Postoperative bleeding from cardiopulmonary bypass.
- Diaphragmatic dysfunction from damage to phrenic nerve.
- Vocal cord palsy from damage to recurrent laryngeal nerve.

Early graft dysfunction

- Presents in first week post-transplant.
- Related to organ harvest and ischaemia–reperfusion injury.
- Characterized by marked hypoxaemia, diffuse pulmonary infiltrates, and diffuse alveolar damage on biopsy.
- Clinical spectrum from mild acute lung injury to ARDS.
- Treatment is supportive with careful fluid balance, ventilation, and expectant treatment of infection.

Bronchial anastomosis

- Complete dehiscence of bronchial anastomosis is rare and requires urgent surgery.
- Partial dehiscence is managed conservatively with drainage of pneumothorax and reduction in steroid dose.
- Bronchial anastomotic stenosis typically occurs weeks to months after transplant. May be managed with balloon dilatation or bronchoscopic stent insertion.
- Excess granulation may be removed at surveillance bronchoscopy.
- Airway collapse may occur at the site of anastomosis.

Infection

Bacterial

- Early infection may come from the donor (from seeding to the blood or mediastinum during explantation of chronically infected lungs), through spread to the lungs from chronic sinus disease in CF patients, or extrinsic ICU-acquired pneumonia.
- Most commonly caused by coagulase-negative staphylococcus and Gram-negative organisms, especially *Pseudomonas aeruginosa* (in both CF and non-CF patients).

Viral

Cytomegalovirus

- CMV is the second commonest infection after bacterial pathogens, with peak incidence 1–6 months post-transplant.
- CMV disease may vary from mild disease, presenting as a febrile illness with leucopenia, to invasive disease usually of the lung or GI tract. CMV pneumonitis presents with fevers and chills, cough, respiratory distress, crackles on auscultation, and diffuse interstitial changes on imaging.
- Asymptomatic shedding of CMV can occur, but isolation of CMV on BAL or trans-bronchial biopsy in clinical context is strongly suggestive of CMV pneumonitis.

- CMV negative recipients who have received lungs from a seropositive donor are at highest risk of CMV disease, with up to 75% affected in the first 6 months, despite postoperative prophylaxis.
- Treatment is with IV ganciclovir for 2–4 weeks.
- CMV may be linked to the development of subsequent bronchiolitis obliterans.

RSV, parainfluenza, influenza, and adenovirus
- There is a risk of severe disease with community respiratory viruses.
- Attention to prevention, with active immunization for influenza, and consideration of passive immunization for RSV (palivizumab).
- Adenovirus may cause an overwhelming illness and death.
- Viral infection may be linked to rapid development of bronchiolitis obliterans.

Pneumocystis jiroveci
- Prophylactic trimethoprim–sulfamethoxazole (TMP-SMZ) has dramatically reduced the burden of pneumocystis disease in post-transplant patients.
- Invasive disease presents with fever, profound hypoxia, crackles, and interstitial infiltrates.
- IV TMP-SMZ is usually effective.

Aspergillus
- Colonization with *Aspergillus* post-transplantation is common although clinical disease is unusual. 50% of previously colonized CF patients and 40% of non-colonized CF patients will have chronic colonization post-transplant despite prophylaxis. 30% of non-CF patients will have chronic colonization post-transplant.
- Infection with *Aspergillus* usually occurs in the first 3 months post-transplant.
- Infection may be detected with surveillance bronchoscopy.
- Spectrum of disease includes tracheo-bronchial lesions with ulceration and necrosis, infection at the anastomosis with potential dehiscence, pneumonitis, and disseminated aspergillosis.
- Invasive disease has high mortality and has been associated with chronic graft rejection.
- Treatment is with IV voriconazole or amphotericin B.

Medication side-effects

Treatment with immunosuppressive therapy aims to strike a balance between the risks of graft rejection and the risks of opportunistic infection. Therapy will need to continue lifelong post-transplantation.

Calcineurin inhibitors
- Headache and sleep disturbance.
- Hirsutism and gingival hypertrophy.
- Hypertension and nephropathy (75% 5 years post-transplant).

Steroids
- Glucose intolerance and diabetes (30% at 5 years post-transplant).

Rejection

Hyperacute rejection

- Rare complication due to circulating recipient antibodies, occurring a few hours post-transplantation.
- Can lead to graft loss.

Acute rejection

- Very common. Usually occurs between 2 and 12 weeks post-transplant. May rarely occur up to 3 years post-transplant.
- Difficult to distinguish from infection. Non-specific signs include malaise, cough, fever, dyspnoea, and hypoxia, with crackles on auscultation. CXR may show non-specific infiltrates. Lung function studies show an obstructive pattern.
- Bronchoscopy with BAL and transbronchial biopsy is indicated. Histology shows perivascular lymphocytic infiltrates with or without airway inflammation.
- Some patients may be asymptomatic.
- Acute rejection is a major risk factor for bronchiolitis obliterans syndrome, and therefore needs to be detected and treated quickly and aggressively. Surveillance bronchoscopy is therefore performed in many centres at 2, 4, 8, and 12 weeks post-transplant.
- Treatment is with pulsed IV methylprednisolone (10mg/kg) daily for 3 days. The majority of patients respond quickly to treatment. Persistent acute rejection may be managed with anti-thymocyte immunoglobulin or modulation of immunosuppression.
- Transplant recipients under the age of 3 years may have fewer episodes of acute rejection.

Chronic rejection and bronchiolitis obliterans syndrome (BOS)

- Chronic rejection is the term used to describe the insidious onset of breathlessness, cough, and worsening airflow obstruction seen in transplant recipients from 6 months post-transplantation.
- The immunological basis to chronic rejection is poorly understood.
- Histology shows bronchiolitis obliterans (BO) with progressive and irreversible bronchiolar stenosis, fibrosis, and airway occlusion. Distribution of disease is patchy and transbronchial biopsy therefore has low sensitivity.
- Bronchiolitis obliterans syndrome (BOS) is the clinical surrogate for BO in the absence of a histological diagnosis. The major criterion for the diagnosis of BOS is an unexplained drop in $FEV_1 > 20\%$ predicted.
- The two major risk factors for BOS are acute rejection and non-compliance with immunosuppressive therapy. Other postulated risk factors include infection with CMV and other respiratory viruses, anastomotic complications, and graft ischaemic time. GOR may also contribute and early fundoplication is used in some centres.
- Treatment is with increased immunosuppression and aggressive treatment of infection.
- BOS is a heterogeneous condition and some forms may be reversible. A drop in FEV_1 should therefore be assessed aggressively for treatable causes of BOS, e.g. endobronchial *Pseudomonas* infection in CF patients, acquired from chronically infected sinuses.

- 60% of paediatric lung transplant recipients have evidence of BO 6 years post-transplant. BO is responsible for > 40% of all deaths after 1 year post-transplantation.
- Aims of treatment are to halt further deterioration in lung function, ameliorate symptoms, and treat infection aggressively. Re-transplantation is the only definitive treatment.

Malignancy

- Incidence 5.7% at 1 year and 8.7% at 5 years post-transplant.
- Post-transplant lymphoproliferative disease (PTLD) accounts for the majority of malignancies.
- PTLD is an EBV-associated lymphoma in an immunocompromised host.
- PTLD is more common in CF patients, in children compared to adults, and in lung compared to other solid organ transplants. This is thought to be due to the increased requirement for immunosuppression in these groups, and to the fact that many children are EBV seronegative at the time of transplant.
- The most common site for post-transplant malignancy is the lung allograft.
- A high index of suspicion is needed since symptoms are non-specific, including cough, fever, and dyspnoea.
- The disease may present with pulmonary nodules on CXR.
- Other sites of disease include lymph nodes, tonsils, skin, and bowel.
- In 80% of cases where disease is detected early, a reduction in immunosuppressant treatment is successful (this approach, however, increases the risk of BOS). Late stage disease is treated with the chemotherapy protocol for non- Hodgkin's lymphoma.

Follow-up and outcome

- Children are generally discharged from hospital 4–6 weeks after transplantation. During this period, they will commence an intensive course of exercise rehabilitation.
- Surveillance bronchoscopy with BAL and transbronchial biopsy may have been performed pre-discharge depending on local protocols.
- At home, patients will document daily spirometry, temperature, and weight.
- They will be followed closely by the transplant centre, but may also visit the referring centre for assessment, spirometry, ECG, radiology, blood tests, and immunosuppressant blood drug levels.
- Advice should be sought from the transplant team if suspicion of complications arises.

Survival

- Survival rates 1990–2002: 75%, 1 year; ~50%, 5 years; ~40%, 10 years. Median survival 3.7 years. Survivors at 1 year have a median survival of 6.7 years.
- Graft failure and infection are the major causes of death in the first year of life.
- After the first year the major cause of death is BO, but infection remains an important cause.
- Lung transplantation in children conveys a clear survival benefit when compared with patients on the waiting list.
- For patients with PPH, 5-year survival is greater for double lung (65%) compared to single lung transplantation (25%).

Functional outcome

- 80% of recipients report no exercise limitation at 1 and 5 years post-transplantation.
- Lung function can return to the normal range in infants and children.
- At 5 years post-transplantation, 75% of recipients will have systemic hypertension, 25% will have renal dysfunction, and 30% will have CF-related diabetes.
- Quality of life assessments are difficult to perform, but suggest a score lower than in the normal population but equivalent to that in children with other chronic diseases such as asthma or juvenile idiopathic arthritis.

Somatic growth

- Growth of children after lung transplantation remains a problem because of chronic poor nutritional status pre-transplant, and chronic steroid treatment thereafter.
- Augmenting and maintaining nutrition is fundamental to good post-transplant outcome.
- Increased GORD or gastroparesis post-transplant may compromise enteral nutrition.
- Studies in young children have shown that, in the absence of BO, lung allograft growth can occur post-transplant (as measured by FVC and TLCO).

Further information

Burch, M. and Aurora, P. (2004). Current status of paediatric heart, lung, and heart–lung transplantation. *Arch. Dis. Child.* **89**, 386–9.

Aurora, P. (2004). When should children be referred for lung or heart–lung transplantation? *Pediatr. Pulmonol. Suppl.* **26**, 116–18.

Radley-Smith, R. and Aurora, P. (2006). Transplantation as a treatment for end-stage pulmonary hypertension in childhood. *Paediatr. Respir. Rev.* **7**, 117–22.

Part III

Supportive care

Use of oxygen

Introduction

Oxygen is the most important drug in the management of hypoxaemia and tissue hypoxia.

- Hypoxaemia is defined as a low level of oxygen in the arterial blood.
  - Baseline hypoxaemia in a normal child is defined as an oxygen saturation (SaO_2) < 92%, which corresponds to a PaO_2 < 8kPa (60mmHg).
  - Episodic hypoxaemia: the most common definition is a drop of oxygen saturation of 4% or more from baseline.
- Hypoxia is defined as the condition whereby the level of oxygen delivered to the tissues is inadequate to meet the metabolic demands of the body. Important factors in oxygen delivery to the tissues are:
  - cardiac output;
  - pulmonary gas exchange;
  - haemoglobin (Hb) level;
  - oxygen saturation of Hb;
  - oxyhaemoglobin dissociation curve (normal temperature, pH, and 2,3-diphosphoglyceride (2,3-DPG levels)).

Causes of hypoxaemia

There are four primary pulmonary causes of reduced PaO_2 in arterial blood, which may occur singly or in combination in disease.

Hypoventilation

- Causes of hypoventilation are shown in the box.
- Oxygen should be given with care to children with hypoventilation; it will relieve hypoxaemia but may abolish hypoxic drive to breathing and result in CO_2 narcosis.

Causes of hypoventilation

- Central causes:
  - primary central hypoventilation
  - depression of the respiratory centre by drugs
  - diseases of the medulla and brainstem
- Peripheral nervous system:
  - high cord lesions
  - anterior horn cell disease (spinal muscular atrophy, polio)
  - diseases of the nerve supply to the respiratory muscles (e.g. Guillain–Barré, diphtheria)
- Muscle disorders:
  - disease of the myoneural junction (myasthenia)
  - disease of the respiratory muscles (e.g. muscular dystrophy)
- Mechanical problems:
  - thoracic cage abnormalities
  - upper airway obstruction

Ventilation/perfusion (V/Q) mismatch

- This is the most common cause of hypoxaemia in children. It occurs in bronchiolitis, asthma, and chronic obstructive lung disease.
- In most children with V/Q mismatch, CO_2 will be normal or low, reflecting increased minute ventilation. Since the CO_2 levels in air are effectively zero, CO_2 levels fall. Hypoxaemia persists because of mixing of blood from well ventilated lung (saturation 100%) with lung with relatively poor ventilation (saturation < 100%).
- Oxygen therapy promptly relieves hypoxaemia in most children with V/Q mismatch because the V/Q mismatch is not complete. This means that increasing the inspired oxygen concentration will increase the alveolar oxygen concentration even in the poorly ventilated lung units. Hypoxaemia from V/Q mismatch is one form of intrapulmonary shunting.

Shunt

- Blood reaches the systemic arterial system without passing through ventilated regions of the lung. The shunt may be extrapulmonary, e.g. in congenital heart disease, or intrapulmonary, e.g. arteriovenous fistulae within the lung.
- Oxygen therapy has some effect, but oxygen saturation cannot be fully corrected.

Diffusion impairment

- The blood–gas barrier is thickened and less efficient for gas exchange. This tends to have a greater effect on oxygen, which diffuses 20 times more slowly through tissues than CO_2.
- It is a rare cause of hypoxaemia in children. Possible causes include interstitial lung disease pneumonia and hypersensitivity pneumonitis.
- Any impairment is exaggerated on exercise because of the reduced contact time between blood in the capillary and oxygen in the alveolus.

Causes of hypoxia

Oxygen delivery depends on:
- the oxygen-carrying capacity of the blood (Hb);
- cardiac output;
- distribution of blood to the periphery.

Oxygen alone is rarely a definitive treatment but it is supportive and used with other strategies, such as supporting blood pressure, restoring blood volume, etc.

The oxyhaemoglobin dissociation curve

- Oxygen combines with haemoglobin (Hb) to form oxyhaemoglobin and this reaction can move in both directions.
- The relationship between oxygen affinity and Hb is described by the oxygen–Hb dissociation curve
- One gram of Hb can combine with 1.34mL O_2. With an Hb of 15g/dL, 20.1mL O_2 per 100mL blood (vol%) can be found to Hb.

- The oxygen content of the blood and therefore the maximum amount of oxygen available to the tissues varies significantly with the Hb level. For example, if PaO_2 is 9.5kPa and SaO_2 is 93%, the oxygen content for a Hb of 5g/dL is 6.3vol% and for a Hb 15g/dL is 18.9vol%.
- On the steep part of the curve (up to 9.5kPa PaO_2) large amounts of oxygen can be released from Hb with small changes in partial pressure of arterial oxygen; thus measuring oxygen saturation is more sensitive than measuring PaO_2 when assessing gas exchange.
- On the upper flat part of the curve PaO_2 may change significantly while Hb saturation remains around 95%.
- Acidosis and increased temperature shift the curve to the right, resulting in a decrease in affinity of Hb for oxygen. This process assists delivery of oxygen to the tissues.
- Prolonged hypoxaemia, such as occurs in chronic lung or heart disease, results in an increase in 2,3-DPG, and a right-shift of the oxyhaemoglobin dissociation curve. This means that, for a given PaO_2 the SaO_2 will be lower.

Assessment of oxygenation

Arterial blood gas (ABG) analysis

- ABG analysis is most reliable when the blood is taken from an indwelling arterial line; crying during an arterial stab procedure has significant effects on gas exchange.
- ABG measurements should be made at 37°C. pH decreases and CO_2 increases with increased temperature.
- 'Arterialized' capillary samples correspond closely to arterial blood if peripheral circulation is good and the sample is not exposed to air.

Oxygen saturation by pulse oximetry

A pulse oximeter uses two light-emitting diodes at different wavelengths (red and infrared) combined with a photodetector unit. The oximeter calculates the oxygen saturation based on the measurement of the ratio between the detected red (R) and infrared (I) signal. The ratio is calculated many times each cardiac cycle and averaged. There are many potential problems that may affect the validity of the displayed saturation result (see box). Two are of particular concern in children.

- Movement artefact. This is largely overcome by modern machines, which use Masimo technology.
- Malpositioning of the probe—a particular problem for sensors that are wrapped around fingers or toes. If the red and infrared light-emitting diodes are not exactly opposite the photodetector there may be a difference in the path length between each diode and detector resulting in an abnormal R:I ratio and a falsely low result. Importantly the pulse plethysmograph signal may look normal but be coming from one wavelength signal only. A high index of suspicion is needed if there is an unexpectedly low saturation result.

Oxygen saturation monitors—potential problems

- Movement artefact
- Decreased pulse pressure, e.g. hypovolaemia
- Increased venous pulsation, e.g. tricuspid incompetence (picks up venous signal)
- Presence of carboxyhaemoglobin or methaemoglobin
- Electromagnetic interference, e.g. surgical diathermy
- Visible light—especially pulsatile visible light
- Physiological dyes, e.g. methylene blue
- Nail varnish
- Variation between instruments

Oxygen therapy in hospital

Headbox

Oxygen is delivered simply by increasing the oxygen concentration in the ambient air within the box. This is an open system and oxygen concentration is monitored within the box by placing a sensor near the infant's face and flow is adjusted to achieve desired concentration. It is difficult to exceed an oxygen concentration of 60%.

Possible problems

- Small box, large baby. There is little leak around the neck and so only low flow rates are required to maintain oxygen concentration. However, this may result in CO_2 build-up within the box. Adequate flow through the headbox is necessary.
- Large box, small baby. There is a large leak and therefore high flow rates required to maintain oxygen concentration. Oxygen from a wall source is dry and cold and may result in significant cooling.

Nasal cannulae

A low flow system providing oxygen at flow rates below the maximum inspiratory flow rate of the patient. The inspired gas is diluted with entrained room air and the inspired oxygen concentration that the child receives is dependent on the relationships between oxygen flow, breathing pattern (rate and inspiratory:expiratory ratio), and inspiratory flow rate. During episodes of breathlessness or exercise the child's inspiratory flow rate will increase. Since the oxygen flow rate will stay the same, there will be greater dilution of oxygen with room air and the oxygen concentration will fall; during sleep the child's inspiratory flow will decrease and the oxygen concentration will increase. It is impossible to accurately determine the delivered oxygen concentration but it is likely to be between 25% and 40%.

Possible problems

- The cannulae are easily displaced.
- There is a limit to the flow rates that can be delivered. Infants can rarely tolerate more than 2L/min; older children 4L/min. Higher flow rates dry the nasal mucosa and are uncomfortable.
- Unpredictable inspired oxygen concentration worsened by nasal obstruction or mouth breathing.

Masks

Low flow, simple face mask

A system providing oxygen at flow rates below the maximum inspiratory flow rate of the child so room air is entrained and, as with nasal cannulae, the inspired oxygen concentration is variable. A flow rate of at least 4L/min is needed to prevent CO_2 build-up in the mask. Inspired oxygen concentration generally achieved is between 25% and 50%.

Close fitting mask with reservoir bag

These masks have one-way valves so that inspiration is augmented from the reservoir bag rather than entrained room air. This allows high concentrations of oxygen to be delivered. A close-fitting mask may be hot and uncomfortable.

- A re-breathing mask has no valve between mask and reservoir, so on exhalation a proportion of expired air enters the reservoir. This constitutes air from the upper airway, which has remained oxygen-rich, so the oxygen concentration in the reservoir remains high. To prevent re-breathing of exhaled CO_2, wall oxygen flow rate needs to exceed patient minute ventilation. These masks can reliably provide 50–60% oxygen if used with an oxygen flow rate of 10–12L/min.
- A non re-breathing mask has a one-way valve fitted between the mask and reservoir to prevent flow of exhaled gas back into the bag, and a one-way valve on the exhalation port to prevent entraining of room air. With a good mask seal, and an oxygen flow rate at 10–12L/min, this mask system can provide an inspired oxygen concentration of up to 95%. For this to be achieved, however, wall oxygen flow rate must be sufficient to ensure that the reservoir does not completely empty on inspiration.

High flow fixed concentration masks (Venturi mask)

A high flow system that aims to deliver oxygen at flow rates above the child's requirements so that the breathing pattern and variable inspiratory flow do not affect the inspired oxygen concentration. These masks entrain air at a constant rate for a preset oxygen flow rate and can deliver a set oxygen concentration. The high flow rate delivered without the 'work' of entrainment makes this type of mask very comfortable in the very breathless child. Delivered levels of oxygen concentration can be set between 25% and 60%. At higher oxygen concentrations the flow rates produced by the masks may fall below peak inspiratory flow rates of older children. These masks are particularly useful in children with chronic CO_2 retention where hypoxic respiratory drive may be lost if high oxygen concentrations are delivered.

Humidification

Oxygen from a piped or cylinder source is cold and dry so that it may dry the airway mucosa and decrease ciliary activity, particularly if delivered at high flow rates. Oxygen from a concentrator is at room temperature and humidity.

- Headbox. Oxygen at low flows; humidification is rarely necessary.
- Nasal prongs. Oxygen at low flows; humidification is rarely needed but a cold water bubble humidifier can be used.
- Masks. Humidification of inspired air is dependent on flow rate. Cold water bubble humidification adequate at low/moderate flows but a heated humidifier is necessary for oxygen delivered at high flow rates for prolonged periods.

Oxygen therapy at home

Children who are stable but likely to require oxygen therapy for weeks or months should be provided with home oxygen—long-term oxygen therapy (LTOT; see box). Oxygen therapy is generally given in order to maintain SaO_2 at or above 92% or PaO_2 above 8kPa.

Conditions requiring LTOT

- Chronic lung disease of prematurity
- Pulmonary hypoplasia
- Thoracic insufficiency syndromes
- Congenital heart disease with pulmonary hypertension
- Pulmonary hypertension secondary to pulmonary disease
- Interstitial lung disease
- End-stage cystic fibrosis and other causes of severe bronchiectasis
- Palliative care for symptom relief

Benefits of LTOT

- In chronic neonatal lung disease LTOT:
  - reduces pulmonary hypertension;
  - reduces reversible obstructive airways disease;
  - improves growth;
  - reduces the frequency of hypoxaemic and apnoeic episodes during sleep.
- In cystic fibrosis LTOT:
  - alleviates nocturnal hypoxaemia;
  - permits continued school/work attendance;
  - improves exercise ability;
  - does not affect frequency of hospitalization;
  - does not affect mortality.
- In pulmonary vascular disease LTOT:
  - reduces pulmonary hypertension;
  - improves survival.

Criteria for discharge with home oxygen

- Oxygen-responsive hypoxaemia
- Stable oxygen requirement
- Home conditions suitable, including a no smoking policy
- Home telephone
- Community support organized
- Primary health care team accepts care plan
- Plan for emergency access to help (including oxygen for transport)
- Home and car insurers notified

Oxygen delivery at home

In the UK the NHS has contracted with specific supplying companies for different regions of the country. The doctor requesting home oxygen fills in a prescription specifying the flow rate needed, the number of hours needed per day, the need for oxygen during mobility, etc., and the company chooses the mode of delivery.

Oxygen concentrators

These are electrically powered devices that extract oxygen from the air and deliver it in concentrations between 93% and 95%. They generate only low flow oxygen (up to 2–3L/min) They cannot therefore be used with Venturi masks or as driving gas for nebulized medication. They are large and tubing outlets are provided in the one or more rooms in the child's home. Back-up cylinder oxygen is needed in case of equipment malfunction or electricity failure.

Cylinder oxygen

Oxygen is provided in aluminium or steel cylinders of various sizes. They are most likely to be used for patients who require low flow oxygen for a limited number of hours per day, such as infants with chronic lung disease of prematurity. Even the small cylinders are heavy; they are awkward to transport and the oxygen supply is limited. For example, a standard small cylinder weighing 5kg will provide 2L/min for only 2.5h. Aluminium cylinders are lighter.

Oxygen-conserving devices

A battery-operated system that delivers a pulse of oxygen during inspiration only greatly extends the duration of oxygen supply in portable cylinders. Using this system the aluminium Oxylight 240 cylinder, which weighs only 2.3kg, can supply oxygen at 2L/min for 14h. These systems are only suitable for older children able to generate a sufficiently high inspiratory flow rate to trigger the oxygen delivery.

Liquid oxygen

This is a low-pressure oxygen system that can be used with any low-flow oxygen delivery device. It is expensive but the most convenient method for patients with continuous flow needs while ambulatory, e.g. whilst going to school. A lightweight portable system can supply a day's oxygen needs in a backpack. There are no advantages for the house-bound patient.

How to assess/reassess oxygen needs

Measurement of oxygen saturation by pulse oximetry is the best and most convenient method of assessing oxygenation. Pulse oximetry does not indicate the adequacy of ventilation and hypercapnia, and acidosis should be assessed by blood sampling if hypoventilation is suspected. Venous samples are usually adequate. Oximeters do not recognize hyperoxia and use of oxygen saturation as a guide to oxygen therapy must be carefully regulated in preterm infants.

- During acute illness in hospital oximetry should be performed within 30min of starting therapy and repeated 2–4 hourly depending on the child's condition. Continuous oximetry is indicated in the severely ill.
- For patients on LTOT assessment should take place in each physiological state:
  - sleep;
  - wakefulness;
  - exercise;
  - feeding (in infants).

This is most easily accomplished with a recording oximeter so that both baseline SaO_2 and desaturation episodes can be evaluated. Miniature SaO_2 recording devices are available for overnight recording in the child's home. For complex problems additional channel recording, e.g. chest and abdominal movement or airflow, may be necessary and most often such sleep studies are done in hospital.

- A recent RCT (the 'BOOST' trial) in 358 premature infants still requiring oxygen at 32 weeks postmenstrual age showed that maintaining SaO_2 at 95–98% had no advantage over 91–94% in terms of growth and neurodevelopment assessed at 1 year of age. This study used N-3000 Nellcor oximeters.[1]

When to stop oxygen therapy

- In an acute condition such as asthma or bronchiolitis maintenance of $SaO_2 > 92\%$ in air permits cessation of oxygen therapy.
- In infants with chronic lung disease of prematurity a room air challenge may be used. $SaO_2 > 92\%$ after 40min in room air predicts readiness for oxygen cessation. Infants whose oxygen was stopped on these criteria maintained normal growth over the following 6 months.[2] Some infants who successfully stop oxygen may need further short periods of oxygen during respiratory infections.
- In many children, e.g. those with CF or pulmonary hypertension, oxygen treatment will be needed either until the child has a lung transplantation or until death.

1 Askie, L.M., Henderson-Smart, D.J., Irwig, L., et al. (2003). Oxygen-saturation targets and outcomes in extremely preterm infants. N. Engl. J. Med. **349**, 959–67.

2 Simoes, E.A., Rosenberg, A.A., King, S.J., et al. (1997). Room air challenge: prediction for successful weaning of oxygen-dependent infants. J. Perinatol. **17**, 125–9.

Further information

Balfour-Lynn, I.M., Primhak, R.A., and Shaw, B.N. (2005). Home oxygen for children: who, how and when? *Thorax* **60** (1), 76–81.

Dodd, M.E., Haworth, C.S., and Webb, A.K. (1998). A practical approach to oxygen therapy in cystic fibrosis. *J. R. Soc. Med.* **91** (S34), 30–9.

Inhalers and nebulizers

Introduction

- Aerosol therapy is used to deliver drugs directly to the respiratory tract.
- The commonest aerosol therapies are used in the treatment of asthma and there has been great investment in development of high specification portable metered dose and dry powder inhalers.
- Other medications that may be delivered by aerosol include adrenaline, drugs to improve secretion clearance such as dornase alfa or hyperosmolar saline, antibiotics such as colomycin, tobramycin, and gentamicin, and antiviral and antifungal therapies such as ribavarin and amphotericin. Specialist treatments like these lack funding for specific inhaler development and are generally administered using generic nebulizer devices.
- To reach the lower airways, particles delivered by aerosol need to pass through the protective filtering mechanisms of the upper airway. The convoluted structure of the nasal airways, posterior oropharynx, and larynx causes angular flow. Particles settle and stick to the mucus-secreting epithelium, from where they may be removed from the airway by effective mucociliary mechanisms. Large particles settle in the upper airway and oropharynx on inhalation. Very small particles remain suspended and are exhaled without sedimentation in the airways.
- Optimal particle size for targeting deposition in the lower airways is 1–5µm. Smaller particle sizes (1–2µm) are deposited in a more uniform pattern within the lung. Larger particles (3–5µm) tend to deposit in a more heterogeneous distribution that has to do with airway geometry. The non-uniform deposition is more marked in children with airways disease.
- Effective particle size (or aerodynamic particle diameter) is dependent not only on particle size, but also on particle mass and the shape of particles produced by the inhaler.

Metered dose inhalers and valved holding chambers

- Metered dose inhalers (MDIs) consist of a pressurized chamber that holds a propellant and the drug. The propellant is a liquid under pressure that vaporizes on exposure to atmospheric pressure suspending the drug as small particles.
- Before each use, the canister needs to be shaken to ensure that propellant and suspended drug are evenly dispersed. Within the canister is a fixed volume chamber that refills after each inhaler actuation, in preparation for the next dose. If the canister is not shaken between actuations, the drug concentration may vary above or below the recommended dose depending on the relative amount of propellant and drug that collects in the fixed volume chamber.
- Propellants were historically chlorofluorocarbons (CFCs), but recently CFC-free propellants have replaced these products. Some CFC-free propellant MDIs have been shown to emit drugs with a smaller effective particle size, and this is likely to increase drug dose delivery to the peripheral lung.
- Aerosolized drug is ejected at a velocity of 25–30m/s. Coordinating inspiration, inhaler actuation, and breath-holding requires a high degree of skill. Even when used optimally, an MDI held directly between the lips will result in significant upper airway particle compaction and sub-maximal delivery of drug to the lower airways. Particle compaction in the upper airway from steroid inhalers may result in oropharyngeal thrush or a hoarse voice.
- Using a valved holding chamber (VHC) into which the MDI actuation is delivered enables the child to breathe in from a static suspension of drug particles. This dramatically improves distal airway drug delivery and reduces particle compaction in the upper airway. VHCs also significantly reduce systemic absorption of drug from the GI tract.
- Drug deposition data shows great variability between different approaches to drug delivery. MDI alone delivers < 15% of the drug to the lungs even in highly coordinated well trained adults. MDI with VHC delivers on the order of 30% of the drug. In infants, pulmonary deposition is of the order of 2% using MDI with VHC and mask.
- VHC use should be encouraged in children of all ages. Older children should be trained to take a single slow deep inspiration and hold their breath to maximize drug sedimentation in the distal airways. Tidal volume breathing in younger children means that several breaths may be needed to clear the VHC of suspended drug.
- VHCs (e.g. Volumatic, Aerochamber) are most effective if they are large, non-static (especially metal), and used with a mouthpiece rather than a mask. A mouthpiece should be used whenever possible.
- For children under the age of 4 years, a mask covering mouth and nose is usually used with the VHC. Great care must be taken with the mask–VHC combination as even a small facemask leak results in little if any drug being delivered to the airways.

- Cooperation remains the major difficulty in effective drug delivery. For young children, we train parents to take a position sitting on the floor leaning against a wall. The child lies down with their head on the floor between the parent's thighs. In this position, the parent has control of the face position and can ensure an effective mask seal.
- VHCs are rather bulky and can be unwieldy to use. They are rarely used by older children outside the home. Breath-actuated MDIs (e.g. Autohaler, Easybreathe) theoretically improve drug deposition compared to traditional MDIs by reducing the coordination needed for successful use. Upper airway drug deposition is still very high compared to MDI used with VHC. A more effective alternative for this age group is a dry-powder inhaler (DPI).

Dry powder inhalers

- Dry powder inhalers (DPI) contain small drug particles fixed to larger inert binding molecules such as lactose with a diameter of 30–60μm. These particles have better flow characteristics, and are easier to disperse than small particles, which bind each other through electro-static interactions. Upon inspiration, the particles pass through an aperture that generates high turbulence and this disperses the drug from the binding molecule. Suspended drug particles enter the lung and the binding molecules are deposited in the pharynx. Common devices use blister packs (e.g. Diskhaler) or fixed volume chambers (e.g. Turbohaler, Clickhaler, Easyhaler, Accuhaler). The priming manoeuvre either pierces the blister or deposits the correct drug volume in the outflow channel.
- DPIs rely on the patient to generate sufficient inspiration to disperse and deliver the drug. Generation of flow rates of 30L/min or higher are needed to effectively use a DPI. DPIs are not therefore recommended for children under the age of 5 years.
- Deposition data suggest that DPIs and MDIs plus VHC deliver equivalent doses to the distal airways.
- DPIs are often preferred by older children and adolescents as they are compact and easily portable.
- Because there is significant upper airway deposition with a DPI, children using steroid preparations may develop a hoarse voice or oropharyngeal thrush and should be encouraged to gargle with water after administration.

Nebulizers

- The standard jet nebulizers used by most children are relatively inefficient devices with < 10% of the starting dose reaching the lungs with significant oral and gastric deposition. This compares poorly with an MDI and VHC and, where available, the latter is usually preferred.
- Nebulizers can be driven by oxygen and, where a child needs oxygen, nebulizers can allow drug to be given without interrupting oxygen flow. There are also a number of drugs, particularly antibiotics and proteins such as DNAase, that are only available as solutions for nebulization. For these drugs there is no choice in delivery device. Dry powder versions of some of these drugs are being developed and, once available, will provide a useful alternative.

Methods of nebulization

Jet nebulizers

- This is the simplest form of nebulization. Compressed air is passed through a small orifice to generate a high velocity jet of air. The air pressure around the jet falls (the Bernoulli effect) forcing the solution in the surrounding reservoir towards the jet. Droplets that are pulled into the jet path are fragmented into tiny particles and aerosolized. A wide distribution of particle sizes is produced (range 0.1–30µm).
- Particle size is principally determined by the flow rate of jet of air and each unit will have a specified flow rate for optimal use (between 4 and 8L/min). In general, higher flow rates increase output, decrease mean particle size, and reduce particle size distribution.
- A baffled exit to the nebulizer catches larger aerosolized particles that sediment out quickly and rain back into the reservoir. This reduces the size distribution of particles leaving the device and increases the proportion of nebulized particles in the respirable range. Most devices aim at particle size with a diameter equal or less than 5µm.
- The large shearing forces generated by a jet nebulizer may damage complex molecules.

Ultrasonic nebulizers

- A piezoelectric crystal rapidly vibrates the nebulizing solution from below, causing droplets to detach from the liquid surface. A flow of air across the surface directs the nebulized solution to the patient.
- Particle size distributions are generally larger than with jet nebulizers.
- Disadvantages include a large residual volume and wastage of drug, heat generation and potential denaturing of proteins in the solution, and damage to complex molecules from large shearing forces.

High frequency vibrating mesh nebulizers

- Aerosol is generated by forcing the nebulizer fluid from a reservoir beneath the membrane, through holes of fixed diameter in the vibrating membrane.
- Particle size is defined by diameter of holes in the membrane and the viscosity of nebulized fluid. An extremely narrow particle size distribution is achieved, thereby increasing the percentage of particles in the respirable range.

- There is no requirement for residual volume and consequently these nebulizers are highly cost-efficient when using expensive therapies.
- Increased efficiency translates to reduced nebulizer times.

Methods of delivery

Constant output nebulizers

These nebulizers deliver a constant flow of nebulized particles through inspiration and expiration (e.g. Sidestream jet nebulizer (Medic-Aid), eFlow vibrating mesh nebulizer (Pari)).

Breath-enhanced (Venturi) nebulizers

- These devices aim to maximize delivery during inspiration and minimize loss of drug during expiration (jet nebulizers—Pari LC plus, Pari LC star, Pari LC sprint, Ventstream (Respironics)).
- As the child inhales from the device, air is entrained through the nebulizer bowl resulting in increased output of aerosol. The increased output is thought to be due to drying of droplets (thereby reducing their size) prior to impaction on the baffle, thus allowing a higher proportion of nebulized droplets to exit the nebulizer. The increased aerosol output during inspiration means that shorter nebulization times are required to deliver the same dose of drug. Also, since the proportion of aerosol generated during inspiration is greater than during expiration, there are smaller total losses to the atmosphere.

Dosimetric nebulizers

Automated sensing devices or manual triggering are used to restrict release of aerosol to inspiration only (e.g. I-neb vibrating mesh nebulizer (Respironics), Akita jet nebulizer). Dose/inhalation is controlled and environmental losses are minimized. The Akita dosimeter also controls inspiratory flow rate, which further improves deposition.

Deposition data

- Many variables contribute to final quantity of drug deposited in the distal airways, including method of nebulization, particle size distribution, method of delivery, timing of delivery, and flow dynamics of inspiration.
- Up to 50% of the drug dosage will be left in a jet nebulizer as residual volume that cannot be effectively nebulized. Vibrating mesh nebulizers can effectively nebulize all the filled dose.
- Constant output devices result in 25–30% loss of drug to the environment. Effective breath-enhanced devices may reduce these losses to 15–20%. Dosimetric devices theoretically have no environmental losses.
- Jet nebulizers vary on the particle size distribution of their output, largely dependent on the complexity of the baffle system used, e.g. for the Pari LC Plus the percentage of particles under 5μm is 50%, whereas for the Pari LC star it is 65–75%.
- Vibrating mesh nebulizers have an extremely narrow particle size distribution and therefore deliver a larger proportion of particles in the respirable range.

- Deposition studies have generally been performed using jet nebulizers. 10% of starting dose is deposited in lungs using the Pari LC Plus breath enhanced jet nebulizer. This is a little better than constant output devices, with the additional benefit that the dose is delivered more quickly—8min versus 12min for a 3mL fill.
- 20% of starting dose is deposited using the Pari LC Star jet nebulizer. This increase in efficiency is due to a combination of a higher total dose output and a better particle size distribution.
- For the Pari LC Plus and LC Star, total lung deposition is in the range of 30–50% of the output of the nebulizer (50–70% being lost either during expiration or as residual volume).
- For the Pari LC Star plus jet nebulizer used with the Akita dosimetric delivery unit, lung deposition reaches 80% of the output of the nebulizer. The Akita ensures nebulization only on inspiration and controls the rate of inspiration so that linear airflow is optimized. New developments combining the Akita2 with Pari vibrating mesh technology deliver 75% of the filled dose. The Akita is particularly useful when using high dose therapy, expensive medication, and drugs with a small therapeutic window.

Which nebulizer?

The requirements placed on a nebulizer should dictate the choice of system.

- For emergency treatment of asthma with salbutamol and ipratropium or for croup with budesonide and adrenaline, simple disposable constant output jet nebulizers are adequate.
- For expensive medication, consider breath-enhanced Venturi systems such as the Pari LC Plus, LC Star, or Ventstream, or vibrating mesh nebulizers with low residual volumes such as the eFlow and I-neb. The I-neb has the additional advantage of being dosimetric.
- For chronic treatment and where size, portability, noise levels, and speed of nebulization all affect compliance, the vibrating mesh nebulizers offer big advantages.
- For high doses and measured doses consider more complex delivery systems such as the dosimetric Akita plus Pari LC Star.

Further information

Wilson, D., Burniston, M., Moya, E., Parkin, A., Smye, S., Robinson, P., and Littlewood, J. (1999). Improvement of nebulised antibiotic delivery in cystic fibrosis. *Arch. Dis. Child.* **80**, 348–52.

Devadason, S.G., Everard, M.L., Linto, J.M., and Le Souef, P.N. (1997). Comparison of drug delivery from conventional versus 'Venturi' nebulizers. *Eur. Respir. J.* **10**, 2479–83.

Airway clearance techniques

The value of physiotherapy

The goal of chest physiotherapy is to clear airway secretions from the small airways that they are partially obstructing to the large airways where they can be expelled by coughing or huffing. Many different techniques are available and they are applied to many different clinical situations. Occasionally there is clear-cut and immediate benefit from physiotherapy, e.g. in assisting the re-inflation of a collapsed lobe of the lung in a child on a ventilator. More often improvements are harder to identify immediately and success is measured in volumes of airway secretions expelled as a proxy for genuine clinical benefit. Physiotherapy has not been rigorously studied by clinical trial, partly because the treatment predates evidence-based medicine, partly because trial design is difficult, and partly because it seems self-evident that, when thick green secretions are expelled during a physiotherapy session, it must be a good thing.

Cystic fibrosis

Most studies of the effectiveness of chest physiotherapy have been carried out in children with CF. Studies in the 1970s and 1980s demonstrated that chest physiotherapy using percussion and postural drainage improved outcomes, including lung function, compared to directed coughing. More recent studies have been comparative and, in the short term, most techniques appear to be equivalent, as assessed by volume of expelled secretions and improvement in lung function during an exacerbation. There are fewer longer-term studies and results are more variable. We do not know whether it is critical that well children with CF undertake daily physiotherapy routines, or how long or how frequent these routines should be. In practice daily physiotherapy can be used both as a therapy and as an early indication for the family when there is an increase in secretions so that other interventions, such as the use of antibiotics, can be used before the child becomes unwell.

Asthma

Chest physiotherapy is not helpful in the management of acute exacerbations of asthma. Occasionally, when there is mucus retention and collapse of part of the lung, physiotherapy may be considered, particularly in the ventilated child. Vigorous physiotherapy may worsen bronchoconstriction.

Pneumonia

Chest physiotherapy does not improve outcomes of otherwise healthy children with acute lobar pneumonia.

Bronchiolitis

Chest physiotherapy does not improve outcomes in infants with acute viral bronchiolitis.

Inhaled foreign body

Chest physiotherapy is contraindicated in children with suspected foreign body. If the foreign body is dislodged but not expelled from the airway it may re-impact in a different airway (e.g. shift from right main bronchus to left main bronchus). Since the first airway may be oedematous, the shift may result in life-threatening airways obstruction.

Neuromuscular weakness

Although there are no trials showing the benefit of secretion clearance in children with neuromuscular weakness, practical experience with children who have weak ineffective coughs makes it clear that secretion clearance techniques form an essential part of improving survival in this group of children.

Specific techniques

- All airway clearance techniques combine secretion mobilization, where airway secretions are detached from the airway wall and moved to the large airways, with an expiratory manoeuvre to expel the secretions from the large airways into the mouth. Carrying out secretion mobilization without the clearance step will be ineffective.
- The choice of technique will depend on the local physiotherapy service and the preference of the child and the family. There are limited comparative trials, almost exclusively in children with CF, and most suggest equivalence. Some techniques work well for some children, but are ineffective or associated with poor compliance by others.

Percussion and postural drainage

This method is appropriate in infants and young children.
- Standard therapy uses 6 positions:
  - sitting up, leaning forward 30° (infants can recline against a carer) to percuss upper part of front of chest;
  - sitting up, leaning backwards 30° to percuss upper part of back of chest;
  - reclining head down 30° (infants horizontal) on left side to percuss right side of chest;
  - reclining head down 30° (infants horizontal) on right side to percuss left side of chest;
  - reclining head down 30° (infants horizontal) prone to percuss lower part of back of chest;
  - reclining head down 30° (infants horizontal) supine to percuss lower part of front of chest.
- The head down positions are not used in infants since they can exacerbate gastro-oesophageal reflux. Data from adults with CF also indicate that the head down position can be associated with some undesirable consequences, including worsening of GOR, decreased expiratory flow rates, and decreased oxygenation. Many CF centres now advise against head down positioning during physiotherapy.
- The different positions can be achieved using the parent's lap, pillows, a physiotherapy wedge, or a tipping bed. In each position gentle percussion, using a cupped hand, is used to loosen and mobilize airway secretions.
- In infants chest vibration and compression are used to drive the secretions towards the large airways where they may be cleared by coughing. Older children are encouraged to carry out huffing manoeuvres to do the same thing. It takes 2min for each position, so a full session takes around 12–15min. Older children can carry out the percussion to some parts of the chest themselves.

Active cycle of breathing technique (ACBT)

This technique is useful for older children and can be performed without assistance. The subject starts with relaxed tidal breathing. The next phase involves taking 3–4 slow maximum inspirations with inspiratory hold, followed by passive exhalation. It is thought that this phase opens up smaller airways and gets air in behind any airway secretions. The final phase involves one or two forced expirations, with an open glottis, to push the secretions into the large airways. This step should be carried out at mid- to low lung volumes. Any secretions in the proximal airways can then be cleared by huffing or coughing at high lung volume.

Autogenic drainage

This technique also uses cycles of breathing. It can be harder to learn than ACBT. The subject starts with a slow deep inspiration with inspiratory hold for 3–4s with an open glottis. This is followed by a rapid exhalation. This should be a fast as possible, with a wide open glottis, without causing airway compression, as indicated by audible wheezing. Once down at a low lung volume, the subject starts tidal breathing. This phase is thought to un-stick secretions from the peripheral airways. The lung volume is then increased to mid-volume and tidal breathing is continued, allowing the secretions to move proximally. Lung volumes are increased again, continuing tidal breathing that should move the secretions into the large airways when they can be cleared by huffing or coughing.

Positive pressure techniques

This technique may be useful in older children with evidence of airflow obstruction on spirometry. When obstruction is present it may be difficult to clear distal secretions. Applying positive expiratory pressure (PEP), using a mask with a variable resistor, during expiration can splint open the airways and improve secretion clearance. The correct resistance is selected using a manometer attached to the mask; during mid-expiration the subject should generate pressures of 10–20cmH_2O. Treatment is then carried out in the sitting position. 10 tidal breaths are made. Expiration should not be forced or prolonged. Secretions are then cleared by huffing or coughing. The cycle is then repeated. In short-term studies, PEP appears to be as effective as percussion and postural drainage for clearing secretions in patients with CF, and in a long-term study it was superior in maintaining pulmonary function.

Acapello, RC-Cornet, and Flutter devices

These devices provide oscillating positive pressure. It is believed that this causes the airway walls to vibrate, loosens mucus, and promotes its clearance. The oscillations may also decrease spinnability and viscoelasticity of the secretions, which some patients find effective and easier to perform than mask PEP. In children with CF, these devices appear to be effective in the short term for clearing airway secretions. Longer-term studies suggest that, when used as the only form of physiotherapy, they may be less effective than other techniques at preserving lung function.

Vibrating vests

High frequency chest wall oscillation can be achieved using pressure vests such as the Hayek jacket (Medivent RTx) and the Vest Airway Clearance system (Hill-Rom). These can be very effective at mobilizing secretions. Their use needs to be combined with a forced expiratory manoeuvre, such as huffing, to expectorate any secretions. These devices are expensive and have not been shown to improve long-term outcomes in CF.

Intrapulmonary percussive ventilation

The Percussionaire (Percussionaire Corp, Sandpoint, Idaho, USA) delivers percussive pressure waves via a mouthpiece or facemask. Mobilized secretions need to be cleared from the airway by coughing or huffing. It has been used in children with mild neuromuscular weakness and shown to be beneficial although the comparison arm was incentive spirometry rather than any established cough assistance technique.

Assisted coughing

- An effective cough requires a cough peak flow of 160L/min. A normal 15-year-old will produce a cough peak flow of over 700L/min. Children with neuromuscular weakness may be unable to generate sufficient flows because:
  - they are unable to take in a sufficiently large breath;
  - they are unable to generate sufficient expiratory force;
  - they have glottic weakness.
- Generating sufficient inspiratory lung volumes can be augmented either manually with a resuscitation bag, or mechanically with either a ventilator or a cough-assist machine. Breath-stacking and glossopharyngeal or 'frog' breathing, in which the glossopharyngeal muscles are used to push air into the lungs, can also be used to augment lung volumes in motivated older children. In some children, once adequate insufflation has been achieved, the child's own cough can be effective at clearing secretions.
- Expiratory flows during coughing can be improved manually by compressing the upper abdomen or chest wall as the child coughs. Mechanical cough-assist devices are also available. These devices use a face mask to deliver a relatively high pressure (+25 to +40cmH$_2$O) insufflation of 2–3s followed by a similar high pressure exsufflation of 1–2s as the child attempts to cough. Airway secretions are then either expelled into the mask or suctioned from the oropharynx. The timings of insufflation and exsufflation can be manual or automated. If these devices are used it is important to finish the session with 2 or 3 good inflations to try and restore a good functional residual volume. The value of these devices has not been subject to clinical trials but, at an anecdotal level, they appear to be a very useful addition to secretion clearance techniques, particularly during infective exacerbations.

Further information

Flenady, V.J. and Gray, P.H. (2002). Chest physiotherapy for preventing morbidity in babies being extubated from mechanical ventilation. *Cochrane Database Syst. Rev.* 2002 (2), CD000283.

Hofmeyer, J.L., Webber, B.A., and Hodson, M.E. (1986). Evaluation of positive expiratory pressure as an adjunct to chest physiotherapy in the treatment of cystic fibrosis. *Thorax* **41**, 951–4.

Konstan, M.W., Stern, R.C. and Doershuk, C.F. (1994). Efficacy of the flutter device for airway mucus clearance in patients with CF. *J. Pediatr.* **124**, 689–93.

Main, E., Prasad, A., and Schans, C. (2005). Conventional chest physiotherapy compared to other airway clearance techniques for cystic fibrosis. *Cochrane Database Syst. Rev.* **2005** (1), CD002011.

McCarren, B. and Alison, J.A. (2006). Physiological effects of vibration in subjects with cystic fibrosis. *Eur. Respir. J.* **27**, 1204–9.

McIlwaine, P.M., Wong, L.T.K., Peaccck, D., and Davidson, A.G.F. (1997). Long-term comparative trial of conventional postural drainage and percussion versus positive expiratory pressure physiotherapy in the treatment of cystic fibrosis. *J. Pediatr.* **131**, 570–4.

McIlwaine, P.M., Wong, L.T., Peacock, D., and Davidson, A.G. (2001). Long-term comparative trial of positive expiratory pressure versus oscillating positive expiratory pressure (flutter) physiotherapy in the treatment of cystic fibrosis. *J. Pediatr.* **138**, 845–50.

McIlwaine, M. (2007). Chest physical therapy, breathing techniques and exercise in children with CF. *Paediatr. Respir. Rev.* **8**, 8–16.

Perrotta, C., Ortiz, Z., and Roque M. (2007). Chest physiotherapy for acute bronchiolitis in paediatric patients between 0 and 24 months old. *Cochrane Database Syst. Rev.* **2007** (1), CD004873.

Reardon, C.C., Christianser, D., Barnett, E.D., and Cabral, H.J. (2005). Intrapulmonary percussive ventilation vs incentive spirometry for children with neuromuscular disease. *Arch. Pediatr. Adolesc. Med.* **159**, 526–31.

Reisman, J.J., Rivington-Law, B., and Corey, M. (1988). Role of conventional physiotherapy in cystic fibrosis. *J. Pediatr.* **113**, 632–6.

van der Schans, C., Prasad, A., and Main, E. (2000). Chest physiotherapy compared to no chest physiotherapy for cystic fibrosis. *Cochrane Database Syst. Rev.* **2000** (2), CD001401.

Immunization

Introduction

- Children with lung disease are more likely to become unwell with intercurrent infection. It is important that they are protected against infection by immunization where this is possible. This guidance refers to children with the following conditions:
  - cystic fibrosis;
  - bronchiectasis;
  - chronic lung disease of prematurity;
  - persistent asthma;
  - interstitial lung disease;
  - children undergoing home ventilation or with neuromuscular disorders.
- Children with these conditions should receive:
  - routine childhood immunizations, including live vaccines;
  - pneumococcal vaccine;
  - annual influenza vaccination from age 6 months.
- Immunization schedules will differ between countries. The following comments apply largely to the UK.
- The evidence that influenza vaccine reduces risk of exacerbation in children with asthma is not robust.

Pneumococcal vaccine

- At risk children between the age of 2 and 12 months should be given the 7-valent pneumococcal conjugate vaccine (PCV) according to the routine immunization schedule at 2, 4, and 13 months of age. They should also receive one dose of the 23-valent pneumococcal polysaccharide vaccine (PPV) after their second birthday.
- Unimmunized at risk children between the ages of 12 months and 5 years of age should receive two doses of PCV separated by 2 months and a single dose of PPV after their second birthday and at least 2 months after their last dose of PCV.
- Unimmunized at risk children over the age of 5 years should receive one dose of PPV only.

Influenza vaccine

- While most viruses are antigenically stable, the influenza viruses A and B (especially A) are constantly altering their antigenic structure as indicated by changes in the haemagglutinins (H) and neuraminidases (N) on the surface of the viruses.
- It is essential that influenza vaccines in use contain the H and N components of the prevalent strain or strains. Every year the WHO recommends which strains should be included in that year's vaccine.
- The recommended strains are grown in the allantoic cavity of chick embryos (therefore contraindicated in those hypersensitive to eggs).
- Since influenza vaccines will not control epidemics they are recommended only for persons at high risk.

- Annual immunization is strongly recommended for individuals aged over 6 months with the conditions listed above and, in addition, in children with asthma on chronic corticosteroid therapy, and those previously admitted to hospital with lower respiratory tract disease.
- As part of the winter planning, NHS employers should offer vaccination to healthcare workers directly involved in patient care.
- Studies have shown that 2 doses of inactivated vaccine are required to achieve adequate antibody levels in children aged < 13 years, as they may never have been exposed to influenza or been vaccinated before. Thus, children aged < 13 years should receive a second dose 4–6 weeks after receiving influenza vaccine for the first time. Children aged > 13 years are given a single dose.
- Vaccination in children aged < 6 months is not recommended.
- There are a number of different formulations available. All contain inactivated influenza virus. Dosage is age- and manufacturer-dependent and should be taken from the manufacturer's summary of product details.
- Contraindications. Most vaccines have some basic contraindication to their use, and the product literature should be consulted for details. In general, vaccinations should be postponed if the individual is suffering from an acute illness. Minor infections without fever or systemic upset are not contraindications. The influenza vaccine should not be given to those who have a confirmed anaphylactic reaction to a previous dose of the vaccine, any component of the vaccine, or a confirmed anaphylactic hypersensitivity to egg products as these vaccines are prepared in hen's eggs.

Passive immunization against respiratory syncytial virus (RSV)

- Monthly injections of monoclonal antibody (palivizumab) against RSV will provide 40–50% protection against severe disease (defined as disease requiring hospital care).
- In the UK, where there is a clear RSV season injections are usually given from October to February.
- Effectiveness has been shown in infants born prematurely, in those who have chronic lung disease, and in those with haemodynamically significant or cyanotic congenital heart disease
- Palivizumab should be prescribed under specialist supervision. The specific groups of children who receive the drug will vary according to local policy. This reflects the high cost of the treatment.

Further information

Department of Health (2007). *Immunisation of individuals with underlying medical conditions*, Department of Health Green Book. Department of Health, London.
British National Formulary for Children (2007).

Dealing with non-adherence to therapy

Introduction
- Non-adherence to paediatric medical treatment regimens may occur in up to 50% of cases. This problem becomes particularly prominent in adolescence where the adolescent agenda of self definition, social exploration, and independence naturally conflicts with the demands of treatment for chronic disease.
- Chronic disease and complex treatment regimens impact on both patient and family, and ensuring good adherence to treatment therefore necessitates the cooperation of both patient and parents. This requires acceptance both of the disease itself, and the validity of the proposed treatment.
- A well-organized household with a well structured daily routine will tend to promote adherence to medical treatment.
- Chaotic households are more likely to struggle with adherence, with difficulty incorporating new tasks into the daily routine, especially time-consuming treatments such as physiotherapy. They are more likely to fail on lifestyle advice such as dietary guidance, rules about smoking in the house, or situations and activities to avoid, and are more likely to default on tasks that require planning ahead such as refilling prescriptions or attending hospital appointments.
- A cohesive family where the climate is supportive and responsive, rather than critical and disengaging will be more successful at accommodating the additional pressures and change in family dynamic that chronic disease may impose.

Approach to non-adherence to therapy
- It is important first to clarify whether the parents and patient have a clear understanding of what treatments have been implemented. Treatment compliance is unlikely to be successful if reasons for treatment have not been made clear.
- A written treatment plan is an essential part of any treatment regimen, providing all carers within the family as well as the patient with a clear guideline. It helps avoid confusion that may occur during a short consultation with the health carer. It should be user friendly for the family.
- For children with chronic disease, copies of clinic letters forwarded to the family can provide a clear progress report and help re-clarify any changes made to treatment.
- Non-adherence to treatment in adolescence is very common. Teenagers > 14 years of age (depending on the child's maturity) should be seen alone in clinic consultations as well as with their parents, so they have an opportunity to express themselves in confidence.
- The setting and the quality of the physician–patient relationship may be important in improving treatment adherence, and teenagers with poor compliance should be seen by the same physician over time so that a trusting relationship can develop.
- Information regarding the disease should be given at a level appropriate to the maturational stage of the patient.

- Difficulties in adhering to the treatment strategy should be discussed openly and sympathetically, rather than in a disappointed or paternalistic manner. Teenagers are more likely to be truthful about compliance in a non-judgemental environment.
- Evidence indicates that adherence to one aspect of the treatment does not necessarily mean adherence to all aspects of the regimen. All components of treatment should therefore be discussed. What compliance is demonstrated should be praised.
- Asking for proposals from the patient may help engage them in treatment plans. Within reason, treatment should be simplified as much as possible and be open to negotiation. Therapy should be adapted to the teenager's lifestyle.

Further information

Michaud, P.A., Suris, J.C., and Viner, R. (2004). The adolescent with a chronic condition. Part II: healthcare provision. *Arch. Dis. Child.* **89**, 943–9.

Non-invasive ventilation

Need for non-invasive ventilation

- Non-invasive ventilation (NIV) is a technique that increases alveolar ventilation without the use of an endotracheal tube or tracheostomy tube.
- The increased availability of appropriate ventilators and mask systems means that many children who would previously have needed a tracheostomy can now be supported with a non-invasive ventilator. See box for pros and cons of NIV versus tracheostomy.
- Children who benefit from NIV are those with respiratory failure who are able to self-ventilate for variable periods of time. Most commonly this group of children requires support during sleep only.
- For those needing long-term 24h/day support ventilation via a tracheostomy is preferred.
- Children with neuromuscular conditions form the largest group of children using NIV. Other possible conditions are given in the box. Further details of all of these conditions can be found in the relevant chapters elsewhere in the book.

NIV versus tracheostomy ventilation

Pros

- Speech function preserved
- Increased mobility
- Swallowing function preserved
- Decreased cost

Cons

- Pressure sores on the face, discomfort
- Nasal dryness, irritation
- Eye irritation
- Possible increased risk of aspiration

Conditions that can lead to chronic ventilatory failure

- Central hypoventilation:
  - trauma/surgery
  - congenital central hypoventilation syndrome
  - Arnold–Chiari malformation
  - post-encephalitis
  - brainstem tumour
- Neuromuscular disease:
  - Duchenne muscular dystrophy
  - spinal muscular atrophy
  - congenital muscular dystrophies and myopathies
  - demyelinating neuropathies
- Chest wall disease:
  - scoliosis
  - restriction secondary to lung resection
- Obesity including Prader–Willi syndrome
- Airway disease:
  - cystic fibrosis
  - chronic lung disease of prematurity

Methods of non-invasive ventilation

NIV can be delivered using positive or negative pressure and via a number of different interfaces between the child and the ventilator. For positive pressure ventilation, the choices of interface are:
- nasal mask;
- face mask;
- nasal prongs;
- mouthpiece.

For negative pressure ventilation, the interface is a Perspex cuirass that fits over the child's chest and abdomen.

Positive pressure ventilation

Positive pressure ventilators can be either volume- or pressure-cycled.

Pressure cycled (often known as BIPAP machines)
- These are by far the most commonly used ventilators in children.
- In pressure support mode the ventilator delivers a preset inspiratory pressure to assist a patient-triggered breathing effort. Time-cycled inspiratory and expiratory pressures are delivered.
- Some ventilators offer a pressure support mode in which the length of the inspiration is controlled by the patient, with a preset maximum (e.g. 3s). The ventilator cycles to expiration when there is a fall in inspiratory flow below a threshold level—an expiratory trigger. Some weak infants and children may not be able to decrease the flow sufficiently to activate the trigger and this can result in a prolonged and uncomfortable inspiratory time. For these children (and most others), the pressure control mode, in which the inspiratory time can be set, is more suitable.
- The ventilator delivers air flow to achieve the set pressure independently of small/moderate leak (and thus ventilation delivered to the patient is relatively stable even with variable leak).
- Most machines are light, portable, and relatively inexpensive. Examples are: BIPAP (Respironics); Nippy (B&D Electromedical).
- The ideal ventilator for use in mask ventilation would have the following characteristics:
  - user-friendly;
  - portable/quiet;
  - reliable and robust;
  - low cost/low maintenance;
  - battery option;
  - low pressure, high pressure, and power alarms.

Volume-cycled

- A volume cycled ventilator is generally set in assist-control mode for home ventilation and delivers set volumes of air triggered by the patient's inspiratory effort with a backup rate for inadequate triggering.
- The volume delivered to the ventilator circuit remains constant regardless of the amount of leak and/or changes in airway resistance or pulmonary compliance. The volumes delivered to the lungs may therefore change from breath to breath and over time.
- These ventilators can deliver high volumes and high pressures and are most useful in individuals with poor lung compliance. They are generally larger, heavier, more expensive, and more complicated than pressure cycled machines but permit mouthpiece sip ventilation and air-stacking, which may be particularly useful for individuals who require some daytime support as well as nocturnal ventilation.
- Examples are: PLV-Continuum (Respironics); LP 10 (Puritan Bennett).

CPAP or BIPAP?

- Continuous positive airway pressure (CPAP) reduces the work of breathing by increasing functional residual capacity. It provides a constant flow of positive pressure to prevent alveoli collapse. CPAP can be used in children with chronic lung disease to improve poor ventilation and oxygenation. It is also effective in preventing upper airway obstruction in patients with obstructive sleep apnoea by splinting the upper airway.
- BIPAP combines the benefits of pressure support ventilation and CPAP, and provides support during the entire respiratory cycle. It is required for children with hypoventilation.

Positive pressure ventilation interfaces

- *Nasal masks* are by far the commonest interface and there is a very large variety of shapes and styles available for adults and large children. The range is much more limited for infants and small children but is improving. The correct size of mask is dependent on nose size and face shape. It is important where possible to permit the child to try several different mask and head piece combinations to see which feels most comfortable for them. The newer gel masks will last for 6–12 months before replacement. The companies Resmed, Respironics, and Sleepnet Corporation are major mask suppliers.
- *Face masks* cover the nose and mouth. They are useful in some weak children where the mouth hangs open during sleep and are sometimes preferred to a nasal mask with chin strap in these situations. Again there is a variety of different types available.
- *Nasal prongs* or *nasal pillows* are available in increasing variety for adult use but there are few in child appropriate sizes.
- *Mouthpieces* are useful for daytime sip ventilation but rarely used overnight. Some adults use a mouthpiece with an additional lip-seal device.

How to initiate mask ventilation

- Initially, efforts should be taken to familiarize the child and family with the mask and the apparatus.
- A CPAP or BIPaP machine provides a constant flow of gas to the mask to create a pressure during both inspiration and expiration. Flow rates are high. *Any nasal mask system must have an inbuilt leak*. Always make sure you know where the leak is and that it is not obstructed before a patient is put on a mask system.
- The mask should be well fitting but not too tight. Poor mask fit contributes to skin and eye irritation. It may be responsible for leaks around the mask. A mask leak is acceptable as long as it does not alter the ventilator's capability to cycle from expiration to inspiration and back again and does not cause irritation to the child (particularly likely if the leak is directed towards the eyes).
- The child should be introduced to the mask and machine gradually and the amount of time that the apparatus is used should be built up, starting with just a few minutes with mask on without ventilation. When the ventilator is first used, low pressures may improve tolerability. The pressures can then be increased gradually until the target pressures are reached. Most children take to using the machine and mask very quickly, usually because they feel physically better after their night's sleep and therefore realize the benefits of using the apparatus.
- Occasionally, young children will either refuse to wear the mask or take it off after only a few minutes' use. Before NIV is abandoned, it is worth trying again using clonidine as a non-respiratory depressant sedative. If this is successful, sedation should be used until ventilation has been established for 5 nights after which the clonidine can be weaned over 3 days. A protocol for the use of clonidine in this way has been published.[1]
- A repeat sleep study will be needed to assess adequacy of the ventilation once the child has become established on a particular regime.

Negative pressure ventilation

Negative pressure ventilation started with the 'iron lung', which saved many lives during the polio epidemics of the 1950s. These devices enclosed the entire body, apart from the head, in a sealed chamber. A bellows then provided the negative pressure to initiate inspiration and expiration was either passive or augmented with positive bellows pressure. The iron lung has now been superseded by cuirass ventilators with light weight, and sometimes custom-made jackets that deliver negative pressure to the chest and abdomen. The cuirass is attached to a power unit that actively controls both phases of the respiratory cycle.

---

1 Bhatt, J.M., Primhak, R.A., and Mayer, A.P.T. (2006). Oral clonidine as a sedative agent to establish children on non-invasive ventilation. *Chest* Electronic letter, 6th December. See *www.chestjournal.org/cgi/eletters/130/5/1369*

Medivent Hayek RTx (Medivent International)

- One of the most common cuirass ventilators available for children is the Medivent RTx (previous generation known as Hayek oscillator).
- It consists of a light-weight flexible cuirass (11 sizes) which fits snugly over the front of the chest and well down on the abdomen. The fit over the abdomen is important to ensure proper diaphragmatic descent when the negative pressure is applied. The operator sets the frequency, end inspiratory and expiratory chamber pressures, and inspiratory/expiratory ratio with the control unit. The control unit adjusts the performance of the power unit by feedback from internal pressure transducer connected to the cuirass with pressure sensor tubing.
- Ventilation is achieved by rapidly decreasing and then increasing the pressure within the cuirass chamber around a negative mean chamber pressure. The applied negative pressure pulls the chest and abdomen out thus transmitting the decreased pressure to the airways and generating inspiration. Expiration, by increasing the cuirass pressure, is also active.
- As with all negative pressure devices, a stable patent upper airway is essential. It is not suitable for patients with bulbar palsy. The RTx is suitable for both hospital and home use but is expensive.

Equipment maintenance and monitoring

- All home equipment needs to be maintained in accordance with the manufacturer's instructions. For most home non-invasive ventilators this means an annual service. Consumables such as masks and tubing generally need 6 monthly replacement. Most children on NIV can breathe spontaneously for some time and therefore need access to replacement machine within 24h in case of breakdown. For those more dependent on respiratory support, a back-up machine at home may be necessary.
- Most children using NIV have a stable condition and therefore, once set up on ventilation at appropriate settings, only need a check study to ensure ventilation is satisfactory every 6–12 months. The most important parameters are assessment of oxygenation and CO_2. For assessment of patient/ventilator interaction, recordings of chest, abdominal, and body movement and ECG in addition are needed. A change in the child's symptoms should generate earlier reassessment.

Further information

Bach, J.R. (ed.) (2002). *Noninvasive mechanical ventilation*. Hanley and Belfus, Philadelphia.
For useful patient advice: International Ventilator Users Network (*http://www.post-polio.org/ivun*)

Tracheostomy

Reasons for a tracheostomy

The underlying goal of tracheostomy is to maintain an open airway. There are many reasons for a tracheostomy including the following.

- Structural airway problems:
  - subglottic stenosis;
  - subglottic haemangioma;
  - tumours, such as cystic hygroma;
  - severe syndromic upper airway obstruction, e.g. Apert's syndrome;
  - severe tracheomalacia;
  - injury to the larynx or mouth.
- Lung problems:
  - chronic lung disease needing prolonged respiratory support;
  - to reduce anatomical dead space (this may be sufficient to allow a child who is otherwise ventilator-dependent to self-ventilate).
- Neurological problems:
  - neuromuscular disease (combination of problems with secretion clearance and hypoventilation);
  - high spinal cord injury;
  - vocal cord paralysis;
  - diaphragmatic dysfunction;
  - bulbar palsy.

Types of tracheostomy tube

- There are several different types of tracheostomy tube. Selection is primarily on basis of size (related to age) of diameter and length. It is important to remember that tracheostomy tubes are sized by internal diameter but external diameter can vary between manufacturers (see Table 62.1).
- Diameter. A relatively large tube keeps airways resistance and work of breathing low and permits clearance of airway secretions. Too large a tube will damage airway mucosa. A small diameter tube permits translaryngeal airflow past the tube and hence speech. Common practice is that tube diameter should not exceed 2/3 tracheal diameter.
- Length. The tracheostomy tube should end 1–2cm above the carina. In general, infants < 1 year should have a neonatal length tube and older children paediatric length. Custom-made tubes are available for children with unusual anatomy (e.g. Bivona tubes).
- Tube connector. All tubes should have the standard 15mm connector to allow connection to bag or ventilator. The few that do not, e.g. the GOS tube, need an adaptor.
- Some tubes (e.g. the Bivona Flextend) have a fixed flange mounted partway along the shaft leaving a longer external component to the tube . This is particularly useful for children with short necks or soft tissue under the chin that could potentially cover the tracheostomy.

- Cuffed tubes (a cuff is a soft balloon around the distal end of the tube) have limited use in children. They are more difficult to change and if left inflated too long can damage the tracheal mucosa. They are used occasionally, particularly in older children, if:
  - the child has chronic aspiration (suction above the cuff can protect the lower airways);
  - ventilation with high positive pressure is needed (the cuff prevents loss of pressure around the tube).
- A tight-to-shaft cuff minimizes airflow obstruction around the tube when the cuff is deflated and is ideal for those needing only intermittent cuff inflation. It also makes tracheostomy tube change easier. Cuffs must be deflated regularly to minimize trauma to the airway wall.
- Fenestrated tubes allow the patient to breath around and through the tube and promote translaryngeal airflow. They are ideal for use with speaking valves. There may be one large fenestration at the tube angle or multiple fenestrations on the shaft. Care must be taken that suction catheters do not go through a large fenestration and cause damage to the airway wall and granulation formation. Some tubes are available with dual cannula—an outer fenestrated tube for use during the day to permit speech and an inner non-fenestrated tube for overnight ventilation. The smallest such dual tube is size 5mm internal diameter.

Table 62.1 Examples of size, diameter, and length of tracheostomy tubes*

Size	ID	OD	Length Neonatal	Length Paediatric
Portex				
3.0	3.0	5.2	32	36
3.5	3.5	5.8	34	40
4.0	4.0	6.5	36	44
Bivona				
3.0	3.0	4.7	32	39
3.5	3.5	5.3	34	40
4.0	4.0	6.0	36	41

* All sizes are in mm. ID, Internal diameter; OD, external diameter.

Tracheostomy care

General care

- Daily care is needed to prevent infection and skin breakdown, especially under the tracheostomy tube and ties. The skin needs to be inspected on a daily basis to ensure that there are no sores or signs of infection. Rubbing of the tracheostomy tube and secretions can irritate the skin around the stoma. Infection around the stoma should be treated with topical antibiotics.
- Tapes should be tight enough to prevent accidental decannulation yet loose enough to allow for the increased neck size during laughing, crying, and feeding. The correct size is when one finger can be slipped beneath the tape at the back of the neck.

Suctioning

- The tracheostomy tube and the trachea must be kept clear of secretions. The child will often clear their secretions with cough but suction may be required when:
  - there is noisy breathing with air bubbling through secretions;
  - there are visible secretions at the tracheostomy tube opening;
  - child is coughing and there are audible secretions in the tube;
  - child has increased respiratory rate and/or is working hard to breathe.
- A child with a tracheostomy should have two suction machines; one electric and one battery for transport. Every suction unit should be set to a standard pressure (usually 140mmHg or 20kPa). If the pressure is set above this it may cause trauma to the trachea and upper airways.
- It is important to use the correct size of suction catheter. Usually the catheter is double the size of the tracheostomy tube, e.g. for a size 4 tube a size 8 suction catheter would be appropriate. To minimize trauma to the trachea the catheter should only be passed as far as the tip of the tracheostomy tube. A template showing the length of the tracheostomy tube can be used to ensure that the catheter is not inserted too far.
- Suctioning should last only a few seconds. Prolonged suctioning may result in hypoxia.
- When secretions are very sticky a small amount (0.5mL) of sterile normal saline can be instilled in the tracheostomy tube directly before suctioning.

Changing a tracheostomy tube

- Safe changing of the tracheostomy tube is most important. Usually the tube is changed once per month unless there are increased secretions or suspicion that the tube is blocking.
- It is important that parents or carers feel confident and competent in tube changing before they leave hospital.
- For more details see ⊞ Chapter 66.

Types of suction pump

- SAM 12: uses mains electricity. The filter should be changed monthly or earlier if it becomes discoloured
- LAERDAL: portable suction unit with transformer. It takes 36h to recharge fully and has a battery life of 4h if used continuously
- VACU-AIDE: lightweight portable suction unit with carrying case, power cord, and battery charger. It takes only 24h to become fully recharged
- AMBU HAND/FOOT PUMP does not require electricity and is used as an emergency back-up if other suction units are broken

Humidification

- Air entering through a tracheostomy bypasses the warming, moistening, and filtering effect of the nasal passages.
- When a tracheostomy is first inserted, good humidity from a heated humidifier is essential to ensure there is no build-up of secretions and to prevent tube blockage.
- Once the tracheostomy is established, a passive humidifier 'Swedish nose' can be used. These devices pick up heat and moisture during exhalation and partly return it during inspiration. They do add resistance and dead space. Different devices are available depending on child's tidal volume.

Speech

- If there is a leak past the tracheostomy tube some soft vocalization may be possible. In older children a fenestrated tube will increase that airflow over the vocal cords.
- A speaking valve placed at the end of the tracheostomy tube allows air flowing through the valve into the tracheostomy tube during inspiration. During exhalation the valve closes, directing exhaled air through the larynx and vocal cords. Speaking valves can be used for children who require mechanical ventilation.
- Benefits of speaking valve:
  - permits natural voice, uninterrupted phonation, louder vowel intensity, and normal speech patterns;
  - reduces secretions and makes them easier to manage requiring less suctioning;
  - facilitates cough and oral expectoration;
  - facilitates swallowing by increasing the pharyngeal pressures needed to move the food bolus down the pharynx and into oesophagus;
  - restores sense of smell and taste, increasing appetite and facilitating nutritional intake.
- Contraindications to using a speaking valve:
  - no leak around tracheostomy tube;
  - tenacious pulmonary secretions;
  - decreased cognitive status.

Tracheostomy complications

Accidental decannulation

- This can occur at any time. It is more likely in a mobile ventilated child because of the weight of the ventilator tubing.
- It is less likely with a well placed, appropriately sized tracheostomy and well fitting tracheostomy ties.

Blockage of the tube

- This is one of the most frequent complications.
- It is more likely in preterm or young infants because of small tube diameter. It is less likely with careful tracheostomy care.
- If the tube is blocked and does not clear with suctioning, it will need to be removed. The same tube can be cleaned using tap water and replaced if necessary.

Bleeding

Small amounts of bleeding (pink or red streaked mucus) can occur as a result of:

- too frequent or vigorous suctioning;
- suction pressure that is too high;
- lack of humidity to the airway;
- infection.

Infection

- Children with tracheostomies are at higher risk for respiratory infections.
- Colonization with *Staphylococcus aureus* or *Pseudomonas aeruginosa* is frequent and requires treatment only when the child is symptomatic. Topical antibiotics may be effective.

Granuloma formation

- These can occur just above the stoma on the anterior tracheal wall and are probably related to frictional trauma from the tube .They are often small, asymptomatic, and require no treatment unless decannualtion is being considered. Topical steroids are usually effective.
- Granulation tissue around the external stoma site is also common and can be treated with topical steroid cream or with topical silver nitrate.
- Granulomata may also occur within the trachea at the site of the tube tip caused by a poor tube position or by suction trauma. They may cause partial obstruction. If they persist after topical steroid treatment they may require surgical treatment.

Essential training and equipment

A box containing essential equipment (see boxes) should accompany the child at all times. Everyone looking after a child with a tracheostomy must:

- know what to do if there is an accidental decannulation, including knowing whether the child has a patent airway above the tracheostomy stoma. If that is the case and the tube cannot easily be replaced, then the bag and mask ventilation will be effective. This avoids the risk of forming false tracts during traumatic and panicky attempts to replace the tracheostomy tube;

- know what to do if there is a tube blockage;
- be able to perform safe suction;
- be able to change a tracheostomy tube;
- have been trained in resuscitation.

Home equipment needs

- Tracheostomy tubes: normal size and one size smaller
- Tracheostomy tube ties
- Dressing supplies
- Gauze or cotton wool
- Sterile water or boiled water
- Container for holding water
- Electric suction machine
- Portable suction machine with charger
- Suction catheters
- Suction connecting tubing
- Sterile normal saline and syringes
- Scissors

Travel kit

- Portable suction unit fully charged
- Tracheostomy tubes: normal size and one size smaller
- Size 12 suction catheter (to be used in the event of tracheostomy stoma closing up)
- Normal saline
- Scissors

Further information

Mini-symposium (2006). Tracheostomy in children. *Paediatr. Respir. Rev.* **7**, 161–85.

Part IV

Practical procedures

Airway management

The paediatric airway

- Respiratory failure may rapidly progress to hypoxic cardiopulmonary arrest in children. Outcome of properly managed respiratory arrest is good. Outcome of cardiorespiratory arrest is poor.
- Resistance to laminar airflow is inversely proportional to the *fourth* power of the airway radius. Airflow resistance and work of breathing therefore increase exponentially with small reductions in airway radius. The paediatric airway in particular is compromised by relatively small amounts of oedema.
- Resistance to turbulent airflow is inversely proportional to the *fifth* power of the airway radius. Turbulent airflow may be minimized by keeping the child calm and quiet.
- Posterior displacement of the tongue may cause severe airway obstruction in children as the tongue is proportionally larger than in adults, and the position of the larynx is more cephalad.

The spontaneously breathing child with respiratory distress

Alert children should be left to take a comfortable position. The semi-conscious or unconscious child who is breathing spontaneously may experience upper airway obstruction as a result of loss of pharyngeal muscle tone and posterior displacement of the tongue. Airway patency should be optimized using the head tilt–chin lift manoeuvre (or the jaw thrust if cervical spine injury is suspected).

Oxygen

Oxygen should be delivered to all children with respiratory difficulty. If spontaneous ventilation is effective, oxygen may be given by oxygen mask, nasal cannulae, or headbox. Humidified oxygen should be given as soon as possible to prevent airway obstruction from dried secretions.

Oxygen may be delivered by:
- simple face mask;
- face mask with reservoir bag;
- a Venturi mask;
- nasal cannulae;
- headbox.

These devices are discussed in 📖 Chapter 56.

Airway adjuncts
Oropharyngeal airway (Guedel airway)
- An oropharyngeal airway is designed to hold the tongue away from the posterior pharyngeal wall and is indicated in the spontaneously breathing unconscious patient where airway patency cannot be maintained with normal positional manoeuvres.
- An oropharyngeal airway should be avoided in a conscious or semi-conscious child as it may cause gagging and vomiting.
- The Guedel airway consists of a flange, a bite block, and an ergonomic curved body designed to hold the tongue anterior to the oropharynx when correctly sited.
- The airway provides an air channel and suction access through the mouth.
- Sizing the oropharyngeal airway is essential as a poor fit will exacerbate obstruction. If the oropharyngeal airway is too large, the epiglottis is pushed down obstructing the glottic opening, and laryngeal structures may be damaged. If the airway is too small, the tongue will be pushed posteriorly into the oropharynx thereby worsening obstruction.
- The correct size can be estimated by measuring oropharyngeal airway against the face. If flange is positioned at the mouth, tip of the airway should just reach angle of jaw. Airway sizes vary from 4cm to 10cm. Guedel airways are size–colour-coded (sizes range from 000 to 4).
- An oropharyngeal airway should be inserted using a tongue depressor. If this is unavailable, in the older child the airway may be inverted for insertion, and rotated back 180° to its proper orientation as it enters the posterior oropharynx.

Nasopharyngeal airway

- A nasopharyngeal airway provides a conduit for airflow between the nares and the posterior oropharynx. Nasopharyngeal airways are available in sizes 12F to 36F but a shortened soft endotracheal tube (ETT) is commonly used. A 3mm ETT corresponds approximately to the calibre of a 12F nasopharyngeal airway and will fit down the nasopharynx of a term infant.
- Nasopharyngeal airways are usually used in the non-acute setting, in the management of infants with upper airway obstruction secondary to micrognathia and other structural abnormalities of the oropharynx.
- Nasopharyngeal airways also have a role in acute resuscitation and may be better tolerated than oropharyngeal airways in semi-conscious children with airway compromise.
- The correct length for a nasopharyngeal airway can be estimated as the distance from the tip of the nose to the tragus of the ear. A term infant is likely to need a 6–6.5cm tube.
- Before inserting the nasopharyngeal airway, drip 1mL of 1% lignocaine down the larger nostril. Lubricate the nasopharyngeal airway with lignocaine gel and advance it in an inferoposterior direction, perpendicular to the face and along the floor of the nasopharynx. Laceration may cause bleeding from the nasal mucosa or adenoidal tissue. The tube is too large if the skin of the nostril remains blanched.
- The ideal position is for the tip of the nasopharyngeal tube to lie just behind the edge of the soft palate (in children with intact palates). A laryngoscope may be used to visualize the tip of the nasopharyngeal airway as it advances beyond the soft palate. It should then be withdrawn until it just disappears from view. In child with cleft palate the tip of the tube is sited at the estimated position where the intact palate would have reached. Irritation of the vocal cords, epiglottis, and vagal nerve from a long tube may cause reflex coughing, vomiting, and laryngospasm.
- If an ETT is used as a nasopharyngeal airway, the 15mm diameter adapter must be firmly re-inserted into the shortened tube to prevent accidental advancement beyond the nostril. For children with chronic nasopharyngeal airway insertion, the shortened ETT may be sutured to wings, which can be neatly fixed to the face with tape.
- When the tube is first placed there are likely to be lots of secretions and regular assessment of patency with suctioning is necessary. Secretions will settle. If an infant feeds with the tube *in situ*, milk will initially reflux up the tube. With time most infants learn to feed with the tube in position with little milk reflux. Withdrawing the tube back slightly (0.5cm) during feeds may be helpful.
- CPAP may be administered via a nasopharyngeal airway in cases of severe upper airway obstruction.

Suction

- A suction force of 80–120mmHg is required to adequately remove secretions from the airway. Wall-mounted vacuum suction units provide airflow of 30L/min corresponding to a maximum suction force of 300mmHg. Portable units do not provide comparable suction power but are easy to transport.
- Flexible plastic suction catheters may be used to suction thin secretions from the upper airway, from oropharyngeal airways, nasopharyngeal airways, and ETTs. Large-bore rigid catheters (e.g. yanker catheter) are more effective for thick secretions, blood, and vomitus in the oropharynx.
- Suctioning should be performed with sterile technique. It may produce vagal-induced bradycardia and should always be performed with adequate monitoring. Patients should be pre-oxygenated and each suction attempt should not exceed 5s. Flexible suction catheters should not be inserted > 1cm beyond the end of an ETT as trauma to the carina or bronchi may cause significant granulation tissue. Suction should only be applied on withdrawing the catheter.

Respiratory failure or arrest

In the case of respiratory failure, basic life support should be commenced:
- open AIRWAY;
- support BREATHING;
- assess CIRCULATION.

Bag-valve mask ventilation

Ventilation face masks need to create an airtight seal if administration of high oxygen concentrations and assisted pressure ventilation are to be effective. Bag-valve systems can also be used with an oropharyngeal or nasopharyngeal airway.

When sizing the mask, the correct size should reach from the bridge of the nose to the cleft of the chin, forming a tight seal around both mouth and nose, but without compression of the eyes. Mask volume should be small, particularly in infants, so that rebreathing of exhaled gases is minimized.

Bag size and tidal volume

- Tidal volume should be 10–15mL/kg and should dictate which size of bag to use. Neonatal-size bags (250mL) are generally inadequate for a term infant.
- Lung compliance may be assessed during bag mask ventilation. This is most easily done when the size of the bag is appropriate for the child. Sudden decrease in lung compliance should alert the user to the possibility of airway displacement, airway obstruction, or pneumothorax.

Airway positioning

- The mask is held on the face with 1 hand, which also positions the airway correctly with a head-tilt–chin-lift manoeuvre (2nd hand compresses the ventilation bag). In infants, the mandible is supported with the base of the middle finger without pressure. In older children, fingers 3–5 are placed on the ramus of the mandible and used to lift the jaw forward.
- Ventilation is usually most effective for infants and toddlers with the head in a neutral position without hyperextension of the neck, but it may be necessary to gently move the head and neck to determine the position of maximum airway patency and optimum mask ventilation. Hyperextension of the neck may cause airway obstruction in infants and should be avoided. In children > 2 years, airway patency may be improved by placing a small support (e.g. a folded towel) under the head and neck.
- If ventilation is ineffective, reassess the face mask seal, the airway position, and the need for suction and check equipment.

Nasogastric tube

- An NG tube should be passed as gastric dilatation is common with mask ventilation, may precipitate vomiting and aspiration, and will prevent optimal ventilation.
- Gastric inflation and regurgitation in an unconscious child may be minimized by applying pressure to the cricoid cartilage with the thumb and index finger (the Sellick procedure) to occlude the oesophagus.

Self-inflating bag-valve mask ventilation

Ventilation may be supported with or without an oxygen supply, as the elastic recoil of the bag results in spontaneous reinflation between administered breaths irrespective of whether or not there is a pressurized oxygen supply in the circuit.

The bag has three valves: the gas intake valve; the mask valve; and an exhalation valve near the mask. During bag compression, the mask valve opens allowing flow from bag to mask, and the gas intake valve closes. During patient exhalation, through the exhalation valve, the valve mask closes preventing accumulation of exhaled gases in the bag, and the gas intake valve opens allowing entrained room air (and/or oxygen if connected) to refill the bag.

Oxygen supply and reservoir

Oxygen connected to a bag-valve mask ventilation system at 10L/min can provide 30–80% oxygen. In older children with larger tidal volumes, oxygen flow may be rate-limiting and room air as well as oxygen may be entrained into the bag during re-inflation. Bag valve mask devices fitted with a reservoir and run with high flow oxygen at 10–15L/min can provide higher oxygen concentrations.

Ventilation pressures

Most self-inflating bags may have a pressure-limited pop-off valve. In situations of poor lung compliance or high airway resistance, high pressures may be necessary for adequate ventilation. A pop-off valve in this situation may limit the tidal volume delivered. The pop-off valve may be twisted closed or the pressure limit altered to an upper limit of $035–40cmH_2O$.

Positive end expiratory pressure (PEEP)

PEEP may be provided by a bag-valve mask system if a spring-loaded or magnetic ball or disk PEEP valve is sited at bag-valve outlet. PEEP valves only open with compression of the bag and cannot be used in the self-ventilating patient to administer CPAP.

Self-ventilating patients

Bag-valve-mask systems should not be used to deliver oxygen to self-ventilating children. Valves within the system may result in inadequate oxygen flow if the bag is not compressed with each inspiration.

Anaesthesia ventilation systems

- An anaesthesia bag (Ayre's bag, A-bag, Jackson Rees circuit) consists of a standard face mask and 15–22mm connector to which a T-piece is connected. The T-piece has a gas inflow port and an overflow port leading to a latex reservoir bag with an open tail. High flow oxygen enters the circuit through the inflow port and, if the face mask seal is good, it leaves via the overflow port and out of the reservoir bag tail. The reservoir bag is held with the tail sitting between the 4th and 5th finger. Partial occlusion of the tail increases resistance to gas flow and the reservoir bag will inflate. This generates a pressure within the circuit. Compression of the reservoir bag with ongoing resistance at the tail will increase circuit pressure and generate an inspiratory breath. Maintaining some resistance at the reservoir tail will generate PEEP during expiration. Full occlusion of the tail can generate dangerously high pressures.

- This is a closed system so oxygen concentrations are predictable but, as it is a rebreathing system, flow rates need to be high to wash out exhaled gases. A high flow rate at the wall is needed to ensure that these gases are washed out even while circuit flow is restricted to generate PEEP during expiration.
- Run oxygen at 2L/min in infants and 4–6L/min in children.
- Bag sizes: 500mL for infants; 1000–2000mL for children.
- CPAP can be administered to the spontaneously ventilating patient using the T piece because there are no high resistance flow valves to overcome on inspiration.

Endotracheal airway

- Endotracheal intubation is the most effective approach to assisted ventilation, as the circuit to the airway is secure, ensuring complete control of ventilation and oxygenation. The tube also protects the airway from potential aspiration of gastric contents.
- Elective intubation of self-ventilating children is generally after gas induction of anaesthesia using volatile anaesthetic agents such as halothane or sevofluorane.
- Rapid sequence induction of anaesthesia is used in the acute setting when children will be at risk of aspiration.

Preparation

- Call anaesthetist early.
- Check laryngoscope (straight blade age < 2 years; curved blade in older children).
- Check suction is working.
- ETT sizing: (age in years/4) + 4 (uncuffed, age < 8 years; cuffed in older children).
- Endotracheal length estimate: (age in years/2) + 12.
- Monitor heart rate, saturations, and BP. IV access is mandatory.
- Pre-oxygenate in 100% oxygen using self-inflating bag-valve-mask with reservoir and high flow oxygen (or A-bag circuit).
- Pass an NG tube and empty stomach contents.
- Apply cricoid pressure before giving sedative drugs. If there is concern about cervical cord injury place 1 hand behind the neck to provide additional support when applying cricoid pressure.
- Give:
  - atropine (prevents vagal-induced bradycardia during laryngoscopy);
  - sedative/hypnotic such as a combination of benzodiazepine and opiate or propofol or thiopentone (Watch for hypotension!);
  - a rapid-onset short-acting muscle relaxant such as suxamethonium.

Intubation technique

- The child should be lying flat. In suspected cervical spine injury, the child is maintained in the neutral position with manual cervical stabilization. Otherwise, in children aged < 2 years, chin is lifted to sniffing position. In children aged > 2 years, chin is lifted to sniffing position and cervical spine displaced anteriorly with small pillow placed under head.
- Using laryngoscope in left hand, and standing at patient's head, the laryngoscope is placed to the right of the tongue and advanced.
- Suction may be necessary (yanker).
- With a curved laryngoscope, the blade is inserted into the vallecula (which lies between the root of the epiglottis and the base of the tongue). Upward pressure in the direction of the laryngoscope handle elevates the jaw and the glottic opening becomes visible. A straight laryngoscope is used in younger children because the epiglottis in this age group is relatively larger. The tip of the straight blade may be placed distal to the epiglottis, which is then displaced with the same upward pressure manoeuvre. Cricoid pressure may help visualize the glottic opening. Care should be taken not to damage teeth and gums.
- Insert the ETT gently through the vocal cords under direct vision. With cuffed tubes, the cuff should be placed just below the vocal cords.
- Remove the laryngoscope. inflate the cuff on cuffed tubes, and check position of ETT looking for symmetrical chest movements and listening for equal breath sounds on auscultation. Monitor end-tidal CO_2 if possible. A simple colour change CO_2 detector can be used to confirm ETT is in airway.
- If doubt exists regarding the tube position, deflate the cuff, remove the tube and re-oxygenate before trying again.
- Secure the tube. Document position at the lips. Continue ventilation with a self-inflating bag with oxygen and reservoir.
- Confirm ETT position on CXR.

Cricothyroidotomy

Percutaneous needle cricothyroidotomy may be needed in children with complete acute upper airway obstruction, although it has rarely been perfomed successfully in this age group. This temporary surgical airway is sufficient for oxygenation but usually inadequate for ventilation so ENT surgeons will need to perform a formal surgical cricothyroidotomy. Causes of acute complete airway obstruction include foreign body, severe laryngeal infection, severe orofacial injuries, or laryngeal fracture. Call for anaesthetic and ENT help immediately.

Needle cricothyroidotomy

- Place a roll of towels under the child's shoulders to maximally displace the larynx anteriorly (check there is no possibility of cervical injury before extending the neck).
- Locate the cricothyroid membrane (extending from the thyroid cartilage caudally to the cricoid cartilage). Palpate with a fingernail of left index finger (cartilage is only 1mm wide in infants).

- Stabilize the trachea with the left-hand middle finger and thumb while locating the cricothyroid membrane with the index finger.
- Clean with aseptic swab.
- Define the path by first introducing a small bore needle attached to a syringe (20–22 gauge) in the midline directed 45° caudally (towards the feet). If air is aspirated, repeat the procedure with a cricothyroidotomy cannula-over needle if available or a large IV cannula (14 or 16 gauge).
- Once the membrane is punctured (air is aspirated), remove the needle, advance the cannula caudally, and check air can still be aspirated.
- Connect high-flow oxygen to the cannula using a Y connector. Set the flow rate to the child's age in years. Occlude the outflow limb of the Y connector for 1s and assess for chest movement. If there is no chest rise, turn up the oxygen by 1L/min until it is observed. Inflate for 1s and allow passive deflation for 4s. If a Y connector is not available, a hole can be made in the oxygen tubing and intermittently occluded.
- Note the following.
  - Expiration must occur via the upper airway. It cannot occur through the cannula since the resistance is too high. If the upper airway is completely occluded, the oxygen flow should be reduced to 1–2L/min, which will provide some oxygenation but little ventilation.
  - Bag and mask devices will be ineffective at driving gas through the cannula. They cannot generate sufficient pressure.

Surgical cricothyroidotomy
- Risk of injury to vital structures is significant and this procedure should only be carried out by those with appropriate surgical training, usually an ENT surgeon.
- The skin is cleaned and infiltrated with local anaesthetic.
- A small vertical midline skin incision is made.
- A transverse cricothyroid membrane incision is made.
- The tract is dilated and an appropriately sized endotracheal or tracheostomy tube is inserted.

Further information
Advanced Life Support Group (2005). *Advanced paediatric life support: the practical approach*, 4th edn. Blackwell BMJ Books, Oxford. See also www.alsg.org.

Bronchoscopy

Types of bronchoscope

The airways can be examined using either a flexible bronchoscope, which is a fibreoptic instrument, or by using a rigid bronchoscope, which is a hollow metal tube down which instruments and optics can be passed. Figure 64.1 shows the major bronchi and bronchopulmonary segments.

Flexible bronchoscopy

Flexible bronchoscopy permits dynamic examination of the nose, pharynx, larynx, and tracheobronchial tree to the second or third airway generation and sampling of secretions and mucosal tissue from the lower airways. The child has to breathe past the bronchoscope during the procedure. Flexible bronchoscopy can be performed under sedation or general anaesthesia and is most commonly performed by a paediatric respiratory physician.

Rigid bronchoscopy

Rigid laryngoscopy and bronchoscopy permit visualization and operative manipulation of larynx and major airways. It is performed under general anaesthesia, usually with laryngeal suspension. The child is ventilated through the bronchoscope during the procedure. Rigid bronchoscopy is most commonly performed by ENT surgeons.

Indications for bronchoscopy

Flexible bronchoscopy

Indications are mainly diagnostic and occasionally therapeutic and include the following.
- Stridor (especially biphasic).
- Isolated/unusual/unresponsive wheeze.
- Chronic cough.
- Recurrent/persistent radiological changes:
  - consolidation;
  - atelectasis;
  - hyperinflation.
- Suspicion of foreign body aspiration (foreign body removal should be by rigid bronchoscopy, which allows safer control of the airway during the procedure).
- Investigation of haemoptysis.
- Suspected alveolar disorder:
  - pulmonary haemorrhage;
  - alveolar proteinosis.
- Evaluation tracheostomy.
- Procedures including:
  - broncho-alveolar lavage;
  - bronchial brushings;
  - bronchial/transbronchial biopsy;
  - local administration of drugs.

Rigid laryngoscopy/bronchoscopy

- Laryngeal inspection. Some defects, particularly type 1 laryngeal clefts, are difficult to detect using the flexible instrument.
- Laryngeal operative procedures, such as aryepiglottoplasty and cyst removal.
- Foreign body removal.
- Laser treatment or injection of granulomata, haemangiomata, and papillomata.

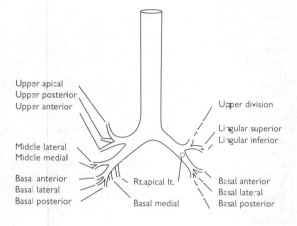

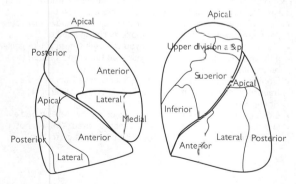

Fig. 64.1 The major bronchi and bronchopulmonary segments.

Flexible bronchoscopy: procedure

- Flexible bronchoscopy can be performed on any age or size of child from a preterm infant to an adolescent.
- It can be performed in a variety of locations, such as ICU or neonatal units, as well as in dedicated procedure rooms or operating theatres and under conscious sedation or general anaesthesia.
- The clinical status of the child and the indication for the procedure will influence the choice of sedation or anaesthetic.
- In general, the more compromised child will be examined under general anaesthesia.
- Bronchoscopes come in varying sizes (Table 64.1). In the smallest preterm infant even the smallest scope will block the airway and apnoea must be assumed. Several passes of the scope with interval ventilation may be necessary to obtain the information required. In larger infants and children on ICUs the scope may be passed through an ETT if necessary.
- Most information is obtained by examining dynamic movements of the airway during spontaneous breathing, when both the upper airway and lower airways can be examined, e.g. vocal cord movements can be observed as can dynamic closure of malacic airways on expiration.
- If sedation is used the scope is passed through the nose. During general anaesthesia, the anaesthetic may be given by facemask or through a nasopharyngeal airway so that the larynx as well as the lower airways can be examined. If the lower airways alone are to be examined then a laryngeal mask gives good lower airway access.
- It is more difficult to manipulate the scope if it has been passed through a long ETT before reaching the airways.
- Sedation is generally with a combination of midazolam and pethidine (both reversible agents).
- General anaesthesia, if used, is often with propofol or sevofluorane.
- Local anaesthesia, particularly to the vocal cords, is very important regardless of the other agents used.
- Technically bronchoscopy is not a difficult skill to learn. Knowing what you are looking at is much more difficult. Here are a few tips.
  - You only know where you are in the airway if you know how you got there; one bronchial division looks much like another.
  - Don't advance down the airway if you can't see where you're going.
  - If the image is upside down, straighten out the bronchoscope to re-orientate yourself.
  - Don't be tempted to squeeze through a narrowed airway—the trauma to the mucosa may result in oedema and catastrophic airway narrowing.
  - Don't be tempted to carry out biopsies or remove foreign bodies in a child who is sedated rather than anaesthetized. You will not have sufficient control of the airway if things don't go to plan.

Table 64.1 Common paediatric flexible bronchoscope sizes

Maximum external diameter	Suction/working channel diameter	ETT size scope can pass through
2.2mm	—	3mm
2.8mm	1.2mm	3.5mm
3.6mm	1.2mm	4.0mm
4.9mm	2.2mm	5.5mm

Patient management for flexible bronchoscopy

- Fast for 4h
- Establish IV access
- If the child has a history of asthma or bronchospasm pre-treat with a bronchodilator
- Administer sedation or general anaesthesia
- Monitor ECG and oxygen saturation throughout procedure. Monitor CO_2 by capnography if using general anaesthesia
- The child should be observed and monitored by an experienced nurse and/or anaesthetist throughout
- Topical anaesthesia: 1–2% lignocaine should be used in the nose and larynx, especially on the vocal cords and in the lower airway
- Oxygen should be given throughout the procedure
- Observation should continue throughout recovery period
- The child should not be allowed to eat or drink until at least 1h after the procedure as local anaesthesia (and sedative agents) will blunt upper airway protective reflexes

Bronchoalveolar lavage (BAL)

- BAL is usually performed to examine the cellular content and to culture secretions from the lower airways and alveoli. Less commonly it may be performed as a therapeutic manoeuvre in an attempt to encourage a collapsed lobe to re-inflate or, very rarely, in the management of a child with alveolar proteinosis.
- The bronchosope is passed to the lung segment of interest and advanced until it becomes wedged in the airway. The suction channel of the bronchoscope is separate from the optical channels and often the best position for efficient lavage technique will mean that the operator does not have a view of the airway during the lavage procedure.
- Lavage is carried out with pre-warmed non-bacteriostatic normal saline. Up to 3 aliquots of 1mL/kg can be used (maximum 60mL). Each aliquot is given as a rapid bolus followed by suctioning. The fluid is aspirated into a suction trap over 10–20s using negative pressures of 100–150mmHg. The wedge must be maintained throughout. The returns for the first aliquot will be the lowest, around 20–30% of the volume instilled. For the 2nd and 3rd aliquots the return should be around 50%.
- If the main purpose is to identify airway pathogens, e.g. in a child with CF, 1–2 aliquots will be sufficient. If the main purpose is to examine the cellular content and microbiology of the alveolar space, 1st aliquot should be discarded and only 2nd and 3rd used for analysis.
- Once the lavage fluid has been obtained, a proportion needs to be sent for bacterial, fungal, viral, and mycobacterial culture and PCR as appropriate. A separate portion needs to be prepared for microscopy, using a cytospin, to examine the cellular content and also to allow special stains for fungal hyphae and for pneumocystis. Special stains can also be used to assess fat-laden or haemosiderin-laden macrophages.
- Anaerobic cultures are not usually done on BAL specimens because the swirling and sucking involved in collecting the specimen expose the specimen to lots of air.
- Quantitative bacterial cultures of BAL fluid are most informative. Bacterial colony counts of 10^5/mL or more are generally considered to represent true LRTI and to correlate, e.g. with infiltration of the airway by neutrophils. Lower counts may be significant for unusual organisms.
- Normal values for the cellular content of BAL fluid have been published. Although total cell counts should be assessed the issue of correcting for dilution is still problematic and percentage cell counts are sufficient for most clinical purposes. In normal children, the percentage cell counts are:
  - macrophages, 90% (84–94%)
  - lymphocytes, 8% (4.7–12.8%)
  - neutrophils, 2% (0.6–3.5%)
  - eosinophils, 0.1% (0.0–0.3%)
  - ratio of CD4:CD8 T-cells, 0.6 (0.4–1).

Complications of flexible bronchoscopy

- Common:
  - epistaxis;
  - minor oxygen desaturation;
  - transient laryngospasm;
  - post-procedure cough;
  - post-procedure wheeze;
  - if BAL undertaken, minor fever within 24h.
- Uncommon:
  - haemoptysis;
  - significant desaturation;
  - significant laryngospasm/stridor;
  - prolonged sedation;
  - respiratory depression.

Care of the flexible bronchoscope

- The bronchoscope contains glass fibres and must be handled gently. It must not be kinked or forcibly twisted as the glass fibres will break.
- It is important that bronchoscopes are cleaned and disinfected between patients to prevent any cross-infection.
- The suction channel should be rinsed immediately post-procedure and then brushed through with a (disposable) cleaning brush. Suction valves should be disassembled, brushed, and cleaned (some are disposable). The outside of the instrument should be wiped clean. Most commonly automated cleaning machines are used for disinfection, rinsing, and drying after use.
- Bronchoscopes should be stored hanging to prevent kinking of the fibres. After storage they should be cleaned and disinfected again before use.

Further information

Midulla, F., deBlic, J., Barbato, A., Bush, A., Eber, E., Kotecha, S., Haxby, E. Moretti, C., Pohunek, P., and Ratjen, F. (2003). Flexible endoscopy of paediatric air-ways. *Eur. Respir. J.* **22**, 698–708.

Riedler, J., Grigg, J., Stone, C., Taurc, G., and Robertson, C.F. (1995). Bronchoalveolar lavage cellularity in healthy children. *Am. J. Respir. Crit. Care Med.* **152**, 163–8.

Chest drains

Indications

- Tension pneumothorax (after immediate needle decompression).
- Symptomatic primary pneumothorax with failed resolution after aspiration.
- Symptomatic secondary pneumothorax.
- Complicated parapneumonic effusion and empyema.
- Malignant pleural effusion (for symptomatic relief or pleurodesis).
- Haemothorax.
- Chylothorax.

Types of chest drain

Most clinical problems in children requiring a chest drain can be managed with a relatively small pigtail catheter generally between 8F and 14F in size, inserted using a Seldinger technique. These are easier and safer to insert than large bore trocar drains, less painful, better tolerated, and consequently allow the child to be mobile and active during treatment.

Position of chest drain

Complicated parapneumonic effusion or empyema

- Optimal position for drain insertion should be evaluated with ultrasound. If the drain is not inserted at the time of the ultrasound, with direct ultrasound guidance, the clinician who plans to insert the drain should be present at ultrasound evaluation of the effusion. It is important that the ultrasound exam is performed with child in the same position as they will be in for the drain insertion procedure. The position of the child, the thickness of the chest wall, the depth of the pleural effusion, and the presence of fibrinous septi should be noted. The site where the effusion is deepest is marked with a cross for later guidance.
- The recommended site for drain insertion is the mid-axillary line, specifically anterior to the lateral aspect of latissmus dorsi. In some cases where the effusion is posterior, it may be necessary to insert the chest drain in the posterior chest wall. Pigtail catheters are surprisingly well tolerated in this position even when lying down. Care must be taken to avoid positions close to the inferior border of the scapula, and placement towards the midline posteriorly should be avoided as the intercostal space narrows significantly and intercostal vessels assume a more central position between ribs.

Pneumothorax

Most cases of spontaneous pneumothorax will be due to rupture of an apical bleb. Full re-expansion of the lung is most likely if a chest drain is sited towards the apex of the lung. This can be achieved by inserting the drain in the anterior chest wall, in the second intercostal space in the mid-clavicular line.

Insertion of a Seldinger pigtail catheter

- The patient should be kept nil by mouth for 5h prior to the procedure.
- Sedation: pethidine 1mg/kg IV; midazolam 0.2mg/kg IV. In some centres the procedure is carried out using general anaesthesia.
- Give oxygen and monitor with pulse oximetry.
- Using sterile technique, instil 2mL of 2% lignocaine advancing the needle to infiltrate muscle and parietal pleura, and to define the path for the drain insertion. A green needle (21G) should be long enough to reach the pleural space in most children. Drain insertion should not proceed if fluid (in empyema) or air (in pneumothorax) cannot be aspirated from the pleural space at this stage.
- Make a small incision with a scapula blade at the site of insertion. Insert a large bore grey cannula (16G) with syringe attached, following the track previously defined. In cases of empyema, ultrasound estimations of chest wall thickness and pleural fluid depth are a useful guide to determining how far to advance the cannula and at what depth to expect successful aspiration of fluid. It may not always be possible to aspirate much fluid, particularly in heavily loculated small effusions.
- Remove the needle from the cannula and gently insert the guide wire through the cannula until at least 2–3cm is estimated to have passed into the chest. In practice the wire can be passed until resistance is felt. If the wire does not thread easily, the cannula may have kinked on a rib and another cannula may need to be sited.
- After successful wire insertion, remove the cannula from the guide wire. Employ an assistant so that the guide wire is always held.
- Slide sequential dilatators over the guide wire to enlarge the track through the chest wall.
- Slide the drain over the guide wire (with trocar removed but hollow stiffener still *in-situ*). Advance drain over the guide wire and through the chest wall. Once the tip of the drain is in the pleural space, remove the guide wire so that it doesn't curl up in the pigtail tip as the stiffener is removed. Introduce the drain and simultaneously withdraw the stiffener in small increments until all the side-ports of the drain are within the pleural space. Some pigtail catheters have a nylon thread running inside the lumen that can be used to pull the pigtail tighter. This thread should be removed before inserting the drain as it can become stuck within the organizing pleural fluid and complicate drain removal.
- Once drain is in position, attach a 3-way tap and aspirate from the drain. Attach the drain to an underwater seal bottle via the 3-way tap and tubing, and observe for swinging with respiration.
- The drain may be fixed without sutures using an adhesive dressing (e.g. niko drain fix, Niko Surgical Ltd). Attach a flag (a small piece of tape) to the drain so that accidental outward movement of the drain can be easily detected.

- For pleural effusions, the underwater seal bottle may be attached to wall suction (set at 20cmH$_2$O) to encourage drainage. Where there is significant mediastinal displacement, drainage should be gradual to prevent rapid shifts in mediastinal position. If > 20mL/kg fluid is drained in the 1st hour, discontinue suction and consider clamping the drain for a short period.
- In cases of pneumothorax with significant lung collapse, re-expansion pulmonary oedema (RPO) may occur if re-inflation of the lung is very rapid. Applying negative pressure to the drain may increase this risk. Suction for the first 24h should therefore be avoided, but may be applied thereafter if complete re-inflation of the lung has not been achieved. RPO is rare with drainage of pleural fluid.

General points
- Children with chest drains should be managed by specialist nursing staff.
- Good analgesia is essential to encourage mobilization. This is especially important in empyema where movement helps to break down fibrinous septations. Paracetamol with diclofenac is an effective oral treatment for pleuritic pain. Intrapleural marcaine 0.25% (0.5–1.0mL/kg) may be instilled into the drain at the same time as urokinase in the treatment of empyema. Pain may increase immediately after drainage of empyema, as pleural friction increases.
- Chest drains may kink or become occluded. If the drain is not swinging, check for drain displacement or kinking, and flush the drain with 5mL normal saline.
- A bubbling drain should never be clamped as there is a risk of tension pneumothorax.
- Consider tension pneumothorax in any patient with a drain *in situ* who has an acute respiratory deterioration. Consider insertion of a second drain even if the first drain is bubbling as small gauge drains may be insufficient for large air leaks.

Complications of the procedure
- Excessive sedation with decreased respiratory effort.
- Pain.
- Broncho-pleural fistula.
- Haemorrhage from intercostal vessels after traumatic insertion.
- Organ damage (e.g. liver, spleen).
- Re-expansion pulmonary oedema in cases of large pneumothorax.

Changing a tracheostomy tube

Important considerations

- Anyone caring for children with tracheostomies should be able to change the tube. This includes parents and carers who look after children at home and nurses and doctors who care for children in hospital. The following are indications for changing a tracheostomy tube.
  - Routine tube change. The frequency of tube change depends on the type of tube used, the amount and nature of airway secretions, and local practice. In general, tracheostomy tubes are routinely changed every 2–4 weeks.
  - Urgent tube change because of new or worsening respiratory distress, which may be caused by an obstructed tube or because of tube displacement.
- Everyone caring for a child with a tracheostomy must know whether or not the child has a patent upper airway. Some children will have tracheostomies placed as an interface with a ventilator and will have normal upper airways. Others will have a tracheostomy because their upper airway is compromised. If a tracheostomy tube has become blocked and cannot be replaced easily, a child with a patent upper airway can be supported, if necessary, with bag-valve mask ventilation, or by ventilation via an oral ETT. This approach is likely to be simpler and safer than prolonged attempts to resite the tracheostomy tube. In a child without a patent upper airway, urgent assistance of someone expert in tracheostomy care should be sought if difficulty is encountered.
- A tracheostomy stoma in a child is usually formed by simply cutting the skin and the trachea. If the tube is removed the stoma will contract and heal spontaneously. In some children, if the tube is out of the stoma for more than a few minutes, it will be difficult to replace the tube. Having said that, children can breathe quite easily through the stoma whilst the tube is changed, and the procedure should be carried out in a calm and unhurried manner.
- Bigger children (> 5 years) may have an outer and inner tracheostomy tube. The inner tube can be removed and cleaned without disturbing the child. The outer tube, which is often fenestrated to permit speech, will need to be changed less frequently than a single lumen tube, and sometimes only once every 1–2 months.

The procedure

Changing a tracheostomy tube is usually a straightforward and simple procedure. Occasionally difficulties are encountered but these can be minimized with good preparation.

- For most children, two people should be available to change a tracheostomy tube. In older cooperative children with a well-established tract, the procedure can be carried out by one carer. Explain the procedure to the child if appropriate.
- Suction the tracheostomy tube, taking care not to pass the catheter beyond the end of the tracheostomy tube.
- Lie the child down and extend the neck with a neck roll under the shoulders to maximize access to the tracheostomy site. Older children can sit up during the procedure if they prefer.

- An assistant holds the current tube *in situ*. Remove the ties and clean the site. If the ties are dirty, new ties can be placed around the neck in readiness for the new tube. When ready, gently remove the tube following the curve of the tube.
- Before the clean tube is inserted, the stoma and trachea can be suctioned to remove thick secretions that will otherwise be pushed down the trachea by the new tube. This is not usually necessary during routine tube changes.
- Hold the new tube by the flanges with the introducer in place (if this is to be used) and gently advance it into the stoma again following the curve of the tube so as not to damage the trachea. Remove introducer if this has been used.
- Hold the new tube securely by the flanges. The procedure can cause child to cough, which will displace an unsecured tube. Allow coughing to settle. Check for air movement through the tracheostomy tube.
- Clean the skin around the tube. The ties should be fastened so that only a little finger can be placed between the ties and the neck. Loose ties may lead to accidental extubation. Tight ties may be uncomfortable and cause sores.

Equipment required

- New or clean tracheostomy tube. Check the size is correct and that the tube is intact and in good order. If an introducer is to be used, make sure this fits snugly and can be removed easily
- A smaller sized tracheostomy tube to be used if the normal tube cannot be re-sited
- A size 12 suction catheter with suction machine or wall suction
- Tracheostomy tape
- Round-ended scissors
- Water based lubricant
- Introducer, if this has been recommended

Tips if there are problems

Where difficulty arises, several approaches to recannulation may be attempted.

- Lubrication of the tracheostomy site and tracheostomy tube will help tube insertion.
- A smaller tracheostomy tube may be inserted (later replaced with the appropriate size).
- A well lubricated size 12 suction catheter may be inserted into stoma. It should pass without resistance into the trachea. The catheter can then be used as a guide to assist placement of the tracheostomy tube. In the hospital setting, a bronchoscope may also be used as a guide.
- If a tracheostomy tube is not available, an ET may be inserted into the stoma in an emergency.

Ciliary brush biopsy

Purpose

The main indication for a ciliary brush biopsy is evaluation of ciliary activity and ultrastructure as a means of diagnosing primary ciliary dyskinesia (PCD). More rarely, brush biopsy samples of the lower airway may be used for microbiological culture where some clinicians feel they provide additional sensitivity for detection of endobronchial infection. Finally, airway epithelial cells collected by brush biopsy may be used for research.

Nasal brushing technique

- The aim of the procedure is to remove small strips of ciliated epithelium from the inferior turbinate of the nose.
- It is a good idea to visualize the turbinates before brushing, using an auroscope, to make sure they are as free from mucus as possible. If there is a lot of mucus and if the child can cooperate, they should be asked to blow their nose. In infants it may be possible to carry out simple nasal suctioning.
- A small cytology brush is then advanced into the nostril and ideally passed under the inferior turbinate. In practice it is difficult to hold the auroscope and brush and, with experience, it is possible to get a good sample without direct visualization. The sample is collected using a backwards and forwards and rotational brushing action.
- The key is to make sure the child is firmly held and continue the brushing action for a count of 5s.
- It is important to try and avoid the septum as contact here will cause bleeding.
- Once the sample is collected the brush should be placed into pre-warmed tissue culture medium. Any basal medium will do (e.g. RPMI and DMEM) and will be available from most hospital laboratories (cytology or virology labs are most likely have this type of medium).
- The samples are stable for several hours. Analysis should be carried out the same day. If necessary they can be sent by courier at room temperature to a centre with expertise in ciliary analysis. In England 3 centres are funded to provide a national service. These are:
  - Leicester: Glenfield Hospital, University Hospitals of Leicester NHS Trust;
  - Southampton: Southampton General Hospital, Southampton University Hospitals NHS Trust;
  - London: Royal Brompton Hospital, Royal Brompton and Harefield NHS Trust.

Notes

- Respiratory viral infections cause secondary dyskinesia and will affect ciliary beat frequency and ultrastucture. *It is essential that the child has been free of an acute respiratory tract infection for 6 weeks prior to the nasal biopsy.* This can be difficult in young children, particularly those with PCD who will have a persistently runny nose. In these children the biopsy should be carried out when nasal discharge is at the 'basal level'.

- Although high doses of lignocaine can inhibit ciliary activity *in vitro*, doses used for topical local anaesthesia do not appear to affect subsequently measured ciliary beat frequency. In practice, the brush biopsy is usually well tolerated and lignocaine is not usually required.

Tracheal brushing technique

- Tracheal samples are less affected by secondary dyskinesia associated with URTI. Taking samples from the trachea tends to produce better quality material in children with persistent nasal discharge. Thus, if a child with suspected PCD is undergoing bronchoscopy, that opportunity should be used to collect a brush biopsy sample.
- It is inevitable that lignocaine will be used during bronchoscopy and, as noted above, at doses used for topical local anaesthesia it does not appear to affect ciliary activity.
- Most children requiring brush biopsy for investigation of possible PCD will be of a size that will require the use of a small bronchoscope (e.g. the 3.6mm paediatric Olympus bronchoscope, which has a 1.2mm instrument channel). The instrument channels on these bronchoscopes are too small for the sheathed cytology brush used in larger instruments. Instead the unsheathed cytology brush is passed directly through the instrument channel of the bronchoscope until it is seen protruding into the airway lumen. The bronchoscope is then positioned so that the brush is pressed against the tracheal wall. The brush is then pushed backwards and forwards 3–4 times.
- The brush should *not* be withdrawn through the bronchoscope. This will result in most of the sample being lost inside the instrument channel. Instead, the bronchoscope with the brush *in situ* (i.e. still protruding out the distal end of the scope) should be removed from the airway. The brush should then be placed into tissue culture medium as above and the epithelium removed from the brush by agitation, using a pipette. It is worth taking a few minutes to do this thoroughly.

Lower airway samples

Induced sputum

- This method is used for collecting lower airway secretions, both for identification of infection and for assessing cellular content. It is generally used when children are unable to spontaneously expectorate sputum. Although it is more commonly used in adults and older compliant children, it can be used in infants.
- Ideally the child will brush their teeth and rinse out their mouth prior to the procedure to minimize upper respiratory tract contamination.
- Salbutamol (5 puffs via spacer) is given to minimize bronchoconstriction.
- Hypertonic (3–5%) saline is given, either with a jet or an ultrasonic nebulizer, using a face mask or mouthpiece to induce coughing. Typically the nebulization is continued for 15–20min. Cooperative children can be encouraged to cough and to expectorate sputum into a specimen pot. For infants a session of physiotherapy is carried out using chest percussion, and sputum is then collected from the nasopharynx by suctioning.
- Expectorate can be analysed for cell counts, soluble mediators, and for pathogens by PCR and culture.

Non-bronchoscopic lavage

- Non-bronchoscopic BAL is generally used in intubated patients to collect lower respiratory secretions for culture or cytology. It is usually performed in acutely unwell patients on paediatric ICU, but may be performed under short elective anaesthesia.
- Sterile technique should be used.
- If the child is lightly sedated or anaesthetized, 1mL of 1% lignocaine is instilled into the trachea via the ETT to minimize coughing.
- Pre-oxygenation with high inspired oxygen concentrations for a few minutes will reduce any desaturation in children with unstable lung disease.
- An 8F end-hole suction catheter is passed through the ETT until a wedge in a small airway is established. This is likely to be in the right lower lobe. It is important to use appropriate end-hole catheters. Side-hole catheters will not work, and cutting these catheters to produce a single end hole will leave sharp edges that will damage the airway.
- 1mL/kg of normal saline is instilled into the suction catheter followed by 5mL of air to clear the tube of fluid. The fluid can then either be aspirated using wall suction into a suction trap (usually via a 3-way tap), over 10–20s using negative pressures of 100–150mmHg, or aspirated back into the syringe. The procedure is repeated to collect 3 sequential samples that are analysed separately. For more details on BAL fluid analysis see 📖 Chapter 64.

Early morning gastric aspirates

- Infants and young children do not expectorate respiratory secretions and tend to swallow them instead. Aspiration or lavage of the gastric contents is the best approach to obtaining respiratory secretions for culture. Early morning gastric aspirates or lavage taken before gastric emptying are favoured as the sample taken will represent accumulation of secretions from overnight.
- The procedure is performed principally for *Mycobacterium tuberculosis* culture. Children with primary tuberculous chest disease produce few organisms and sampling accumulated secretions increases the likelihood of obtaining organisms for culture. Use of induced sputum is an alternative.
- The child should be kept nil by mouth on waking up in the morning. Overnight feeds in infants should be omitted. Before the child gets out of bed and ideally shortly after waking, an NG tube is passed and gastric contents aspirated. If less than 5mL can be aspirated, 10–20mL of sterile water is instilled and re-aspirated. Specimens should be delivered immediately to the laboratory for Ziehl–Neelsen staining and culture.

Further information

Zar, H.J., Hanslo, D. Apolles, P., Swingler, G., and Hussey, G. (2005). Induced sputum versus gastric lavage for microbiological confirmation of pulmonary tuberculosis in infants and young children: a prospective study. *Lancet* **365**, 130–4.

Exercise testing

Physiology of exercise

- DO_{2max} (mL O_2 per kg) is the maximum rate of oxygen delivery that can be physiologically achieved in an individual during exercise.
- VO_{2max} is the maximum level of oxygen consumption and is limited and equal to DO_{2max}. Above VO_{2max}, greater exercise will induce anaerobic respiration and lactic acidosis production and is therefore non-sustainable.
- Maximum breathing capacity (MBC) is defined as the maximum minute volume of ventilation that may be sustained by an individual for 15s. In children with moderate to severe lung disease, VO_{2max} is limited by a decreased MBC.
- Airways resistance through the nose restricts the high flows needed during exercise and mouth breathing is required. This means that the air entering the lungs is cooler and drier than at rest, and these changes can lead to bronchospasm in susceptible children.
- Exercise testing is generally performed in children:
  - to assess cardiorespiratory endurance in the context of a chronic lung disorder;
  - to reproduce reported exercise-induced symptoms (cough, wheeze, noisy breathing, breathlessness), which can help identify the reason for the symptoms and allow assessment of response to treatments.

Monitoring progress of chronic disease

The time-standardized walk and the 10-metre modified shuttle walk are tests of cardiorespiratory endurance designed to measure symptom-limited maximum performance, which may be used to monitor disease progress. These tests are commonly carried during the annual review of children with CF.

Time-standardized walk tests

- Walk tests of 2, 6, and 12min have been validated in children with CF. Short walks may not truly measure symptom-limited performance. Primary outcome is the distance walked in the given time and this has been shown to correlate with VO_{2max}.
- The walk is performed on level ground. Children are asked to cover as much distance as possible at their own pace with the opportunity to stop and rest at any point. Children are informed of the time at 30s intervals but are given no verbal encouragement.
- A pulse oximeter is used during the test to monitor heart rate and oxygen saturations. Stable measurements may be obtained by placing the patient's arm in a sling. Walk distance, peak heart rate, and lowest saturations are recorded. Peak heart rate achieved in these tests is lower than that achieved using the treadmill test outlined below.

10 metre modified shuttle walk test

- The individual walks up and down a 10m course at times dictated by a pre-recorded audio signal on a cassette deck.
- Walking speeds increase incrementally by 0.17m/s each minute. Walking speed starts at 0.5m/s in minute 1, escalating to 2.37m/s in minute 14. More shuttles are performed per minute as walking speed is increased.

- The test to completion lasts 15min. The audio signal standardizes the increments in walking speed and motivates the individual.
- This test is probably a more robust way of assessing cardiorespiratory endurance than the time-standardized tests, but requires motivated children to carry it out effectively.

Assessment of exercise-induced symptoms

- In normal children, lung function may initially improve after exercise. This is followed by a post-exercise fall in lung function, with a drop in FEV_1 of up to 8%. Full spontaneous recovery occurs after 30–45min.
- A drop in FEV_1 > 10% on exercise, which is reversible with bronchodilator therapy, is consistent with asthma, although some children will be asymptomatic. Exercise-induced symptoms occur in up to 80% of children with asthma. Using a free running exercise test on a monthly basis over the course of a year, 50% of school children aged 8–10 years were shown to have at least 1 post-exercise fall in FEV_1 of 15%.
- Not all exercise-induced symptoms are due to asthma. Formal exercise testing may precipitate reported symptoms and allow alternative diagnoses to be made.
- Lung function pre-exercise, post-exercise, and after bronchodilator therapy will help to:
  - confirm or exclude the diagnosis of asthma as the cause for the exercise induced symptoms. If a child with exercise-associated symptoms does not have a fall in FEV_1 during an exercise test that reproduces those symptoms, asthma is not the cause of the symptoms;
  - assess the severity of bronchial obstruction after exercise;
  - evaluate treatment interventions in children with poorly controlled asthma;
  - exclude reversible airways disease in children with other chest disorders (e.g. children with CF, primary ciliary dyskinesia, bronchiolitis obliterans, tracheo-bronchomalacia);
  - identify children who are breathless for other reasons, such as lack of fitness, hypoxia (in the rare child with pulmonary hypertension or a diffusion defect), or vocal cord dysfunction.

Six minute treadmill test

- Formal exercise testing aims to achieve a level of exercise that will precipitate symptoms due to underlying disease. One standardized test is a 6min run on a treadmill at a speed of 3–5 mph with a slope of 10%. In general, this has been shown to result in a heart rate of 170–180bpm and an oxygen consumption of 60–80% VO_{2max}; it is usually adequate to precipitate clinically important symptoms.
- Children should avoid exercise for at least 3h prior to exercise testing.
- Anti-asthma treatment may modify response. Slow- and long-acting beta-agonists should be stopped 6 and 12h before the test, anti-cholinergics 8h before, and cromolyns 24h before the test.

- In cases where the diagnosis of asthma is in doubt, all anti-asthma therapy including corticosteroids should be stopped 2–4 weeks prior to testing, so that asthma may be unambiguously excluded if reversibility is not demonstrated.
- Physical examination, lung function, oxygen saturation, and pulse rate should be documented before exercise. The child may be monitored during exercise for heart rate, oxygen saturations, and respiratory rate.
- The child should stand on the treadmill platform with the belt stationary. A handrail should be available. Instructions are given to take long strides as the belt starts to move. A safety strap is attached from the patient to the front of the treadmill. If strap contact is broken, the treadmill will slow to a halt. Modern treadmills have a large safety button in easy reach of the patient.
- The child runs for 6min on the treadmill at a speed of 3–5 mph with a slope of 10%. They may be given encouragement and are given the chance to stop at any point should they request to do so.
- Heart rate and saturations should be measured immediately after exercise. If the heart rate is less than 170 beats/min, exercise should continue for a further 2min and pulse rate reassessed.
- Lung function should be measured at 2, 5, and 10min post-exercise.
- Bronchodilators (2–4 puffs salbutamol via spacer) should then be administered and lung function rechecked 2min later to assess for bronchodilator reversibility.

Oxygen destauration with exercise: a surrogate kCO

During exercise, pulmonary blood flow is increased. Patients with a reduced diffusion capacity (kCO) due to interstitial lung disease may show oxygen desaturation with exercise as the supply of deoxygenated blood to the lungs surpasses capacity for gas transfer and oxygenation of blood. Desaturation on exercise should therefore lead to assessment of formal lung function including gas transfer studies.

Further information

Powell, C.V., White, R.D., and Primhak, R.A. (1996). Longitudinal study of free running exercise challenge: reproducibility. *Arch. Dis. Child.* **74**, 108–14.

Exhaled and nasal NO measurement

Exhaled nitric oxide

- The measurement of NO concentration in exhaled air is a reproducible non-invasive method of assessing airway inflammation.
- Levels < 18ppb are defined as normal. In practice, baseline levels vary between individuals and change in level is more informative than a single measurement.
- NO levels are increased in the nasal, sinus, and oral cavities. There is also the possibility of ambient NO contamination. True lower airway levels are defined as the plateau level achieved through mid-expiration.
- To minimize contamination from the nasal cavity and sinuses, exhalation is carried out against a fixed pressure, causing the soft palate to close off the nasopharynx. Contamination from the atmosphere is minimized by inspiring air with a very low NO concentration (< 5ppb). This is achieved in some devices by inhaling through the device.
- The single-breath online measurement method is the preferred method in all children who can cooperate. The child is required to inhale to near TLC and then exhale at a constant flow rate against a resistance for 6–10s. Audiovisual aids can assist in these manoeuvres, but they can still be difficult for some children. Wearing a nose clip is not recommended since it may affect nasal contamination.
- An offline method can also be used, again with the child exhaling at a constant flow rate. The child exhales into an inert balloon. NO concentrations can be stable for several hours. With the newer hand-held portable NO devices (such as the NIOX® MINO), offline methods have largely been superseded by constant flow methods
- Whichever device is used, the analyser will measure fractional exhaled NO (FENO) in parts per billion.
- Exhaled NO levels are elevated in patients with asthma, suppressed in patients with primary ciliary dyskinesia, and relatively low in children with CF. Exhaled NO levels for other conditions are shown in Table 70.1.
- In the short term exhaled NO levels are reduced by exercise, spirometry, and sputum induction manoeuvres. These should therefore be avoided before NO measurement.
- Measurements of FENO can be made during tidal breathing in very young children. The values obtained are not equivalent to single breath measurements and age-related normal values have yet to be established. The use of FENO by this method is currently of use only as a research tool.

Procedure for measurement of FENO using NIOX® MINO

- The NIOX® MINO is ready to use when the blue top light is on.
- Ask the patient to fully empty the lungs.
- With lips sealed around the mouthpiece, inhale deeply to total lung capacity. During inhalation the blue top light turns off.
- Exhale slowly back through the filter.
- Listen to the sound signals and view the top blue light.
  - A continuous sound and steady blue light mean the exhalation pressure is correct.

- An intermittent high sound and flickering light mean exhalation is too hard.
- A flickering light and intermittent low sound mean exhalation is too weak.
- The sound ceases and the light turns off after successful exhalation.

Table 70.1 Effect of various diseases on fractional exhaled NO

Disease	FENO*
Asthma	↑
Cystic fibrosis	↓; ↑ with respiratory exacerbations
Primary ciliary dyskinesia	↓
Pulmonary hypertension	↓ or ↔
Bronchiectasis	↔ or ↑
Viral infection	↔ or ↑
Allergic rhinitis	↔ or ↑
Alveolitis	↑
Lung rejection post-transplant	↑
Sarcoidosis	↑
Chronic cough	↑
Smoking	↓
Bronchospasm	↓
Caffeine	↓
Alcohol	↓
Exercise	↓

*↑, Increased; ↓, decreased; ↔, normal.

Nasal nitric oxide
- Levels of NO in the nasal cavity and paranasal sinuses are several-fold higher than those found in the lower airways.
- The exact source of the gas is not known.
- For most conditions, such as cystic fibrosis or allergic rhinitis, the significance of the level of nasal NO is not clearly understood.
- In children with primary ciliary dyskinesia (PCD), nasal NO levels are consistently lower than in control subjects and measurement of nasal NO can assist in the diagnosis of this condition (see 🔲 Chapter 34).
- Unlike measurements of exhaled NO there are no simple to use commercially available portable devices for measuring nasal NO. Measurement of nasal NO is only available in specialist centres.

- The preferred method of measuring of nasal NO requires air to be aspirated from one nostril at a constant rate (0.25–3L/min), whilst it is entrained through the other nostril. To prevent contamination from ambient air, the nostrils are plugged with olives through which the sampling catheters are passed. To prevent contamination from the lower airways, the child must exhale against a fixed resistance of at least 10cmH$_2$O to close the soft palate. NO levels take 15–30s to plateau.
- The requirements of the test mean that it can only be used on cooperative older children (generally > 5 years of age).
- Normal values range between 150 and 1000ppb. Values in PCD are usually less than 100ppb. Low values are also seen in children with blocked noses, sinus disease, or cystic fibrosis.

Further information

American Thoracic Society; European Respiratory Society (2005). ATS/ERS recommendations for standardized procedures for the online and offline measurement of exhaled lower respiratory nitric oxide and nasal nitric oxide, 2005. *Am. J. Respir. Crit. Care. Med.* **171**, 912–30.

Skin prick testing

Introduction

- Skin prick testing is most commonly used as an *in vivo* test for assessment of antigen-specific allergy. It is performed with aqueous solutions of allergens available for common inhaled, occupational, and food allergens, e.g. house dust mite, grass pollen, cat dander, dog hair, latex, antibiotics, egg, milk, fish, shellfish, tree nuts, and ground nuts.
- Skin prick testing is usually performed in the clinic setting.
- Children having skin prick tests must omit antihistamine treatments for at least 48h prior to testing.
- Note that skin prick testing is different from patch testing. The patch test is used specifically in the diagnosis of contact dermatitis, and can help discriminate between irritant and allergic contact dermatitis. It is not used as part of the diagnosis of atopy or allergic sensitization.

The procedure

- Arrange all allergens to be tested in sequence.
- Clean the forearm with alcohol. This is particularly important in children using emollients for atopic dermatitis.
- Label the forearm for each allergen to be used.
- For each test, a drop of allergen solution is placed by its marker, and a sterile lancet is used to prick the skin through the solution. This is painless and care must be taken to ensure that the skin is actually breached by the lancet. The excess solution is removed using an absorbent paper tissue, and the size of the wheal is read after 15min. The site may itch and the patient must be encouraged not to scratch.
- Disposable lancets should have a 1mm point with a blunt shoulder to prevent excessive trauma. A needle should not be used since the variable depth of penetration will affect the response.
- The test is performed with a standardized positive control (histamine 10mg/mL) and negative control (allergen diluent).
- The test is read at 15min and again at 30min. The greatest response is recorded. A positive result is defined as a wheal 2mm greater than the negative control. The wheal is the raised area in the centre of a reaction and not the redness surrounding it (this is called the flare).
- Itching after testing may be alleviated with topical 1% hydrocortisone cream.
- Skin prick tests are very safe. There is however a small chance of systemic reaction and even anaphylaxis, particularly with food allergens. Testing for food allergy should only be performed in specialist centres. Adrenaline and resuscitation equipment must be available.

Interpretation

- Many children with a positive result on skin prick testing will not have symptoms of overt allergy and results must be considered in the context of the history.
- A strong history of allergic symptoms associated with a specific allergen that gives a negative result on skin prick testing should be reassessed with a repeat skin prick test and serum antigen-specific IgE levels.
- The size of the wheal does not correlate with the severity of the clinical problem.

Contraindications to skin prick testing

If there is a history of anaphylaxis to the test allergen, skin prick testing should be avoided and a serum RAST test used instead.

Relative contraindications

- Severe eczematous dermatitis and dermatographism both make interpretation difficult.
- Infants under 6 months have a higher incidence of systemic reactions.
- If the child is unwilling to discontinue antihistamines.
- Poorly controlled asthma (peak expiratory flow < 75%) at the time of the test.

For these groups of children serum RAST tests are preferred.

Further information

Sporik, R., Hill, D.J., and Hosking, C.S. (2000). Specificity of allergen skin prick testing in predicting positive open food challenges to milk, egg and peanut in children. *Clin. Exp. Allergy* **30**, 1540–6.
Morris, A. (2006). ALLSA position statement: Allergen skin-prick testing. *Curr. Allergy Clin. Immunol.* **19**, 22–5.

Appendices

Blood gases and acid–base balance

Blood gas analysis

Blood gas analysis in children is generally achieved using arterialized capillary blood samples or venous blood samples. Attempts at arterial sampling are painful and tend to result in crying and hyperventilation, with consequent difficulty in blood gas interpretation. Venous and capillary testing provide information regarding ventilation and metabolic compensation, but cannot provide information regarding oxygenation.

Ventilation and oxygenation

- PCO_2 taken from venous or arterialized capillary sampling is an adequate representation of arterial $PaCO_2$ and can therefore be used in the assessment of ventilation.
- Pulse oximetry is used to detect percentage oxyhaemoglobin and provides an easy non-invasive assessment of oxygenation. Normal oxygen saturation levels range between 96% and 100%. Children with intercurrent respiratory infection should be provided with oxygen to maintain oxygen saturations above 92%.
- Transcutaneous CO_2 measurements provide a non-invasive continuous assessment of plasma CO_2 levels. In order to obtain absolute CO_2 levels, frequent correction to arterial blood gas measurements is necessary. Continuous CO_2 monitoring in the ITU setting can serve as a useful adjunct in ventilated patients. It can also be used in sleep studies where trends in ventilation (rather than absolute CO_2 levels) may be monitored and correlated with other measured parameters.

Acid–base balance

- Venous or arterialized capillary blood gas measurement provides information regarding the acid–base balance of the blood.
- Raised $PaCO_2$ from ventilation failure produces a respiratory acidosis.
- Reduced $PaCO_2$ either from spontaneous or mechanical hyperventilation produces a respiratory alkalosis.
- If these changes in ventilation are rapid, they will be reflected in the pH of the blood, which is measured on blood gas analysis (normal range is pH 7.35–7.45). A child with acute asthma who has ventilation failure with a raised $PaCO_2$ may therefore also have an acidaemia.
- In chronic ventilation failure, metabolic compensation by physiological buffers in the blood prevents longstanding acidaemia. The main blood buffering system is the bicarbonate system, where CO_2 and water are in equilibrium with bicarbonate and hydrogen ions. In respiratory acidosis that is prolonged, CO_2 and water accumulate and shift the buffer equilibrium towards bicarbonate and hydrogen ions. Hydrogen ions are then excreted in the kidneys. The result is a respiratory acidosis with a compensatory metabolic alkalosis, with normal pH and no acidaemia.

- Bicarbonate can therefore be used to assess the degree of metabolic compensation secondary to a respiratory acidosis and give insight into the duration of respiratory compromise. Children with chronic lung disease may run high $PaCO_2$ levels with full metabolic compensation, raised bicarbonate, and a normal pH.
- Chronic hyperventilation (e.g. at altitude due to hypoxia) producing a drop in $PaCO_2$ will generate a respiratory alkalosis and compensatory metabolic acidosis through the same blood buffers.
- In primary metabolic acidosis (most commonly caused by sepsis in children) hydrogen ions accumulate and shift the buffer equilibrium towards water and CO_2. A compensatory respiratory alkalosis through hyperventilation is therefore established to maintain normal pH. This is called Kussmaul's breathing.
- Primary metabolic alkalosis (e.g. associated with hypokalaemia) will also act through the buffer system but can only produce a limited compensatory respiratory acidosis through hypoventilation, as hypoxic drive will maintain ventilation at a certain threshold.
- The base excess (BE) is the bicarbonate relative to the normal value of 25meq/L. A positive BE therefore represents metabolic alkalosis, and a negative BE represents a metabolic acidosis.

Fitness to fly

Introduction

- Cabins of commercial aircraft are pressurized to an atmospheric partial pressure equivalent to an altitude of 8000 feet (2348m). This is equivalent to breathing approximately 15% oxygen at sea level.
- In a healthy adult, PaO_2 at 8000ft will fall to 7.0–8.5kPa (53–64mmHg) and oxygen saturation will be 85–91%.
- In healthy children the figure is probably higher, and the limited studies that are available suggest that at 8000ft oxygen saturations would not normally fall below 90%.
- For children with chronic lung disease symptomatic hypoxaemia may occur, which may cause headaches, sleepiness, or, more rarely, acute increases in pulmonary pressure and right heart failure.
- It is difficult to assess the risk of flying in children with lung disease. Longer flights are likely to carry higher risk because of more prolonged hypoxaemia and the increased chance that the child will sleep during the flight with consequent worsening of hypoxaemia.
- Children who are hypoxic at rest because of respiratory disease will already be receiving supplemental oxygen. This will need to be increased during the flight.

Who needs assessment?

- Current British Thoracic guidelines[1] suggest that children with chronic lung disease (the study was on children with CF[2]) who have an FEV_1 of less than 50% should undergo a hypoxic challenge and those children whose saturations drop below 90% during the test should be provided with in-flight oxygen.
- Infants and children < 5 years of age who are unable to carry out simple spirometry and who have a history of chronic lung disease, particularly if there was previous oxygen-dependency, may also desaturate whilst breathing 15% oxygen and may need to be assessed by hypoxic challenge before flying. These children may have oxygen saturations at rest > 95%.

Hypoxic challenge test

- The ideal test of exposing a subject to hypoxia in a hypobaric chamber, is not widely available.
- The alternative assumes that breathing hypoxic gas mixtures at sea level (normobaric hypoxia) equates to the hypobaric hypoxia of altitude.

1 BTS guideline: Managing passengers with respiratory disease planning air travel. www.brit-thoracic.org.uk/guidelines.html

2 Buchdahl, R.M., Babiker, A., Bush, A., et al. (2001). Predicting hypoxaemia during flights in children with cystic fibrosis. Thorax 56, 877–9.

- Subjects are usually asked to breathe the 15% oxygen diluted in nitrogen hypoxic gas mixture using a mouthpiece or tight-fitting face mask for 20min or until equilibration. Saturation is monitored throughout. Cylinders of 15% oxygen are commercially available (e.g. from British Oxygen Corporation).
- An alternative, suitable for younger children, is to fill a body plethysmography box with 15% oxygen to provide the hypoxic environment. This can be achieved by diluting out the oxygen with nitrogen passed into the box at 50L/min for 5min. The advantage of using the body box is that, if de-saturation occurs, the amount of oxygen to correct the hypoxaemia can be titrated accurately using nasal prongs to supply oxygen within the body box.
- The level of oxygen saturation during the hypoxia test at which supplemental oxygen is recommended for flying is arbitrary. In children the value, based on very limited data, is 90%. In adults the figure is 85%.

Other groups to consider

- It is prudent to wait for at least 1 week after an infant in born before flying to ensure that they are healthy.
- The BTS also recommends that infants who are born prematurely should not fly for 6 months because of the risk of apnoea.
- Children who have had pneumothorax should not fly within 2 weeks of a CXR confirming complete resolution. The risk of recurrence is small and is not increased by flying. Small pneumothoraces present before flying will enlarge with increasing altitude. Pneumothoraces that occur at altitude will become smaller as the aeroplane descends.

Further information

Buchdahl, R., Bush, A., Ward, S., and Cramer, D. (2004). Pre-flight hypoxic challenge in infants and young children with respiratory disease. *Thorax* **59**, 1000.

Lee, A.P., Yamamoto, L.G., and Relles, N.L. (2002). Commercial airline travel decreases oxygen saturation in children. *Paed. Emerg. Care* **18**, 78–80.

Polysomnography

Introduction

Polysomnography, also called sleep study, refers to the process by which several physiological parameters are measured and recorded during sleep. The information provided by a sleep study is helpful in the diagnosis and management of children with sleep-disordered breathing.

Indications for polysomnography

Investigation of suspected:
- obstructive sleep apnoea
- hypoventilation associated with neuromuscular weakness
- hypoventilation associated with abnormal respiratory control
- infant apnoea
- narcolepsy

Monitoring of children:
- using non-invasive ventilation
- using night-time oxygen
- being considered for removal of tracheostomy
- with progressive neuromuscular weakness

Recorded information

- The amount and type of data recorded during a sleep study vary both from centre to centre and depending on the purpose of the study. The box on the next page indicates the full range of parameters that can be assessed. Current technology means that each measurement requires the detection device to be attached to the child and associated wires to be attached to a data recording box. In general, the more monitoring attached to the child, the less likely they are to have a typical night's sleep. Wireless technology is being developed.
- Sleep-staging is important when interpreting the data. During active or REM sleep (also called dream sleep) there is diminished respiratory drive and loss of tone in the intercostal and pharyngeal muscles. This means that many forms of sleep-disordered breathing are more pronounced during this phase of sleep. Precise sleep staging requires EEG recording. The distinction between active and non-active sleep can also be made in the majority of children without the need for an EEG, by assessing heart-rate variability (increased during active sleep) and by the relative contribution of the chest and abdominal movement during breathing (relative loss of chest contribution during active sleep). This form of sleep-staging is sufficient for most clinical purposes. Sleep stages using these parameters are harder to identify in older children (> 10 years of age).

- Obstructive sleep apnoea can be accurately identified and graded in most children using the following parameters:
  - ECG (heart rate);
  - pulse oximetry (heart rate and oxygen saturation);
  - movement monitor (usually attached to the toe);
  - chest band (to assess chest movement);
  - abdominal band (to assess chest movement).
- To assess children with suspected hypoventilation, CO_2 should also be measured, either by using transcutaneous or end-tidal devices.
- To assess infants with suspected apnoea, where seizures are a possible cause, EEG and infrared video recording should be included.

Possible measured parameters during polysomnography

- EEG: minimum of 3 leads
- Electro-oculograms: left and right to detect eye movements
- Electromyogram (EMG) of the genioglossal muscle to help with sleep staging (activity is decreased in active sleep)
- EMG of the diaphragm
- ECG
- Nasal airflow
- Mouth airflow
- End-tidal CO_2
- Transcutaneous CO_2
- Pulse oximetry
- Chest excursion
- Abdominal excursion
- Leg movement
- Infrared camera recording child throughout the study
- Microphone to detect snoring

Interpretation

- Data from polysomnography need to be analsyed carefully. Although software is available to interpret much of the data in an automated fashion, it is not sufficiently robust to be relied upon, and visual inspection of the waveforms is always required. This is time-consuming and requires experience and skill.
- Often there is obvious abnormality, e.g. recurrent episodes of desaturation. It may also be obvious that these are associated with paradoxical chest and abdominal movements and arousal suggesting that obstruction is present. What can be missed, unless care is taken, is that there may be additional events, such as central pauses, mixed in with the more prominent obstructive events.
- Like any recording, artefacts can occur, and experience is required to identify when this has happened. For example, an apparent desaturation is not likely to be real if there is no associated change in respiratory movement, heart rate, or arousal , and if the pulse oximetry signal is of low amplitude.
- Reference values for sleep studies are given on 📖 p. 816.

Figure A3.1 shows a typical multichannel recording from a normal 5-year-old boy.

Respiratory rate and heart rate

- High respiratory rates are seen in children with underlying heart or lung disease.
- Low respiratory rates are seen in children with respiratory control disorders, including congenital central hypoventilation syndrome and brainstem compression (by Arnold–Chiari malformation, brain tumour, or bony compression in children with craniosynostosis).
- Central respiratory pauses are common in infants.
- High heart rates are associated with fever, lung disease, and heart disease. Heart rate will usually increase in response to hypoxia (may go down in early infancy). Heart rate will also increase with seizure activity and, in contrast, this will occur *before* any associated hypoxia.
- Bradycardia in infants is usually associated with apnoea.

Oxygenation

- Chronic hypoxia is associated with lung or heart disease.
- Episodic hypoxia usually reflects changes in minute ventilation which can be central or obstructive.
- Normal central pauses in young infants, especially infants who were preterm, can be associated with brief de-saturation to the mid-80s. Oxygen saturation can also fluctuate during normal periodic breathing.

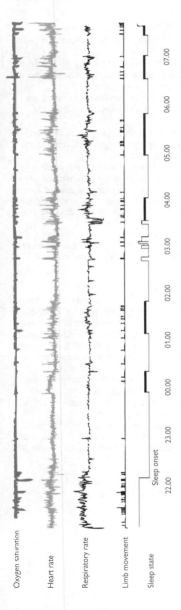

Fig. A3.1 Typical multichannel recording from a normal 5-year-old boy. The recording shows that over the 9 hours of the study, he remained well oxygenated and had 5 episodes of active sleep (solid black bars), scored according to changes in heart rate and respiratory pattern.

Carbon dioxide

- CO_2 levels are largely unaffected by age, with mean values of end-tidal CO_2 of 5.3kPa (40mmHg).
- Peak levels of CO_2 are very variable and tend to be higher in children < 5 years of age. Occasional values above 50mmHg are seen in normal children but will often prompt further investigation.
- Absolute values of CO_2 measured with transcutaneous devices are liable to artefact, although changes in CO_2 levels can be detected accurately.
- CO_2 increases of 2–7mmHg are seen at sleep onset in all children. This increase may be exaggerated in those with lung disease, respiratory control disorders, or neuromuscular weakness.
- Interpretation of elevated CO_2 levels seen during a sleep study depends on the clinical context, the nature of the increase, and any associated changes in oxygen saturation, heart rate, or state of arousal.
- Episodic increases in CO_2 associated with active sleep in a child with neuromuscular weakness or with a respiratory control disorder are very likely to represent episodes of hypoventilation.
- In children with diminished respiratory drive, CO_2 can increase progressively through the night. This needs to be distinguished from artefact caused by a drifting baseline on the measurement device.

Respiratory movements

- These are assessed with the chest and abdominal leads.
- If inductance devices are used, the size of the signal may correlate with the size of the excursion. This is not the case for impedance bands.
- Normal inspiration is generated by outward movement of the chest and abdomen. If there is resistance to expansion of the lungs (caused by reduced compliance or increased airways resistance) the abdomen will still move out as the diaphragm descends, but the outward movement of the chest will be retarded. In its most extreme form there will be paradoxical inward movement of the chest during the early phase of inspiration. When loss of phase occurs intermittently during a study, particularly if the episodes are associated with active sleep, the cause will be upper airways obstruction.
- Out of phase respiratory movements are usually sufficient to identify obstructive events, especially if they are associated with arousal and desaturation. They cannot distinguish between obstructive breaths and obstructive apnoea. To make this distinction airflow monitoring is required. Airflow measurement is felt by some sleep specialists to be essential for accurate polysomnography. Others have found that the measurements are difficult to make and disturb the child, and feel clinical decisions can be made without information on airflow.

Some examples

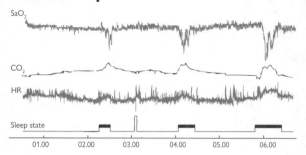

Fig. A3.2 Sleep study from a 5-year-old boy with muscle weakness showing 6h of data, with 3 episodes of hypoxia and hypercapnia associated with periods of active sleep. HR = heart rate; CO_2 = transcutaneous CO_2; SaO_2 = oxygen saturation.

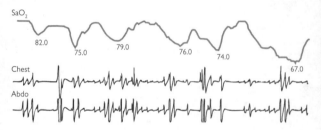

Fig. A3.3 Expanded section from study in Fig. A3.2, showing 2min of data from a period of active sleep. The signals from the abdominal and chest bands show synchronous activity of reduced amplitude with pauses, consistent with hypoventilation without obstruction. Chest = signal from chest band; Abdo = signal from abdominal band.

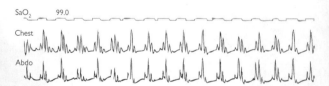

Fig. A3.4 Two minutes of data from a 3-month-old infant showing periodic breathing with short pauses, associated with small changes in oxygen saturation. This pattern of breathing is normal at this age.

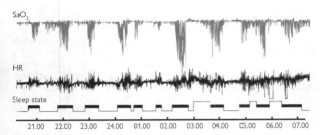

Fig. A3.5 Sleep study from a 2-year-old girl with large tonsils and adenoids and obstructive sleep apnoea. The study shows 11h of data with 11 periods of active sleep (solid bars). Desaturation occurs in each active sleep period.

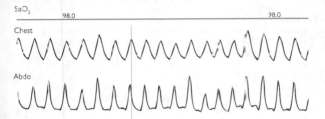

Fig A3.6 Expanded section from study in Fig. A3.5, now showing 1.5min of data from a period of quiet sleep. The vertical line through the chest and abdominal signals shows that the chest and abdominal movements are synchronized.

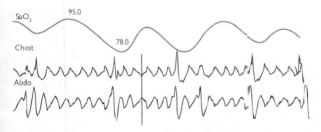

Fig A3.7 Expanded section from study in Fig. A3.5 showing 1.5min of data from a period of active sleep. This shows asynchronous chest and abdominal movements associated with desaturation. The oxygen saturation recovers during brief arousals during which a larger more synchronous and more effective breath is taken. This pattern is typical for obstructive sleep apnoea.

Reference values

There are several papers describing normal values of physiological variables during sleep (see further information). For the purpose of providing a quick easy to use reference source, we have rounded some values across age ranges. Heart rate and respiratory rate vary considerably with age and several age-related values are given (Table A3.1). Other sleep parameters show less age dependency and overall figures for childhood are given (Table A3.2). Notes are provided to assist with interpretation of the data.

Notes

- For the variables in Table A3.2, apart from the central apnoea index, the effect of age is relatively small.
- Obstructive apnoeas are rare at all ages and in most children none or only 1 event will be seen in the whole study.
- Central apnoeas are common and most children will have at least 1 pause of 10s every night. Central apnoeas > 20s have been regarded as abnormal, but can be seen occasionally in normal children of all ages including adolescents. They are more common in early infancy. Whether they are regarded as abnormal will depend on the context and the severity of any associated desaturation or heart rate change.
- High or low ambient temperature, outside the child's preferred temperature (thermoneutral range), will cause increases in the heart rate and respiratory rate. In infants the proportion of periodic breathing increases as the ambient temperature approaches the upper end of the infant's thermoneutral range.

Table A3.1 Respiratory rate (RR) and heart rate (HR) during sleep according to age*

Age	RR (breaths/min)[†]	HR (beats/min)[†]
0–6 weeks	40 (30–70)	130 (80–160)
6 weeks–6 months	34 (25–45)	122 (92–140)
1–3 years	25 (20–29)	100 (70–120)
4–6 years	23 (18–27)	84 (65–105)
7–10 years	20 (16–24)	75 (55–93)
11–18 years	16 (12–20)	62 (45–80)

* Note that values refer to quiet sleep. Some of the data were derived from quiet and relaxed but awake children.

† The mean and values ± 2SD (in brackets) are given.

Table A3.2 Selected sleep parameters in children

Parameter	Mean	Values ± SD
Sleep time spent in REM or active sleep (%)	20	5–35
Obstructive apnoea index*	0.1	0–0.5
Central apnoea index 1[†]	0.8	0–3
Central apnoea index 2[‡]	0.3	0–1
Saturation index[§]	0.5	0.2–3.0
Lowest recorded saturation during sleep (%)	92	86–98

* The number of obstructive apnoeas (2 respiratory cycles with effort but no airflow) per hour.

† The number of central apnoeas (cessation of effort and airflow for > 10s) per hour.

‡ Central apnoea index when apnoea is > 20s or > 10s + desaturation of 3% or more.

§ Number of desaturations of 4% or more per hour.

Further information

Iliff, A. and Lee, V.A. (1952). Pulse rate, respiratory rate, and body temperature of children between two months and eighteen years of age. *Child Dev.* **123**, 237–45.

Katona, P.G and Egbert, J.R. (1978). Heart rate and respiratory rate differences between preterm and full-term infants during quiet sleep: possible implications for sudden infant death syndrome. *Pediatrics* **62**, 91–5.

Montgomery-Downs, H.E., O'Brien, L.M., Gulliver, T.E., and Gozal, D. (2006). Polysomnographic characteristics in normal preschool and early school-aged children. *Pediatrics* **117**, 741–53.

Richards, J.M., Alexander, J.R., Shinebourne, E.A., de Swiet, M., Wilson, A.J., and Southall, D.P. (1984). Sequential 22-hour profiles of breathing patterns and heart rate in 110 full-term infants during their first 6 months of life. *Pediatrics* **74**, 763–77.

Traeger, N., Schultz, B., Pollock, A.N., Mason, T., Marcus, C.L., and Arens, R. (2005). Polysomnographic values in children 2–9 years old: additional data and review of the literature. *Pediatr. Pulmono'.* **40**, 22–30.

Uliel, S., Tauman, R., Greenfeld, M., and Sivan, Y. (2004). Normal polysomnographic respiratory values in children and adolescents. *Chest* **125**, 872–8.

Verhulst, S.L., Schrauwen, N., Haentjens, D., Van Gaal, L., De Backer, W.A., and Desager, K.N. (2007). Reference values for sleep-related respiratory variables in asymptomatic European children and adolescents. *Pediatr. Pulmonol.* **42**, 159–67.

Measuring lung function

Introduction

Lung function

- The function of the lungs is to maintain normal arterial oxygen, arterial CO_2, and arterial pH.
- Pulmonary function tests are used to measure lung volumes, airflow resistance patterns, and efficiency of gaseous exchange.
- Three main approaches can be used in the compliant older child.
  - Spirometry is the mainstay of most paediatric lung function protocols and is used to measure dynamic lung volumes and flow rates during forced ventilatory manoeuvres.
  - Plethysmography is used to measure static lung volumes, in particular total lung capacity and residual volume. Effort-independent measures of airway obstruction may also be generated.
  - Gas diffusion techniques can be used to measure static lung volumes and to determine the efficiency of gaseous exchange.

Indications for pulmonary function testing in children

- Diagnosis:
  - characterization of impairment in physiological function;
  - quantification of impairment in physiological function.
- Monitoring of chronic disease:
  - cystic fibrosis;
  - asthma;
  - neuromuscular disease.
- Establishing the effectiveness of therapeutic intervention:
  - asthma;
  - cystic fibrosis.
- Assessing risk of an intervention:
  - anaesthetic;
  - chemotherapy;
  - fitness to fly.

Lung volumes and capacities

Figure A4.1 shows the various lung volumes and capacities.

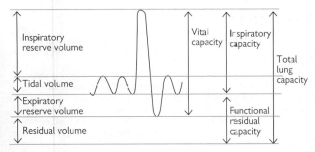

Fig. A4.1 Lung volumes and capacities.

Spirometry

- Spirometry is the easiest and most commonly performed measure of lung function. It uses forced ventilatory manoeuvres to assess maximal flow rates and dynamic lung volumes.
- As the patient performs forced inspiratory and expiratory manoeuvres through the mouthpiece of the spirometer, flow rates and time are measured. Volumes are calculated from these parameters. Flow is derived either using a pneumotachometer, which measures pressure change across a fixed resistance, or from the speed of a rotating fan.
- Two plots are generated: volume against time and flow against volume. The latter is usually more informative.

The flow–volume loop (Fig. A4.2)

The forced inspiratory manoeuvre

- The forced inspiratory manoeuvre starts from a point of maximal expiration. The lung at this point is at residual volume (RV). As forced inspiration commences, lung volumes are low, airways are relatively collapsed, and so flow rates start slowly and increase as airway calibre increases. As inspiration progresses, inspiratory muscle strength tails off and flow rates again slow until total lung capacity (TLC) is achieved.
- Maximum flow rates are seen around mid-inspiration giving the inspiratory limb of the flow–volume loop a domed appearance.
- The forced inspiratory flow rate at a point when 50% of VC has been reached (FIF_{50}) should be about equal to the forced expiratory flow rate at the same point (FEF_{50}).

The forced expiratory manoeuvre

- To keep the lungs at TLC, a negative pleural pressure is maintained by contraction of the inspiratory muscles. Supportive structures of the lung transmit this negative pressure to the airways, which are therefore held maximally patent and supported.
- On expiration, as lung volume decreases, airway support decreases and the airway becomes progressively more susceptible to narrowing or closure. This volume-dependent property of the airway is called dynamic compliance, and airway narrowing that occurs as a consequence of this is termed dynamic compression.
- Dynamic compression does not occur during quiet expiration in the normal lung but becomes particularly important in a forced expiratory manoeuvre.
- During forced expiration, a large positive pleural pressure is applied to intrathoracic structures by contraction of expiratory muscles.
- Dynamic compression of the airway is at its minimum at TLC and consequently flow rates are at their highest. The peak expiratory flow rate (PEFR) is therefore seen at the beginning of forced expiration.
- As lung volume decreases through forced expiration, maximal flow rates also decrease because of increasing dynamic compression of the airway. In fact, as lung volumes fall, a dynamic compression-wave occurs along the airway, starting in the proximal airway and extending towards the bronchial periphery (see box on 📖 p. 858).

- Dynamic compression of the airway rather than effort actually limits the maximum expiratory flow rate that can be achieved during forced expiration. Bronchial flow limitation from dynamic compression occurs at relatively modest pleural pressures. The consequence is that flow rates become effort-independent, can be taken as a true measure of airflow resistance, and are relatively reproducible. This phenomenon is the great advantage of using the forced expiratory manoeuvre.
- It is important to note that, because children aged < 5–7 years are generally unable to perform a forced expiratory manoeuvre where bronchial flow limitation is achieved, the direct relationship between measured flow rates and airflow resistance is lost so interpretation of spirometry in this age group may be difficult.
- The pattern and degree of dynamic compression (and therefore airflow resistance) seen on forced expiration will depend on intrinsic properties of the airway, including the stability of the bronchial walls, the degree of airway inflammation, airway wall thickness, and smooth muscle tone. The forced expiratory manoeuvre is therefore invaluable in the assessment of obstructive airways disease.
- The end of the forced expiratory manoeuvre in young healthy lungs occurs when expiratory muscles can contract no further. In diseased or older lungs, dynamic compression of small distal airways at the end of expiration may actually completely close the airways and further deflation becomes impossible. The remaining lung volume at the end of forced expiration is called the residual volume (RV) and can be measured using plethysmography. This may be elevated in obstructive small airways disease.

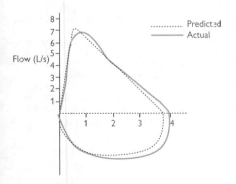

Fig. A4.2 The flow–volume loop plots inspiratory and expiratory flow rates against lung volume for maximal forced expiratory and inspiratory manoeuvres.

Flow limitation theory

- At all lung volumes below around 90% of vital capacity, the speed at which air can be expelled by the lungs is flow limited at relatively modest pleural pressures—around 20cmH$_2$O. It is this phenomenon that makes forced expiratory manoeuvres relatively reproducible.
- Understanding the basis of flow limitation is important not only in interpretation of lung function tests, but also in understanding diseases in which airflow obstruction occurs.
- The driving force for air to leave the lung during a forced expiratory manoeuvre is the pleural pressure plus the pressure generated by the elastic recoil of the lung. Any gas travelling through a tube will meet a resistance that is inversely proportion to the surface area of the tube and directly proportional to its length. Thus the airways of the lung provide a resistance to the flow of air. As a consequence, the pressure inside the lumen of the airway falls. When the intraluminal pressure falls below that in the pleura (the *equal pressure point*), airway narrowing starts to occur, causing a further fall in intraluminal pressure and further airway narrowing. The existence of the equal pressure point neatly explains how increased expiratory effort might have an equal effect on both the driving force for exhalation and on airway narrowing. It does not fully explain why there is flow limitation. This turns out to be a physical property of all elastic tubes.
- Flow in elastic tubes, such as the airways, is limited by the ability of elastic tubes to propagate pressure waves. Bulk flow cannot occur at speeds above which pressure driving the flow can be propagated along the tube—the tube wave speed. Bulk flow will be limited when it approaches the tube wave speed— this is known as the choke point. Increasing the driving pressure once the choke point has been reached does not lead to increased flow. Maximal flows are proportional to the density of the gas, the airway wall compliance, and the surface area of the airway lumen.
- Total small airways cross-sectional area is large at high lung volumes and decreases as lung volume diminishes. Peripheral airway resistance thus increases, the equal pressure point moves towards the alveoli, and the proportion of airways that are dynamically compressed increases. The reduction in surface area of these airways increases the number of airways that are choked or flow limited. As lung volume decreases further, the number of flow limited airways increases exponentially giving the typical expiratory flow–volume loop.

Flow–volume loop patterns (see Fig. A4.3)
- In patients with healthy lungs there is a predictable linear reduction in maximal flow rate as lung volumes decrease.
- In children with obstructive small airways disease, flow rates fall quicker than anticipated as the lungs deflate, and the expiratory limb of the flow–volume loop appears 'scooped out'.
- In children with restrictive lung disease, either because of chest wall deformity, weakness, pulmonary hypoplasia, or stiff lungs, there will be reduced volumes with a near normal shape to the flow–volume curve. This pattern is often indistinguishable from that caused by inadequate inspiratory effort and interpretation needs to take this into account.
- The effect of fixed large airways obstruction or flow dynamics can also be seen clearly on the flow–volume loop. The peak expiratory flow rate achievable will be limited by the fixed airways obstruction and this will produce a plateau to the expiratory limb of the flow–volume loop. As lung volumes continue to decrease during the expiration, maximal flow rates will eventually decrease to beneath the threshold defined by the obstruction, and at this stage the flow–volume loop assumes its normal dynamic. The same clipped appearance is seen in the inspiratory limb giving the classic square box appearance to the flow–volume loop.
- Mobile lesions causing upper airways obstruction may be more prominent in either inspiration or expiration. Mobile extrathoracic obstructions, such as vocal cord paralysis, have a more prominent effect during inspiration, and classically result in a square inspiratory limb and a normal expiratory limb on the flow–volume curve. The FEF_{50} is larger than the FIF_{50}. Mobile intrathoracic large airway obstructions (such as a bulky mobile granuloma) may have a more prominent effect during expiration when the thorax is compressed, and may show a square expiratory limb and a normal inspiratory limb.

Measurements in spirometry
- The central measurements taken from a forced expiratory manoeuvre are the forced vital capacity (FVC) and the forced expiratory volume in one second (FEV_1). Normative data from cross-sectional studies are available for children (see Appendix 5).
- FVC is reduced in restrictive lung defects. This may be due to poorly compliant lungs, e.g. interstitial lung disease, to pulmonary hypoplasia, to respiratory muscle weakness, or to structural abnormalities of the thoracic cage. Children with muscle weakness, e.g. Duchenne's muscular dystrophy, will generally be unable to achieve bronchial flow limitation in forced expiration but should be able to perform a slow vital capacity (VC) manoeuvre that can be used to assess the degree of ventilatory restriction.
- FEV_1 is reduced in obstructive small airways disease and is seen with scooping of the expiratory flow–volume loop. The degree of scooping is usually expressed as the ratio $FEV_1/VC\%$ or $FEV_1/FVC\%$. Although FVC may also be reduced in more severe obstructive airways disease where full expiration is limited by closure of small airways, FEV_1 will be more affected and so the ratio will always be reduced. The normal range for the ratio $FEV_1/FVC\%$ is > 80%.

- FEF_{25-75} is defined as the average forced expiratory flow rate between 25% and 75% lung capacity. A reduction in this parameter may be a more sensitive index of obstructive small airways disease than $FEV_1/FVC\%$ as it reflects flow rates once the dynamic compression-wave has reached the small diseased airways.

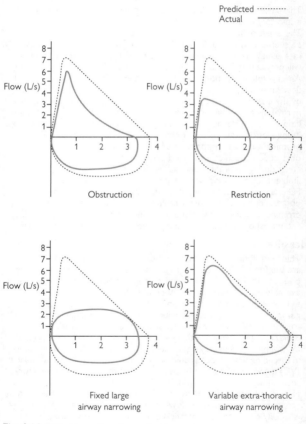

Fig. A4.3 Typical low-volume loop patterns.

Application of spirometry

- The forced expiratory manoeuvre requires inspiration to total lung capacity followed by a maximal hard and fast forced expiration that continues to residual volume. Children as young as 5 years of age may be able to perform useful spirometry and peak flow measurements if given a child-friendly environment, good training, and breath-activated visual animated incentives, available on most electronic spirometers.
- Older school children and adolescents may be able to perform satisfactory flow–volume loops with instruction alone, but breath-activated visual animated incentives, available on most electronic spirometers, should be used in the younger age group.
- A nose clip should be used where possible but this may prove difficult in younger children. The technician must always give encouragement throughout the test.
- Performance in younger children will improve as they become familiar with the process. Children with chronic lung diseases should be introduced to the spirometer at an early age.
- Flow–volume loops should be analysed in detail. Blows that are taken before total lung capacity is achieved, where maximal effort is not given, or where the child coughs or ends short of residual volume should be rejected. The child should perform at least 3 manoeuvres. The best result is used.
- Assessment for reversibility using bronchodilator therapy should be performed if the history or flow–volume loop is suggestive of obstructive airways disease. Five puffs of salbutamol via spacer may be given in clinic, with repeat testing 10min after administration. An increase in FEV_1 of greater than 10%, with a supportive history and flow–volume dynamic, is highly suggestive of reversible airways disease.

Plethysmography

Plethysmography is used to measure static lung volumes, in particular, functional residual capacity (FRC), total lung capacity (TLC), and residual volume (RV). Effort-independent measures of airway obstruction may also be generated (sRAW, sGAW).

Measurement of static lung volumes (TLC, RV)

- Calculations from plethysmography are based on Boyle's law, which states that, for a given mass of gas, the gas pressure × gas volume is a constant (at fixed temperature). Therefore changes in pressure measured during the procedure may be used to calculate lung volumes.
- Measurements are made using a box of known volume. The child sits in the box and is asked to breathe normally through a mouthpiece, breathing air from outside the box. It takes about a minute for box temperature to stabilize. To measure FRC, an external occlusion is created by a shutter in the mouthpiece at the start of the test inspiration. Flow is occluded, but chest expansion still occurs as thoracic gas is rarefied.
- Since the box is sealed, the air around the patient will be compressed slightly during this inspiratory manoeuvre and there will be a reduction in air volume in the box that is equal to the increase in thoracic gas volume (ΔV). This volume can be calculated using Boyle's law using the pressure change observed in the box.
- During the same inspiration, pressure changes within the lung are also measured using the pressure transducer in the mouthpiece. Volume at the start of inspiration during tidal breathing is the functional residual capacity (FRC) of the lung, and this can be calculated, again using Boyle's law, using the pre- and post-inspiration airway pressures and the change in lung volume (ΔV) as measured using the external box measurements outlined above.
- FRC measured using this technique includes all the gas in the lung, including any that is trapped. Any gas in the stomach can also affect the results. The measurement is a close approximation of the thoracic gas volume and is referred to as FRCtgv.
- Once FRCtgv is known, full inspiration and full expiration with the shutter released can be used to determine values for total lung capacity (TLC) and residual volume (RV), respectively. These final manoeuvres are only possible in compliant children, usually those aged > 6y.

Measurement of airways resistance

sRAW and sGAW

- Plethysmography can be used to measure airways resistance and is particularly useful in younger children who cannot perform a reliable forced expiratory manoeuvre for spirometry. Measurements are made during normal tidal breathing, requiring only passive cooperation from the child.
- Inspiration and expiration occur through generation of negative and positive alveolar pressure, respectively. If this occurs against complete resistance (as described above) there is rarefaction and compression of

intrathoracic gas, respectively. In contrast, in a system of no resistance, flow will occur across the pressure difference between alveolus and mouth instantaneously and there will be no rarefaction or compression of intrathoracic gas. Change in lung volume here is in complete phase with observed flow, and this situation approximates to the normal lung.

- In the lung with high airways resistance, the volume to flow relationship becomes out of phase with a delay seen between the change in lung volume and the corresponding change in flow. In other words, intrathoracic gas becomes slightly rarefied in inspiration and slightly compressed in expiration.

- To measure airways resistance using plethysmography, a pneumotachometer in the mouthpiece is used to measure flow rates during tidal breathing, while lung volume changes are simultaneously calculated using changes in box pressures as described above. By plotting volume change against flow, an s-shaped resistance loop can be generated. The long axis of the resistance loop is close to vertical in normal airways, and deviates towards the horizontal with increased airways resistance. This deviation is quantified as the parameter sRAW, the specific airways resistance. sGAW (airway conductance) is the reciprocal of sRAW.

The interrupter technique (R_{INT})

- Airways resistance may also be measured using the interrupter technique. This may be performed using standard plethysmograph equipment or with portable devices. Central to this technique is the indirect measurement of alveolar pressure during transient occlusion of the airway at the mouth. This relies on the assumption that alveolar pressure equilibrates with mouth pressure during airway occlusion so that measurements taken using a pressure transducer in the airway mask genuinely represent alveolar pressure. Airflow is measured at the mouth using the pneumotachometer just prior to occlusion, and inferences regarding airway resistance can be made from the pressure–flow relationship observed.

- Optimal timing of the occlusion within the breathing cycle remains unresolved. How best to measure the airway pressure from the post-occlusion oscillatory wave also remains contentious.

- R_{INT} measurements have proved difficult to standardize, although reference data have been published for healthy children. Some centres have incorporated R_{INT} measurements into routine lung function procedure, but a role in the clinical setting remains limited.

Application of plethysmography

- Residual volume (RV) is raised in moderate to severe obstructive small airways disease. The RV/TLC ratio generated using plethysmography is an important marker of disease progress in asthma and cystic fibrosis and should be documented regularly.

- Only passive cooperation is required for successful plethysmography so, generally speaking, children of all ages can be tested, although apparatus may be different for different age groups. However, because the child needs to remain still during measurements, sedation is required for younger children and infants.

- In the younger age group, the need to use a nose clip, to form a seal around the mouthpiece, and to prevent inflation of the cheeks during the manoeuvre makes repeatable acceptable results difficult to obtain. Using a face mask that covers the nose and mouth, with a built in flexible tube that keeps the mouth open and prevents nasal breathing, improves results in this age group.
- In uncooperative children, tests may be attempted with an adult accompanying the child inside the box, although technically this is more difficult. The adult can prevent mouth bulging by stabilizing the cheeks with their hands.
- In older fully compliant children, measurements may be made during panting rather than tidal breathing as this ensures that the vocal cords are open and do not contribute to measured airways resistance.
- sRAW measurements are highly repeatable.
- sRAW and sGAW may help in the assessment of lung function in children as young as 2 years of age.
- Normative data exist for healthy school and pre-school children.
- Abnormal sRAW values are seen in pre-school children with cystic fibrosis and asthma. Cold air bronchial challenge studied in 2–5 year old asthmatic children and healthy pre-school controls showed an increase in sRAW of > 20% in 68% of asthmatics and only 7% of healthy controls. In a study of reversibility using beta-agonist therapy, a 25% decrease in sRAW provided good discrimination between pre-school asthmatic and healthy children.

Gas dilution techniques

Gas diffusion techniques can be used to measure static lung volumes and to determine the efficiency of gaseous exchange.

Multiple-breath closed circuit helium dilution

- This technique is based on dilution of helium in a re-breathing closed circuit.
- Volume of the circuit is known, initial helium concentration in the circuit is measured, and amount of helium in the system calculated.
- The closed circuit is connected to a spirometer and mouthpiece via a 3-way tap. Patient breathes through the mouthpiece with a nose-clip on and tight seal around the mouth, with 3-way tap initially connected to room air. Tidal volume is observed from the spirometer readings.
- At the start of the procedure, the patient is connected to the closed circuit at the end of a tidal expiration (FRC), and breathes through the circuit until helium is equally distributed through circuit and lungs. This point is marked by a levelling off of helium concentration in the system at a new lower level. This may take up to 10min. Because helium is water insoluble and will not diffuse into the blood during the procedure, the total amount of helium in the system remains constant so the new volume of distribution is simply calculated from the final helium concentration. CO_2 is continuously absorbed by soda lime and oxygen continuously added so that the volume of the system remains constant.
- At the end of the procedure, patient is asked to take a maximal inspiration and maximal expiration so that TLC and RV may also be derived. TLC derived using this technique is called alveolar volume (V_A).

Single-breath helium dilution

- TLC may also be calculated by comparing helium concentration provided in inspired air with that in expired air.
- The patient takes a single inspiration to total lung capacity and holds the breath for 10s during which time approximate helium equilibration occurs throughout the lung. The volume of inspired gas and the helium concentration in inspired air is known, so V_A can be calculated from the helium concentration in expired air.
- Prerequisites for a successful test are the ability of the child to hold inspiration for 10s, and a VC of at least1.5L, as the first 750mL is discarded for washout of airways and apparatus dead space. Younger children will therefore find this test difficult. Children with severe restrictive lung disease and therefore a low VC will also be unable to perform this test successfully.
- Volumes measured using gas dilution techniques are generally marginally less than those measured using plethysmography. This discrepancy provides a measure of the degree of air trapping and is useful in the assessment of obstructive airways disease and particularly in CF.

Carbon monoxide transfer

- TLCO and kCO are measures of gas diffusion capacity of the lung.
- CO crosses the alveolar–capillary membrane and is taken up by red blood cells. If a gas mixture containing a known amount of CO is inhaled and held for 10–15s and then exhaled, the difference in the amount of CO seen in inspired and expired air is the amount of CO that has diffused across the gaseous exchange surface of the lung. A vital capacity of at least 1.0L is required for the test.
- The total amount of CO transferred is called the total lung CO (TLCO). If the V_A is measured at the same time using single-breath helium dilution, then the TLCO/V_A ratio can be used to generate a measure of gas transfer per unit lung volume called the transfer factor or kCO.
- kCO will be reduced where there is a barrier to diffusion, usually due to some form of interstitial lung disease, such as those barriers in connective tissue disease or those related to drug-associated hypersensitivity pneumonitis.
- kCO may be increased in the following cases.
  - Alveolar haemorrhage.
  - Restrictive lung disease from neuromuscular disease or deformed chest disease. These patients have essentially normal lungs that are poorly expanded. They may therefore have proportionally more gaseous exchange area per unit volume. This can be normalized by calculating predicted kCO using actual TLC rather than TLC predicted for height.
  - Children with increased pulmonary blood flow, e.g. during exercise or in children with left to right shunts.
- kCO will usually be normal in asthma and cystic fibrosis. TLCO may well be low, but this is corrected by a low alveolar volume (measured by gas diffusion).

Application of gas dilution techniques

- The older school-age child should be able to perform single-breath helium dilution techniques and measurements for transfer factor.
- In younger children, or those with a severe restrictive defect, multiple-breath methods where the child inhales a mix of CO and helium while tidal breathing for several minutes can be used as an alternative. As kCO measurements using this technique are measured at FRC plus half tidal volume, as opposed to TLC for the single breath measurement, results using the two approaches are not directly comparable.
- Normative data for kCO levels in children exists for both single-breath and re-breathing methods. In both cases these values correlate well with V_A and height.
- Children with decreased alveolar diffusing capacity, who cannot be formally tested, will demonstrate desaturation on exercise as pulmonary blood supply exceeds alveolar diffusing capacity. This test is sometimes called the 'poor man's kCO'.

Lung function test findings

Restrictive lung disease

- Restrictive lung disease is defined as a TLC < 80% predicted using plethysmography or gas dilution techniques. This remains the gold standard.
- A reduction in VC below 80% predicted seen on spirometry may also be used to define restriction. FEV_1/FVC% ratio is classically elevated in restrictive lung disease.
- FVC may also be reduced in obstructive lung disease or after a short expiration. If there is any doubt, static lung volumes should be measured formally.
- FVC is effort-dependent and may not be possible in children with muscle weakness. A slow VC in these situations is used to monitor disease progress
- A homogeneous drop in VC, RV, and TLC is seen in parenchymal restrictive lung disease, such as that seen with interstitial lung disease, hypoplasia or post-resection. In restriction from a hypodynamic state such as that seen in early neuromuscular disease, VC is reduced, RV may be increased, and TLC may be normal.
- The inspiratory capacity (IC), the volume from FRC to TLC, needs to be 15mL/kg to maintain adequate spontaneous ventilation. As postoperative pain may reduce IC by 50%, a value of less than 30mL/kg is commonly used as an indicator of patients who may require prolonged postoperative ventilation.

Obstructive airways disease

- Spirometry is the central tool for defining obstructive airways disease. Children from 5 years of age may be able to peform reliable spirometry.
- Reduced FEV_1, FEF_{25-75}, and FEV_1/FVC% ratio, with a scooped expiratory limb of the flow–volume loop, all suggest obstructive small airways disease. A clipped flow–volume loop suggests upper airway obstruction.
- Plethysmography or gas dilution techniques may reveal increased RV and RV/TLC% ratio in moderate to severe obstructive small airways disease. RV can generally only be measured in compliant children above the age of 5 years.
- In pre-school children, the airways resistance measures sRAW and sGAW obtained from plethysmography may be useful when a forced expiratory manoeuvre is unsuccessful.
- In infants and pre-school children, R_{INT} and measures of airways resistance obtained through impedance techniques are being clarified but have limited clinical application at present.
- If an abnormality consistent with obstructive small airways disease is observed, improvement may be seen with bronchodilators and this should be attempted.

- Bronchial hyperresponsiveness may be seen after direct bronchial challenge (histamine or methacholine) or indirect challenge (exercise or cold air). This is a useful tool if asthma is suspected despite normal lung function testing. In direct bronchial challenge with methacholine or histamine, increasing doses are nebulized between which spirometry is performed. The PC_{20} is defined as the provocative concentration that results in a 20% fall in FEV_1. A PC_{20} of less than 1mg/mL indicates moderate to severe bronchial hyperresponsiveness, suggestive of asthma.

Infant lung function testing

- Most lung function tests that are available have been modified for use in infants. However, infant lung function testing is still principally a research tool with little application in the clinical setting.
- Infants need to be sedated.
- Tests are labour-intensive, technically demanding, and time-consuming.
- The majority of infants with respiratory disease have obstructive small airways disease, either from virally induced transient wheeze or from persistent wheeze. Other important groups include infants with chronic lung disease, tracheobronchomalacia, and cystic fibrosis. Monitoring disease progression and drug responses is relevant to all these conditions.
- Obstructive airways disease can be assessed in this age group using several methods. A forced expiratory manoeuvre for spirometry can be simulated using the rapid thoracic compression technique where bronchial flow limitation is achieved by rapid almost instantaneous inflation of a jacket wrapped around the infant's chest.
- sRAW from body plethysmography is also a useful marker of airways resistance in this age group
- Multi-breath gas diffusion techniques may be used in non-sedated infants. Ventilation inhomogeneity is seen in patients with obstructive airways disease and can be assessed if breath-by-breath measurements of gas composition in expired air are recorded. Wash-out dynamics are generally delayed if ventilation is inhomogeneous.

Further information

Hammer, J. and Eber, E. (eds.) (2005). *Respiratory research: paediatric pulmonary function testing.* Karger, Basel.

Lung function: normal values

Introduction

- There are over 100 sets of reference values for lung function in children derived from populations of different ethnicity, with different sample sizes, and collected at different times.
- The strongest predictor of lung function parameters is standing height. Ethnicity, age, and weight also contribute. In general, children of White European descent have higher lung volumes (by around 10–15%) compared to those of children with African or Asian origin. This probably reflects differences in chest wall shape in different populations, e.g. African children tend to have a shorter trunk to leg length ratio. Using values predicted by sitting height can compensate for some of these differences. There is no evidence for differences in lung function among different White European populations.
- For some sets of data predictive equations have been derived. These equations are used by lung function analysis software to produce the predicted values from which the percent predicted scores are given.
- It is important to know which set of reference values your own lung function measurement software uses and to make adjustments for children of different ethnic origin when appropriate. This is particularly the case when comparing predicted values measured on 2 different machines. This can create the impression of a change in lung volumes when none exists. This problem can be avoided if the actual lung volumes or other data are reported as well as the percent predicted.
- Regression equations are generally accurate at predicting most lung function parameters and usually take the form:

  $\log_e$ (lung function parameter) $= k_1 + (k_2 + k_3 \times age) \times height$

- By using a combination of age and height the effects of the adolescent growth spurt can be reasonably accommodated.
- None of the equations accurately deal with the effect of puberty. In general, for girls and taller boys (> 160cm), for a given height, more advanced puberty is associated with an increase in lung function by up to 1 standard deviation. The situation in shorter boys is more complicated. Pre-pubertal boys tend to have slightly greater lung function than those in early puberty of the same height.
- In most clinical situations the shape of the flow–volume curve (as a sensitive indicator of airways obstruction) and the change of lung function parameters with time are more important than the actual values, providing they are within 20% of the expected value. Thus relatively minor variations such as the effects of puberty will not normally influence interpretation of lung function tests.

- In children where it is difficult to obtain an accurate standing height, e.g. children with neuromuscular weakness and scoliosis, arm span or ulnar length can be used to estimate height.[1,2] Of these ulnar length is often the easiest to measure accurately. The regression equations derived from White and Asian children are:

  Boys: height (cm) = 4.605U + 1.308A + 23.003

  Girls: height (cm) = 4.459U + 1.315A + 31.485

where U is ulnar length in cm and A is age in years.

1 Gauld, L.M., Kappers, J., Carlin, J.B., and Robertson, C.F. (2004). Height prediction from ulna length. *Dev. Med. Child Neurol.* **46** (7), 475–80.

2 Gauld, L.M., Kappers, J., Carlin, J.B., and Robertson, C.F. (2003). Prediction of childhood pulmonary function using ulna length. *Am. J. Respir. Crit. Care Med.* **168** (7), 804–9.

Normal values

- The following graphs are taken from references 3 and 4 and based on White British children. They are reproduced here as a quick reference source for those occasions when you may be presented with some data without predicted values and are not quite sure if it sounds about right or not. The graphs at this resolution can only provide approximate values.
- Each of the graphs has 3 lines. The middle line is the mean value and the outer lines are the values ± 2 standard deviations from the mean.
- Reference 5 gives useful regression equations for FEV_1 and FVC derived from children from 5 different European populations and these give similar values to those of references 1 and 2. The relevant regression equations are:

   Girls' FEV_1: $\log_e FEV_1 = -1.5974 + (1.5016 + 0.0119 \times age) \times height$

   Girls' FVC: $\log_e FVC = -1.4507 + (1.4800 + 0.0127 \times age) \times height$

   Boys' FEV_1: $\log_e FEV_1 = -1.2933 + (1.2669 + 0.0174 \times age) \times height$

   Boys' FVC: $\log_e FVC = -1.2782 + (1.3731 + 0.0164 \times age) \times height$

3 Rosenthal, M., Bain, S.H., Cramer, D., Helms, P., Denison, D., Bush, A., and Warner, J.O. (1993). Lung function in white children aged 4 to 19 years: I. Spirometry. *Thorax* **48**, 794–802.

4 Rosenthal, M., Cramer, D., Bain, S.H., Denison, D., Bush, A., and Warner, J.O. (1993). Lung unction in white children aged 4 to 19 years: II. Single breath analysis and plethysmography. *Thorax* **48**, 803–8.

5 Quanjer, P.H., Borsboom, G.J., Brunekreff, B., Zach, M., Forche, G., Cotes, J.E., Sanchis, J., and Paoletti, P. (1995). Spirometric reference values for white European children and adolescents: Polgar revisited. *Pediatr. Pulmonol.* **19**, 135–42.

FEV₁

Boys

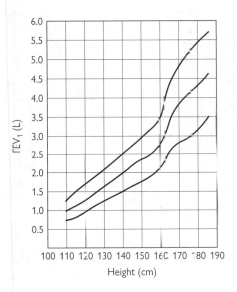

Girls

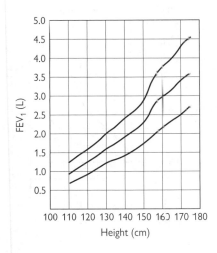

FVC

Boys

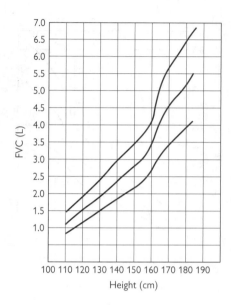

Girls

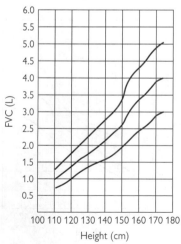

PEFR

Boys

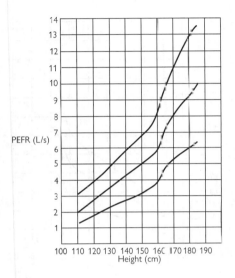

Girls

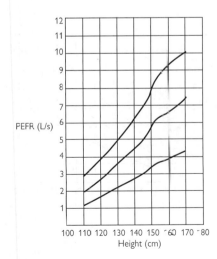

PIFR

Boys

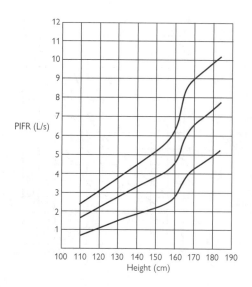

Girls

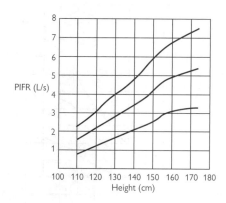

TLC

Boys

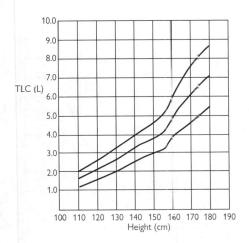

Girls

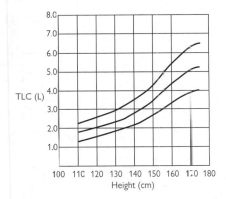

FRC

Boys

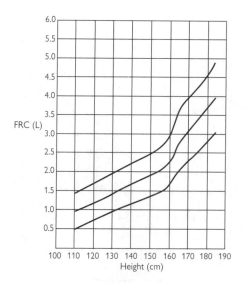

Girls

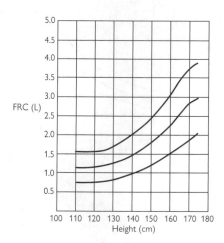

RV

Boys

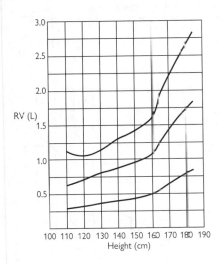

Girls

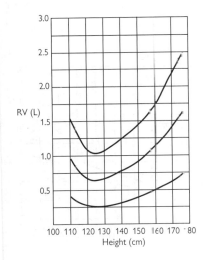

Transfer factor/diffusing capacity

The diffusing capacity of the lung for CO, also known as the transfer factor, is referred to by the abbreviations TLCO or DLCO. When it is corrected for alveolar volume (V_A) it is known as the kCO.

TLCO

Boys

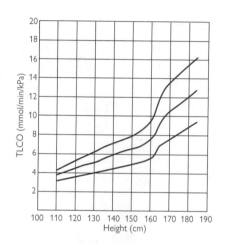

Girls

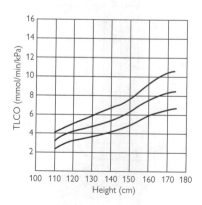

kCO

Boys

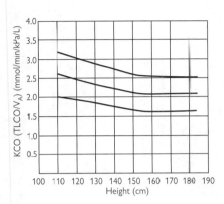

Girls

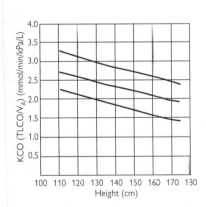

Index